THE
SPERMATOZOON

Proceedings of the Third International Symposium on the Spermatozoon held at the American Academy of Arts and Sciences, Boston, and the Swope Conference Center of the Marine Biological Laboratories, Woods Hole, Massachusetts May 2–5, 1978

THE SPERMATOZOON

Maturation, Motility,
Surface Properties
and Comparative Aspects

Edited by

Don W. Fawcett, M.D.
Hersey Professor of Anatomy
Harvard Medical School
Boston, Massachusetts

and

J. Michael Bedford, Vet. M.B., Ph.D.
Professor of Reproductive Biology
Cornell University Medical College
New York, New York

Urban & Schwarzenberg • Baltimore–Munich   1979

Urban & Schwarzenberg, Inc.
7 E. Redwood Street
Baltimore, Maryland 21202
U.S.A.

Urban & Schwarzenberg
Pettenkoferstrasse 18
D-8000 München 2
GERMANY

© 1979 by Urban & Schwarzenberg, Inc., Baltimore-Munich

All rights including that of translation, reserved. No part of this publication may be reproduced, stored in a retrieval system, or transmitted in any other form or by any means, electronic, mechanical, recording or otherwise without the prior written permission of the publisher.

Library of Congress Cataloging in Publication Data

International Symposium on the Spermatozoon, 3d, Boston and Woods Hole, 1978.
   The spermatozoon.

   Includes index.
   1. Spermatozoa—Congresses.   I. Fawcett, Don Wayne, 1917–   II. Bedford, John Michael, 1932–
III. Title.   [DNLM: 1. Spermatozoa—Congresses. 2. Spermatozoa—Physiology—Congresses.   W3 IN924NS 3d 1978s/WJ834 I617 1978s]
QP255.I58 1978   591.1'66   79-9196

ISBN 0-8067-0601-5   (Baltimore)
ISBN 3-541-70601-5   (München)

Printed in the United States of America

This volume is dedicated to the memory of *Dr. Jean Dan*. Long a major figure among biologists interested in spermatozoa, her works on the acrosome, its response and role during fertilization, and her analysis of the factors that influence it, are classical studies. Her scholarly attitude and her friendly, modest approach to colleagues and students alike provided an example to countless investigators.

CONTENTS

Participants x
Preface xv

PART I *MATURATION* 3

Symposium Papers

Evolution of the Sperm Maturation and Storage Functions of the Epididymis 7
    J.M. Bedford
Biochemical Environment of Sperm Maturation 23
    D.E. Brooks
The Fluid Environment of the Maturing Spermatozoon 35
    S. Howards, C. Lechene, and R. Vigersky
Evidence for a Role for a Forward Motility Protein in the Epididymal Development of
Sperm Motility 43
    D.D. Hoskins, D. Johnson, H. Brandt, and T.S. Acott

Contributed Paper

Some Characteristics of Salt and Water Transport in the Rat Epididymis 57
    P.Y.D. Wong, C.L. Au and H.K. Ngai

PART II *MOTILITY* 65

Symposium Papers

Interpretations of the Pattern of Sperm Tail Movements 69
    D.M. Woolley
Basis of Flagellar Motility in Spermatozoa: Current Status 81
    P. Satir
Studies on the Mechanism of Flagellar Movement 91
    B.H. Gibbons
Advances in the Ultrastructural Analysis of the Sperm Flagellar Axoneme 99
    R.W. Linck

Contributed Papers

Localization of Dynein in Sea Urchin Sperm Flagella 119
    H. Mohri, K. Ogawa, and T. Miki-Noumura
Phosphorylation of Microtubules of Rat Spermatozoa During Epididymal Maturation ... 129
    D. Tongkao and M. Chulavatnatol
A Specific Selenopolypeptide Associated with the Outer Membrane of Rat Sperm
Mitochondria 135
    H.I. Calvin and G.W. Cooper

A Peculiar Cysteine-Rich Polypeptide Related to Some Unusual Properties of Mammalian
Sperm Mitochondria.. 141
    V. Pallini, B. Baccetti, and A.G. Burrini
Asymmetrical Oscillation of Sea Urchin Sperm Flagella Induced by Calcium........... 153
    C.J. Brokaw and G.F. Goldstein
Disassembly of the Guinea Pig Sperm Tail....................................... 157
    D.S. Friend, P.M. Elias, and I. Rudolf
Elimination of the Adverse Effect of Dilution on Hamster Sperm Motility *In Vitro*....... 169
    B.D. Bavister

PART III   *SURFACE PROPERTIES*.. 173

Symposium Papers

Appearance and Partitioning of Plasma Membrane Antigens during Mouse
Spermatogenesis... 177
    C.F. Millette
Cell Surface Changes Associated with the Epididymal Maturation of Mammalian
Spermatozoa... 187
    G.L. Nicolson and R. Yanagimachi
Changes in Sperm Surface Properties Correlated with Capacitation.................. 195
    M.G. O'Rand
Characterization of Sperm Surfaces Using Physical Techniques..................... 205
    R.H. Hammerstedt

Contributed Papers

Persistence of Sperm Surface Components in the Early Embryo..................... 219
    C.A. Gabel, E.M. Eddy, and B.M. Shapiro
Serological Analysis of the Expression of T/t Locus Antigens on Spermatogenic Cells of
the Mouse.. 231
    G.B. Dooher

PART IV   *COMPARATIVE ASPECTS*.. 239

Symposium Papers

Sperm Structure in Relation to Phylogeny in Lower Metazoa....................... 243
    B.A. Afzelius
An Overview of Atypical Spermatozoa in Insects................................. 253
    R. Dallai
Structural, Comparative, and Functional Aspects of Spermatozoa in Urodeles.......... 267
    B. Picheral
Special Features of Sperm Structure and Function in Marsupials.................... 289
    H.R. Harding, F.N. Carrick, and C.D. Shorey
Evolution of the Acrosomal Complex... 305
    B. Baccetti

Contributed Papers

Ultrastructural Study of Spermiogenesis of the Anuran Amphibian *Bombina Variegata*.... 333
    R. Folliot

Classification of Abnormalities in Human Spermatids Based on Recent Advances in
Ultrastructure Research on Spermatid Differentiation 341
    A.F. Holstein and C. Schirren
The Ultrastructure of the Prospermium of *Ornithodoros* Ticks and its Relation to Sperm
Maturation and Capacitation 355
    B. Feldman-Muhsam and B.K. Filshie

APPENDIX 371

WORKSHOP ONE   *Isolation and Biochemical Characterization of Germ Cells and their Structural Components* 373

Separation of Male Germ Cells by Sedimentation Velocity 375
    L.J. Romrell
Isolation of Mammalian Spermatogenic Cells and Characterization of Chromosomal
Proteins 379
    A.R. Bellvé and D.A. O'Brien
Isolation of Stable Structures from Rat Spermatozoa 387
    H.I. Calvin
Separation of the Head and Tail of Mammalian Spermatozoa by Primary Amines:
Evidence for their Junction by Schiff Bases 391
    R.J. Young and G.W. Cooper
Isolation of the Fibrous Sheath and Perforatorium of Rat Spermatozoa 395
    G.E. Olsen
Isolation of Mitochondria from Bull Epididymal Spermatozoa 401
    V. Pallini

WORKSHOP TWO   *Quantitative Assessment of Sperm Motility* 411

Biophysical Aspects of Human Sperm Movement 413
    D.F. Katz and J.W. Overstreet
A Review of the Spectrophotometric Quantitation of Spermatozoon Motility 421
    R.W. Atherton
Measurement of Human Sperm Motility Based on an Optical Doppler Effect 427
    P. Jouannet
Computerized Measurements of Sperm Velocity and Percentage of Motile Sperm 431
    R.P. Amann

Index 437

PARTICIPANTS

Dr. Bjorn Afzelius
Wenner Gren Institute
S-11345, Stockholm
Sweden

Dr. Rupert Amann
Dairy Breeding Research Center
Pennsylvania State University
University Park, Pennsylvania
 16802
U.S.A.

Dr. Jean André
Université de Paris XI
S1405, Orsay
France

Dr. Robert Atherton
Department of Zoology and
 Physiology
University of Wyoming Station
Laramie, Wyoming 82070
U.S.A.

Dr. C.R. Austin
Department of Physiology and
 Animal Reproduction
University of Cambridge
Cambridge, CB2 3EG
England

Dr. Baccio Baccetti
Instituto di Zoologia
53100 Siena
Italy

Dr. A.H. Barr
Rensselaer Polytechnic Institute
Troy, New York 21281
U.S.A.

Dr. Claudio Barros
Embryology Laboratory
Institute of Biological Science
Catholic University of Chile
C, Santiago
Chile

Dr. Barry Bavister
Department of Pathology
Harbor General Hospital
Torrance, California 90509
U.S.A.

Dr. J. Michael Bedford
Department of Obstetrics and
 Gynecology
Cornell University Medical College
New York, New York 10021
U.S.A.

Dr. Anthony R. Bellvé
Laboratory of Human
 Reproduction and Reproductive
 Biology
Harvard Medical School
Boston, Massachusetts 02115
U.S.A.

Dr. Miguel Berrios
Department of Obstetrics and
 Gynecology
Cornell University Medical College
New York, New York 10021
U.S.A.

Dr. Charles Brokaw
Division of Biology
California Institute of Technology
Pasadena, California 91125
U.S.A.

Dr. David Brooks
Department of Animal Physiology
Waite Agricultural Research
 Institute
University of Adelaide
Glen Osmond
South Australia 5064

Dr. Giselda A. Burrini
Instituto di Zoologia
53100 Siena
Italy

Dr. Harold Calvin
Columbia University College of
 Physicians and Surgeons
New York, New York 10032
U.S.A.

Dr. Marina Camatini
Instituto di Zoologia
20133 Milano
Italy

Dr. Edmund Casillas
Department of Chemistry
New Mexico State University
Las Crucas, New Mexico 88001
U.S.A.

Dr. M.C. Chang
Worcester Foundation for
 Experimental Biology
Shrewsbury, Massachusetts 01545
U.S.A.

Dr. Hector Chemes
Centro de Investigaciones
 Endocrinologicas
Hospital General de Niños
 "R. Gutierrez"
Buenos Aires
Argentina 1425

Dr. Montre Chulavatnatol
Department of Biochemistry
Faculty of Science
Mahidol University
Bangkok
Thailand

Dr. Eric D. Clegg
3-230 Life Sciences
Purdue University
West Lafayette, Indiana 47907
U.S.A.

Dr. Jack Cohen
Department of Zoology
University of Birmingham
Birmingham
England

Dr. G.W. Cooper
Department of Obstetrics and
 Gynecology
Cornell University Medical College
New York, New York 10021
U.S.A.

Dr. Marie-Paul Cosson
Kervalo Marine Laboratory
Honolulu, Hawaii 96813
U.S.A.

Dr. R.I. Coubrough
Faculty of Veterinary Science
University of Pretoria
Onderstepoort 0110
Pretoria
South Africa

Mr. Thomas Craig
Department of Physics
University of Guelph
Guelph, Ontario N1G 2W1
Canada

Dr. Jean-Pierre Dadoune
C.H.U. Broussais-Hotel-Dieu
Laboratoire d'Histologie
75270 Paris, CEDEX 06
France

Dr. Romano Dallai
Instituto di Zoologia
53100 Siena
Italy

Dr. George David
Laboratoire d'Histologie
Université de Paris-Sud
94270 Kremlin-Bicêtre
France

Dr. Jean C. Dan
832 Koyatsu
Tateyama (294-03)
Japan

Dr. Gerald B. Dooher
Memorial Sloan-Kettering Institute
New York, New York 10021
U.S.A.

Dr. Martin Dym
Department of Anatomy
Harvard Medical School
25 Shattuck Street
Boston, Massachusetts 02115
U.S.A.

Dr. Edward Eddy
Department of Biological Structure
University of Washington
Seattle, Washington 98195
U.S.A.

Dr. M.A. Fain-Maurel
Laboratoire Biologie Cellulaire
75270 Paris, CEDEX 05
France

Dr. Don Fawcett
Department of Anatomy
Harvard Medical School
Boston, Massachusetts 02115
U.S.A.

Dr. Feldman-Muhsam
Hebrew University
Medical School
Jerusalem
Israel

Dr. J.E. Fléchon
Station de Physiologie Animal
  INRA
78350 Jouy-en-Josas
France

Dr. R. Folliot
Laboratoire de Biologie Generale
Université de Rennes
Rennes
France

Dr. Åke Franzen
Institute of Zoology
Uppsala University
S-75122 Uppsala
Sweden

Dr. Dan Friend
Department of Pathology
University of California
San Francisco, California 94143
U.S.A.

Dr. Barbara Gibbons
Kervalo Marine Laboratory
Honolulu, Hawaii 96813
U.S.A.

Dr. I.R. Gibbons
Kewalo Marine Laboratory
Honolulu, Hawaii 96813
U.S.A.

Dr. Folco Giusti
Instituto de Zoologia
53100 Siena
Italy

Dr. Jacques Gonzales
Laboratoire d'Histologie et
  d'Embryologie
Faculté de Medecine
75634 Paris, CEDEX 13
France

Dr. Rodrigo Guerrero
Universidad del Valle
Cali
Colombia

Dr. Ralph B. Gwatkin
Merck Institute
Rahway, New Jersey 07065
U.S.A.

Dr. D. Hahn
Ortho Pharmaceutical Corporation
Rahway, New Jersey 07065
U.S.A.

Dr. G.L. Hahn
Department of Biochemistry
University of Massachusetts
School of Medicine
Worcester, Massachusetts 01605
U.S.A.

Dr. Roy Hammerstedt
Department of Biochemistry and
  Biophysics
Pennsylvania State University
University Park, Pennsylvania
  16802
U.S.A.

Dr. Mary A. Handel
Department of Zoology
University of Tennessee
Knoxville, Tennessee 37916
U.S.A.

Dr. H.R. Harding
Department of General Studies
University of New South Wales
Kensington
2033 N.S.W.
Australia

Dr. Norman Hecht
Department of Biology
Tufts University
Medford, Massachusetts 02155
U.S.A.

Dr. Jose Hib
Rodriguez Pena 1015-Piso 1
1020 Buenos Aires
Argentina

Dr. Anita Hoffer
Department of Anatomy
Harvard Medical School
Boston, Massachusetts 02115
U.S.A.

Dr. A.F. Holstein
Anatomisches Institut der
  Universität
2 Hamburg 20
West Germany

Dr. Dale Hoskins
Oregon Regional Primate Center
Beaverton, Oregon 97005
U.S.A.

Dr. R. L. Hughes
Department of Anatomy
University of Queensland
St. Lucia, Brisbane
Queensland 4067
Australia

Dr. P. Jouannet
Laboratoire d'Histologie-
 Embryologie
Université de Paris-Sud
C.H.U. Bicêtre 94270
Kremlin–Bicêtre
France

Dr. David F. Katz
Department of Mechanical
 Engineering
University of California
Berkeley, California 94720
U.S.A.

Dr. James Koehler
Department of Biological Structure
University of Washington
School of Medicine
Seattle, Washington 98195
U.S.A.

Dr. Wylie Lee
Department of Biological Structure
University of Washington
School of Medicine
Seattle, Washington, 98195
U.S.A.

Dr. Richard Linck
Department of Anatomy
Harvard Medical School
Boston, Massachusetts 02115
U.S.A.

Mr. Bernard Marchand
Faculté des Sciences
Laboratoire de Zoologie
Université de Dakar
Dakar
Senegal

Dr. Mazzini Massimo
Instituto di Zoologia
Universita de Siena
53100 Siena
Italy

Dr. X. Mattei
Department de Biologie Animale
Faculté des Sciences
Université de Dakar
Dakar
Senegal

Dr. Charles Metz
Institute for Molecular and Cellular
 Evolution
University of Miami
Coral Gables, Florida 33134
U.S.A.

Dr. Clark Millette
Laboratory of Human
 Reproduction and Reproductive
 Biology
Harvard Medical School
Boston, Massachusetts 02115
U.S.A.

Dr. Hideo Mohri
Department of Biology
University of Tokyo
Komaba, Meguro-ku
Tokyo 153
Japan

Dr. Diana Myles
Laboratory of Reproductive Biology
Harvard Medical School
Boston, Massachusetts 02115
U.S.A.

Dr. Garth Nicolson
Department of Developmental and
 Cell Biology
University of California
Irvine, California 92717
U.S.A.

Dr. Deborah O'Brien
Laboratory of Human
 Reproduction and Reproductive
 Biology
Harvard Medical School
Boston, Massachusetts 02115
U.S.A.

Dr. G. Okuno
Division of Biology
California Institute of Technology
Pasadena, California 91125
U.S.A.

Dr. Patricia Olds-Clarke
Department of Biology
Bryn Mawr College
Bryn Mawr, Pennsylvania 19010
U.S.A.

Dr. Gary Olsen
Department of Anatomy
Vanderbilt University
Nashville, Tennessee 37232
U.S.A.

Dr. Michael G. O'Rand
Department of Anatomy
University of Florida
Gainsville, Florida 32601
U.S.A.

Dr. Marie C. Orgebin-Crist
Department of Obstetrics and
 Gynecology
Vanderbilt University
School of Medicine
Nashville, Tennessee 37232
U.S.A.

Dr. Vitaliano Pallini
Instituto de Zoologia
53100 Siena
Italy

Dr. Lauri Pelliniemi
Laboratory of Electron Microscopy
University of Turkee
Turkee
Finland 52

Dr. M.E. Perotti
Instituto di Istologia
7-20129 Milano
Italy

Dr. David M. Phillips
Population Council
Rockefeller University
New York, New York 10021
U.S.A.

Dr. Bertrand Pichéral
Faculté des Sciences Biologiques
Laboratoire de Biologie Cellulaire
35031 Rennes
France

Dr. Leif Ploen
Department of Anatomy
College of Veterinary Medicine
Swedish University of Agricultural
 Sciences
S-75007 Uppsala
Sweden

Dr. Kenneth Polakoski
Department of Obstetrics and
 Gynecology
Washington University
St. Louis, Missouri 63110
U.S.A.

Dr. M.R.N. Prasad
Special Program on Human
 Reproduction
World Health Organization
1211 Geneva 27
Switzerland

Dr. M. Rajalakshimi
Department of Zoology
Delhi University
Delhi
India 11007

Dr. Tommasa Renieri
Instituto di Zoologia
53100 Siena
Italy

Dr. R. Rikmenspoel
Department of Biology
State University of New York
Albany, New York 12222
U.S.A.

Dr. Lynn Romrell
Department of Anatomy
College of Medicine
University of Florida
Gainesville, Florida 32610
U.S.A.

Dr. Edward Roosen-Runge
Department of Biological Structure
University of Washington
School of Medicine
Seattle, Washington 98195
U.S.A.

Dr. A. Rosado
Biochemistry Division
Instituto Mexicano del Seguro
 Social
Mexico 12, D.F.
Mexico

Dr. R.G. Saacke
Department of Dairy Science
Virginia Polytechnic Institute
Blacksburg, Virginia 24060
U.S.A.

Dr. William Sadler
Center for Population Research
National Institute of Child Health
 and Human Development
National Institutes of Health
Bethesda, Maryland 20014
U.S.A.

Dr. Daniel Sandoz
67 Rue Maurice Gunsbourg
34200 Ivry
France

Dr. Peter Satir
Department of Anatomy
Albert Einstein College of Medicine
Bronx, New York 10461

Dr. Sheldon Segal
The Population Council
Rockefeller University
New York, New York 10017
U.S.A.

Dr. Bennett N. Shapiro
Department of Biochemistry
University of Washington
Seattle, Washington 98195

Dr. Pierre Soupart
Department of Obstetrics and
 Gynecology
Vanderbilt University
School of Medicine
Nashville, Tennessee 37232
U.S.A.

Dr. Z. Swiderski
University of Geneva
Comparative Anatomy and
 Physiology
CH-1211, Geneva 4
Switzerland

Dr. Maria Vegni Talluri
Instituto di Zoologia
53100 Siena
Italy

Dr. Toby M. Tamblyn
Department of Biochemistry and
 Nutrition
Virginia Polytechnic Institute
Blacksburg, Virginia 24061
U.S.A.

Dr. P. Veriyapanick
Department of Obstetrics and
 Gynecology
Cornell Medical College
New York, New York 10021
U.S.A.

Dr. Joseph Voglmayr
Worcester Foundation for
 Experimental Biology
Shrewsbury, Massachusetts 01545
U.S.A.

Dr. J. Wais
Department of Anatomy
Albert Einstein College of Medicine
Bronx, New York 10461
U.S.A.

Dr. Ian G. White
Department of Veterinary
 Physiology
University of Sydney
2006 Sydney
Australia

Dr. Joelle Wiels
Laboratoire Immunohematologie
Hospital St. Louis
75475 Paris, CEDEX 10
France

Dr. George Witman
Department of Biology
Princeton University
Princeton, New Jersey 08540
U.S.A.

Dr. P.Y.D. Wong
Department of Physiology
University of Hong Kong
Hong Kong

Dr. David Woolley
Department of Physiology
The Medical School
University of Bristol
Bristol BS8 1TD
England

Dr. Lewis Tilney
Joseph Leidy Laboratory of Biology
University of Pennsylvania
Philadelphia, Pennsylvania 19174
U.S.A.

Dr. R. Yanagimachi
Department of Anatomy and
 Reproductive Biology
University of Hawaii
Honolulu, Hawaii 06822
U.S.A.

Dr. R.J. Young
Department of Obstetrics and
 Gynecology
Cornell Medical College
New York, New York 10021
U.S.A.

PREFACE

In 1969, on the initiative of Professor Baccio Baccetti, an international group of scientists met at the Accademia Nazionale dei Lincei in Rome and at the Universita di Siena to discuss the contributions of electron microscopy, histochemistry, and cell physiology to our understanding of spermatozoa and to explore the possible contributions of comparative investigations of spermatozoa in systematics and studies of phylogeny. The proceedings of that meeting were published in *Comparative Spermatology* (B. Baccetti, ed.), Academic Press. Four years later, in 1973, a second International Symposium was organized by Professor Bjorn Afzelius and held at the Wenner-Gren Center in Stockholm, Sweden. The emphasis of this meeting was on the correlation of structure and function of the spermatozoon in the events leading to fertilization. The participants included zoologists, morphologists, immunologists, biochemists, individuals interested in the breeding of animals for food and fiber, and investigators interested in the control of human fertility. The proceedings were published in *Functional Anatomy of the Spermatozoon* (B. Afzelius, ed.), Pergamon Press.

Fertilization requires physiological maturation of the spermatozoon, vigorous motility and fusion of the membranes of the gametes. In the past five years, there has been major progress in our understanding of the cell surface and significant methodological advances in studying the surface properties and molecular organization of biological membranes. In the same period compelling evidence has accumulated in support of a sliding-microtubule mechanism of flagellar locomotion of muscle contraction. There has also been a growing awareness that spermatozoa only gradually acquire fertilizing capacity during a long period of biochemical and physiological maturation after they leave the testis. These changes are dependent upon environmental factors to which they are exposed in the course of their transport and storage in the epididymis and are finally completed during their ascent of the female reproductive tract.

A better understanding of the surface properties, locomotion, and maturation of spermatozoa might lead to identification of vulnerable steps in the reproductive process that could be the focus of new methods of fertility control. Therefore in planning the third International Symposium on the Spermatozoon held at the American Academy of Arts and Sciences, Boston, and the Swope Conference Center of the Marine Biological Laboratories, Woods Hole, Massachusetts, these three areas were selected for special emphasis. All of the papers presented were of high quality, but regrettably, as the duration of the meetings and the number of participants have increased, it has become impractical to publish the proceedings in full. Many contributed papers have had to be omitted, in spite of their merit.

The present volume includes the invited symposium papers on the main themes of the meeting and on the comparative aspects of sperm structure which has been a continuing interest of the group. Also included are selected contributed papers relevant to these topics. Concise resumes of methods discussed in the workshops "Isolation and Biochemical Characterization of Germ Cells and Their Structural Components" and "Quantitative Assessment of Sperm Motility" are presented in an appendix in the belief that broader application of the methods described may accelerate progress in the field.

The meeting and publication of the proceedings would not have been possible without financial assistance from several sources. It is a pleasure to acknowledge generous support from the Center for Population Research of the National Institute of Child Health and Human Development, the Population Council, The Josiah Macy Foundation, the World Health Organization and the Needmor Fund. Additional contributions were received from the Upjohn Company and Ortho Pharmaceutical Corporation.

THE SPERMATOZOON

PART I
MATURATION

Although it has long been recognized that spermatozoa emerging from the mammalian testis are not fertile, only in recent years has much attention been paid to the nature of the process whereby they mature and are stored in the epididymis. As a consequence of this neglect, there is little conceptual understanding of the factors responsible for the evolution of these functions as they exist in present day mammals, including man. Neither is there enough factual knowledge about the maturation process itself, nor about the special quality of the environment in the epididymis that supports maturation or sperm storage. Moreover, even where particular macromolecules or electrolytes have been identified in unusual concentration in the epididymal milieu it has been difficult to interpret their role. Beside the possible place of the epididymis in syndromes of human subfertility, the epididymis is currently seen as a potentially promising target for development of acceptable methods for interruption of male fertility, and for this reason alone it is deserving of more intense efforts to elucidate its functions. This section addresses these questions from the viewpoints of the evolution and biological significance of epididymal function; the character of the epididymal milieu; the methodology required for its investigation; and the nature of the biochemical events involved in a key aspect of sperm maturation—acquisition of the potential for independent progressive motility.

SYMPOSIUM PAPERS

EVOLUTION OF THE SPERM MATURATION AND SPERM STORAGE FUNCTIONS OF THE EPIDIDYMIS

J.M. Bedford

Departments of Obstetrics and Gynecology and Anatomy, Cornell University Medical College, New York, New York 10021 USA

INTRODUCTION

It is well established that spermatozoa of eutherian mammals undergo important changes in that part of the Wolffian duct designated as the ductus epididymidis. These changes are expressed in the fact that spermatozoa emerging from the testis cannot yet fertilize, and only acquire this ability during their transit from the caput to the cauda epididymidis, where they are stored and whence they can be expelled at ejaculation. Both maturation and storage of eutherian spermatozoa appear to depend, moreover, on a special environment created by androgen-dependent activities of the epithelium of the epididymis. Something is now known of the biochemical attributes of the environment of the epididymis and of the subcellular changes in epididymal spermatozoa which probably reflect their maturation; and when viewed within the confines of the present mammalian literature the biology of the epididymis appears conceptually straightforward. Placed in a comparative setting, on the other hand, the apparent complexity of epididymal function in eutherian mammals becomes an enigma. Biologists interested in fertilization in teleost fish use spermatozoa released from the testis since these are fertile and support normal embryonic development (Henderson, 1962), and the same practice has long been applied in studies of fertilization in cyclostomes and frogs. In such vertebrates, therefore, the excurrent duct makes no essential contribution to the maturation of spermatozoa. Important evolutionary modifications appear to have taken place also in the system that modulates sperm storage. The rooster, for example, displays no evident dependence on androgenic support of the testis for storage of spermatozoa in the epididymis (Munro, 1938a), whereas withdrawal of testicular androgen reduces drastically the longevity of spermatozoa in the cauda epididymidis in therian mammals (Orgebin-Crist et al., 1975). Although this prelude to conception thus appears more complex in eutherian mammals, there is no understanding of its adaptive significance nor of the advantage gained by such a transfer of the final maturation of spermatozoa from the testis to a duct whose function in this respect, as well as for sperm storage, has become highly androgen-dependent.

It seems important that epididymal research should be based, if possible, on some understanding of the wider biological significance of the phenomena being investigated. However, the paucity of information about the maturation and storage of spermatozoa in most vertebrates has precluded hypotheses about the significance of the features of epididymal function for reproduction in mammals, although further comparative information in itself will not necessarily assure an explanation. The author and colleagues have begun a systematic investigation of the main features of epididymal function in sub-eutherian vertebrates by probing the phylogenetic appearance or onset of certain aspects that seem to characterize epididymal function in most Eutheria. Transit of eutherian spermatozoa through the epididymis is accompanied by change in their metabolic profile and so the capacity for motility, in the molecular character of the surface, and in the structural quality of both head and tail organelles; and, morphologically, in loss of the droplet of spermatid cytoplasm from the sperm tail and in some by a reduction in size and/or a remolding of the rostral region of the acrosome (Bedford, 1975). Accordingly, those parameters have been used as guides to evaluate the events occurring in the male excurrent duct in different submammalian vertebrates. Similar studies on maturation and in some cases on storage have been conducted in prototherian, metatherian, and in a few ascrotal eutherian mammals—the last on the basis of the suggestion that descent to a scrotum bears on the endocrine dependence of sperm storage (Munro, 1938a), and the idea that scrotal evolution may have been influenced primarily by the sperm storage function of the epididymis (Bedford, 1978a, b).

Thanks are expressed to Dr. Jeffrey Kerr and other members of the Department of Anatomy at Monash University, and to the Howard Florey Institute for Experimental Medicine, Melbourne University, for facilities and help in connection with observations made on the echidna; to Dr. D. Kroodsma of Rockefeller University for help in obtaining specimens of *Melospizia melodia;* and to Drs. George W. Cooper and Gil Dryden for reading the manuscript. Technical assistance was provided by Miu Ying Fong and Angela Cantone; and financial support by the South Branch Foundation, the Ford Foundation and by the National Institutes of Health (HD-07257).

© 1979 Urban & Schwarzenberg, Inc. Baltimore-Munich *The Spermatozoon,* edited by D.W. Fawcett and J.M. Bedford

Table 1. Species Studied*

Subtheria
    Xiphophorus maculatus   (platyfish)
    Poecilia reticulata   (guppy)
    Raja eglanteria   (skate)
    Natrix sipedon   (water snake)
    Anolis carolinensis   (lizard)
    Pseudemys scripta   (turtle)
    Gallus gallus   (rooster)
    Mergus serrator   (duck)
    Columba domestica   (dove)
    Melospizia melodia   (song sparrow)
Protheria
    Tachyglossus aculeatus   (echidna)
Theria
  Metatheria
    Trichosurus vulpecula   (brush-tailed possum)
    Didelphis virginiana   (opossum)
  Eutheria
    *Procavia capensis***   (hyrax)
    *Dasypus novemcinctus***   (armadillo)
    *Octodon degus***   (degu)
    *Suncus murinus***   (musk shrew)

This table does not include the common scrotal mammals investigated by the author and by many others.
**Ascrotal.*

This chapter brings together the general findings obtained thus far from this approach. Different phases of the study have involved collaboration with P.D. Temple-Smith, G.W. Cooper, R.P. Millar, G. Dryden, and J. Rifkin. Accounts dealing with some marsupials and ascrotal eutherians have been published, and more detailed descriptions of the maturation and storage functions of the male reproductive tract of Elasmobranchii, reptiles, birds, and a monotreme—the echidna—will appear in due course.

OBSERVATIONS

Sperm Maturation

Sperm Motility Because it is known that the spermatozoa of mammals develop the ability to swim as they pass along the epididymis, the character of the motility of spermatozoa released into a variety of physiological solutions from successive regions of the excurrent duct of different vertebrates has been followed in a phase contrast microscope for varying periods from several minutes to 24 h. The general outcome of these observations is depicted in Figure 1. As can be inferred from their immediate ability to fertilize, spermatozoa of cyclostomes, teleosts, and anuran amphibia develop the capacity for optimal motility in the testis. However, testicular spermatozoa of the cyprinodont teleosts *Xiphophorus maculatus* and *Poecilia reticulata* in which fertilization is internal (Amoroso, 1960) also were highly motile when suspended in Tyrode's solution of 60-80% normal concentration. By contrast, in the skate *Raja eglanteria*, a member of the Elasmobranchii, all of which display internal fertilization, spermatozoa from the testis and proximal segments of the excurrent duct exhibited little or no movement in Tyrode's solution, sea water, or other physiological media. Vigorous swimming activity in Tyrode's was manifested only by spermatozoa released from a region approximately two-thirds along the excurrent duct and beyond. In the course of their swimming activity, these highly active spermatozoa often appeared to shed a sheath from the posterior midpiece, and those released from the terminus often swam together in clumps because their heads were embedded in a mucus matrix.

A similar maturation of the capacity for motility in the excurrent duct was seen in the water snake *Natrix sipedon*. Spermatozoa collected from the testis and upper part of the excurrent duct during active spermatogenesis and passage of spermatozoa into the excurrent duct (in September and October) were not motile. Potentially motile spermatozoa were present at such times approximately one-third along the duct and more distally where a great majority displayed the capacity for prolonged progressive motility if released into Tyrode's solution at 23°C (see, however, section on Sperm Storage). A similar picture was presented also in reptiles from other orders, specifically the turtle *Pseudemys scripta* and the lizard *Anolis carolinensis*.

There was a marked difference in the sperm motility profile in the excurrent duct of the rooster, pigeon, and drake on the one hand, and in the passerine song sparrow *Melospizia melodia* on the other. In the former group some 2-5% of spermatozoa released directly from the testis into Tyrode's solution maintained progressive vigorous motility for the 2-3 h in which they were observed, though a majority did not swim actively unless released from some point (in pigeon and drake approximately one-fifth and in rooster two-thirds) along the excurrent duct. Thus, in these three birds this aspect of sperm maturation does not necessarily require the environment created in the excurrent duct, but it does occur there for a majority of sperm. In the sparrow, the gross morphology of the male tract differs from its simple form in the rooster, drake, and pigeon (Fig. 2); and spermatozoa collected from the sparrow testis, from the long ciliated duct and from the proximal portion of the coiled terminal region are quite immotile at 23-37°C in Tyrode's and Ringer's solutions or in M 199. These observations negate the suggestion of Middleton (1974) that mature spermatozoa are flushed from the passerine

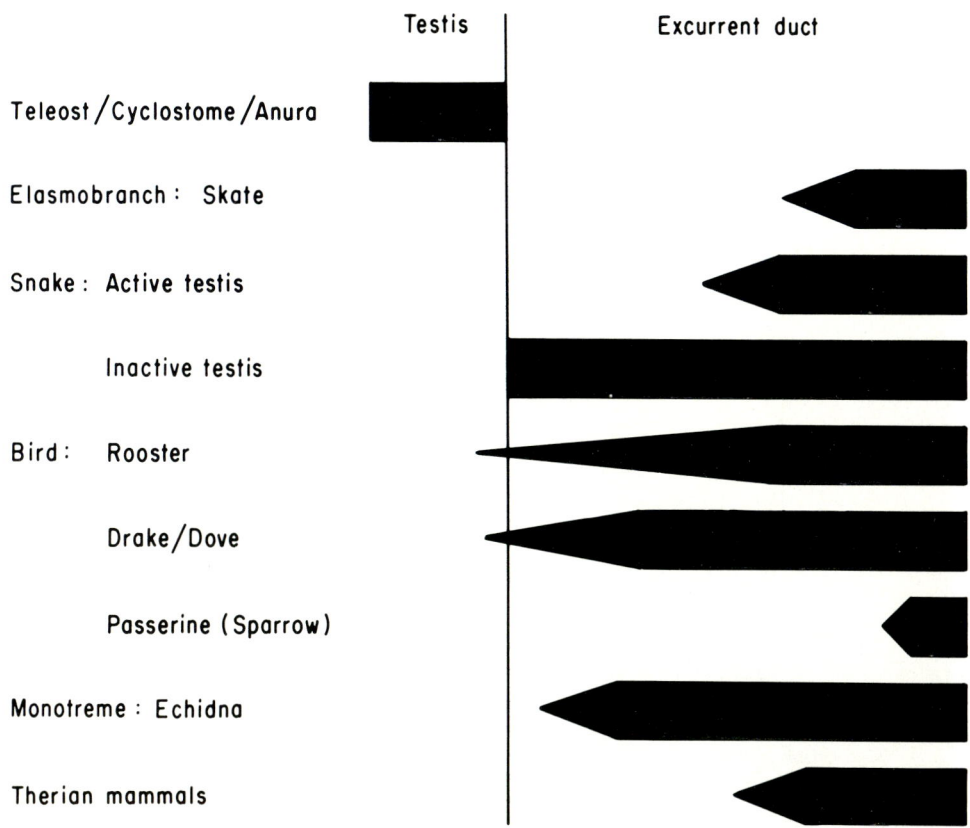

Figure 1. The potential for motility of sperm populations taken from testis and different levels of the excurrent duct in representative species. This indicates in a general way the point at which this capacity is acquired as the sperm move along the duct (here left to right). Note particularly the contrast between the teleost/anuran/cyclostome group and the remainder in which fertilization is consistently internal; and the fact that some motile spermatozoa exist in the testis of the birds studied.

testis and pass rapidly to the seminal sac. For the capacity for sustained progressive motility in such passerines seems not to be acquired until spermatozoa reach the mid-portion of the paracloacal coiled mass of tubules which protrudes in the fashion of a scrotum. This distal region may therefore make some special contribution to this aspect of maturation in the passerine bird.

The pattern of maturation of the capacity for motility displayed by the sauropsid-like spermatozoa of the echidna *Tachyglossus aculeatus* resembled that seen in the snake during spermiation. None released from the echidna testis or from proximal regions of the excurrent duct, displayed any movement when released into a variety of the standard physiological media; the capacity for this being evident first in those collected from an approximate midpoint of the tract. While spermatozoa from the more distal regions of the echidna duct did flagellate actively in Ringer's solution, none of the media used (NaCl, M199, Tyrode's, Ringer's) elicited a coordinated progressive motility in spermatozoa from any level of the tract, suggesting that this may require conditions different from those afforded by the standard physiological media.

The pattern found in the Theria differs from that in most of the birds studied in that therian spermatozoa have developed an absolute dependence upon the epididymal environment for maturation of the capacity for optimal motility. Some of the spermatozoa released from the eutherian testis already have the potential for a twitching nonprogressive activity which may be heightened somewhat if they are retained there by efferent duct ligation (O'Shea and Voglmayr, 1970; Cooper and Orgebin-Crist, 1977) or are stored *in vitro* at 1°C in testicular fluid for a short period (Setchell et al., 1969). But in none of the eutherians studied can spermatozoa ripen in the testis to a point at which their activity resembles that of mature spermatozoa (see also Hoskins et al., 1979). Ligation of the mid or distal region of the eutherian epididymis has shown that the

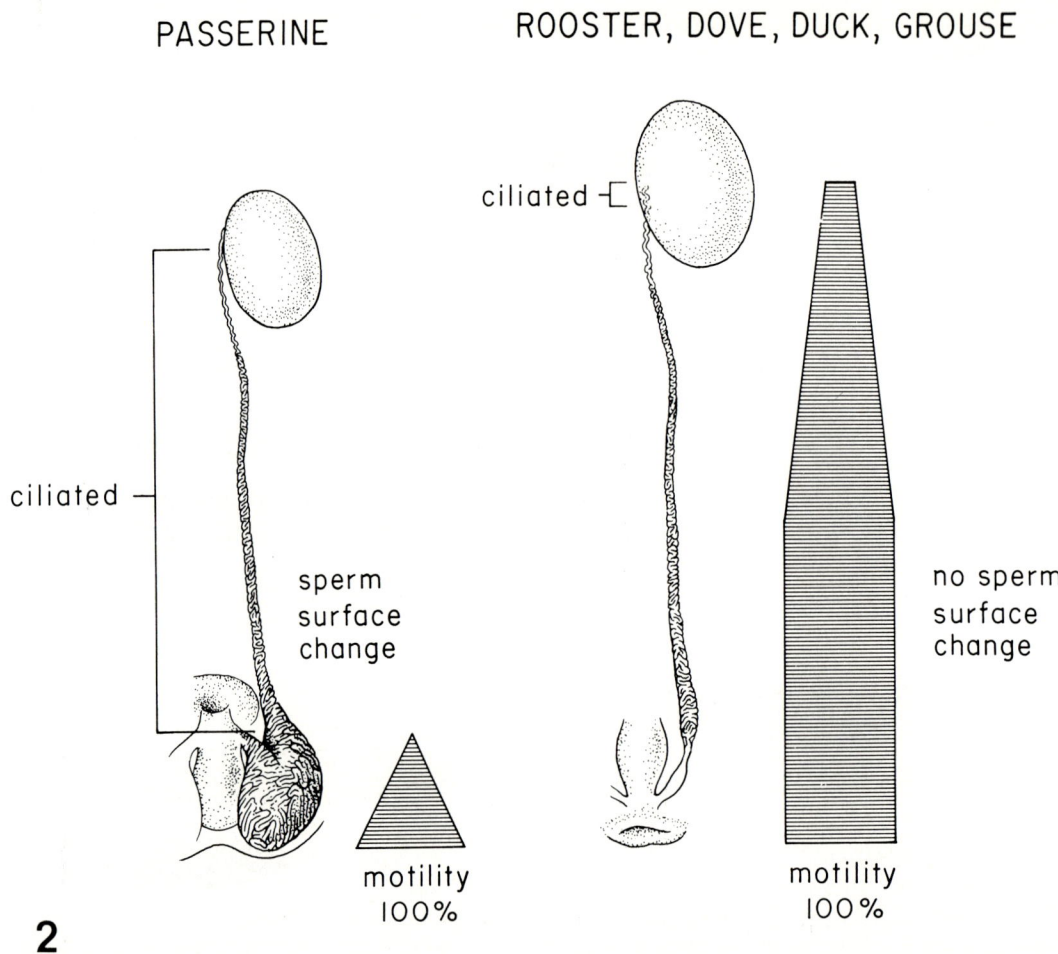

Figure 2. The male excurrent duct in the passerines as compared with that of many other birds. The maturation/storage function has become relatively more complex in the former, in some ways approaching that of the Therians, and the coiled terminal "epididymis" occupies a quasi-scrotal location in the para-cloacal protuberance.

normal pattern can be altered considerably in the rabbit (Gaddum and Glover, 1965; Bedford, 1966; Orgebin-Crist, 1967), but not as successfully in some rodents (Horan and Bedford, 1972).

Surface Change in the Excurrent Duct Change in the surface of the plasmalemma of the spermatozoon during its transit through the epididymis has been demonstrated in all eutherian mammals studied in this respect with one exception, *Suncus* (see Bedford, 1975; Cooper and Bedford, 1976). It has been revealed through observation of microelectrophoretic behavior, autoagglutination, response to fixatives, and more recently by use of visible surface markers having an affinity for anionic groups or for specific oligosaccharide (Bedford and Cooper, 1978). In the present series three surface markers, cationized colloidal ferric oxide and two fluorescein isothiocyanate-conjugated lectins, wheat germ agglutinin (WGA) and concanavalin A (Con A) have been used. The ferric colloid, used at a pH between 1.8 and 3.2 is visualized on the surface of spermatozoa in the electron microscope, and its binding reflects the existence of charged cationic groups there. The binding patterns of WGA and Con A were assessed subjectively in a light microscope with fluorescent optics. The details of the methodology of these techniques are given by Temple-Smith and Bedford (1976).

Binding of either ferric colloid and of one or both lectins was apparent on restricted regions and sometimes the whole surface of spermatozoa from all the vertebrate species studied. However, as can be seen from the summary in Table 2, with the one exception of the passerine bird *Melospizia melodia*, there was no consistent change in the pattern of binding of any of the markers as a concomitant of sperm passage from the proximal to the distal segment of the excurrent duct in subtherian species. In marked contrast, spermatozoa of the Theria examined—that is the metatherian (marsupial) and eutherian mammals—whether scrotal or not (Bedford and Millar, 1978), express distinct changes in the sur-

Table 2. Characteristic Changes in Spermatozoa of Different Vertebrate Groups during Transit through the Excurrent Duct, and their Dependence for Storage on Testicular Androgen

	Motility	Sperm Surface[1]	-S-S Dependent Structural Change	Acrosomal Modification	Androgen-Dependent Storage
Subtheria					
Cyclostome	−		−		
Teleost fish	−	−	−		−?
Anuran amphibian	−	−	−	−	−?
Elasmobranch Fish–*Raja*	+	+	?	−	?
Reptiles–*Natrix*	+	−	−	−	−?
Anolis	+	−	−	−	−?
Pseudemys	+	−	−	−	−?
Birds–Rooster	+	−	−	−	−
Duck	+	−	−	−	−?
Pigeon	+	−	−	−	−?
Sparrow	+	+	−	−	+?
Protheria					
Monotreme–Echidna	+	−	−	−	?
Theria					
Metatheria					
Marsupial–*Trichosurus*	+	+	+[2]	+	+
Didelphis	+	+	+[2]	−	+
Eutheria					
Scrotal	+	+	+	+[3]	+
Ascrotal–Hyrax	+	+[4]	+	+	+
Armadillo	+	+	+	+	+?
Degu	+	+	+	−	+
Suncus	+	−	+	−	−

[1] As judged by change in affinity for Fe^{+++} colloid or lectins (Con A or WGA)
[2] Tail structures only
[3] Variable
[4] Head only
±?: Anticipated result, but not yet shown by acute experiment
?: Not known

face of spermatozoa taken from successive regions of the epididymis. The one apparent exception in this group is seen in a soricid insectivore *Suncus murinus* (Cooper and Bedford, 1976).

Morphological and Structural Change Passage of spermatozoa through the epididymis of eutherian mammals is known to be accompanied by migration and eventual shedding of a droplet of residual spermatid cytoplasm from the tail midpiece, and sometimes also by modification of the form of the rostral region of the acrosome. Droplet migration appears at least as early as the amphibian stage in vertebrate evolution. In the snake studied in late September during the period of spermiation, most spermatozoa collected from the testis displayed neck droplets as did those from the proximal part of the excurrent duct, though in many of these it had migrated away from the neck. By contrast, droplets were absent from a majority of spermatozoa in the midregion and from 95% in the terminal region of the duct. A similar picture was presented in the turtle *Pseudemys* and lizard *Anolis* in individuals possessing motile spermatozoa in the terminal segment of the excurrent duct, in the birds studied, and in the echidna. Transformation and loss of the droplet are also features of epididymal maturation in marsupial spermatozoa (Temple-Smith and Bedford, 1976). In these, however, the droplet initially invests most of the head excepting the acrosome in immature spermatozoa, and subsequently passes to and remains in an eccentric position in the anterior neck region from whence it is discarded.

Posttesticular change in the form of the acrosome as a concomitant of sperm passage through the excurrent duct has not been observed in any of the subtherian species studied here, including the prototherian echidna. Change in the eutherian acrosome ranges from a major reorganization expressed in the guinea pig and chinchilla (Fawcett and Phillips, 1969) to the more modest change seen for instance in the rabbit, elephant, hyrax, and some primates (Bedford and Nicander, 1971; Bedford, 1974; Bedford and Millar, 1978; Jones et al., 1974). It occurs also in some rodents, e.g., in *Mystromys albicauda* (Fig. 3), but not in the ground squirrel *Citellus lateralis* (Fawcett, 1979) nor in the musk shrew *Suncus murinus* (Cooper and Bedford, 1976) both of which have a prominent acrosome. Nor does it occur in man (Bedford et al., 1973). Such changes are exhibited by some Metatheria (Harding et al., 1979), and spermatozoa of the brush-tailed possum *Trichosurus vulpecula* display perhaps the most radical reorganization seen in any species so far (Fig. 4). This reorganization begins as a withdrawal of flimsy acrosomal extensions followed by sloughing in the form of vesicles of the excess plasmalemma overlying the acrosome (Temple-Smith and Bedford, 1976; Harding et al., 1976). As in the Eutheria, this aspect does vary among marsupials, and is absent in several (Harding et al., 1979) including the Virginia opossum.[1] Nonetheless, many marsupials stand out from the eutherians studied with respect to the complexity of other visible structural changes that accompany sperm passage through the epididymis. Besides acrosomal changes, these may include a reorientation of the nucleus upon the neck, change in the membrane configurations in the neck region, condensation of the mitochondrial cristae, visible change both within and without the midpiece surface membrane (Phillips, 1970; Olson and Hamilton, 1976; Harding et al., 1975, 1976; Temple-Smith and Bedford, 1976) and in New World species a pairing of spermatozoa which in *Didelphis* is established in the lower corpus epididymis.[1] It is of interest, finally, that maturational changes in the acrosome of the guinea pig at least, depend on regional androgen-dependent characteristics of the luminal environment (Blaquier et al., 1972).

In so far as nonvisible structural changes are concerned, recent attention has been focused on the obvious stabilization in eutherian sperm chromatin and perinuclear material in the head, and in dense fibers, sheath, and mitochondrial shell in the tail, all engendered by oxidation of protein-bound —Sh to —S—S— during epididymal passage. Such studies, performed by evaluation of the effects of sodium dodecyl sulfate (SDS) or SDS plus dithiothreitol at the ultrastructural level (Calvin and Bedford, 1971; Bedford and Calvin, 1974a, b) show that significant stabilization of the head structures by —S—S— bonds in the posttesticular phase is limited largely to eutherian mammals, excluding even marsupials. While the author's observations on skate spermatozoa are, in this respect, incomplete, it is apparent that in none of the reptiles, birds, marsupials, or the monotreme studied do spermatozoa display comparable changes in passing through the Wolffian duct. Posttesticular stabilization of the structural components of the sperm tail also stands out primarily as a therian feature. For, with the exception of the sparrow, the tail organelles of mature reptile or the bird spermatozoa studied displayed little or no resistance to SDS, though this can be enhanced in some species by artificial promotion of—SH oxidation (Bedford and Calvin, 1974a). A notable exception is seen in urodele amphibians where the undulating membrane and tail skeletal elements are so stabilized. And, by contrast with other birds, the dense fibers of the passerine sperm tail seem largely stabilized by —S—S— bonds already as they pass from the testis, though their mitochondria show no stability when exposed to SDS. Thus the unusual stability of the outer membrane of the sperm mitochondrion engendered by —S—S— bonds seems a truly therian characteristic, for this does not occur even in monotreme spermatozoa.[2] The significance of this development for the function of therian sperm mitochondria, which presumably depends on the SH—rich mitochondrial protein discussed by Pallini in this volume, is at present quite obscure.

Sperm Storage

The importance of testicular androgen for maturation and for the viability of mature spermatozoa in the eutherian epididymis has long been recognized (see Orgebin-Crist et al., 1975). It is not clear, however, at what point in evolution the secretions of the testis become important in this respect, nor has much attention been paid to the reason for the development of this dependent relationship. The limited information suggests that, with the possible exception of passerine birds, this has appeared coincidentally with evolution of therian mammals. Past studies of the effects of the testis on the lizard excurrent duct epithelium (e.g., Takewaki and Fukuda, 1935) and those of recent vintage (Dufaure and Gigon, 1975; Gigon-depeiges and Dufaure, 1977) show clearly that testicular hormones modulate its secretory activity. Furthermore, although not clear-cut in all (e.g., Fox, 1952), there is little question that this epithelium responds to androgen in other reptiles and in birds. Nonetheless, potentially motile spermatozoa were obtained from the duct of a turtle 74 days after castration, which also brought a reduction in the height of the epithelium and thus probably a reduced metabolic/secretory contribution to the environment of the duct (Hansen, 1938). Somewhat compara-

---

[1] Temple-Smith, P.D.; Bedford, J.M.: Sperm Maturation in the North American Opossum *Didelphis virginiana*, in prep

[2] Bedford, J.M.; Rifkin, J.M.: An Evolutionary View of the Male Reproductive Tract and Sperm Maturation in a Monotreme Mammal, *Tachyglossus aculeatus*. Am J Anat, in press

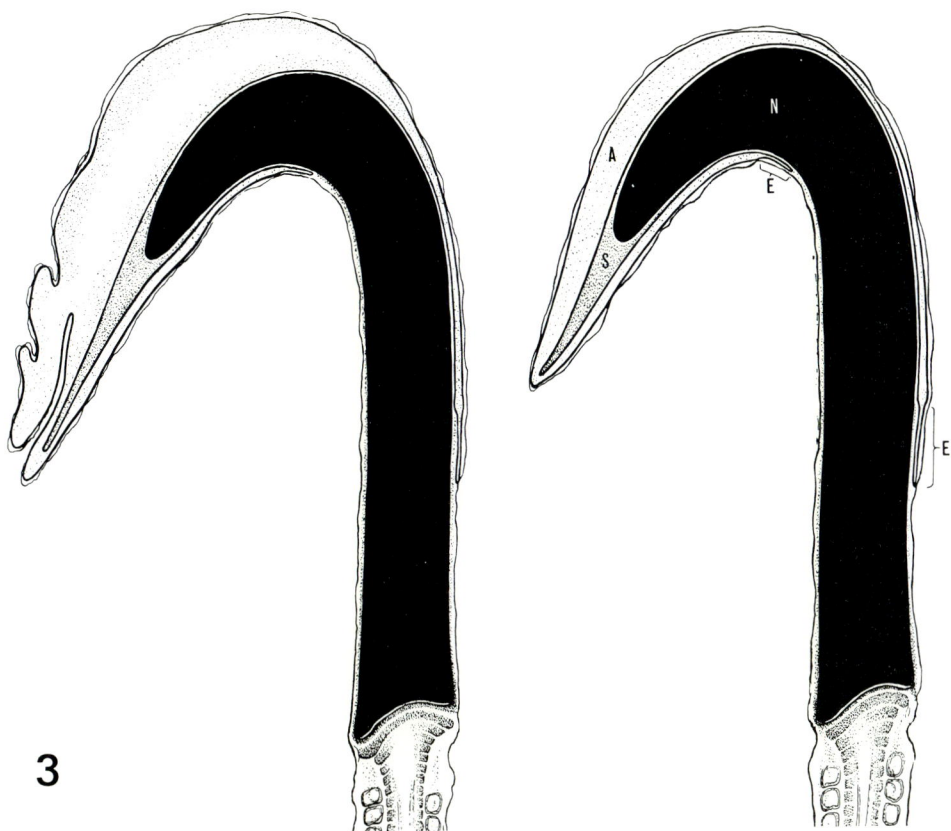

Figure 3. Sagittal section of the sperm head of the white-tailed rat *Mystromys albicauda*. These structures, constructed from different thin sections observed in the electron microscope, illustrate the way that, in passing through the epididymis, the acrosome of the immature spermatozoon in the caput epididymidis (left) becomes modified and eventually adopts the more discrete form displayed typically by mature spermatozoa (right) in the cauda epididymidis. A: acrosome S: subacrosomal material of the perforatorium N: nucleus E: equatorial segment of the acrosome.

ble results were obtained in the garter snake *Thamnophis*, in which hypophysectomy failed to impair the potential motility of spermatozoa released from the site of storage up to five months later (Tsui and Licht, 1974). This is in accord with experience in the snake *Natrix sipedon*. For although its testes were inactive in late April and early May as judged by an absence of spermatogenesis and a low Wolffian duct epithelium, the stored spermatozoa that filled its excurrent duct throughout, displayed a high grade of progressive motility for more than 20 h when released into Tyrode's solution at room temperature. Although there seems to be little information about the androgen-dependence of sperm survival in the excurrent duct of other reptiles, the implication of these sparse results for the turtle and snake, *i.e.*, that testicular androgen does not modulate the survival of their spermatozoa is echoed clearly by the findings of Munro (1938a) in the chicken. For his observations suggest that in this bird at least, androgens do not prolong the survival of its spermatozoa either.

In contrast to these submammalian species, removal of the marsupial testis (*Trichosurus*, *Didelphis*) brings a precipitous loss of viability of spermatozoa in the cauda epididymidis at an approximately similar rate to that seen after orchidectomy of the rabbit.[3] An exception in this respect among therian mammals is the cryptorchid musk shrew *Suncus murinus*. At 21 days after castration, a time verging on the limit of sperm viability in the normal male, there is no significant difference in the motility of spermatozoa retained in the cauda epididymidis of the castrate *Suncus* as compared with that in testosterone-treated or unilaterally castrated males.[4] Why *Suncus* should be an exception in this respect is not clear. Because Munro laid great emphasis on the difference created by the scrotal condition, and since *Suncus* is a natural cryptorchid, it was first suspected that descent to a scrotum might have some bearing on the relationship between androgen and

---

[3]Temple-Smith, P.D.; Bedford, J.M.: unpublished
[4]Bedford, J.M.; Dryden, G.L.: unpublished

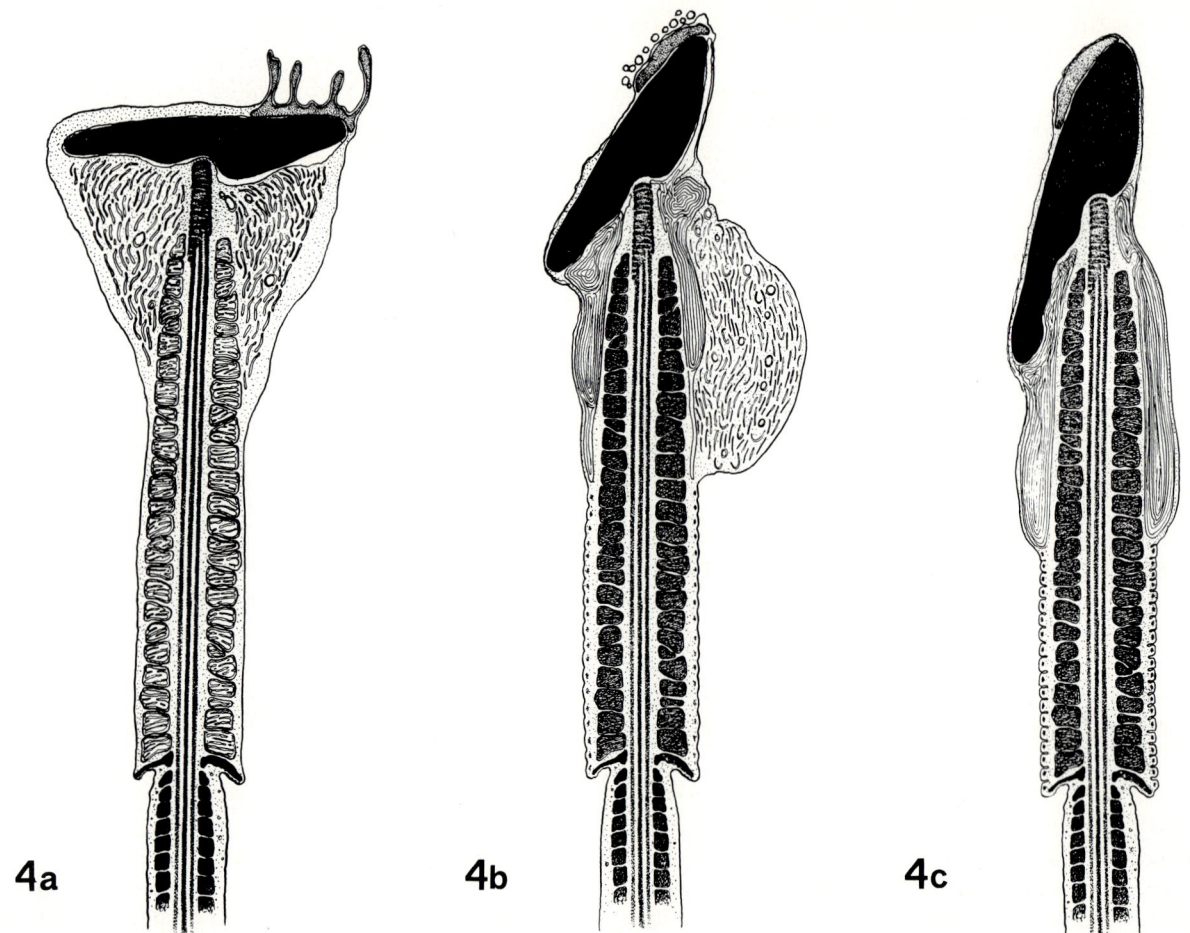

Figure 4a-c. Ultrastructure, in sagittal section, of the spermatozoon of the brush-tailed possum *Trichosurus vulpecula* at different stages of its maturation in the epididymis. Figure 4a depicts the immature spermatozoon in the head of the epididymis, characterized by: a nucleus set at 90° to the axis of the tail, filamentous immature acrosome, the cytoplasmic droplet which essentially envelops the head and neck, and the absence of electron-density in the mitochondrial matrix. In 4b, typical of spermatozoa found in the mid-lower corpus epididymidis, the head has begun to rotate toward the long axis of the spermatozoon, the acrosomal extensions have withdrawn and the excess plasmalemma is seen as a series of peri-acrosomal vesicles in this section. The droplet has migrated to an eccentric position in the upper midpiece from where it is shed, membrane whorls begin to occupy the neck region, and sub-plasmalemmal fibrous bands surround the now dense mitochondria in the posterior half of the midpiece. The mature spermatozoon in 4c displays a modest asymmetrically placed acrosome, voluminous membrane sheets in the neck region, and regular plasmalemmal invaginations along the posterior of the midpiece (from Temple-Smith and Bedford, 1976).

sperm storage. Recent studies in the testicondid hyrax show, however, that spermatozoa were always dead 25 days after bilateral castration, whereas approximately 80% remained viable in the cauda of the ipsilateral duct in unilateral castrates.[5] Similarly, all epididymal spermatozoa were dead 15 days after bilateral castration of the ascrotal degu, yet 50% remained potentially active in the ipsilateral cauda of the unilateral castrate. These results indicate that both hyrax and degu have a clear dependence on androgen for sperm storage in the cauda, and it is unlikely therefore that the exceptional situation in *Suncus*, or indeed the difference between subtherian and therian mammals studied in this respect, can depend on factors associated with the presence or absence of a scrotum.

In considering sperm storage in the male, it should be noted finally that the regional specialization for this in therian mammals probably does not exist to the same extent in either the snake or in nonpasserine birds. It is striking how soon spermatozoa retained in proximal part of the eutherian duct lose all potential for motility even where the epithelium remains intact (Gaddum and Glover, 1965; Bedford, 1967; Paufler and Foote, 1968), whereas this capacity is retained for weeks in the

---

[5] Millar, R.P.; Bedford, J.M.: unpublished

cauda epididymidis (Hammond and Asdell, 1926; White, 1933). By contrast, present observations show that during the period of testicular regression, spermatozoa carrying the potential for optimal motility are stored for some months throughout the excurrent duct of *Natrix*. Further, as noted previously, spermatozoa of potentially optimal motility exist throughout the tract of chicken, duck, and pigeon, if only in small numbers in the upper regions. But careful reading of the results of Munro (1938a) suggests that rarely does the capacity for optimal motility persist in most spermatozoa for more than 6-12 days even in the distal segments of the intact rooster.

DISCUSSION

A wider appreciation of the details of the maturation and storage of spermatozoa in the epididymis in recent years has not removed the conceptual vacuum that surrounds its function, and the question "why is there an epididymis" cannot yet be answered fully. Nothing is known, for instance, of the adaptive significance of the surface and metabolic changes in spermatozoa that appear to be key elements in their epididymal maturation, nor why this and sperm storage have come to depend acutely on androgens emanating from the testis. The difficulty in resolving such questions has been compounded in part by the narrowness of an approach confined almost exclusively to mammals. As a consequence of this legacy, there is a paucity of comparative information about spermatozoa in the male tract, about the relationship of spermatozoa within the female (Thibault, 1973), and about the mode of fertilization itself. This is unfortunate, for the evolution of epididymal function may have been determined or at least influenced by either or both of the last, it being unlikely that this function evolved in isolation and independently of other developments in the reproductive process.

The present comparative studies were undertaken in an attempt to begin to trace the pattern of evolution of the features that characterize sperm maturation and sperm storage in most eutherian mammals. As yet, they provide only a rather incomplete picture gained from a very few species. However, while the assumption that findings in one or two species necessarily reflect the situation of the whole group may prove misleading at times, these results and those of others already point to certain conclusions, and have uncovered exceptions which may allow further insights. It appears that epididymal function has indeed become considerably more complex with the evolution of therian mammals, as regards both the changes occurring in the spermatozoa and their dependence on the androgen-modulated environment of the duct. There is no critical posttesticular maturation in the cyclostomes, teleosts, or anuran amphibians studied. The urodele amphibians are not investigated here, but form an interesting subject in view of the unusual complexity of the spermatozoon and the fact that many species practice internal fertilization. The possibility that there is a posttesticular maturation process in this group is suggested by the negligible fertilization rate versus a 70% fertilization rate when testicular and vas deferens spermatozoa were used, respectively, to inseminate Notophthalmus females (McLaughlin and Humphries, 1978).

The first signs of posttesticular maturation in lower vertebrates have been detected in development of the capacity for optimal motility. This seems to be the major and perhaps only facet in elasmobranch fish, in reptiles, in many birds, and in monotreme mammals. It is noteworthy, moreover, that this seems to be a consistent feature of sperm physiology in species in which *all* members of the larger group are viviparous or ovoviviparous. Thus it may have arisen in response to demands imposed on spermatozoa deep within the female tract, particularly perhaps the need to survive there as active cells for hours and often for much longer. The coincidence of internal fertilization and the appearance of some degree of posttesticular maturation is not absolute. Spermatozoa of both *Xiphophorus* and *Poecilia* display good motility when released directly from the testis, and incidentally it has not been possible to demonstrate other post-testicular changes in the (but *cf* Bertin, 1958). It would be of interest to know more about the natural history of spermatozoa in the female tract of cyprinodont and perciform teleosts, whether they are activated before storage in the ovary, and how long they can swim there when active?

There seem to be distinct differences between therian and most subtherian vertebrates in respect of the specificity and the hormonal dependence of the environment needed for maturation of motility and the maintenance of this capacity during storage. Therian spermatozoa apparently cannot reach their potential for optimal motility in the testis (O'Shea and Voglmayr, 1970; Cooper and Orgebin-Crist, 1977), and although this may, but does not necessarily require a restricted specific region of the duct (Bedford, 1967; Orgebin-Crist, 1967), mature spermatozoa cannot survive for more than a brief period other than in a defined terminal region—the cauda epididymidis. Finally, acquisition of the capacity for optimal motility in therian spermatozoa, and its maintenance during storage, are highly dependent on androgen-mediated activities of the duct epithelium.

Although Munro (1938b) recorded that the motility

of testicular spermatozoa in the rooster is uniformly poor, in the present studies a small proportion of spermatozoa definitely displayed optimal and persistent progressive motility on their release directly from the testis in three nonpasserine birds. In view of the brief time required for their epididymal passage (de Reviers, 1975), the capacity for this must be acquired within a relatively few hours of spermiation in the cockerel. Studied carefully in fact the early results of Munro (1938b) suggest that chicken spermatozoa can mature to a fertile state within the testis on occasion. Thus the belief of Young (1931) that maturation may merely involve aging in a suitable but rather nonspecific environment, rejected now for mammals (Orgebin-Crist, 1969), could be true for some subtherian species. Such an inference challenges a suggestion of great seniority by Van der Stricht (1893), recently reiterated by Dufaure and Gigon (1975), that products from the secretory epithelium have a specific role in maturation of spermatozoa in the epididymis of the lizard *Lacerta vivipara*. As noted by Fox (1952), differences may exist between lizards and snakes in this respect, and it may be invalid to consider all reptiles as one group. However, the possibility that the relationship between reptilian spermatozoa and the epididymis is generally neither androgen-dependent nor highly specific in a regional sense is raised by the present observation that viable spermatozoa are stored throughout the excurrent duct during testicular regression in *Natrix sipedon*, that they exist there 74 days after castration in the turtle (Hansen, 1938), and finally that *Thamnophis* spermatozoa are motile when released up to five months after hypophysectomy (Tsui and Licht, 1974). The extent of the dependence of monotreme spermatozoa on androgen support of the epididymis remains to be established. It can only be noted here that they have retained the sauropsid form,[6] and that their maturation seems simpler than that in therian mammals[2] (Table 2).

An interesting exception among the subtherians as far as motility is concerned, is the small passerine bird. For the abrupt advent of the capacity for motility only at a point approximately half way through the nonciliated coiled duct (Fig. 2), and the dependence of this terminal region on testicular androgen for its very existence (Bailey, 1953), suggests that it may have a specific influence on the state of the spermatozoa within it. The sparrow is equally interesting for the unusual change in the affinity of the sperm head surface for visible markers. For while such expression of surface change is nearly ubiquitous among the therians, and is probably due in part to the acquisition of an acidic glycoprotein (Lea *et al.*, 1978; Olson and Hamilton, 1978), this does not seem to occur in other subtherians. The functional significance of surface change remains obscure. Since passerine birds comprise the only known example among subtherians where the epididymis is, in a sense, scrotal (Wolfson, 1954) and the one exception to this among the Eutheria studied (*Suncus murinus*) is a natural cryptorchid (Cooper and Bedford, 1976), it seemed possible that this might have been influenced by descent to a scrotum. That this is unlikely, however, is indicated first by the fact that the maturation process seems no different from the usual therian mode in the hyrax and the armadillo (Bedford and Millar, 1978), nor in the cryptorchid degu *Octodon degus*.[7] Furthermore, while sperm storage is suppressed by subjection of the epididymis to abdominal temperatures, this does not interrupt maturation (Bedford, 1978b).

Ultimately, attempts to understand the significance of epididymal function may profit from consideration of the problems facing spermatozoa in the female tract. For instance, as surface sialoglycoproteins influence the survival and fate of red cells and lymphocytes in the vascular system (Woodruff and Gesner, 1967; Marikovsky and Danon, 1969), it is possible that the surface modifications occurring in therian spermatozoa may relate to their ability to deal with the environment of the female tract. This particular question is complicated, however, by the need to consider also the further changes that may accompany capacitation in the female; for neither the exact nature of these, nor indeed the biological significance of the need for capacitation are established. A great deal may be gained by study of the features of conception in exceptions to the general pattern, notably here the passerine bird and the musk shrew *Suncus murinus*. It is intriguing how the character of sperm maturation in the sparrow (surface, motility change, and probable regionality and androgen-dependence), and its specialized sperm store placed in a scrotal environment, have come to mimic the therian condition so closely. It is also particularly striking how much the structure of passerine spermatozoa differs from that of other birds and indeed the monotreme mammals, which retain the reptilian form (Figs. 5 and 6). This and the relative complexity of the post-testicular maturation process merit serious study of their natural history within the female, as well as the character of the egg vestments and mode of fertilization in passerines.

It may be significant that in *Suncus* where epididymal

---

[6]Carrick, R.N.; Hughes, L.: Aspects of the Structure and Development of Monotreme Spermatozoa and their Relevance to the Evolution of Mammalian Sperm Morphology. Cell Tiss Res, submitted

[7]Bedford, J.M.: unpublished

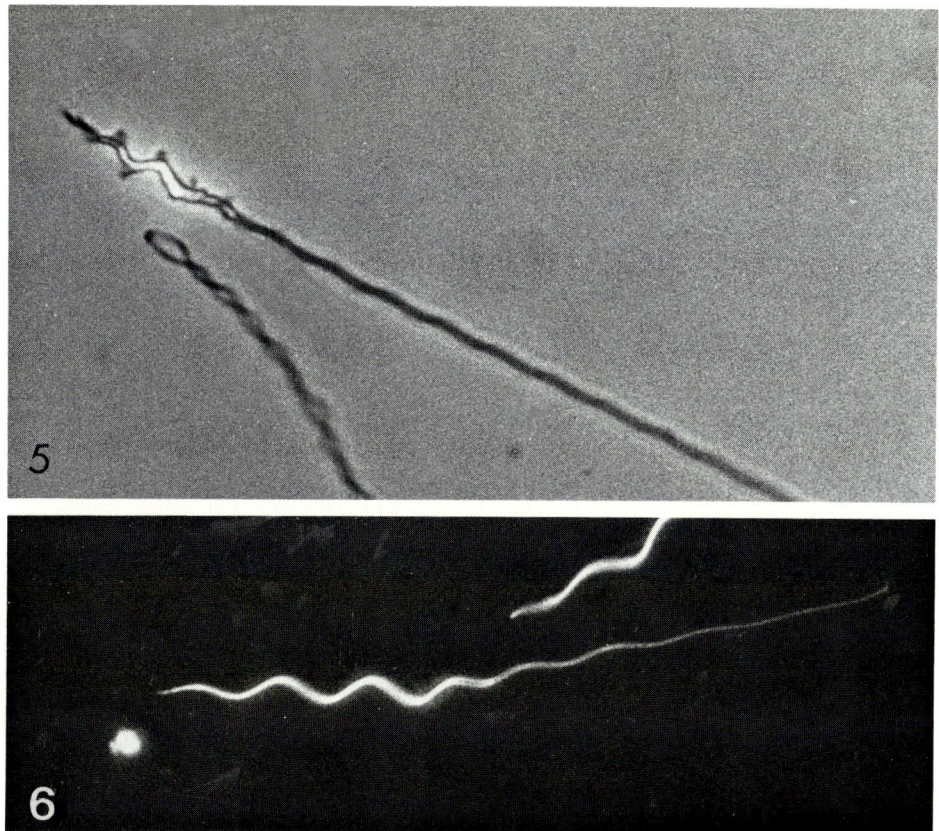

Figure 5. Phase contrast of spermatozoon of the song sparrow *Melospizia melodia*. It differs from the sauropsid pattern retained by many other birds in its corkscrew-like head—expressed in the shaping of the nucleus itself—and in the dispersed mitochondria which spiral down and around the sperm tail, an impression of which is given in this light photomicrograph. The tail itself is stabilized by thick dense fibers. X1500

Figure 6. Spermatozoon from the excurrent duct of the echidna. Although monotremes are mammals, their spermatozoa seem to have retained the sauropsid pattern in all major respects. Dark field. X950

function deviates from the normal eutherian pattern, the egg has an unusual follicular cell vestment stabilized by specialized intercellular junctions that make it insensitive to hyaluronidase.[8] For one obvious correlate of reproduction that is relevant to sperm function and which separates the Theria from the reptiles, birds, and even monotremes is the form of the female gamete. Other than a reduction in size, the ovum appears to have changed little in the evolutionary transition to the monotreme state (Hughes, 1977), and perhaps in keeping with this, monotreme spermatozoa seem to exhibit *none* of the structural or maturational features that distinguish those of the Theria from the sauropsid pattern. In the Theria, by contrast, not only is the egg much smaller than that of subtherian vertebrates, but in Eutheria especially it has come to be invested by an unusually thick, resilient zona pellucida and a follicular cell vestment that often persists throughout fertilization

(Austin and Bishop, 1958; Austin, 1961). Moreover, the way that spermatozoa are incorporated by the eutherian egg (Yanagimachi and Noda, 1970; Bedford, 1972) is very different from that which may typify subtherian vertebrates as represented by species as diverse as the lamprey (Nicander and Sjoden, 1971) and the chicken (Okamura and Nishiyama, 1978). Thus, evolutionary change in the ovum could possibly have ordained not only the unique mode of sperm/egg interaction in Eutheria, but also certain features of sperm structure (Bedford and Calvin, 1974b; Bedford *et al.*, 1979) and epididymal function.

There is at present no explanation of the functional significance, if any, of the movement and loss of the cytoplasmic droplet or the visible modification in the form of the therian acrosome after spermiation, though the latter may possibly reflect a need for further organization of the complex array of enzymes that exist within the acrosome (see Morton, 1976). Before this can be considered, more information is needed about the di-

---

[8]Bedford, J.M.; Cooper, G.W.; Dryden, G.L., in preparation

versity of the enzyme content of the subtherian acrosome, and thus whether this has changed significantly in the transition to the therian condition.

Turning finally to the question of storage, the evolutionary co-appearance of an androgen-dependent regional storage function and a heightened complexity of maturation in most Theria (and in passerines?) seem highly significant. As yet, however, the advantage conferred by these developments has not been explained. For instance, the rooster may achieve multiple matings (Munro, 1938a; Brantas et al., 1972) yet it has no obvious specialized storage capacity nor is sperm life prolonged by androgen. The key to the question may lie in a causal relationship or inverse correspondence between the complexity of epididymal maturation and a rate of transport through the duct that is compatible with this. For consideration of testicular output, excurrent duct capacity, and sperm longevity in the androgen-deficient and androgen-supported situation in relation to the kinetics of sperm transport along the duct suggests that *androgen-dependent prolongation of sperm viability acts to maximize the number stored.* The point is illustrated by comparison of events in the chicken on the one hand and the rabbit on the other. The testes of the rooster produce approximately 2×10^9 sperm per day, and the average capacity of its whole duct system is about 7×10^9 spermatozoa or sufficient to accommodate perhaps 4-5 days production (de Reviers, 1975). Since they are expelled after such a short period, there can be no advantage to extension of the intrinsic or androgen-dependent fertile life of some 7-12 days suggested by the data of Munro (1938a). On the other hand, rapid transport of 24-48 h permitted by a simple maturation process and which can be hastened by ejaculation, together with a high production rate, allows continuous rapid renewal of the available population. Rabbit spermatozoa also have an androgen-dependent functional life in the cauda of only about 6-8 days (Orgebin-Crist et al., 1975), but their testis-to-cauda transit requires 8-10 days. This prolonged transit in the absence of androgen clearly would preclude storage of viable spermatozoa in the cauda. Further, (for average figures from the literature see Moore and Bedford, 1978) even if transported *immediately* from testis to cauda in an androgen-free system, this life span and a testicular production of approximately 1.2×10^8 sperm per day would together allow an accumulation of only about $8-9 \times 10^8$ viable spermatozoa. This compares unfavorably with the $10-20 \times 10^8$ actually housed by the cauda of the sexually rested male rabbit.

Thus, extension of the functional life of the rabbit spermatozoon beyond the limits of its 6-8 day androgen-independent period to about 35 days in the androgen-supported tract (Hammond and Asdell, 1926) can be seen to provide a means whereby they may be stored as viable cells and so increase substantially the functional capacity of the caudal sperm reserve. The advantage of this for multiple fertile matings in any one brief period is readily apparent; for, unlike the chicken, the slow intrinsic transport in eutherians fails to respond significantly to ejaculation (Koefoed-Johnson, 1960; Orgebin-Crist, 1962; Amir and Ortavant, 1968). Our results in the ascrotal hyrax and degu show that androgen prolongation of sperm survival and scrotal evolution are not functionally linked. Nonetheless, since a cooler scrotal situation in some way optimizes the volumetric capacity of the cauda epididymidis (Fig. 7a-c)[9] it is possible that the androgen-prolongation of sperm life and the scrotum are both factors that maximize the capacity for storage of functional spermatozoa (Bedford, 1978b).

CONCLUDING REMARKS

Phylogenetic analysis of the character of spermatozoa from successive regions of the male tract of different vertebrates suggests that there has been a considerable increase in the complexity of epididymal function coincidental with the evolution of therian mammals. There appears to be no posttesticular maturation or storage of spermatozoa among the vertebrate groups in which all or most species practice external fertilization. The first sign of a maturation phase in the excurrent duct, reflected primarily in a development of the capacity for optimal motility, occurs in subtherian groups in which internal fertilization is the rule, *i.e.,* elasmobranch fish, reptiles, birds, and monotreme mammals. A further increase in complexity of epididymal function with the evolution of therian mammals is suggested in the coincidental occurrence of additional posttesticular modifications of the sperm surface, of the structural quality of head and tail organelles, in some cases of the form of the acrosome, in regional specialization for maturation and storage, and in clear evidence of an acute dependence of both maturation and storage on testicular androgen. Interesting exceptions that may help to illuminate the reasons for this occur in passerine birds where these functions seem almost as complex, and in at least one insectivore *Suncus murinus* where they appear unusually simple.

While the adaptive significance of this apparent progression to a greater complexity of the function of the male excurrent duct in therian mammals cannot be

---

[9]Bedford, J.M.: Effects of the Abdominal Environment on the Sperm Storage Capacity of the Rat Cauda Epididymidis, in prep

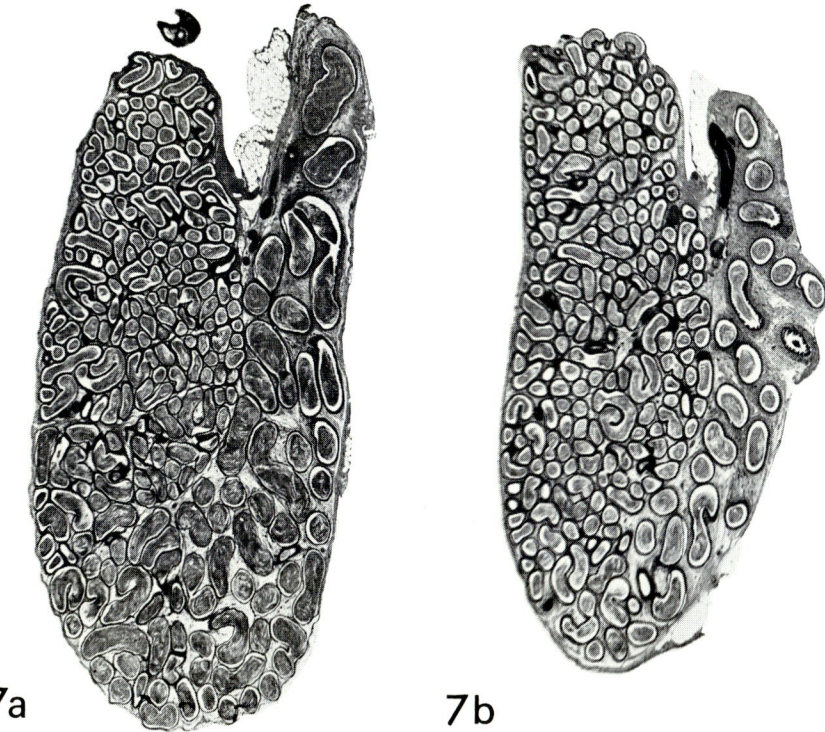

Figure 7a and b. Longitudinal sections of the left and right cauda epididymidis from the same white Norway rat, aged 8 months. The cauda in 7a is the normal scrotal control. That in 7b had been reflected to the abdomen for 5 months, but remained attached to a functioning testis of normal size retained in the scrotum (see Bedford, 1978b). Exposure to the temperature of the abdomen for such a prolonged period reduced the volumetric capacity of the cauda (compare the number and also size of cross section of large-diameter tubules) and the number of spermatozoa within it.[9]

explained with any confidence, a number of possible correlates can be considered. In the first place, there seems little relationship between the pattern of function in the epididymis and that in the testis. As can be gleaned from the discussion of Roosen-Runge (1977), the species that comprise the three broad groups defined here according to the character of their excurrent duct function (subtherians with external fertilization, those with internal fertilization, and the Theria) cannot be classified in the same groups on the basis of the mode of their spermatogenesis or spermiation. The character of epididymal function does not vary either according to the different patterns of seasonal breeding, nor does the increased complexity of sperm maturation and the dependence on androgen in the therian epididymis have any direct connection with the fact that, in many, this descends to a cooler situation in the scrotum. In seeking to understand the adaptive significance of epididymal function, it may be most rewarding to consider the possibility that several facets of epididymal function have been ordained largely by problems that face spermatozoa in the female tract. It seems significant that the advent of the initial and most obvious feature of post-testicular maturation—sperm motility—appears to coincide with the situation in which internal fertilization has been adopted by all members of the larger group. The subsequent appearance of other aspects in therian mammals could reflect the appearance of special problems of survival as a consequence of some evolutionary change in the milieu of the female tract, or equally those created by change in the vestments of the egg.

Although present evidence is limited, it suggests at least that therian spermatozoa may be much more dependent for their storage on androgen-mediated characteristics of the duct than are those of subtherians. The reasons for this also are uncertain. However, from comparison of testicular output, the androgen-independent and androgen-dependent life span of spermatozoa, and also storage capacity in relation to the rate of testis-to-cauda transit in chicken and rabbit, respectively, it can be seen that androgen-mediated prolongation of the viable life of spermatozoa increases enormously the number that can be stored in the cauda epididymidis; and this may be maximized further by the situation of the cauda in the scrotum. Such developments may be of particular advantage for the Theria. For, notwithstanding a relatively slow and complex phase of sperm maturation in the epididymis, they tend toward polygyny and so to the potential need for multiple fertile ejaculation over a brief period.

REFERENCES

Amir, D.; Ortavant, R.: Influence de la Fréquence des Collectes sur la Durée du Transit des Spermatozoides dans le Canal Epididymaire du Bélier. Ann Biol Anim Biochem Biophys 8(1968)195-207

Amoroso, E.C.: Viviparity in Fish. Symp Zool Soc Lond 1(1960)153-181

Austin, C.R.: The Mammalian Egg. Blackwell Oxford (1961)

Austin, C.R.; Bishop, M.W.H.: Role of the Rodent Acrosome and Perforatorium in Fertilization. Proc R Soc Lond [Biol] 149(1958)234-240

Bailey, R.E.: Accessory Reproductive Organs of Male Fringillid Birds: Seasonal Variations and Response to Various Sex Hormones. Anat Rec 115(1953)1-20

Bedford, J.M.: Development of the Fertilizing Ability of Spermatozoa in the Epididymis of the Rabbit. J Exp Zool 163(1966)312-329

Bedford, J.M.: Effect of Duct Ligation on the Fertilizing Ability of Spermatozoa from Different Regions of the Rabbit Epididymis. J Exp Zool 166(1967)271-282.

Bedford, J.M.: An Electron Microscope Study of Sperm Penetration into the Rabbit Egg after Natural Mating. Am J Anat 133(1972)213-254

Bedford, J.M.: Biology of Primate Spermatozoa. In: Reproductive Biology of the Primates. Contributions to Primatology. Vol. 3, pp. 97-139, ed. by W.P. Luckett Karger, Basel, 1974

Bedford, J.M.: Maturation, Transport and Fate of Spermatozoa in the Epididymis. In: Handbook of Physiology: Endocrinology. Vol. V., pp. 303-317, ed. by R.O. Greep and D.W. Hamilton. American Physiological Society, Washington, D.C., 1975

Bedford, J.M.: Anatomical Evidence for the Epididymis as the Prime Mover in the Evolution of the Scrotum. Am J Anat 152(1978a)483-508

Bedford, J.M.: Influence of Abdominal Temperature on Epididymal Function in the Rat and Rabbit. Am J Anat (1978b)509-522

Bedford, J.M.: Nicander, L.: Ultrastructural Changes in the Acrosome and Sperm Membranes during Maturation of Spermatozoa in the Testis and Epididymis of the Rabbit and Monkey. J Anat 108(1971)527-544

Bedford, J.M.; Calvin, H.I.; Cooper, G.W.: The Maturation of Spermatozoa in the Human Epididymis. J Reprod Fertil Suppl 18(1973)199-213

Bedford, J.M.; Calvin, H.I.: Changes in —S—S—linked Structures of the Sperm Tail during Epididymal Maturation, with Comparative Observations in Sub-mammalian Species. J Exp Zool 187(1974a)181-204

Bedford, J.M.; Calvin, H.I.: The Occurrence and Possible Functional Significance of —S—S— Crosslinks in Sperm Heads with Particular Reference to Eutherian Mammals. J Exp Zool 188(1974b)137-156

Bedford, J.M.; Cooper, G.W.: Membrane Fusion Events in the Fertilization of Vertebrate Eggs. In: Cell Surface Reviews: Membrane Fusion. Vol. 5, pp. 65-125, ed. by G. Poste and G.L. Nicolson. Elsevier/North Holland, Amsterdam, 1978

Bedford, J.M.; Millar, R.P.: The Character of Sperm Maturation in the Epididymis of the Ascrotal Hyrax, *Procavia capensis* and Armadillo, *Dasypus novemcinctus*. Biol Reprod 19(1978)396-406

Bedford, J.M.; Moore, H.D.M.; Franklin, L.E.: Significance of the Equatorial Segment of the Acrosome of the Spermatozoon in Eutherian Mammals. Exp Cell Res. 119(1979)119-126

Bertin, L: Sexualite et fecondation. In: Traite de Zoologie. Vol. XIII, part 2, pp. 1584-1662, ed. by P.-P. Grasse. Masson, Paris (1958)

Blaquier, J.A.; Cameo, M.S.; Burgos, M.H.: The Role of Androgens in the Maturation of Epididymal Spermatozoa in the Guinea Pig. Endocrinology 90(1972)839-842

Brantas, G.C.; Dennert, H.G.; Dennert-Distelbrink, A.L.: The Influence of the Number of Cocks on the Conception Rate among White Leghorns. Arch Geflugel K 36(1972)16-28

Calvin, H.I.; Bedford, J.M.: Formation of Disulphide Bonds in the Nucleus and Accessory Structures of Mammalian Spermatozoa during Maturation in the Epididymis. J Reprod Fertil Suppl 13(1971)65-76

Cooper, G.W.; Bedford, J.M.: Asymmetry of Spermiation and Sperm Surface Charge Patterns over the Giant Acrosome in the Musk Shrew *Suncus murinus*. J Cell Biol 69(1976)415-428

Cooper, T.G.; Orgebin-Crist, M-C.: Effect of Aging on the Fertilizing Capacity of Testicular Spermatozoa from the Rabbit. Biol Reprod 16(1977)258-266

de Reviers, M.: Sperm Transport and Survival in Male Birds. In: The Biology of Spermatozoa. INSERM, Nouzilly pp. 10-16, ed. by E.S.E. Hafez and C.G. Thibault. Karger, Basel. 1975

Dufaure, J.P.; Gigon, A.: Action des Hormones Androgenes sur l'Epididyme de Reptile *Lacerta vivipara* Jacquin. Gen Comp Endocrinol 25(1975) 112-120

Fawcett, D.W.: Comparative Aspects of the Organization of the Testis and Spermatogenesis. In: Animal Models for Research on Contraception and Fertility, in press

Fawcett, D.W.; Phillips, D.H.: Observations on the Release of Spermatozoa and on Changes in the Head during Passage through the Epididymis. J Reprod Fertil Suppl 6(1969)405-418

Fox, W.: Seasonal Variation in the Male Reproductive System of Pacific Coast Garter Snakes. J Morphol 90(1952)481-542

Gaddum, P.; Glover, T.D.: Some Reactions of Rabbit Spermatozoa to Ligation of the Epididymis. J Reprod Fertil 9(1965)119-130

Gigon-depeiges, A.; Dufaure, J.P.: Secretory Activity of the Lizard Epididymis and its Control by Testosterone. Gen Comp Endocrinol 33(1977)473-479

Hansen, I.: Studies on Reproductive Tract of Box Turtle. Anat Rec 72(1938)121

Hammond, J.: Asdell, S.A.: The Vitality of Spermatozoa in the Male and Female Reproductive Tract. J Exp Biol 4(1926)155-185

Harding, H.R.; Carrick, F.N.; Shorey, C.D.: Special Features of Sperm Structure and Function in Marsupials. In: *The Spermatozoon*, ed. by D.W. Fawcett and J.M. Bedford. Urban and Schwarzenberg, Baltimore, 1979

Harding, H.R.; Carrick, F.N.; Shorey, C.D.: Ultrastructural Changes in Spermatozoa of the Brush-tailed Possum, *Trichosurus vulpecula* (Marsupialia) during Epididymal Transit. I. The Flagellum. Cell Tiss Res 164(1975)121-132

Harding, H.R.; Carrick, F.N.; Shorey, C.D.: Ultrastructural Changes in Spermatozoa of Brush-tailed Possum, *Trichosurus vulpecula* during Epididymal Transit. II. The Acrosome. Cell Tiss Res 171(1976)61-73

Henderson, N.E.: The Annual Cycle in the Testis of the Eastern Brook Trout, *Salvelinus fontinalis* Mitchill. Can J Zool 40(1962)631-641

Horan, A.H.; Bedford, J.M.: Development of the Fertilizing Ability of Spermatozoa in the Epididymis of the Syrian Hamster. J Reprod Fertil 30(1972)417-423

Hoskins, D.D.; Johnson, D.; Brandt, H.; Acott, T.S.: Evidence for a Role for a Forward Motility Protein in the Epididymal Development of Sperm Motility. In: The Spermatozoon, ed. by D.W. Fawcett and J.M. Bedford. Urban and Schwarzenberg, Baltimore, 1979

Hughes, R.L.: Egg Membranes and Ovarian Function during Pregnancy in Monotremes and Marsupials. In: Reproduction and Evolution, pp. 281-291, ed. by J.H. Calaby and C.H. Tyndale-Biscoe. Australian Academy of Science, Canberra, 1977

Jones, R.C.; Rowlands, I.W.; Skinner, J.D.: Spermatozoa in the Genital Ducts of the African Elephant *Loxodonta africana*. J Reprod Fertil 41(1974)189-192.

Koefoed-Johnson, H.H.: Influence of Ejaculation Frequency on the Time Required for Sperm Formation and Epididymal Passage in the Bull. Nature 185(1960)49-50

Lea, O.A.; Petrusz, P.; French, F.S.: Purification and Localization of Acidic Epididymal Glycoprotein (AEG): A Sperm-coating Protein Secreted by the Rat Epididymis. Int J Androl Suppl 2(1978)592-607

Marikovsky, V.; Danon, D.: Electron Microscope Analysis of Young and Old Red Blood Cells with Colloidal Iron for Surface Charge Evaluation. J Cell Biol 43(1969)1-7

McLaughlin, E.W.; Humphries, A.A.: The Jelly Envelopes and Fertilization of Eggs of the Newt, *Notophthalmus viridescens*. J Morphol 158(1978)73-90

Middleton, A.L.A.: Spermiation and Sperm Transport in Passerine Birds. J Reprod Fertil 40(1974)31-37

Moore, H.D.M.; Bedford, J.M.: Fate of Spermatozoa in the Male. I. Quantitation of Sperm Accumulation after Vasectomy in the Rabbit. Biol Reprod 17(1978)784-790

Morton, D.B.: Lysosomal Enzymes in Mammalian Spermatozoa. In: Lysosomes in Biology and Pathology. Vol. 5, pp. 203-255, ed. by J.T. Dingle and R.T. Dean. North Holland, Amsterdam, 1976

Munro, S.S.: The Effect of Testis Hormone on the Preservation of Sperm Life in the Vas Deferens of the Fowl. J Exp Biol 15(1938a)186-196

Munro, S.S.: Functional Changes in Fowl Sperm during their Passage through the Excurrent Ducts of the Male. J Exp Zool 79(1938b)71-92

Nicander, L.; Sjoden, I.: An Electron Microscopical Study of the Acrosomal Complex and its Role in Fertilization in the River Lamprey, *Lampetra fluvialis*. J. Submicros Cytol 3(1971)309-317

Okamura, F.; Nishiyama, H.: Penetration of Spermatozoa into the Ovum and Transformation of the Sperm Nucleus into the Male Pronucleus in the Domestic Fowl, *Gallus gallus*. Cell Tiss Res 190(1978)89-98

Olson, G.; Hamilton, D.W.: Morphological Changes in the Midpiece of Woolly Opossum Spermatozoa during Epididymal Transit. Anat Rec 186(1976)387-404

Olson, G.; Hamilton, D.W.: Characterization of the Surface Glycoproteins of Rat Spermatozoa. Biol Reprod 19(1978)26-35

Orgebin-Crist, M-C.: Recherches Experimentales sur la Durée de Passage des Spermatozoides dans l'Epididyme du Taureau. Ann Biol Anim Biochem Biophys 2(1962)51-108

Orgebin-Crist, M-C.: Sperm Maturation in Rabbit Epididymis. Nature 216(1967)816-818

Orgebin-Crist, M-C.: Studies on the Function of the Epididymis. Biol Reprod 1(1969)155-175

Orgebin-Crist, M-C.; Danzo, B.J.; Davies, J.: Endocrine Control of the Development and Maintenance of Sperm Fertilizing Ability In the Epididymis. In: Handbook of Physiology: Endocrinology. Vol. V, pp. 319-338, ed. by R.O. Greep and D.W. Hamilton American Physiological Society, Washington, D.C., 1975.

O'Shea, T.; Voglmayr, J.K.: Metabolism of Glucose, Lactate and Acetate by Testicular and Ejaculated Spermatozoa of the Ram. Biol Reprod 2(1970)326-332

Pallini, V.: A Peculiar Cystein-Rich Polypeptide Related to Some Unusual Properties of Mammalian Sperm Mitochondria. In: The Spermatozoon, ed. by D.W. Fawcett and J.M. Bedford. Urban and Schwarzenberg, Baltimore, 1979

Paufler, S.K.; Foote, R.H.: Morphology Motility and Fertility of Spermatozoa Recovered from Different Areas of Ligated Rabbit Epididymides. J Reprod Fertil 17(1968)125-137

Phillips, D.H.: Ultrastructure of Spermatozoa of the Woolly Opossum, *Caluromys philander*. J Ultrastruct Res 33(1970)381-397

Roosen-Runge, E.C.: The Process of Spermatogenesis in Animals. Cambridge University Press, Cambridge, 1977

Setchell, B.P.; Scott, T.W.; Voglmayr, J.K.; Waites, G.M.H.: Characteristics of Testicular Spermatozoa and the Fluid Which Transports Them into the Epididymis. Biol Reprod 1(1969)40-66S

Takewaki, K.; Fukuda, S.: Effect of Gonadectomy and Testicular Transplantation on the Kidney and Epididymis of a Lizard, *Takydromus takydromoides*. J Faculty Sci Imp Univ Tokyo Sect 4 Zool 4(1935)63-76

Temple-Smith, P.D.; Bedford, J.M.: The Features of Sperm Maturation in the Epididymis of a Marsupial, the Brush-Tailed Possum *Trichosurus vulpecula*. Am J Anat 147(1976)471-500

Thibault, C.: Sperm Transport and Storage in Vertebrates. J Reprod Fertil Suppl 18(1973)39-53

Tsui, H.W.; Licht, P.: Pituitary Independence of Sperm Storage in Male Snakes. Gen Comp Endocrinol 22(1974)277-279

Van der Stricht, O.: La Signification des Cellules Epitheliales de l'Epididyme de *Lacerta vivpara*. C R Soc Biol (Paris) 45(1893)799-801

White, W.E.: The Duration of Fertility and the Histological Changes in the Reproductive Organs after Ligation of the Vasa Efferentia in the Rat. Proc R Soc Lond [Biol] 113(1933)544-550

Wolfson, A.: Sperm Storage at Lower than Body Temperature Outside the Body Cavity in some Passerine Birds. Science 120(1954)68-71

Woodruff, J.; Gesner, B.M.: Lymphocytes: Circulation Altered by Trypsin. Science 161(1967)176-8

Yanagimachi, R.; Noda, Y.: Electron Microscope Studies of Sperm Incorporation into the Golden Hamster Egg. Am J Anat 128(1970)429-462

Young, W.C.: A Study of the Function of the Epididymis. III. Functional Changes Undergone by Spermatozoa during their Passage through the Epididymis and Vas Deferens in the Guinea Pig. J Exp Biol 8(1931)151-162

BIOCHEMICAL ENVIRONMENT OF SPERM MATURATION

D.E. Brooks

Department of Animal Physiology, University of Adelaide, Waite Agricultural Research Institute, Glen Osmond, South Australia 5064 Australia

In the epididymis, spermatozoa are bathed in the fluid or epididymal plasma that fills the lumen of the duct. Epididymal fluid is derived from the rete testis fluid, but the latter is modified by the epididymal epithelium which is active both in absorption and secretion.

A comprehensive account of the composition of rete testis fluid can be found in a number of reviews (*e.g.* Setchell *et al.*, 1969; Setchell, 1970; White, 1973; Setchell and Waites, 1975). In general terms, rete testis fluid has a higher potassium content than blood plasma but contains little protein. It contains little reducing sugar but substantial quantities (7mM) of inositol (Setchell, 1970). Although most amino acids are present in lower concentration than in blood plasma, several amino acids, including those that can be formed by transamination reactions, are more concentrated in rete testis fluid and there is good evidence that these are formed as a result of glucose metabolism in the testis (Setchell *et al.*, 1967; Mushahwar and Koeppe, 1973).

In the proximal regions of the epididymis there occurs substantial resorption of fluid which must be accompanied by, and may be consequent upon, the removal of ions because the ionic composition remains relatively unchanged (Levine and Marsh, 1971; Turner *et al.*, 1977). This fluid resorption results in the spermatozoa being concentrated 20-fold or more. Further down the epididymal canal, sodium chloride is removed while the concentration of potassium increases. The replacement of sodium chloride by organic molecules maintains the osmotic pressure and a degree of hyperosmolality exists (Johnson and Howards, 1977).

One of the questions relating to the chemical environment of spermatozoa in the epididymis is the nature of the metabolic fuel(s) used by the sperm during their maturation and storage. Although a number of papers have speculated on this topic, there appears to have been no real attempt to support such speculation with quantitative evaluation. It is one of the purposes of this chapter to draw together some of the data available in the literature and to formulate some estimates of the possible contribution of various substrates toward maintaining the metabolism of spermatozoa in the epididymis.

© 1979 Urban & Schwarzenberg, Inc. Baltimore-Munich *The Spermatozoon*, edited by D.W. Fawcett and J.M. Bedford

METABOLIC STATE OF SPERMATOZOA IN THE EPIDIDYMIS

There are no data available concerning the metabolic rate of spermatozoa within the environment of the epididymal lumen. All estimates of metabolic parameters have been derived from spermatozoa removed from the epididymal environment and these estimates must therefore be considered as potential metabolic rates which may or may not coincide with the actual rates *in vivo*.

It is generally accepted that, within the epididymis, spermatozoa are immotile (Bishop and Walton, 1960). While this assumption may be true, definitive experimental proof is lacking. Spermatozoa have either been observed *in situ* but after the normal blood supply has been interrupted or after withdrawal into an environment which excludes the normal exchange of respiratory gases. Calculations based on the respiratory rate of rat epididymal spermatozoa (68 μl $O_2/10^9$ sperm/h at 25°C (Brooks, 1978b), sperm concentration in the cauda (1.74 x 10^9/ml (Brooks *et al.*, 1974a)) and oxygen tension in the epididymal lumen (pO_2 = 24 mmHg (Free *et al.*, 1976)) indicate that, without gaseous exchange, the spermatozoa would totally deplete the oxygen supply within 30 s. Thus the lack of motility observed in specimens collected by devices such as glass capillaries could be due to depletion of oxygen and the induction of motility observed upon subsequent dilution may largely reflect re-oxygenation.

SUBSTRATES FOR EPIDIDYMAL SPERMATOZOA

Reducing Sugars

Little reducing sugar appears to be present in rete testis fluid (Voglmayr *et al.*, 1970; Setchell, 1970; Cooper *et al.*, 1976) or epididymal plasma (Crabo, 1965; White, 1973; Jones and Glover, 1973a). However, isolated measurements of glucose concentration may be misleading. First, the glucose concentration could be reduced due to metabolic activity of the sperm during the collection period. Second, the level of glucose may be low but there may be continual replenishment of the glucose used, by transport from the blood stream. The rate of glucose utilization by testicular bull or ram sperm is approximately 0.2 µmol/10^8 sperm/h (Voglmayr et al., 1967, 1970). Even if glucose levels are as low as 0.1mM, as appears to be the case in rete testis fluid (Setchell, 1970), these could be sufficient to support the metabolism of testicular sperm for 30 min at the normal concentration of 10^8 cells/ml, although at this low glucose concentration the rate of glucose use might be expected to be less due to nonsaturation of the sperm membrane transport systems. In the testis, Setchell and Waites (1975) reported the accumulation of the nonmetabolizable glucose analogue, 3-0-methylglucose, which appeared to have a transport K_m of about 7mM as assessed by competition with glucose. Further evidence for the transport of glucose into testicular fluid and its metabolism by spermatozoa is cited by Voglmayr et al. (1970) as an inverse relation between sperm numbers and glucose concentration in rete testis fluid.

It is less likely that glucose would be a significant substrate for spermatozoa in the epididymis. First, negligible levels of glucose have been reported in epididymal plasma (White and Wales, 1961; White, 1973). Second, the utilization of glucose by the epididymal epithelium is restricted, probably due to limited membrane transport (Brooks, 1978a). Third, the spermatozoa are concentrated about 20-fold or more by fluid resorption in the proximal regions of the epididymis and the glycolytic demand per unit volume of sperm suspension would be much greater than in rete testis fluid. As motile ejaculated sperm have a much greater glycolytic rate than nonmotile testicular sperm (Voglmayr et al., 1967, 1970), the process of concentrating sperm in the epididymis may be of some importance in restricting the metabolic activity of potentially motile epididymal sperm by creating a greater competition for substrates of limited availability.

Lactic Acid

Lactic acid has been found in both rete testis fluid and epididymal plasma (Scott et al., 1963b; Setchell et al., 1969; Setchell, 1970; White, 1973). Moreover, the striking apical location of lactic dehydrogenase—NAD—diaphorase in the epithelial cells of the corpus epididymidis of the mouse might suggest the production and directional transport of lactate into the epididymal lumen (Allen and Slater, 1961). Rat epididymal tissue forms lactic acid from glucose in vitro (about 3 µmol/g/h under aerobic conditions at 30°C) (Brooks, 1978a). As the respiratory activity of rat epididymal sperm is equivalent to about 17 µmol of acetyl units/g/h (Brooks, 1978b) at 30°C and the sperm content of the rat epididymis represents about 4% of the epididymal weight (Vreeburg, 1975), the use of lactate by sperm in the epididymis can be calculated to be of the order of 0.7 µmol/g whole epididymis per hour. The production of lactate by the epididymis could be sufficient, therefore, to meet the needs of the spermatozoa. In addition to lactate resulting from epididymal glycolysis, lactate might also be transported from the blood stream to the epididymal lumen. The oxidation of lactate by spermatozoa would require the presence of oxygen. From the measurements of Cross and Silver (1962), epididymal tissue appears to be reasonably aerobic and this has been confirmed by direct intraluminal measurements of oxygen tension by Free et al. (1976).

Glycerol

It is well established that ejaculated spermatozoa can metabolize glycerol (Mann and White, 1957; White, 1957) but this activity is largely dependent on the presence of oxygen. The requirement for oxygen is undoubtedly related to the fact that spermatozoa contain the flavin-linked mitochondrial enzyme glycerol phosphate dehydrogenase (EC 1.1.99.5) (Mohri et al., 1965; Schenkman et al., 1965; Brooks, 1978b) but contain little of the NAD-linked cytoplasmic enzyme (EC 1.1.1.8) (Geer et al., 1975; Brooks, 1976b).

Somewhat surprisingly, no serious consideration has hitherto been given to the possibility that glycerol might serve as an energy substrate for spermatozoa in the epididymis, where attention has been predominantly focused on the measurement of glycerylphosphorylcholine (GPC). Estimations of GPC have frequently been made using the periodate oxidation method which is unspecific, and a number of compounds including free glycerol react in this procedure (White, 1959). In some instances more specific methods for GPC have been used. These have been based on the determination of acid-labile choline, either by formation of a chemical complex (e.g., Dawson et al., 1957) or by an enzymatic procedure (Brooks et al., 1974a). However, due to the high levels of GPC encountered in the epididymis, a comparison of the concentration of GPC determined by the specific and nonspecific methods could not be expected to show up relatively small amounts of free glycerol. The estimates of total glycerol in the epididymis made by Hodgen (1972) were based on the nonspecific method and would almost certainly reflect GPC rather than free glycerol. Reliable estimates of glycerol in the epididymis therefore, still remain to be made.

Glycerol could pass to the epididymal lumen, either as a result of lipid metabolism in the epididymal epithelium, or by transport from the blood stream in a manner analagous to the accumulation of radioactivity by the epididymis following the administration of radioactive α-chlorohydrin (Crabo and Appelgren, 1972; Edwards et al., 1975).

Glycerol enters the metabolic machinery of the spermatozoon through a phosphorylation step catalyzed by glycerol kinase (EC 2.7.1.30) (Mohri and Masaki, 1967), and is then oxidized to dihydroxyacetone phosphate catalyzed by mitochondrial glycerol phosphate dehydrogenase. Glycerol kinase is apparently not present in spermatozoa from all species, being notably absent from human sperm (Mohri and Masaki, 1967).

It is highly probable that the glycerol analogue, 1-chloro-2,3-propanediol (α-chlorohydrin) exerts its detrimental effect on spermatozoa by entering by the same route (Brooks, unpublished observations). For instance, α-chlorohydrin is a substrate for glycerol kinase (Fig. 1b, d) and also acts as a competitive inhibitor with glycerol for this enzyme (Fig. 1a, c). Furthermore, the phosphorylated product of α-chlorohydrin must act as a substrate for both cytoplasmic and mitochondrial glycerol phosphate dehydrogenases, since the cytoplasmic enzyme was used as a coupling enzyme in the glycerol kinase assay (Fig. 1) and α-chlorohydrin reac-

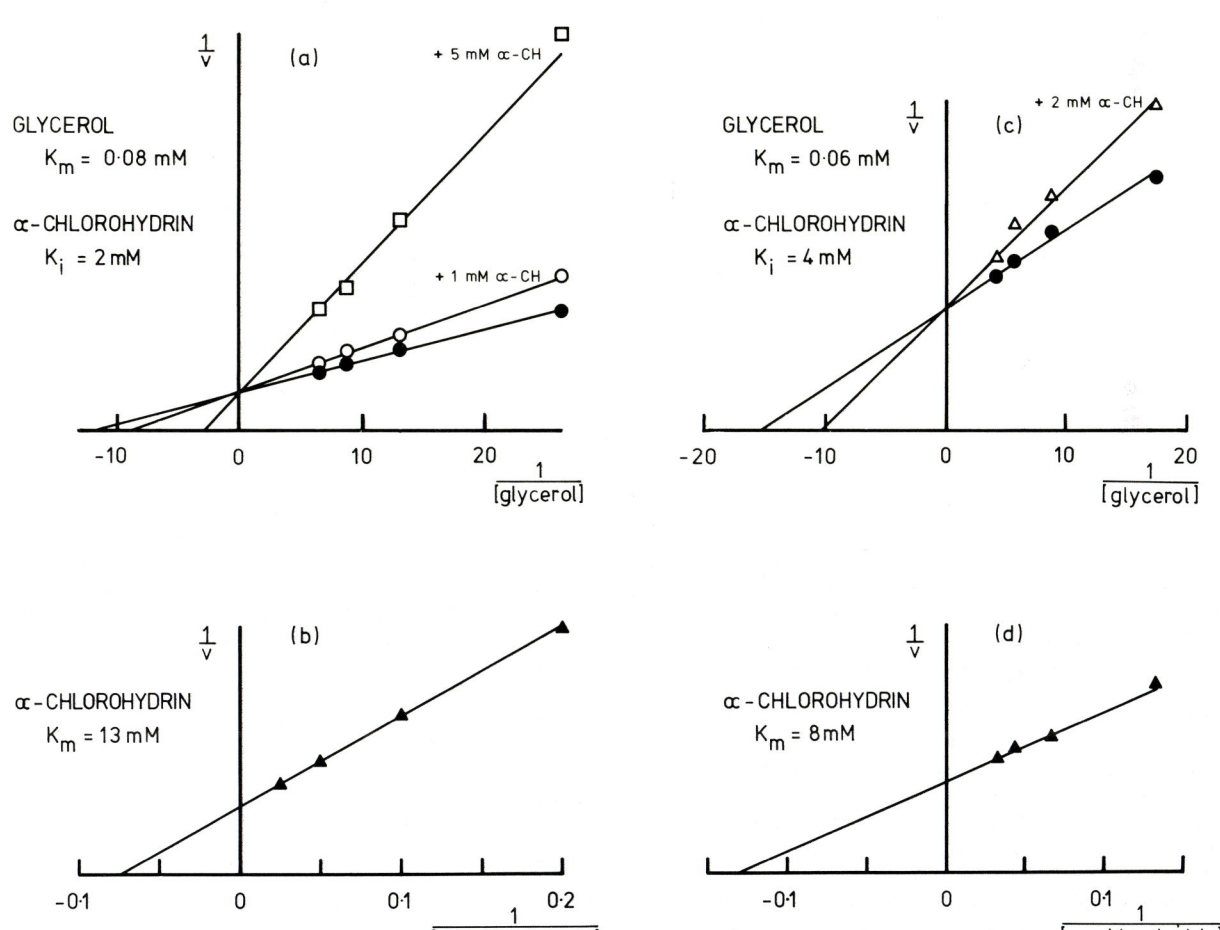

Figure 1. Kinetic behavior of glycerol kinase. A spectrophotometric assay was carried out at 25°C in 1 ml of : 180mM glycine, 3.8M hydrazine hydrate, 2mM MgCl$_2$, 1.4mM ATP, 1mM NAD, 1mM KCN, 1.2 units of glycerol phosphate dehydrogenase (EC 1.1.1.8), and various concentrations of glycerol and α-chlorohydrin. The final pH was adjusted to 9.8 with HCl and all assays were read against blanks in which the substrate was omitted. (a) and (b), purified glycerol kinase from Candida mycoderma (0.007 units per assay); (c) and (d), washed and sonicated ram spermatozoa (2.72 × 10^7 sperm per assay, equivalent to 0.0043 units of glycerol kinase). Although the data are presented as Lineweaver-Burk plots, the kinetic constants were determined by the procedure of Wilkinson (1961).

ted in the assay of the mitochondrial enzyme from rat testis when glycerol kinase and appropriate cofactors were added.

Sufficient evidence has now accumulated to indicate that α-chlorohydrin is not itself the active compound causing disruption of sperm metabolism. For instance, a period of pre-incubation with α-chlorohydrin is required before inhibition of the metabolism of glycerol is noted (Edwards et al., 1976) and α-chlorohydrin is not itself an inhibitor of several glycolytic enzymes in ram sperm (Mohri et al., 1975; Brown-Woodman et al., 1978) or mitochondrial glycerol phosphate dehydrogenase in rat sperm (Brooks, unpublished observations). However, there is strong evidence that a metabolic product of α-chlorohydrin inhibits several enzymes of the glycolytic sequence (Mohri et al., 1975). Mohri et al. also report that DL-1-chloro-1-deoxyglycerol-3-phosphate inhibits glyceraldehyde phosphate dehydrogenase. The results in Figure 1 suggest that conversion of α-chlorohydrin could proceed further to 1-chloro-1-deoxydihydroxyacetone phosphate (Fig. 2), and this latter compound might be expected to accumulate and possibly act as an inhibitor of glycolytic enzymes.

Because GPC is structurally related to both glycerol and α-chlorohydrin it is possible that it might also interact with glycerol kinase. Using 40mM GPC, no reaction could be detected in the spectrophotometric assay for glycerol kinase although some inhibition of the rate of glycerol conversion was noted (K_i for GPC = 54mM) (Brooks, unpublished observations). GPC has been shown not to be a direct substrate for sperm metabolism (Dawson et al., 1957; Storey and Keyhani, 1974) indicating that these cells do not contain the appropriate diesterase.

Inositol

The epididymis contains significant amounts of inositol (Eisenberg and Bolden, 1964) although the testis is the active region of inositol synthesis (Eisenberg and Bolden, 1963) by a mechanism involving cyclization of glucose 6-phosphate followed by liberation of phosphate and inositol (Eisenberg, 1967). Inositol is carried to the epididymis in the rete testis fluid (Setchell et al., 1968) but may also be accumulated from the blood stream (Lewin et al., 1976). Inositol is predominantly present as myoinositol, although some scylloinositol is present in addition to glycerylphosphorylinositol in the rat epididymis (Seamark et al., 1968). Testicular but not ejaculated sperm can carry out some synthesis of inositol from glucose (Voglmayr and White, 1971) but inositol is unable to stimulate sperm respiration (Voglmayr and White, 1971) although the endogenous inositol content of sperm is depleted during incubation without exogenous substrate (Voglmayr and Amann, 1973). The total tissue and epididymal fluid concentration of inositol undergoes marked changes along the epididymis, decreasing from caput to cauda in the bull and rabbit (Voglmayr and Amann, 1973) but increasing in the rat (Voglmayr, 1974; Hinton et al., 1977), with concentrations as high as 50mM having been recorded in plasma from the vas deferens (Hinton et al., 1977). These changes may partly be due to transport across the epididymal epithelium but may also be attributable to epididymal metabolism as the cauda of the rabbit and rat actively incorporate inositol into phosphatidylinositol in vitro (Voglmayr and Amann, 1973; Voglmayr, 1974).

Lipids

Apart from glycolytic substrates, spermatozoa can also oxidize free fatty acids (Flipse, 1960; Mills and Scott, 1969; Payne and Masters, 1970; Casillas, 1972; Casillas and Erickson, 1975a; Hamilton and Olson, 1976) and are also able to degrade exogenous phospholipids (Scott and Dawson, 1968). The oxidation of endogenous phospholipids was first suggested by Lardy and Phillips (1941) and later confirmed by Hartree and Mann (1959, 1961) who identified choline plasmalogen as the principal endogenous lipid oxidized by ram spermatozoa, although this has been questioned by Darin-Bennett et al. (1973). Changes in sperm phospholipids during epididymal transit have been well documented

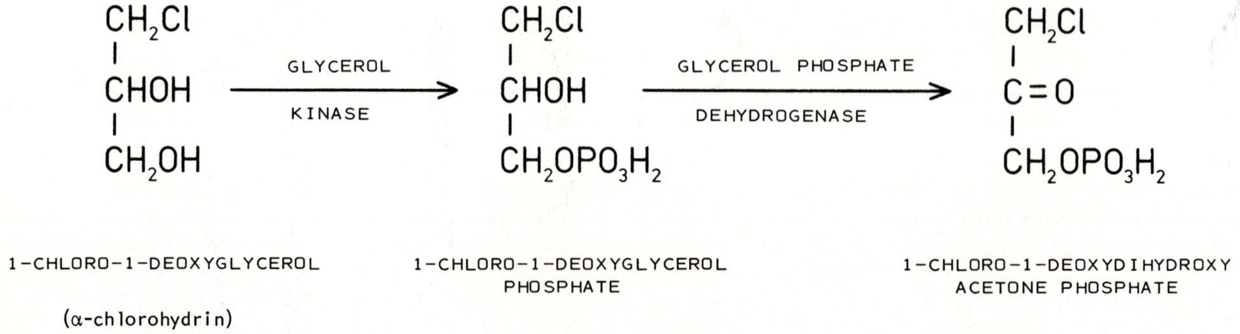

$$\text{CH}_2\text{Cl}-\text{CHOH}-\text{CH}_2\text{OH} \xrightarrow{\text{GLYCEROL KINASE}} \text{CH}_2\text{Cl}-\text{CHOH}-\text{CH}_2\text{OPO}_3\text{H}_2 \xrightarrow{\text{GLYCEROL PHOSPHATE DEHYDROGENASE}} \text{CH}_2\text{Cl}-\text{C}=\text{O}-\text{CH}_2\text{OPO}_3\text{H}_2$$

1-CHLORO-1-DEOXYGLYCEROL (α-chlorohydrin)   1-CHLORO-1-DEOXYGLYCEROL PHOSPHATE   1-CHLORO-1-DEOXYDIHYDROXY ACETONE PHOSPHATE

Figure 2. Possible conversion of α-chlorohydrin to effective metabolic inhibitors in spermatozoa.

(Scott et al., 1963a, 1967; Dawson and Scott, 1964; Grogan et al., 1966; Pickett et al., 1967; Quinn and White, 1967; Lavon et al., 1970; Poulos et al., 1973b, 1975). In general, the phospholipid content of spermatozoa has been found to decrease during epididymal transit, but in the case of the rat and rabbit an accumulation of choline plasmalogen has been noted (Scott et al., 1963a; Dawson and Scott, 1964; Cummins and Teichman, 1974; Teichman et al., 1974).

It has been suggested that the loss of sperm lipids during epididymal transit indicates that these lipids may serve as an endogenous source of metabolic fuel for spermatozoa in the epididymis (Scott and Dawson, 1968). Taking bovine spermatozoa as an example, the respiration rate of both testicular and ejaculated sperm is about 120 μl $O_2/10^9$ sperm/h at 37°C (Voglmayr et al., 1970) which represents a flux through the tricarboxylic acid cycle of 1.8 μmol of acetyl units/10^9 sperm/h. The total loss of lipid in bovine sperm during epididymal transit is about 1.8 mg/10^9 sperm (Lavon et al., 1970). If it is assumed that this lipid is glycerol dipalmitin, this represents 50 μmol of acetyl units/10^9 sperm, which would be sufficient to support sperm respiration for 28 h. Since epididymal transit takes about 14 days, it is clear that endogenous substrates are not sufficient on their own to maintain sperm metabolism.

Fatty acids could be made available for sperm metabolism, either as a result of metabolic activity of the epididymal epithelium or by the transport of fatty acids from the blood stream into the epididymal lumen. Long-chain free fatty acids (principally palmitic, stearic, and oleic acids) have been found in cauda epididymal plasma of the rat at a total concentration of 1mM, about five times the concentration of that found in blood plasma (Brooks et al., 1974a). The pattern of the types of fatty acids was distinctly different from that in blood plasma, and also quite different from that characteristic of spermatozoa, which in general contain substantial amounts of either docosahexaenoic or docosapentaenoic acid (Poulos et al., 1973a, b; Darin-Bennett et al., 1974, 1976, 1977; Evans and Setchell, 1978). The origin of the fatty acids in epididymal plasma is therefore unresolved, although derivation from the epididymal epithelium remains a distinct possibility. In addition to long-chain fatty acids, volatile fatty acids (1.7mM) have been detected in ram epididymal plasma (Scott et al., 1961) but may be only a feature of ruminant animals.

There have now been many reports of the high levels of glycerylphosphorylcholine (GPC) in epididymal plasma (Dawson et al., 1957; Dawson and Rowlands, 1959; White and Wales, 1961; Scott et al., 1963b; Crabo, 1965; Crabo et al., 1967; Quinn and White, 1967; Jones and Glover, 1973a, b; Brooks et al., 1974a; Jones, 1974a, b, 1977; Back et al., 1974, 1975). Although this compound is present in high concentration in the epididymal plasma, it cannot be directly metabolized by spermatozoa (Dawson et al., 1957; Storey and Keyhani, 1974). Moreover, as GPC accumulates in the epididymis in the absence of spermatozoa (Dawson and Rowlands, 1959; Brooks et al., 1974a; Jones 1974a; Brown-Woodman et al., 1976), it is clear that it is derived from the epididymal epithelium. It is most probable that GPC is formed from the degradation of lecithin (Scott et al., 1963b) although Wallace et al. (1966) contend that GPC is formed *de novo*. However, the conclusion of the latter workers is based on the assumption that the total tissue lecithin would act as a single precursor pool for GPC production, an assumption that may not be valid as acknowledged by the authors. GPC is formed principally in the caput epididymidis as evidenced by relatively little change in its concentration between the caput and caudal regions of the epididymis (Dawson and Rowlands, 1959; Crabo, 1965; Riar et al., 1973; Brooks et al., 1974a; Brown-Woodman et al., 1976).

The rate of GPC production in the epididymis can be estimated if it is assumed that the inflow of spermatozoa into the epididymis equals the outflow. Thus in the rat, rete testis fluid contains 32×10^6 sperm/ml (Setchell et al., 1973) and is produced at a rate of 22 μl/g testis/h (Tuck et al., 1970) or 33 μl/testis/h for a testis of 1.5 g (Brooks, 1976a). The concentration of sperm in cauda epididymal fluid is 1.74×10^9/ml (Brooks et al. 1974a) from which it follows that the rate of fluid outflow from the cauda is 0.6 μl/h per epididymis. As the concentration of GPC in fluid from the cauda is 41mM (Brooks et al., 1974a), the rate of production would be 25 nmol/h per epididymis, assuming that GPC is not transferred from the epididymal lumen to the blood. As GPC production is essentially restricted to the caput, which weighs 200 mg (Brooks, 1976a), this corresponds to a production rate of 125 nmol/g/h. Moreover, if dipalmityl phosphatidylcholine was the precursor of GPC, this would provide 16 moles of acetyl units per mole of lecithin and hence the rate of production of acetyl units from lecithin in the caput would be 0.034 μmol/min/g.

In the efferent duct ligated epididymis, the flux of acetyl units through the tricarboxylic acid cycle in the caput would be 0.2 μmol/min/g at 35°C (Brooks, 1978b based on a Q_{10} of 2 and temperature measurements of Brooks, 1973) and two-thirds of this flux is due to the oxidation of lipids (Brooks, 1978a) which therefore amounts to 0.13 μmol/min/g. By comparison with the estimated rate of production of acetyl units from lecithin (see above), it can be seen that lecithin could provide a quarter of the lipid-derived fatty acids for oxidation in the caput with the consequent release of GPC into the epididymal lumen. If some of the GPC escapes into the blood stream, the calculations above would be underestimated and the relative importance of lecithin to epididymal metabolism would be even greater.

Although these calculations indicate that lecithin may be of great importance for the metabolic mainte-nance of the epididymal epithelium, they also indicate that lecithin metabolism *per se* would not be sufficient to provide fatty acids for use by spermatozoa in the lumen. It may be that carnitine plays a role in this context for this is a compound which in other tissues is intimately involved with the oxidation of fatty acids. Like GPC, this compound accumulates to high concentrations in epididymal plasma (63mM in the rat, Brooks *et al.*, 1974a), but differs in that it is derived by transport from the blood stream (Brooks *et al.*, 1973) rather than being synthesized by the epididymis (Casillas and Erickson,

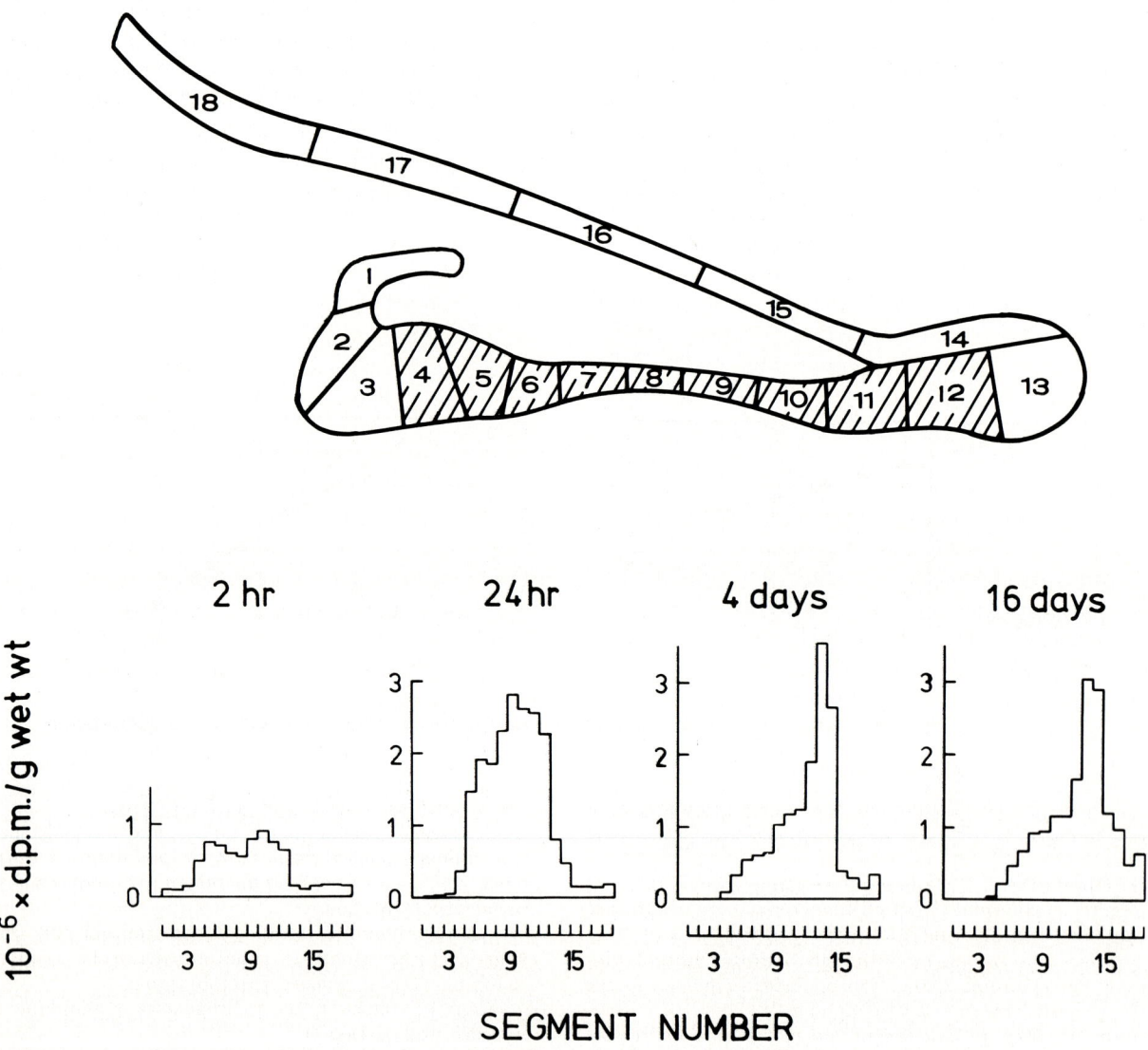

Figure 3. Uptake of radioactivity by the epididymis following an intravenous pulse of L-[methyl-^{3}H] carnitine. The rat excurrent duct system was sectioned into 18 segments as indicated in the upper section of the figure. The segmental distribution of radioactivity (disintegrations per minute) at various times following the pulse administration of radio-active carnitine is shown in the lower section of the figure. Those regions of the epididymis that actively took up carnitine during the pulse period (see segmental distribution of radioactivity at 2 h) are indicated by the cross-hatching in the upper section of the figure. Subsequently the radioactive carnitine migrated distally along the excurrent duct system. The data in this figure are reproduced from Brooks *et al.* (1973) by permission of Academic Press.

1975b). By applying the same calculations as were used to derive the rate of GPC synthesis, the rate of carnitine accumulation by the rat epididymis can be estimated as 38 nmol/h per epididymis. However, in contrast to GPC, the regions involved in carnitine transport are the distal caput, corpus, and proximal cauda (Fig. 3) with the consequence that the concentration of carnitine progressively increases throughout the length of the epididymis (Brooks et al., 1974a). As the total weight of the epididymal segments associated with carnitine accumulation was 250 mg (Brooks et al., 1973), the flux of carnitine into the epididymis is equivalent to 150 nmol/h/g. This high rate of flux is only surpassed by three other tissues, namely the kidney, spleen, and liver (Brooks and McIntosh, 1975).

Although the net transport of carnitine from the blood to the epididymal lumen has been established, the nature of the transport mechanism is entirely obscure. In other tissues carnitine acts as a carrier of fatty acids across the mitochondrial membrane mediated by the enzyme, carnitine palmitoyltransferase. It remains a possibility worthy of investigation that this enzyme, which is quite active in the epididymis (Brooks, 1978b), is partially associated with cell surface membranes such that fatty acylcarnitine is formed at the basal surface of the epithelial cells with the subsequent release of carnitine and fatty acid at the apical surface, thereby providing fatty acids for spermatozoa in the lumen. Alternatively, the fatty acids may be oxidized to acetyl units in the epithelial cells and transported to the epididymal lumen as acetylcarnitine, which is present in substantial concentration in epididymal fluid from the cauda of the rat (6mM, calculated from the data of Brooks et al., 1974a) and be available in this form for oxidation by spermatozoa. If acetyl groups are transported into the epididymal lumen in the form of acetylcarnitine, then the rate of transport would be equivalent to the flux of carnitine as calculated above, namely 0.15 μmol/g epididymis/h for the rat epididymis. However, based on the rate of acetyl group utilization by rat sperm in the epididymis of 0.7 μmol/g epididymis/h (see section on lactic acid), transport of acetylcarnitine would account for only about 20% of the energy requirements of the sperm in those regions of the epididymis which actively accumulate carnitine.

Bull and rat spermatozoa from the cauda epididymidis contain about 1 μmol of total carnitine (i.e. carnitine + acetylcarnitine)/10^9 sperm (Table 1). The vol-

Table 1. Carnitine and Acetylcarnitine Concentration in Spermatozoa and Epididymal Plasma

| | | Sperm | Epididymal Plasma | | |
| | | Carnitine | Carnitine | Acetylcarnitine | |
Species	Location	(μmol/10^9 Sperm)	(mM)	(mM)	Reference
Octopus	Spermatophore	[a]14.6			Brooks et al. (1974b)
Rat	Cauda	0.62	63	6	Brooks et al. (1974a)
Rat	Cauda	[b]0.97			Brooks et al. (1974a)
Rat	Cauda	0.6			Casillas (1972)
Rat	Cauda	[c]0.4	[c]16	[c]1	Marquis and Fritz (1965)
Rabbit	Cauda		[d]69		Jones (1977)
Boar	Cauda	4.4			Casillas (1972)
Bull	Cauda	1.3			Casillas (1972)
Bull	Cauda	1	2		Casillas (1973)
Bull	Cauda	[b]0.8			Casillas & Erickson (1975a)
Bull	Cauda	[b]0.7			Milkowski et al. (1976)
Bull	Cauda	0.6			Van Dop et al. (1977)
Monkey	Cauda	3.3			Casillas (1972)
Monkey	Ejaculated	2.1			Casillas and Erickson (1975a)
Monkey	Ejaculated	[b]3.8			Casillas and Erickson (1975a)
Human	Ejaculated	0.85			Frenkel et al. (1974)
Human	Ejaculated	0.006			Kohengkul et al. (1977)
Human	Cauda		[e]6		Brooks & Howards (unpublished observation)

[a] μmol/g wet wt of sperm packed by hard centrifugation
[b] Total carnitine (i.e. acetylcarnitine plus carnitine)
[c] Calculations were based on the following data and extrapolation of % dry wt and sp. gr. from bull sperm to rat sperm: a) sp. gr. of epididymal bull sperm = 1.1 (Lindahl and Thunqvist, 1965; Lavon et al., 1966) b) % dry wt of bull sperm = 34 (Lavon et al., 1970) c) Volume of rat sperm = 75 fl (Brotherton, 1975) d) sperm concentration in rat cauda epididymidis = 1.74 × 10^9/ml (Brooks et al., 1974a)
[d] Corpus and vas ligated for 35 days
[e] Obtained by micropuncture from a patient aged 65 years after orchidectomy for prostatic carcinoma and without subjection to hormonal therapy.

ume of a bull and rat epididymal sperm is 31 and 75 fl respectively (Brotherton, 1975). If it is assumed that the carnitine distribution space is about one-third of the total sperm volume, then it follows that the intracellular total carnitine concentration is about 100mM and 40mM respectively for the two species. It is now clear that the acetylation state of carnitine can be profoundly influenced by the presence of exogenous substrates (Casillas and Erickson, 1975a; Milkowski et al., 1976; Van Dop et al., 1977) and that acetylcarnitine can act as a ready source of oxidizable acetyl units for spermatozoa (Storey and Keyhani, 1974; Hutson et al., 1977a) in addition to serving as a buffer to acetyl coenzyme A levels. Carnitine depresses the oxidation of acetylcarnitine by bovine epididymal sperm mitochondria (Hutson et al., 1977b) possibly by competing with acetylcarnitine for mitochondrial transport (Calvin and Tubbs, 1976); and it may be for this reason that a significant concentration of acetylcarnitine occurs in epididymal plasma rather than being kept low by the metabolic activity of the spermatozoa.

Reports on the effect of carnitine on palmitate oxidation have been more contradictory. In bovine sperm, carnitine has been shown 1) to enhance the rate of palmitate oxidation by sonicated epididymal sperm (Casillas, 1972), 2) to have no effect on palmitoylcarnitine oxidation by epididymal sperm mitochondria (Hutson et al., 1977b), and 3) to depress oxidation by ejaculated sperm (Hamilton and Olson, 1976), while the mitochondria of rabbit epididymal sperm can oxidize palmitoylcarnitine but not palmitoyl CoA in the presence of carnitine (Storey and Keyhani, 1974).

Amino Acids

Several amino acids are present in rete testis fluid in concentrations greater than in blood plasma, and even higher concentrations are found in luminal fluid from the epididymis and ductus deferens. Quantitatively, glutamate is the most important amino acid in epididymal plasma of the ram, bull, and boar but not the rat; estimates of its concentration have ranged from 12-25mM (Setchell et al., 1967; Sexton et al., 1971; Johnson et al., 1972; Brown-Woodman and White, 1974). In boar epididymal plasma hypotaurine has been reported at a concentration of 45mM and urea at 8mM (Johnson et al., 1972). Of particular interest is the recent demonstration that several enzymes of the γ-glutamyl cycle are active in the epididymis (DeLap et al., 1977). The γ-glutamyl cycle has been proposed as a mechanism for the transport of amino acids across membranes (Meister and Tate, 1976). This mechanism could therefore exist for the uptake of amino acids from the rete testis fluid by the epididymal epithelium, particularly in the proximal regions of the duct where the large resorption of fluid occurs. In this connection, the membrane-bound enzyme γ-glutamyltranspeptidase, which plays a key role in the γ-glutamyl cycle, is particularly active in the caput epididymidis. This enzyme is relatively inactive in spermatozoa but it is present in epididymal plasma, suggesting its origin from the plasma membrane of epithelial cells (DeLap et al., 1977).

The metabolism of glutamate by spermatozoa has been studied in some detail (Setchell et al., 1967; Flipse and Dietz, 1969; Flipse et al., 1969; Sexton et al., 1971). This amino acid can be oxidized by testicular, epididymal and ejaculated spermatozoa to a limited extent (about 2% of the rate at which glucose is used) but does not stimulate endogenous respiration (Setchell et al., 1967; Sexton et al., 1971). The mechanism of oxidation is partly due to transamination and partly due to the activity of glutamate dehydrogenase (Flipse and Dietz, 1969; Flipse et al., 1969). However, the slow rate of oxidation indicates that amino acids are unlikely to form a significant metabolic fuel for spermatozoa in the epididymis.

SUMMARY

Traces of reducing sugar are found in rete testis fluid and it is possible that glucose may, at least in part, contribute to the maintenance of testicular sperm, but it is less likely that glucose is available to spermatozoa in the epididymis. On the other hand, lactic acid occurs in epididymal plasma and the rate of production of lactate resulting from the glycolytic activity of epididymal tissue would be sufficient to support sperm metabolism if this substrate were directed into the epididymal lumen. Alternatively, the possibility exists that free glycerol may be available for oxidation by spermatozoa. Although significant concentrations of inositol are present in the epididymal plasma, this compound is not capable of supporting sperm respiration. Neither would amino acids appear to be important substrates since they are metabolized only slowly by spermatozoa. However, lipids could serve as substrates for epididymal spermatozoa. The oxidation of endogenous sperm lipids may contribute to some extent to the maintenance of spermatozoa, but the amount of lipid oxidized would be insufficient to supply the total energy needs. The epididymal epithelium itself actively oxidizes lipids and it is probable that glycerylphosphorylcholine accumulates in the epididymal lumen as a result of this activity. Fatty acids might be provided by the epididymal epithelium for use by the spermatozoa either as long-chain fatty acids or after conversion to acetylcarnitine. Acetylcarnitine is present in significant concentration in epididymal plasma and can be readily utilized by spermatozoa, although its rate of oxidation by sperm mitochondria is reduced in the presence of free carnitine and this may limit the oxidation of acetylcarnitine by sperm in the epididymis.

Note: Subsequent investigation of the interaction of α-chlorohydrin with glycerol kinase has indicated that the reaction detected in the spectrophotometer was due to the presence of glycerol as a trace contaminant in the preparation of α-chlorohydrin. It has since been found that α-chlorohydrin is not a substrate for glycerol kinase but does act as a competitive inhibitor (K_i of 30 mM) of this enzyme (Brooks, 1979).

REFERENCES

Allen, J.M.; Slater, J.J.: A Cytochemical Analysis of the Lactic Dehydrogenase-Diphosphopyridine Nucleotide-Diaphorase System in the Epididymis of the Mouse. J Histochem Cytochem 9(1961)221-233

Back, D.J.; Shenton, J.C.; Glover, T.D.: The Composition of Epididymal Plasma from the Cauda Epididymidis of the Rat. J Reprod Fertil 40(1974)211-214

Back, D.J.; Glover, T.D.; Shenton, J.C.; Boyd, G.P.: The Effects of α-Chlorohydrin on the Composition of Rat and Rabbit Epididymal Plasma: A Possible Explanation of Species Difference. J Reprod Fertil 45(1975)117-128

Bishop, M.W.H.; Walton, A.: The Physiology of Spermatozoa Within the Male Reproductive Tract. In: Marshall's Physiology of Reproduction. Vol. 1, part 2, 3rd ed. pp. 94-129, ed. by A.S. Parkes. Longmans Green, London, 1960

Brooks, D.E.: Epididymal and Testicular Temperature in the Unrestrained Conscious Rat. J Reprod Fertil 35(1973)157-160

Brooks, D.E.: Changes in the Composition of the Excurrent Duct System of the Rat Testis during Postnatal Development. J Reprod Fertil 46(1976a)31-38

Brooks, D.E.: Activity and Androgenic Control of Glycolytic Enzymes in the Epididymis and Epididymal Spermatozoa of the Rat. Biochem J 156(1976b)527-537

Brooks, D.E.: Androgenic Regulation of Metabolic Pathways in the Rat Epididymis. Biol Reprod 18(1978a)629-638

Brooks, D.E.: Activity and Androgenic Control of Enzymes Associated with the Tricarboxylic Acid Cycle, Lipid Oxidation and Mitochondrial Shuttles in the Epididymis and Epididymal Spermatozoa of the Rat. Biochem J 174(1978b)741-752

Brooks, D.E.: The Interaction of α-Chlorohydrin with Glycerol Kinase. J Reprod Fertil 56(1979)593-599

Brooks, D.E.; McIntosh, J.E.A.: Turnover of Carnitine by Rat Tissues. Biochem J 148(1975)439-445

Brooks, D.E.; Hamilton, D.W.; Mallek, A.H.: The Uptake of L-[methyl-^{3}H]Carnitine by the Rat Epididymis. Biochem Biophys Res Commun 52(1973)1354-1360

Brooks, D.E.; Hamilton, D.W.; Mallek, A.H.: Carnitine and Glycerylphosphorylcholine in the Reproductive Tract of the Male Rat. J Reprod Fertil 36(1974a)141-160

Brooks, D.E.; Mann, T.; Martin, A.W.: The Occurrence of Carnitine and Glycerylphosphorylcholine in the Octopus Spermatophore. Proc R Soc Lond [Biol] 186(1974b)79-82

Brotherton, J.: The Counting and Sizing of Spermatozoa from ten Animal Species Using a Coulter Counter. Androl 7(1975)169-185

Brown-Woodman, P.D.C.; White, I.G.: Amino Acid Composition of Semen and the Secretions of the Male Reproductive Tract. Aust J Biol Sci 27(1974)415-422

Brown-Woodman, P.D.C.; Sale, D.; White, I.G.: The Glycerylphosphorylcholine Content of the Rat Epididymis after Injecting α-Chlorohydrin and Ligating the Vasa Efferentia. Acta Eur Fertil 7(1976)155-162

Brown-Woodman, P.D.C.; Mohri, H.; Mohri, T.; Suter, D.; White, I.G.: Mode of Action of α-Chlorohydrin as a Male Antifertility Agent. Inhibition of the Metabolism of Ram Spermatozoa by α-Chlorohydrin and Location of Block in Glycolysis. Biochem J 170(1978)23-37

Calvin, J.; Tubbs, P.K.: A Carnitine:Acetylcarnitine Exchange System in Spermatozoa. J Reprod Fertil 48(1976)417-420

Casillas, E.R.: The Distribution of Carnitine in Male Reproductive Tissues and its Effect on Palmitate Oxidation by Spermatozoal Particles. Biochim Biophys Acta 280(1972)545-551

Casillas, E.R.: Accumulation of Carnitine by Bovine Spermatozoa during Maturation in the Epididymis. J Biol Chem 248(1973)8227-8232

Casillas, E.R.; Erickson, B.J.: The Role of Carnitine in Spermatozoa Metabolism: Substrate-induced Elevations in the Acetylation State of Carnitine and Coenzyme A in Bovine and Monkey Spermatozoa. Biol Reprod 12(1975a)275-283

Casillas, E.R.; Erickson, B.J.: Studies on Carnitine Synthesis in the Rat Epididymis. J Reprod Fertil 44(1975b)287-291.

Cooper, T.G.; Danzo, B.J.; Dipietro, D.L.; McKenna, T.J.; Orgebin-Crist, M.C.: Some Characteristics of Rete Testis Fluid from Rabbits. Androl 8(1976)87-94

Crabo, B.: Studies on the Composition of Epididymal Content in Bulls and Boars. Acta Vet Scand 6 Suppl 5(1965)1-94

Crabo, B.; Appelgren, L.E.: Distribution of α[^{14}C]Chlorohydrin in Mice and Rats. J Reprod Fertil 30(1972)161-163

Crabo, B.; Gustafsson, B.; Bane, A.; Meschaks, P.; Ringmar, J.E.: The Concentration of Sodium, Potassium, Calcium, Inorganic Phosphate, Protein and Glycerylphosphorylcholine in the Epididymal Plasma of Bull Calves. J Reprod Fertil 13(1967)589-591

Cross, B.A.; Silver, I.A.: Neurovascular Control of Oxygen Tension in the Testis and Epididymis. J Reprod Fertil 3(1962)377-395

Cummins, J.M.; Teichman, R.J.: The Accumulation of Malachite Green Stainable Phospholipid in Rabbit Spermatozoa during Maturation in the Epididymis, and its Possible Role in Capacitation. Biol Reprod 10(1974)555-564

Darin-Bennett, A.; Poulos, A.; White, I.G.: A Re-examination of the Role of Phospholipids as Energy Substrates during Incubation of Ram Spermatozoa. J Reprod Fertil 34(1973)543-546

Darin-Bennett, A.; Poulos, A.; White, I.G.: The Phospholipids and Phospholipid-bound Fatty Acids and Aldehydes of Dog and Fowl Spermatozoa. J Reprod Fertil 41(1974)471-474

Darin-Bennett, A.; Poulos, A.; White, I.G.: The Fatty Acid Composition of the Major Phosphoglycerides of Ram and Human Spermatozoa. Androl 8(1976)37-45

Darin-Bennett, A.; White, I.G.; Hoskins, D.D.: Phospholipids and Phospholipid-bound Fatty Acids and Aldehydes of Spermatozoa and Seminal Plasma of Rhesus Monkeys. J Reprod Fertil 49(1977)119-122

Dawson, R.M.C.; Rowlands, I.W.: Glycerylphosphorylcholine in the Male Reproductive Organs of Rats and Guinea-Pigs. Q J Exp Physiol 44(1959)26-34

Dawson, R.M.C.; Scott, T.W.: Phospholipid Composition of Epididymal Spermatozoa Prepared by Density Gradient Centrifugation. Nature 202(1964)292-293

Dawson, R.M.C.; Mann, T.; White, I.G.: Glycerylphosphorylcholine and Phosphorylcholine in Semen and their Relation to Choline. Biochem J 65(1957)627-634

DeLap, L.W.; Tate, S.S.; Meister, A.: γ-Glutamyl Transpeptidase and Related Enzyme Activities in the Reproductive System of the Male Rat. Life Sci 20(1977)673-680

Edwards, E.M.; Jones, A.R.; Waites, G.M.H.: The Entry of α-Chlorohydrin into Body Fluids of Male Rats and its Effect upon the Incorporation of Glycerol into Lipids. J Reprod Fertil 43(1975)225-232

Edwards, E.M.; Dacheux, J.L.; Waites, G.M.H.: Effects of α-Chlorohydrin on the Metabolism of Testicular and Epididymal Spermatozoa of Rams. J Reprod Fertil 48(1976)265-270

Eisenberg, F.: D-Myoinositol 1-phosphate as Product of Cyclization of Glucose 6-phosphate and Substrate for a Specific Phosphatase in Rat Testis. J Biol Chem 242(1967)1375-1382

Eisenberg, F.; Bolden, A.H.: Biosynthesis of Inositol in Rat Testis Homogenate. Biochem Biophys Res Commun 12(1963)72-77

Eisenberg, F.; Bolden, A.H.: Reproductive Tract as Site of Synthesis and Secretion of Inositol in the Male Rat. Nature 202(1964)599-560

Evans, R.W.; Setchell, B.P.: The Effect of Rete Testis Fluid on the Metabolism of Testicular Spermatozoa. J Reprod Fertil 52(1978)15-20

Flipse, R.J.: Metabolism of Bovine Semen. X. Oxidation of [Carboxy-^{14}C]-labeled Fatty Acids by Bovine Spermatozoa. J Dairy Sci 43(1960)777-781

Flipse, R.J.; Dietz, R.W.: Metabolism of Bovine Semen. XVII. Oxidative Metabolism of Glutamate. J Dairy Sci 52(1969)113-116

Flipse, R.J.; Sexton, T.J.; Dietz, R.W.: Metabolism of Bovine Semen. XVIII. Effect of Keto Acids on Glutamate Metabolism. J Dairy Sci 52(1969)386-389

Free, M.J.; Schluntz, G.A.; Jaffe, R.A.: Respiratory Gas Tensions in Tissues and Fluids of the Male Reproductive Tract. Biol Reprod 14(1976)481-488

Frenkel, G.; Peterson, R.N.; Davis, J.E.; Freund, M.: Glycerylphosphorylcholine and Carnitine in Normal Human Semen and in Postvasectomy Semen: Differences in Concentrations. Fertil Steril 25(1974)84-87

Geer, B.W.; Kelley, K.R.; Pohlman, T.H.; Yemm, S.J.: A Comparison of Rat and *Drosophila* Spermatozoan Metabolisms. Comp Biochem Physiol 50B(1975)41-50

Grogan, D.E.; Mayer, D.T.; Sikes, J.D.: Quantitative Differences in Phospholipids of Ejaculated Spermatozoa and Spermatozoa from Three Levels of the Epididymis of the Boar. J Reprod Fertil 12(1966)431-436

Hamilton, D.W.; Olson, G.E.: Effects of Carnitine on Oxygen Uptake and Utilization of [U-^{14}C]Palmitate by Ejaculated Bull Spermatozoa. J Reprod Fertil 46(1976)195-202

Hartree, E.F.; Mann, T.: Plasmalogen in Ram Semen, and its Role in Sperm Metabolism. Biochem J 71(1959)423-434

Hartree, E.F.; Mann, T.: Phospholipids in Ram Semen: Metabolism of Plasmalogen and Fatty Acids. Biochem J 80(1961)464-476

Hinton, B.T.; Setchell, B.P.; White, R.W.: The Determination of Myoinositol in Micropuncture Samples from the Testis and Epididymis of the Rat. J Physiol (Lond) 265(1977)14P-15P

Hodgen, G.D.: Total Glycerol in the Excurrent Ducts of the Male Rat. J Reprod Fertil 28(1972)277-280

Hutson, S.M.; Van Dop, C.; Lardy, H.A.: Mitochondrial Metabolism of Pyruvate in Bovine Spermatozoa. J Biol Chem 252(1977a)1309-1315

Hutson, S.M.; Van Dop, C.; Lardy, H.A.: Metabolism of Pyruvate and Carnitine Esters in Bovine Epididymal Sperm Mitochondria. Arch Biochem Biophys 181(1977b)345-352

Johnson, A.L.; Howards, S.S.: Hyperosmolality in Intraluminal Fluids from Hamster Testis and Epididymis: A Micropuncture Study. Science 195(1977)492-493

Johnson, L.A.; Pursel, V.G.; Gerrits, R.J.; Thomas, C.H.: Free Amino Acid Composition of Porcine Seminal, Epididymal and Seminal Vesicle Fluids. J Anim Sci 34(1972)430-434

Jones, R.: Absorption and Secretion in Cauda Epididymidis of the Rabbit and the Effects of Degenerating Spermatozoa on Epididymal Plasma after Castration. J Endocrinol 63(1974a)157-165

Jones, R.: The Effects of Artificial Cryptorchidism on the Composition of Epididymal Plasma in the Rabbit. Fertil Steril 25(1974b)432-438

Jones, R.: Effects of Testosterone, Testosterone Metabolites and Anti-Androgens on the Function of the Male Accessory Glands in the Rabbit and Rat. J Endocrinol 74(1977)75-88

Jones, R.; Glover, T.D.: The Collection and Composition of Epididymal Plasma from the Cauda Epididymidis of the Rabbit. J Reprod Fertil 34(1973a)395-403

Jones, R.; Glover, T.D.: The Effects of Castration on the Composition of Rabbit Epididymal Plasma. J Reprod Fertil 34(1973b)405-414

Kohengkul, S.; Tanphaichitr, V.; Muangmun, V.; Tanphaichitr, N.: Levels of L-Carnitine and L-O-Acetylcarnitine in Normal and Infertile Human Semen: A Lower Level of L-O-Acetylcarnitine in Infertile Semen. Fertil Steril 28(1977)1333-1336

Lardy, H.A.; Phillips, P.H.: The Inter-relation of Oxidative and Glycolytic Processes as Sources of Energy for Bull Spermatozoa. Am J Physiol 133(1941)602-609

Lavon, U.; Volcani, R.; Amir, D.; Danon, D.: The Specific Gravity of Bull Spermatozoa from Different Parts of the Reproductive Tract. J Reprod Fertil 12(1966)597-599

Lavon, U.; Volcani, R.; Danon, D.: The Lipid Content of Bovine Spermatozoa during Maturation and Ageing. J Reprod Fertil 23(1970)215-222

Levine, N.; Marsh, D.J.: Micropuncture Studies of the Electrochemical Aspects of Fluid and Electrolyte Transport in Individual Seminiferous Tubules, the Epididymis and the Vas Deferens in Rats. J Physiol (Lond) 213(1971)557-570

Lewin, L.M.; Yannai, Y.; Sulimovici, S.; Kraicer, P.F.: Studies on the Metabolic Role of Myoinositol. Distribution of Radioactive Myoinositol in the Male Rat. Biochem J 156(1976)375-380

Lindahl, P.E.; Thunqvist, L.O.: Specific Gravity of Epididymal and Ejaculated Bull Spermatozoa and of Their Parts. Experientia 21(1965)94-95

Mann, T.; White, I.G.: Glycerol Metabolism by Spermatozoa. Biochem J 65(1957)634-639

Marquis, N.R.; Fritz, I.B.: Effects of Testosterone on the Distribution of Carnitine, Acetylcarnitine, and Carnitine Acetyltransferase in Tissues of the Reproductive System of the Male Rat. J Biol Chem 240(1965)2197-2200

Meister, A.; Tate, S.S.: Glutathione and Related γ-Glutamyl Compounds: Biosynthesis and Utilization. Ann Rev Biochem 45(1976)559-604

Milkowski, A.L.; Babcock, D.F.; Lardy, H.A.: Activation of Bovine Epididymal Sperm Respiration by Caffeine. Its Transient Nature and Relationship to the Utilization of Acetyl Carnitine. Arch Biochem Biophys 176(1976)250-256

Mills, S.C.; Scott, T.W.: Metabolism of Fatty Acids by Testicular and Ejaculated Ram Spermatozoa. J Reprod Fertil 18(1969)367-369

Mohri, H.; Masaki, J.: Glycerokinase and Its Possible Role in Glycerol Metabolism of Bull Spermatozoa. J. Reprod Fertil 14(1967)179-194

Mohri, H.; Mohri, T.; Ernster, L.: Isolation and Enzymic Properties of the Midpiece of Bull Spermatozoa. Exp Cell Res 38(1965)217-246

Mohri, H.; Suter, D.A.I.; Brown-Woodman, P.D.C.; White, I.G.; Ridley, D.D.: Identification of the Biochemical Lesion Produced by α-Chlorohydrin in Spermatozoa. Nature 255(1975)75-77

Mushahwar, I.K.; Koeppe, R.E.: Free Amino Acids of Testes. Concentration of Free Amino Acids in the Testes of Several Species and the Precursors of Glutamate and Glutamine in Rat Testes *in Vivo*. Biochem J 132(1973)353-359

Payne, E.; Masters, C.J.: Fatty Acid Metabolism in Bovine Spermatozoa. Int J Biochem 1(1970)409-421

Pickett, B.W.; Komarek, R.J.; Gebauer, M.R.; Benson, R.W.; Gibson, E.W.: Lipid and Dry Weight of Ejaculated, Epididymal and Post-Castrate Semen from Boars. J Anim Sci 26(1967)792-798

Poulos, A.; Darin-Bennett, A.; White, I.G.: The Phospholipid-bound Fatty Acids and Aldehydes of Mammalian Spermatozoa. Comp Biochem Physiol 46B(1973a)541-549

Poulos, A.; Voglmayr, J.K.; White, I.G.: Phospholipid Changes in Spermatozoa during Passage through the Genital Tract of the Bull. Biochim Biophys Acta 306(1973b)194-202

Poulos, A.; Brown-Woodman, P.D.C.; White, I.G.; Cox, R.I.: Changes in Phospholipids of Ram Spermatozoa during Migration through the Epididymis and Possible Origin of Prostaglandin $F_{2\alpha}$ in Testicular and Epididymal Fluid. Biochim Biophys Acta 388(1975)12-18

Quinn, P.J.; White, I.G.: Phospholipid and Cholesterol Content of Epididymal and Ejaculated Ram Spermatozoa and Seminal Plasma in Relation to Cold Shock. Aust J Biol Sci 20(1967)1205-1215

Riar, S.S.; Setty, B.S.; Kar, A.B.: Studies on the Physiology and Biochemistry of Mammalian Epididymis: Biochemical Composition of Epididymis. A Comparative Study. Fertil Steril 24(1973)355-363

Schenkman, J.B.; Rickert, D.A.; Westerfeld, W.: α-Glycerophosphate Dehydrogenase Activity in Rat Spermatozoa. Endocrinol 76(1965)1055-1061

Scott, T.W.; Dawson, R.M.C.: Metabolism of Phospholipids by Spermatozoa and Seminal Plasma. Biochem J 108(1968)457-463

Scott, T.W.; White, I.G.; Annison, E.F.: Fatty Acids in Semen. Biochem J 78(1961)740-742

Scott, T.W.; Dawson, R.M.C.; Rowlands, I.W.: Phospholipid Inter-relationships in Rat Epididymal Tissue and Spermatozoa. Biochem J 87(1963a)507-512

Scott, T.W.; Wales, R.G.; Wallace, J.C.; White, I.G.: Composition of Ram Epididymal and Testicular Fluid and the Biosynthesis of Glycerylphosphorylcholine by the Rabbit Epididymis. J Reprod Fertil 6(1963b)49-59

Scott, T.W.; Voglmayr, J.K.; Setchell, B.P.: Lipid Composition and Metabolism in Testicular and Ejaculated Ram Spermatozoa. Biochem J 102(1967)456-461

Seamark, R.F.; Tate, M.E.; Smeaton, T.C.: The Occurrence of Syclloinositol and D-Glycerol 1-(L-Myoinositol 1-Hydrogen Phosphate) in the Male Reproductive Tract. J Biol Chem 243(1968)2424-2428

Setchell, B.P.: Testicular Blood Supply, Lymphatic Drainage, and Secretion of Fluid. In: The Testis. Vol. 1, pp. 101-239, ed. by A.D. Johnson, W.R. Gomes and N.L. Van Demark. Academic Press, New York and London, 1970

Setchell, B.P.; Waites, G.M.H.: The Blood-Testis Barrier. In: Handbook of Physiology, Vol. 5, Sect. 7, pp. 143-172, ed. by D.W. Hamilton and R.O. Greep, American Physiological Society, Washington, D.C., 1975

Setchell, B.P.; Hinks, N.T.; Voglmayr, J.K.; Scott, T.W.: Amino Acids in Ram Testicular Fluid and Semen and Their Metabolism by Spermatozoa. Biochem J 105(1967)1061-1065

Setchell, B.P.; Dawson, R.M.C.; White, R.W.: The High Concentration of Free Myoinositol in Rete Testis Fluid from Rams. J Reprod Fertil 17(1968)219-220

Setchell, B.P.; Scott, T.W.; Voglmayr, J.K.; Waites, G.M.H.: Characteristics of Testicular Spermatozoa and the Fluid Which Transports Them into the Epididymis. Biol Reprod 1(1969)40-66S

Setchell, B.P.; Duggan, M.C.; Evans, R.W.: The Effect of Gonadotrophins on Fluid Secretion and Sperm Production by the Rat and Hamster Testis. J Endocrinol 56(1973)27-36

Sexton, T.J.; Amann, R.P.; Flipse, R.J.: Free Amino Acids and Protein in Rete Testis Fluid, Vas Deferens Plasma, Accessory Sex Gland Fluid, and Seminal Plasma of the Conscious Bull. J Dairy Sci 54(1971)412-416

Storey, B.T.; Keyhani, E.: Energy Metabolism in Spermatozoa. II. Comparison of Pyruvate and Fatty Acid Oxidation by Mitochondria of Rabbit Epididymal Spermatozoa. Fertil Steril 25(1974)857-864

Teichman, R.J.; Cummins, J.M.; Takei, G.H.: The Characterization of a Malachite Green-stainable Glutaraldehyde-extractable Phospholipid in Rabbit Spermatozoa. Biol Reprod 10(1974)565-577

Tuck, R.R.; Setchell, B.P.; Waites, G.M.H.; Young, J.A.: The Composition of Fluid Collected by Micropuncture and Catheterization from the Seminiferous Tubules and Rete Testis of Rats. Pfluegers Arch 318(1970)225-243

Turner, T.T.; Hartmann, P.K.; Howards, S.S.: *In Vivo* Sodium, Potassium, and Sperm Concentrations in the Rat Epididymis. Fertil Steril 28(1977)191-194

Van Dop, C.; Hutson, S.M.; Lardy, H.A.: Pyruvate Metabolism in Bovine Epididymal Spermatozoa. J Biol Chem 252(1977)1303-1308

Voglmayer, J.K.: α-Chlorohydrin-induced Changes in the

Distribution of Free Myoinositol and Prostaglandin $F_{2\alpha}$, and Synthesis of Phosphatidylinositol in the Rat Epididymis. Biol Reprod 11(1974)593-600

Voglmayr, J.K.; Amann, R.P.: The Distribution of Free Myoinositol in Fluids, Spermatozoa, and Tissues of the Bull Genital Tract and Observations on Its Uptake by the Rabbit Epididymis. Biol Reprod 8(1973)504-513

Voglmayr, J.K.; White, I.G.: Synthesis and Metabolism of Myoinositol in Testicular and Ejaculated Spermatozoa of the Ram. J Reprod Fertil 24(1971)29-37

Voglmayr, J.K.; Scott, T.W.; Setchell, B.P.; Waites, G.M.H.: Metabolism of Testicular Spermatozoa and Characteristics of Testicular Fluid Collected from Conscious Rams. J Reprod Fertil 14(1967)87-99

Voglmayr, J.K.; Larsen, L.H.; White, I.G.: Metabolism of Spermatozoa and Composition of Fluid Collected from the Rete Testis of Living Bulls. J Reprod Fertil 21(1970)449-460

Vreeburg, J.T.M.: Distribution of Testosterone and 5α-Dihydrotestosterone in the Rat Epididymis and Their Concentrations in Efferent Duct Fluid. J Endocrinol 67(1975)203-210

Wallace, J.C.; Wales, R.G.; White, I.G.: The Respiration of the Rabbit Epididymis and its Synthesis of Glycerylphosphorylcholine. Aust J Biol Sci 19(1966)849-856

White, I.G.: Metabolism of Glycerol and Similar Compounds by Bull Spermatozoa. Am J Physiol 189(1957)307-310

White, I.G.: Studies on the Estimation of Glycerol, Fructose and Lactic Acid with Particular Reference to Semen. Aust J Exp Biol Med Sci 37(1959)441-450

White, I.G.: Biochemical Aspects of Spermatozoa and Their Environment in the Male Reproductive Tract. J Reprod Fertil Suppl 18(1973)225-235

White, I.G.; Wales, R.G.: Comparison of Epididymal and Ejaculated Semen of the Ram. J Reprod Fertil 2(1961)225-237

Wilkinson, G.N.: Statistical Estimations in Enzyme Kinetics. Biochem J 80(1961)324-332

THE FLUID ENVIRONMENT OF THE MATURING SPERMATOZOON

S. Howards*, C. Lechene**, and R. Vigersky

Departments of Urology and Physiology*, University of Virginia School of Medicine, Charlottesville, Virginia 22901 USA; Biotechnology Resource in Electron Probe Microanalysis**, Harvard Medical School, Massachusetts 02115 USA

The fact that spermatozoa mature in the epididymis has been recognized by some, if not accepted by all, for almost a century. Hammar (1897) and Tournade and Regaud (1911) first documented that as spermatozoa traverse the epididymis their potential for motility increases. Young's (1931) classic paper reported similar observations regarding spermatozoan fertility in the guinea pig. In the ensuing years numerous investigations using many species have confirmed these original observations (see Bedford, 1975; Orgebin-Crist, 1975). Although both the extent and mechanism of the epididymal epithelial contribution to the maturation process remains undefined, it must be mediated through the epididymal luminal fluid. This chapter discusses studies of the pH, osmolality, elements, sex steroids, and androgen-binding protein in epididymal luminal fluid. In another chapter in this volume, Dr. Brooks has reviewed the biochemical environment in the epididymal duct. Unfortunately, there is insufficient knowledge to permit more than a few speculations concerning the relationship between the epididymal luminal milieu and spermatozoan maturation.

Before reviewing the available information, it might be worth while to discuss briefly the methods used to collect the data. Since the rete testis cannula technique was described by Voglmayr *et al.* (1966), this method has been adapted for use in many species; therefore uncontaminated rete testis fluid has been extensively analyzed. It should be noted that most investigators ligate the ductuli efferentes for 6-48 h prior to rete testis cannulation, thus creating an unphysiologic situation. Studies of the effects of this obstruction are underway in Free's laboratory. In most species, it is also easy to cannulate the vas deferens and collect fluid from the proximal vas deferens and/or the distal cauda epididymidis. However in order to obtain uncontaminated fluid from the seminiferous tubules (SNT), ductuli efferentes, initial segment, and caput, corpus, or proximal cauda, it is necessary to use micropuncture techniques. In fact even with micropuncture, there has been little success in collecting fluid from the ductuli efferentes and the initial segment, and indeed the samples from the other listed sites are difficult to aspirate in many species. Therefore, many studies of these tissues have utilized minces and homogenates of cystosol rather than luminal fluid. Failure to appreciate these technical difficulties has led to confusion in the field. For example, it is commonly stated that rete testis fluid is slightly modified SNT fluid, although in fact, it is much more like a plasma ultrafiltrate with selected components of SNT fluid such as sperm, inositol, and several proteins. Almost all parameters studied are very different in the two fluids. It will be helpful to keep the preceding discussion in mind while reading the following sections.

pH

There are very few studies of the intraluminal pH in the testis and epididymis. Tuck *et al.* (1970) found the SNT fluid pH to be 7.4 and the luminal pH in the caput to be 6.5. Not until Levine's recent study (Fig. 1) was it determined that the transition from a pH similar to that of blood to a relatively acid pH occurs in the initial segment. The significance of the low pH in most of the epididymis is not known, but the fall in pH takes place in an area where initial maturation occurs.

OSMOLALITY

The results of a study on the osmolality of luminal fluid from the hamster testis and epididymis are summarized in Table 1. The osmolalities were measured by freezing point depression with a nanoliter osmometer (Clifton Technical Physics). The osmolalities in the seminiferous tubule and all regions of the epididymis studied were significantly higher ($p < 0.01$) than the serum osmolality. Rete testis fluid osmolality was not different from serum. The osmolality decreased progressively down the length of the ductus epididymidis. Hyperosmolality of the fluids in the male reproductive tract had been previously mentioned in the literature, but not emphasized or statistically documented until the authors' publication (Johnson and Howards, 1977). Levine and Marsh

---

This work was supported by NIH Grant HD09490-02, NIH Contract NIH-NICHD 72-2770, and NIH Career Development Award 1-K04-HD00108-01.

© 1979 Urban & Schwarzenberg, Inc. Baltimore-Munich *The Spermatozoon*, edited by D.W. Fawcett and J.M. Bedford

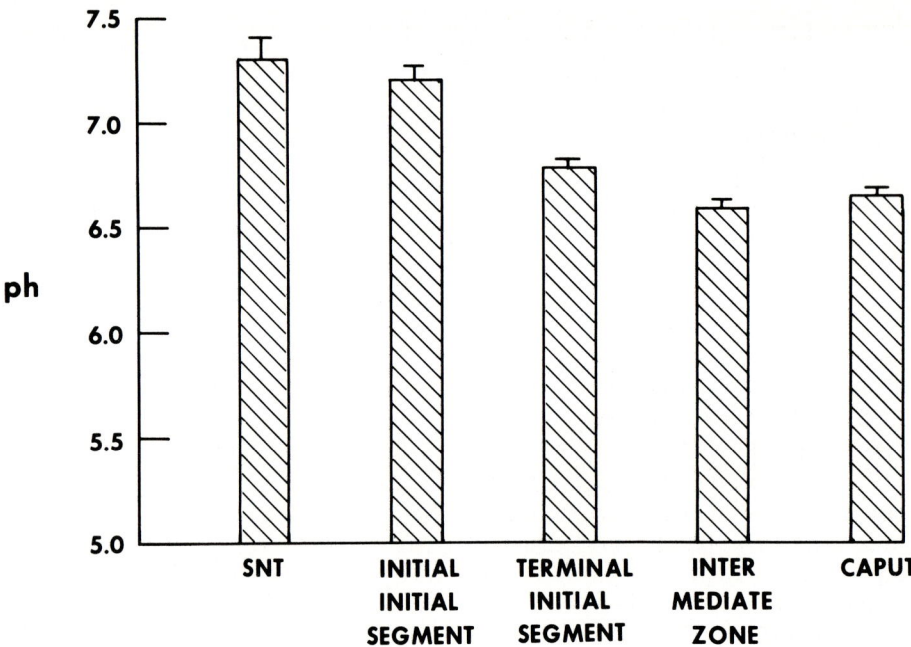

Figure 1. The intraluminal pH in the seminiferous tubule and four sites in the proximal epididymis, adapted from Levine (1978).

(1971) found that SNT fluid was significantly hyperosmolar as compared with plasma, although Tuck et al. (1970) reported no significant difference between the SNT fluid and the plasma in the rat. Jones (1973) using a different collection technique found that the osmolality in the cauda epididymidis of the hamster was 323 ± 27.4 mOsm/kg which is not different from the value of 339.7 ± 3.4 mOsm/kg found in this study. As will become apparent in the following paragraphs, molecules other than Na, K, and Cl—the usual primary osmotic components in physiologic fluids—must be responsible for the hyperosmolality in the male reproductive tract.

It is not clear whether there is a relationship between this hyperosmolality in the male tract and sperm maturation. Orgebin-Crist (1967) did observe that sperm held in the lower corpus epididymidis of the hamster by ligation for three to five days are incapable of fertilization although they do show some improved motility. It is tempting to speculate that spermatozoa acquire fertilizing ability when they are in an environment with an osmolality that is more physiologic, *i.e.* closer to that of plasma, than is present in the proximal epididymis.

ELEMENTS

The initial studies of the concentration of ions in the epididymal fluids were done in the 1950s and 1960s using postmortum specimens from large animals. Many of these reports have not been substantiated; however, the work of Crabo (1965) has held up very well. Levine and Marsh (1971) were the first to use *in vivo* micropuncture techniques to obtain epididymal fluid for analysis. Since then, Jessee and Howards (1976) and Turner, Hartman, Howards (1977) have conducted similar studies in the hamster and the rat. The results of these investigations and several others are summarized in Figure 2 (sodium) and Figure 3 (potassium). Notice that in all of the studies there was a decline in Na concentration along the length of the epididymis from caput concentration of 30 to 120 mEq/L to a caudal level of 5 to 60 mEq/L. K concentrations along the duct were in a range from 20–55 mEq/L and either increased or decreased slightly from the caput to the cauda. The inconsistency in the studies is probably related to tech-

Table 1. Osmolality in the Seminiferous Tubules, Rete Testis, and Five Regions of the Epididymis of the Golden Hamster

Osmolality mOsm	Site
Serum	305
SNT	384*
Rete testis	302
Caput	417*
Corpus	408*
Proximal cauda	359*
Distal cauda	340*
Epididymal vas	332*

*Higher than serum ($p < .05$)
(From Johnson and Howards, 1977)

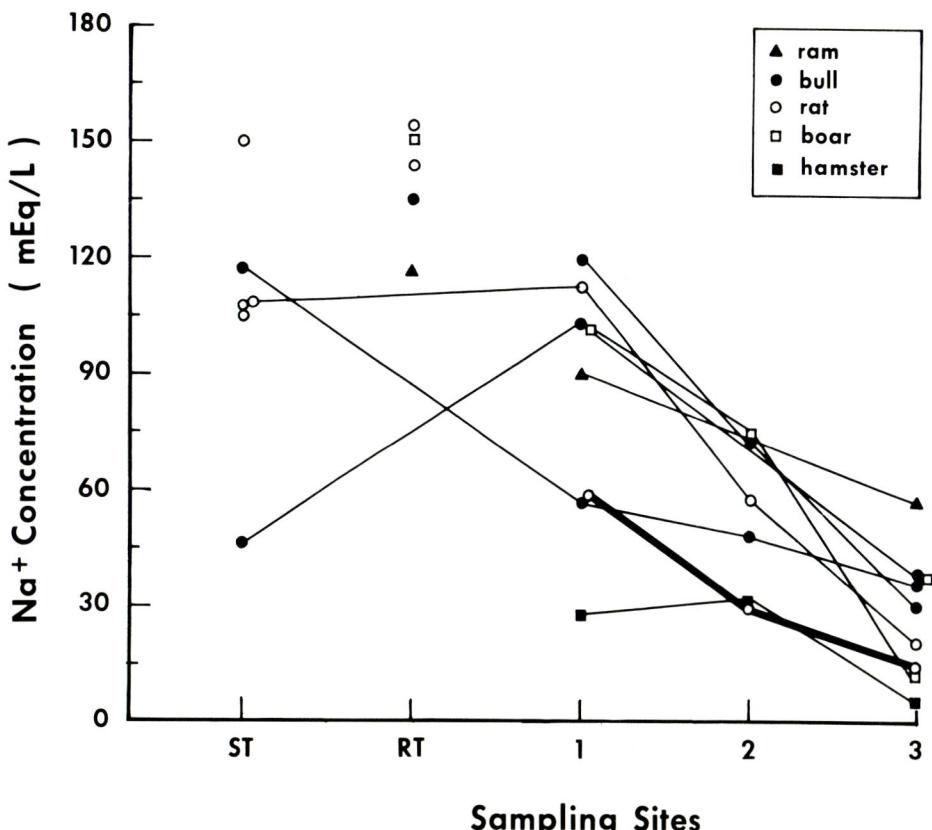

Figure 2. Na concentrations of the male reproductive tract. Data were obtained from previous literature; values from the same study are connected by lines. Results of the present study are indicated by the heavy line. ST, seminiferous tubule; RT, rete testes; (1) caput, (2) corpus, (3) cauda epididymidis. (Reprinted with permission from Fertil Steril 28(2) (1977) 191.

nical difficulties and species variability. Nevertheless, all investigators demonstrated a declining $Na^+:K^+$ ratio along the epididymis. Although the significance of these ionic shifts is not known, they certainly affect spermatozoan membrane function and perhaps play a role in maturation.

To further define the elements in epididymal fluid, the authors have, in collaboration with Dr. Lechene, used electron probe microanalysis to assay the concentration of several elements in epididymal fluid. This technique allows one to analyze picaliter-sized fluid samples for elements with an atomic number greater than five in quantities even lower than $10^{-14}M$. A special ultramicrofiltration method was developed to facilitate analysis with the electron probe of rete testis and epididymal fluid samples obtained by micropuncture. Details of the method and results will be presented in another communication. A summary of preliminary data from the rat is presented in Figures 4 and 5. The findings for Na^+ and K^+ are consistent with the previous studies. The chloride concentration falls from 150 mEq/L in the rete testis to 36 mEq/L in caput and is relatively stable throughout the epididymis. There is a marked increase in P concentration in the distal epididymis which probably represents P incorporated into organic compounds such as glycerolphosphocholine and cyclic AMP. Again, the significance of these findings is uncertain; nevertheless, these alterations may well be related to spermatozoan maturation. Ca^{2+} and Mg^{2+} concentrations are low and relatively stable throughout the epididymis. There is moderate increase in S concentration between the rete testis and the caput and a dramatic elevation in the S concentration in the corpus. Although these data are preliminary, they do document that electron probe microanalysis has the potential to yield exciting new insights into epididymal physiology.

ANDROGENS

The literature on epididymal androgens is too extensive to review in detail in this chapter. All of the available information comes from analysis of tissue homogenates except that from the rete testis, and the data of Ganjam and Amann (1973, 1976) from the bull cauda epididymidis. Although there are variations from study to

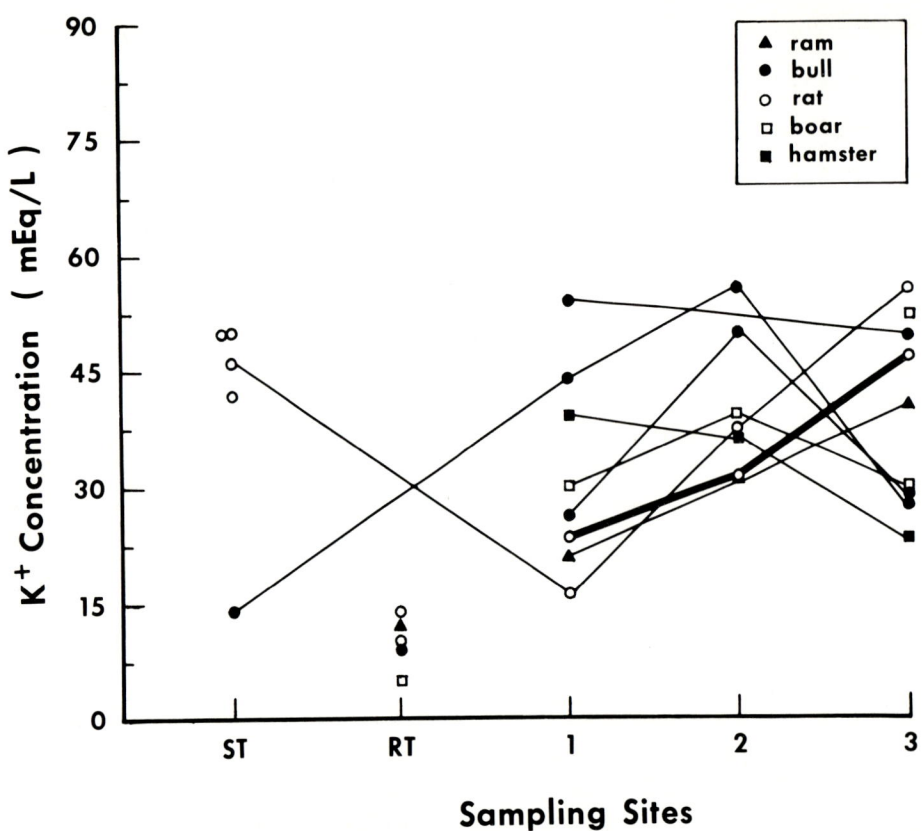

Figure 3. K concentrations of the male reproductive tract. Data were obtained from previous literature; values from the same study are connected by lines. Results of the present study are indicated by the heavy line. Rete testis (RT) and seminiferous tubule (ST) data are included for purposes of comparison. (Reprinted with permission from Fertil Steril 28(2) (1977) 191.

study, the consensus is that: 1) the principle androgen in the testis and the rete testis is testosterone; 2) the testosterone and dihydrotestosterone (DHT) concentrations in the rete testis fluid are approximately 20-30 ng/ml and 0-2 ng/ml, respectively (Ganjam and Amann, 1973, 1976; Harris and Bartke, 1974; Comhaire and Vermeulen, 1976); and 3) DHT is the primary androgen in the epididymis and the concentration of androgens decrease from the proximal to distal epididymis (Granjam and Amann, 1973, 1976; Vreeburg and Aafjes, 1971; Pujol et al., 1976; Vreeburg, 1975; Frankel and Eik-Nes, 1970).

In an attempt to define the intraluminal androgen concentrations at various sites along the epididymal duct fluid collected *in vivo* by micropuncture is being analyzed. The data are too preliminary to publish at this time; however, in general the initial are results are in agreement with previously reported values obtained by analyzing homogenates of epididymal tissue. Careful analysis of the final data may be interesting since subtle differences between epididymal epithelial and luminal androgen concentrations may be physiologically important. There is evidence that exogenous 5α-androstane-3α, 17β-diol is more effective than DHT which in turn is more effective than testosterone in maintaining epididymal sperm maturation (Lubicz-Nawrocki, 1976).

ANDROGEN-BINDING PROTEIN

A complete survey of the work on androgen-binding protein (ABP) in the epididymis is beyond the scope of this chapter. It is generally agreed that in the rat ABP is secreted by the Sertoli cell (Steinberger et al., 1975; Tindall et al., 1975; Fritz et al., 1976) under the influence of follicle stimulating hormone (FSH) (Hansson et al., 1974; Means et al., 1976) and/or androgens (Tindal and Means, 1976). Then ABP travels along the seminiferous tubule to the rete testis and epididymis (French and Ritzén, 1973a, 1973b). The fact that ligation of the ductuli efferentes results in depletion of epididymal ABP (Danzo et al., 1977; French and Ritzén, 1973b), that rete testis fluid contains ABP (Danzo et al., 1977; French and Ritzén, 1973a, 1973b; Vigersky et al., 1976), and Sertoli cell cultures produce ABP (Steinberger et al., 1975; Fritz et al., 1976) support

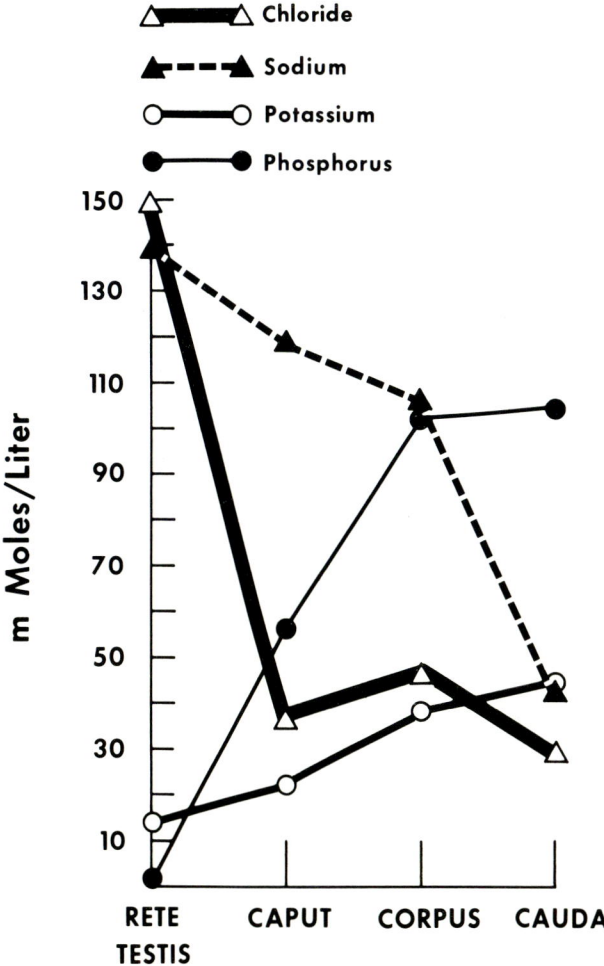

Figure 4. Cl (△), Na (▲), K (○), and P (●), concentrations in mmol/L in the rete testis, caput, corpus, and cauda determined by electron-probe analysis.

these contentions. It is also apparent that there is a progressive decline in the concentration of ABP along the length of the epididymal duct in the rat (Hansson et al., 1974) and the mature rabbit (Danzo et al., 1977).

In collaboration with Dr. Robert Vigersky (1976), this laboratory has used polyacrilamide gel electrophoresis (PAGE) to detect ABP fluid obtained *in vivo* from rat seminiferous tubules, rete testis, and caput epididymidis. Table 2 lists the protein concentrations in the fluid and the minimum volume of fluid and amount of protein necessary to detect ABP. It is noteworthy that either per unit volume or per μg of protein there is significantly less ABP in the SNT fluid than in the caput or rete testis fluid. Using micro PAGE method, Dr. Turner has been able to find ABP in 1-μl samples of SNT fluid. Nevertheless, the activity per unit volume with his system is also less in the SNT fluid than in the caput or rete testis fluid.[1]

[1] Turner, T.T.: Unpublished observation.

To determine whether the ABP in this fluid was the same protein as the ABP in cytosol of rat epididymal homogenates, PAGE was done in gels of 6-14% total gel concentration and K_r-Yo ellipses (Vigersky et al., 1976) were calculated, the centroids of which represented the experimentally determined size K_r) and net charge (Yo) of the proteins. ABP from rat epididymal sperm-free fluid and rat epididymal cytosol were indistinguishable and both were different from human testosterone-estrogen binding globulin (TeBG).

The question of the relevance of ABP to sperm maturation is a difficult one. Recent work by Purvis and Hansson (1978) has demonstrated a high degree of correlation in the rat epididymal distribution of ABP and DHT suggesting that ABP determines rat epididymal DHT concentration which in turn may be essential for epididymal sperm maturation. Fawcett (1978) has shown that the morphologic integrity of the initial segment of the rat epididymis cannot be maintained with exogenous androgens when the flow of fluid from the rete testis is interrupted suggesting the possibility that ABP and intraluminal androgens are required for function of this vital segment of the epididymis.

On the other hand, Lubicz-Nawrocki (1974, 1976) has reported that in the hamster exogenous androgens can maintain the fertilizing capacity of epididymal sperm for 12 days after castration. Indeed, it is not certain that ABP, as distinguished from TEBG, exists in the primate. Vigersky et al. (1976) could not demonstrate ABP in 200 μl samples of monkey rete testis fluid. Several investigators feel that in man ABP cannot be distinguished from TEBG whereas others contend that both proteins are present (Hsu et al., 1977). Perhaps this question will be resolved if the recently developed immunoassay for rat ABP (Gunsalus et al., 1978) can be modified to measure human ABP. This assay will certainly facilitate investigations of the role of ABP in epididymal spermatozoon maturation in the rat. An animal model with absent ABP but normal androgen biosynthesis and steriod secretion would also be a powerful tool to evaluate the role of ABP in epididymal sperm maturation.

Table 2. Minimum Volume of Sperm-Free Fluid and Amount of Total Protein Necessary to Detect Rat ABP

Site	Volume μl	Protein Concentration μg/μl	Total Protein μg
SNT	7.0	52	364
Rete testis	5.0	0.9	45
Caput epididymis	0.3	22.5	67

Adapted from Vigersky et al.: J. Clin. Invest. 58(1976)1061–1068.

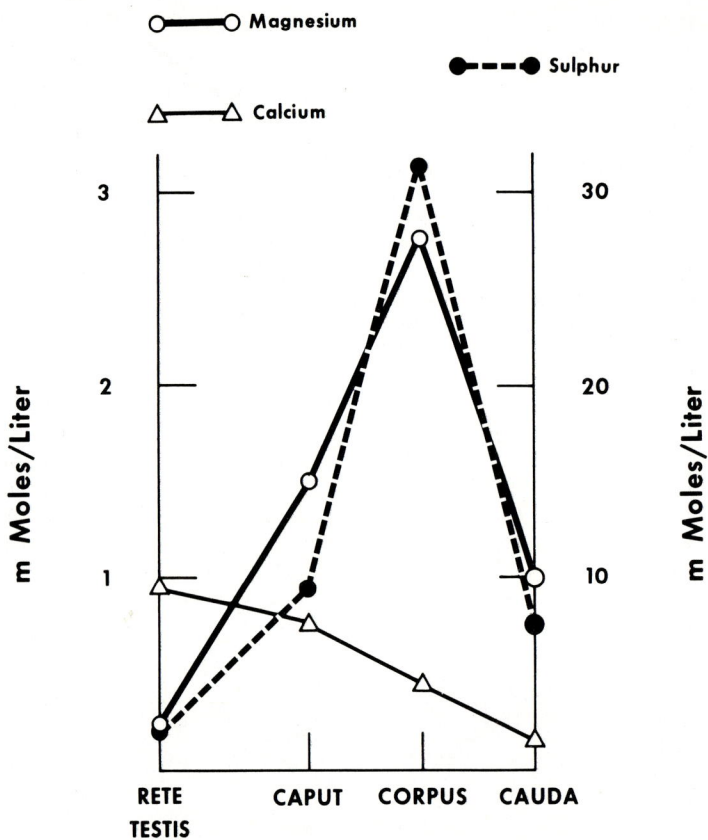

Figure 5. Mg (O), Ca (△), and S (●) concentrations in mmol/L in the rete testis, caput, corpus, and cauda determined by electron-probe analysis. Note scale for Mg^{2+} and Ca^{2+} on left and scale for sulphur on right.

REFERENCES

Bedford, J.M.: Maturation, Transport, and Fate of Spermatozoa in the Epididymis. In: Handbook of Physiology. Vol. 5, sect. 7, Endocrinology, pp. 303-317, ed. by R.O. Greep and D.W. Hamilton. Williams and Wilkins, Baltimore, 1975

Comhaire, F.H.; Vermeulen, A.: Testosterone Concentration in the Fluids of Seminiferous Tubules, the Interstitium and the Rete Testis of the Rat. J Endocrinol 70(1976)229-235

Crabo, B.: Studies on the Composition of Epididymal Content in Bulls and Boars. Acta Vet Scand Suppl 6 5(1965)1-94

Danzo, B.J.; Cooper, T.G.; Orgebin-Crist, M.-C.: Androgen Binding Protein (ABP) in Fluids Collected from the Rete Testis and Cauda Epididymidis of Sexually Mature and Immature Rabbits. Biol Reprod 17(1977)64-77

Fawcett, D.W.; Hoffer, A.P.: Failure of Exogenous Androgen to Prevent Regression of the Initial Segments of the Rat Epididymis after Efferent Duct Ligation or Castration. Biol Reprod, in press

Frankel, A.I.; Eik-Nes, K.B.: Testosterone and Dehydroepiandrosterone in the Epididymis of the Rabbit. J Reprod Fertil 23(1970)441-445

Free, M.: Personal Communication (1978)

French, F.S.; Ritzén, E.M.: Androgen Binding Protein in Efferent Duct Fluid of Rat Testis. J Reprod Fertil 32(1973a)483-497

French, F.S.; Ritzén, E.M.: A High-Affinity Androgen Binding Protein in Rat Testis: Evidence for Secretion into Efferent Duct Fluid and Absorption by Epididymis. Endocrinology 93(1973b)88-95

Fritz, I.B.; Rommerts, F.G.; Louis, B.G.; Dorrington, J.H.: Regulation by FSH and Dibutryl Cyclic AMP of the Formation of Androgen Binding Protein in Sertoli Cell-enriched Cultures. J Reprod Fertil 46(1976)17-24

Ganjam, V.K.; Amann, R.P.: Steroids in Fluids and Sperm Entering and Leaving Bovine Epididymis, Epididymal Tissue, and Accessory Sex Gland Secretions. Endocrinology 99(1976)1618-1630

Ganjam, V.K.; Amann, R.P.: Testosterone and Dihydrotestosterone Concentrations in the Fluid Milieu of Spermatozoa in the Reproductive Tract of the Bull. Acta Endocrinol 74(1973)186-200

Gunsalus, G.L.; Musto, N.A.; Bardin, C.W.: Immunoassay of Androgen Binding Protein in Blood: A New Approach for Study of the Seminiferous Tubule. Science 200(1978)65-66

Hammar, J.A.: Ueber Secretionserscheinungern im Nebenhoden des Hundes Zugleich ein Beitrag Physiologie des Zellenkerns. Arch Anat Entwicklungsgeschichte Suppl (1897)1-42

Hansson, V.; Trygstad, O.; French, F.S.: Androgen Transport and Receptor Mechanisms in Testis and Epididymis. Nature 250(1974)387-391

Harris, M.E.; Bartke, A.: Concentration of Testosterone in Testis Fluid of the Rat. Endocrinology 95(1974)701-706

Hsu, A.-F.; Nankin, H.R.; Troen, P.: Androgen Binding Protein in Human Testis: Effect of Age. In: The Testis in

Normal and Infertile Men, pp. 421-434, ed. by P. Troen and H.R. Nankin. Raven Press, New York, 1977

Jessee, S.; Howards, S.S.: A Survey of Spermatozoa, Sodium, and Potassium Concentrations in the Hamster Epididymis. Biol Reprod 15(1976)626-631

Johnson, A.; Howards, SS.: Hyperosmolality in the Intraluminal Fluids from the Hamster Testis and Epididymis Science 195:492, 1977

Jones, R.: Thesis, University of Liverpool (1973)

Levine, N.; Kelly, H.: Measurement of pH in the Rat Epididymis in Vivo. J. Reprod Fertil 52, 132, 1978

Levine, N.; Marsh, D.J.: Micropuncture Studies of the Electrochemical Aspects of Fluid and Electrolyte Transport in Individual Seminiferous Tubules, the Epididymis, and the Vas Deferens in Rats. J Physiol 213(1971)557-570

Lubicz-Nawrocki, C.M.: Effect of Castration and Testosterone Replacement on Sperm Maturation in the Hamster. J Reprod Fertil 34(1974)315-329

Lubicz-Nawrocki, C.M.: The Effect of Metabolites of Testosterone on the Development of Fertilizing Ability of Spermatozoa in the Epididymis of Castrated Hamsters. J Exp Zool 197(1976)89-96

Means, A.R.; Fakunding, J.L.; Tindall, D.J.: Follicle Stimulating Hormone Regulation of Protein Kinase Activity and Protein Synthesis in Testis. Biol Reprod 14(1976)54-63

Orgebin-Crist, M.C.: Sperm Maturation in Rabbit Epididymis. Nature 216(1967)816-817

Orgebin-Crist, M.C.: Endocrine Control of the Development and Maintenance of Sperm Fertilizing Ability in the Epididymis. In: Handbook of Physiology. Vol. 5, sect. 7, Endocrinology, pp. 319-338, ed. by R.O. Greep and D.W. Hamilton. Williams and Wilkins, Baltimore, 1975

Purvis, K.; Hansson, V.: Androgen and Androgen Binding Protein in the Rat Epididymis. J Reprod Fertil 52(1978)59-63

Pujol, A.; Bayard, F.; Louvet, J.; Boulard, C.: Testosterone and Dihydrotestosterone Concentrations in Plasma, Epididymal Tissues and Seminal Fluid of Adult Rats. Endocrinology 98(1976)111-113

Steinberger, A.; Heindel, J.J.; Lindsey, J.N.; Elkington, J.S.H.; Sanborn, B.M.; Steinberger, E.: Isolation and Culture of FSH-responsive Sertoli Cells. Endocrinol Res Commun 2(1975)261-272

Tindall, D.J.; Vitale, R.; Means, A.R.: Androgen Binding Protein as a Biochemical Marker of Formation of the Blood-Testis Barrier. Endocrinology 97(1975)636-648

Tournade, A.; Regaud, C.: Différences de Motilité des Spermatozoides Recueillis dans Les Différents Segments des Voies Spermatiques. Assoc Anat 13(1911)252-258

Tindall, D.J.; Means, A.R.: Concerning the Hormonal Regulation of Androgen Binding Protein in Rat Testis. Endocrinology 99(1976)809-818

Tuck, R.R.; Setchell, B.P.; Waites, G.M.H.; Young, J.A.: The Composition of Fluid Collected by Micropuncture and Catheterization from the Seminiferous Tubules and Rete Testis of Rats. Eur J Physiol 318(1970)225-243

Turner, T.T.; Hartmann, P.K; Howards, S.S.: *In Vivo* Sodium and Potassium, and Sperm Concentrations in the Rat Epididymis. Fertil Steril 28(1977)191-194

Vigersky, R.A.; Louriaux, D.; Howards, S.S.; *et al.:* Androgen Binding Proteins of Testis, Epididymis, and Plasma in Man and Monkey. J Clin Invest 58(1976)1061-1068

Voglmayr, J.K.; Waites, G.M.H.; Setchell, B.P.: Studies on Spermatozoa and Fluid Collected Directly from the Testis of the Conscious Ram. Nature 210(1966)861-863

Vreeburg, J.T.; Aafjes, J.H.: Dihydrotestosterone in the Epididymis of the Rat in Current Problems. In: Current Problems in Fertility, pp. 203, ed. by A. Ingelman-Sandberg and N.O. Lowell. Plenum Press, New York, 1971

Vreeberg, J.T.M.: Distribution of Testosterone and 5α-Dihydrotestosterone in Rat Epididymis and Their Concentration in Efferent Duct Fluid. J Endocrinol 67(1975)203-210

Young, W.C.: A Study of the Function of the Epididymis. Functional Changes Undergone by Spermatozoa during Their Passage through the Epididymis and Vas Deferens in the Guinea Pig. J Biol 8(1931)151-163

EVIDENCE FOR A ROLE FOR A FORWARD MOTILITY PROTEIN IN THE EPIDIDYMAL DEVELOPMENT OF SPERM MOTILITY

D.D. Hoskins, D. Johnson, H. Brandt, and T.S. Acott

Reproductive Physiology Section, Oregon Regional Primate Research Center, Beaverton, Oregon 97005   USA

It has long been known that mammalian testicular sperm are incapable of motility and that acquisition of this property takes place as sperm move through the epididymis (review: Bedford, 1975). It should be noted that this acquired motility is expressed only after sperm are mixed with male accessory gland secretions at the time of ejaculation or removed from the epididymis and diluted into buffer solutions. The contribution of the epididymis to motility development is that it instills in developing cells the capacity for full motility which may then be expressed when the property of motility is needed to ensure fertilization.

It is also known that the pattern of sperm motility changes during epididymal transit. Thus, sperm taken from the caput epididymidis of various species show a variety of circular twitching or swimming motions. For example, sperm isolated from the caput epididymidis of at least three species, namely the rat, rabbit, and guinea pig show circular swimming patterns (Bedford, 1975) while caput sperm taken from the epididymis of the bull (Igboeli and Foote, 1968), man (Bedford et al., 1973), and nonhuman primates (Hoskins et al., 1975) display a pattern of motion that ranges from near immotility to a weak whiplash-like motion of the tail.

By the time mammalian sperm reach the caudal portion of the epididymis, these ineffective swimming motions have been transformed into a vigorous, unidirectional activity. Although this observation that sperm become progressively motile during epididymal transit was made some 65 years ago by Tournade (1913), we still do not understand the mechanism which brings this about. What is known has led to some controversy. Tournade (1913) originally believed that the process is largely extrinsic to the developing sperm of a number of species (rat, cat, guinea pig, and rabbit); that is, he thought that factors produced by the epididymis are necessary for the development of motility. This view was held until Young (1931) showed that motility of guinea pig sperm retained in the caput epididymidis by simple ligation increases more with time than does the motility of sperm taken from the caput of control, nonligated animals. Young therefore suggested that the development of motility is intrinsic in nature, that is, the process is simply a sperm-aging phenomenon, begun in the testis and completed in the epididymis.

In the last 40 years, many attempts have been made to use this ligation technique to determine whether intrinsic or extrinsic factors are involved in motility development in retained caput sperm. Unfortunately, the picture today is still confused. The primary reasons for this are the variation in experimental conditions such as length or site of ligation, differences in response among species, and the failure of authors to describe in precise terms the pattern of motility observed. Nonetheless, it is quite clear that in almost every species studied, ligation of the corpus for varying lengths of time does, in fact, increase the overall activity of retained caput sperm.

One of the more critical of these studies was carried out by Bedford (1967) who showed that rabbit caput sperm develop a near-normal motility following ligation of lower corpus for a period of 10-12 days. Significantly, however, this capacity for motility was retained by sperm *in situ* for only a few days. Bedford concluded from these observations that acquisition of motility in the rabbit does not require exposure to the more distal portions of the epididymis and that the pattern of motility can be changed by simple retardation of sperm passage (Bedford, 1975). The nature of the changes that must occur in these retained caput sperm and that account for either the change in the pattern of motility or the maintenance of motility, once attained, is not known. Similar increases in caput sperm motility after ligation have been reported for the rabbit (Glover, 1962; Gaddum and Glover, 1965; Orgebin-Crist, 1973), hamster (Horan and Bedford, 1972), and man (Mooney et al., 1972). It is important to emphasize that none of

---

The authors are indebted to Dr. Nancy Alexander, Oregon Regional Primate Research Center, for providing seminal plasma from vasectomized rhesus monkeys.

This work was supported by General Research Support Grant RR00163, Grant for the Operation of the Oregon Regional Primate Research Center, from the Animal Resources Branch, Division of Research Resources, National Institutes of Health; Biochemical Research Grant RR05694 from the National Institutes of Health; and Program Project Grant HD05969 from the Center for Population Research, National Institute of Child Health and Human Development, National Institutes of Health.

© 1979 Urban & Schwarzenberg, Inc. Baltimore-Munich *The Spermatozoon*, edited by D.W. Fawcett and J.M. Bedford

these studies, with the exception of the one described above by Bedford (1967), indicate that simple retention by ligation of caput sperm *in situ* permits the development of the type of motility characteristic of mature caudal sperm; that is, retained sperm do not develop the capacity for vigorous forward progression. In fact, the recent studies of Burgos and Tovar (1974) showed that rat caput sperm retained by ligation of the corpus for 10 days display an identical motility pattern to those obtained from control epididymides, leading these authors to suggest that extrinsic factors produced by the epididymis and located distal to the caput are essential for motility development in this species. The data described below for developing bovine sperm strongly support the view of these authors and suggest that one of these putative extrinsic factors is a glycoprotein that has the ability to instill forward motion in developing bovine spermatozoa.

In those species in which ligation does lead to increased motion in retained caput sperm, the question arises as to what changes in the chemistry of sperm account for the change in motility and whether similar changes occur during normal epididymal sperm transit. Recent studies from the authors' laboratory (Hoskins *et al.*, 1974; Hoskins *et al.*, 1975; Hoskins and Casillas, 1975; Stephens *et al.*, 1978) suggest that one such change during epididymal passage of sperm may be an increase in the content of the nucleotide, cyclic adenosine monophosphate (AMP). The basis for this speculation is that the intrasperm levels of cyclic AMP nearly double in bull sperm during epididymal transit and that a type of twitching motion, without forward progression, can be induced *in vitro* by addition of phosphodiesterase inhibitors to washed caput cells. The pattern of induced motion is similar to what one sees following ligation of the corpus of a number of species, as noted above. Such a stimulation of motion by phosphodiesterase inhibitors was originally reported by Frenkel *et al.*, (1973) for washed guinea pig sperm. This observation has since been confirmed in the rat (Wyler and Howards, 1977) and the rabbit.[1] Although the mechanism responsible for this increase in intrasperm cyclic AMP during epididymal transit is not known, it is of interest that the enzyme cyclic AMP phosphodiesterase, which is responsible for cyclic AMP degradation in cells, is nearly twice as high in immature caput as in mature caudal sperm (Stephens *et al.*, 1978). Thus, it would be very interesting to determine whether ligation of the corpus epididymidis of, for example the rabbit, brings about a simultaneous increase in cyclic AMP levels and a decrease in phosphodiesterase activity.

It is the intent of this chapter to provide evidence that such an epididymal increase in the intrasperm cyclic AMP content, when coupled with the action of specific forward motility glycoprotein, is a necessary part of the process of motility development in the bull. It is emphasized at the onset, however, that motility development in any species undoubtedly involves much more than these two events. For example, the studies of Bedford and his colleagues (Calvin and Cooper, 1971; Bedford and Calvin, 1973; Bedford, 1975) have clearly shown that changes in the oxidation state of sperm sulfhydryl groups occur during motility development in the rabbit epididymis. Since these authors have shown that many structures of sperm, including the segmented connecting piece, coarse outer fibers, outer mitochondrial membranes, and the fibrous sheath of the principal piece become stabilized by disulfide bond formation during epididymal passage, it is likely that motility development involves changes in sperm structure as well as changes in metabolism or chemical content.

It should be clear from the brief preceding account that it is impossible at present to give a detailed biochemical description of how sperm first become motile since this simply is not known. What is offered in this chapter is the description of an *in vitro* model in which immature bovine caput sperm can be activated to a highly motile state in a manner that is believed to mimic, at least in part, the process by which sperm become motile in the bovine epididymis. As noted, studies from the authors' laboratory have demonstrated that the intrasperm levels of cyclic AMP increase during epididymal transit of bovine sperm and that a kind of motility, characterized by vibratory action without forward progression, can be induced in caput sperm by addition of phosphodiesterase inhibitors. It has been possible to show that a wide variety of phosphodiesterase inhibitors induce this kind of motion in bovine caput sperm, and that the observed changes in cyclic AMP precede in time the induction of the observed twitching motion (Hoskins *et al.*, 1975). Attempts to activate these twitching immature sperm to full motility were given considerable impetus by the studies of Lindholmer (1974) who showed that human seminal plasma is capable of inducing forward motion in vibratile human sperm that had been removed from the caput epididymidis of patients with obstructive azoospermia. This observation suggested that the phosphodiesterase-activated motion of bovine caput sperm that had been observed might be converted into forward motion by the simple addition of bovine seminal plasma. This proved to be possible. Thus, the simultaneous addition of a phosphodiesterase inhibitor, for example, theophylline and minute amounts of bovine

---

[1] Casillas, E.R.: personal communication

seminal plasma induce forward progression in nearly 40% of isolated and washed bovine caput sperm within a 10-min period (Hoskins et al., 1974).

This simple observation led to a number of questions, some of which are addressed in this chapter. For example, what is this forward motility inducing factor? Where is it found? How does it work? And, most importantly, is it involved in motility induction in the bovine epididymis?

It first became necessary to develop an assay for this forward motility factor. The method developed (Acott and Hoskins, 1978) is basically a modification of the procedure of Janick and McLeod (1970) in which advantage is taken of the fact that a time exposure of a suspension of moving sperm produces streaks on a photographic plate. From these "tracks" it is possible to calculate the average velocity for a population of moving cells provided only that the dimensions of the system and the exposure time are known. Briefly, the assay is as follows. First, washed immotile bovine caput sperm are activated by addition of a high level of theophylline (33mM) and varying levels of the forward motility factor. After 15 min, the activated cells are diluted to such a degree (final concentration, approximately 5×10^6 sperm/ml) that individual tracks can be identified, the cells placed on a hemocytometer slide at 37°C, and a photograph taken with a 5-s exposure. Protection from inactivation by dilution is provided by the addition of bovine serum albumin. From the number of moving sperm and the lengths of their tracks, a forward motility index may be calculated:

$$FMI = \frac{(\text{No. of moving sperm})(\text{average velocity})(100)}{(\text{total No. of sperm})(0.75)}$$

In simplest terms, the index is a product of the percent of moving cells times their average velocity, with these numbers normalized to a population of 100 cells.

It was soon found that what forward motility factor does is to markedly stimulate the number of moving cells while only marginally increasing the velocity of those few cells that are already moving. Figure 1 shows that increasing concentrations of seminal plasma produce progressively higher forward motility indices until the system becomes saturated at a seminal plasma pro-

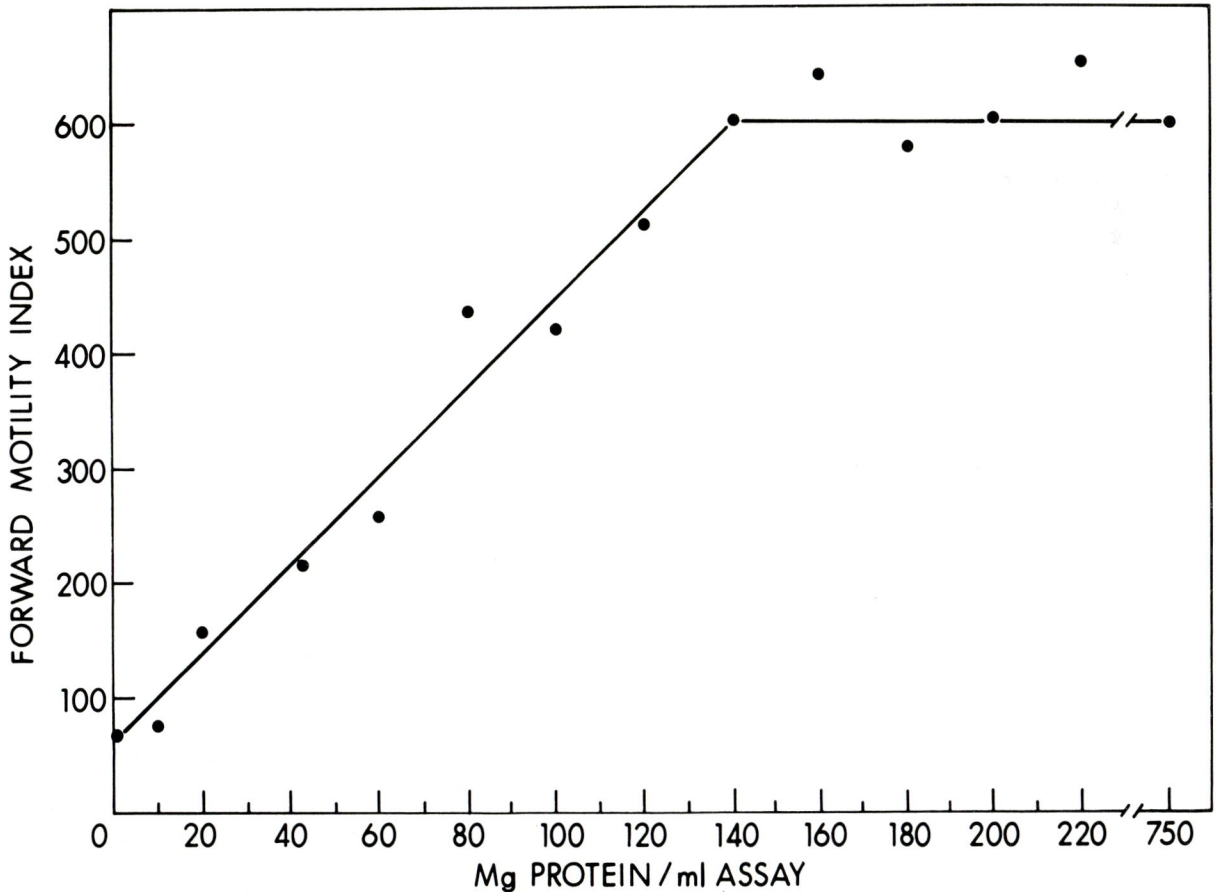

Figure 1. Activation of forward motility in caput spermatozoa by varying levels of seminal plasma protein. Heat-treated (90°C, 10 min) seminal plasma (15 mg/ml) was added to the standard incubation assay.

Table 1. Initiation of Forward Motility in Bovine Caput Spermatozoa by Seminal Plasma from Diverse Mammalian Species

Seminal Plasma Source	FM/μg Plasma Protein[a]	FMI/μl Plasma[a]	FMI_{max}[a]
Bovine	5.97 ± 0.57	359 ± 34	630 ± 30
Monkey (M. mulatta)	3.70 ± 0.17	27.2 ± 1.20	725 ± 41
Elephant	3.60 ± 0.29	7.8 ± 0.90	495 ± 38
Porcine	2.40 ± 0.10	53.3 ± 2.10	570 ± 19
Rabbit	1.80 ± 0.12	16.2 ± 3.80	530 ± 28
Man	1.40 ± 0.11	68.9 ± 5.2	660 ± 26
Dog	0.04 ± 0.03	13.2 ± 1.10	592 ± 71

[a]Values are means ± SEM

tein concentration of about 150 μg/ml. For all comparative data described below, activities reported were taken from linear portions of plots such as the one shown in Figure 1. Values taken from the plateau portion of these curves will be referred to as the maximum forward motility index (FMI_{max}).

One point that should be made is that assay of the forward motility factor by this technique is an exceedingly laborious and time-consuming task. Thus, if the lengths of 30-40 individual sperm tracks on Polaroid pictures are measured in a routine assay and this process is carried out in triplicate, some 90-120 bits of data are generated. One standard curve of the type shown in Figure 1 therefore results from the measurement of the lengths of over 1000 sperm tracks.

This photographic assay has been used to show that a forward motility-inducing activity is present in the seminal plasma of a number of species of mammals (Table 1). The data in the table describe specific forward motility indices in terms of both the volume and protein concentration of seminal plasma as well as in terms of the maximum forward motility index. As might be expected, bovine seminal plasma activates bovine caput sperm to the greatest degree. The absolute specific activity values for the plasma of the other species shown, whether expressed on a volume or protein-concentration basis, should perhaps not be taken too seriously (in terms of absolute values relative to bovine seminal plasma), however, it is well known that the seminal plasma of various mammalian species varies widely with regard to both volume and protein concentration (Mann, 1964). The clearly significant data in the table, however, show that the seminal plasma of every species studied has the potential to induce a maximum forward-motility activity in bovine caput sperm comparable to that shown with bovine seminal plasma, provided only that sufficient amounts are used. This is especially significant since, as will be shown below, only seminal plasma and epididymal fluids, of a large number of body fluids studied, has the potential to attain a forward motility index as high as 600. What the data in the table indicate, then, is that some kind of sperm forward motility-inducing activity is common to the seminal plasma of all mammals.

The data in Table 2 show that the active factor present in bovine seminal plasma has the ability to activate sperm from the caput epididymidis of a number of species provided only, as is always the case, that a phosphodiesterase inhibitor is also present. This is simply the reverse of the experiment shown in Table 1. For simplicity's sake, only relative specific FMI, based on the amount of bovine seminal plasma protein in the

Table 2. Activation of Caput Sperm from Diverse Species by Bovine Seminal Plasma

			Individual Motility Characteristics		
				Average Sperm Velocity (μm/s)	
Sperm Obtained From:	n	Relative Specific FMI[a] (per μg Protein)	% Motile Sperm	Experimental	Literature[b]
Bull	(> 300)	100	40	88	120
Guinea pig	(2)	98	23	46	60
Bear	(1)	73	16	50	—
Cat	(2)	62	14	60	—
Dog	(2)	60	18	42	45
Monkey	(2)	55	19	54	80–100
Rabbit	(3)	12	11	38	—

[a]Assay conditions are those given in text for assay of bovine caput sperm. No attempt has been made to maximize the motility of caput from other species.
[b]A dashed line indicates that values are not available.

assay mixture, are given in the table. The two motility characteristics shown are the percent motile sperm and the average velocity of these cells. Note that, with the exception of studies carried out with the bull, the number of epididymides used was quite small. When taken with the fact that no attempt was made to maximize the assay conditions for determination of the motility of caput sperm from any species other than the bull, the data can only be interpretable as indicating trends rather than absolute values. Nonetheless, what the data show is that bovine seminal plasma does have the ability to stimulate caput sperm from a number of species and that the experimentally induced velocities in several species, specifically, the bull, guinea pig, dog, and monkey approach the velocities reported in the literature for mature ejaculated sperm.

The data shown for the bull are statistically significant (n > 300) and efforts have been made to optimize the motility parameters shown. Thus, 40% of isolated and washed bovine caput sperm are activatable by theophylline and seminal plasma. The induced velocity of these cells is approximately two-thirds that of ejaculated sperm (Nelson, 1975). The percent activatable cells is identical to the value reported by Igboeli and Foote (1968) for the percent of motile sperm taken from the bovine cauda epididymidis. The data provide further support for the idea that a factor found in bovine seminal plasma is involved in epididymal motility initiation in this species and demonstrate that the factor can act on caput sperm of other species.

Using the photographic motility assay the somewhat laborious task of purifying and characterizing the factor from bovine seminal plasma has been begun (Acott and Hoskins, 1978). To date, it has been shown that the factor is a heat-stable glycoprotein that exists in seminal plasma in at least four aggregate equilibrium forms. The glycoprotein nature of the factor, which is henceforth called "forward motility protein" or FMP, was initially indicated by its heat stability and anamolous behavior on molecular sieves and subsequently confirmed by its complete inactivation by trypsin, partial inactivation by a number of carbohydrate-splitting enzymes (including β-galactosidase neuraminidase, galactose oxidase, and α-mannosidase), and most importantly, by the fact that the factor is bound to concanavalin-A columns and eluted off such columns by α-methylmannoside.

FMP exists in seminal plasma as a number of multiple forms as evidenced by three separate protein separation techniques, namely, molecular sieving on Sepharose 6B columns, chromatography on diethylaminoethyl (DEAE) cellulose, and preparative isoelectric focusing. Figure 2 shows the separation obtained when heat-treated bovine seminal plasma is applied to a Sepharose 6B column. Note that four peaks of activity are obtained. This elution profile is reproducible with respect to the relative elution positions of individual peaks but varies from preparation to preparation with regard to the shape of each peak. The multimeric nature of FMP is shown by the fact that molecular sieving on this same Sepharose 6B column in the presence of either sodium dodecyl sulfate (SDS) or urea generates a single peak of activity (Fig. 3). Furthermore, reapplication of the single peak of activity to the same Sepharose column, after removal of SDS or urea, results in the regeneration of the four original peaks of activity. The data shown in Figure 4 indicate that the apparent molecular weight of this monomeric form is approximately 37,000 daltons.

The reproducible way in which these four peaks of activity elute from Sepharose 6B columns provides a tool to study the body fluid origin of FMP. Somewhat parenthetically, it should be noted that the absolute identification of this protein in various biological fluids is by no means an easy task since the photographic assay measures a complex, physiological parameter, that is, the induction of motion in sperm. Nonetheless, the molecular size distribution patterns obtained by elution from Sepharose columns (Figure 2) have been used as fingerprints for FMP identification in various biological fluids. Figure 5 shows the comparative elution profiles off a Sepharose 6B column of forward motility-inducing activity derived from both bovine seminal plasma and from fluid from the cauda epididymidis. Note that four major peaks are obtained in each case and that the elution position of each of these, off the same Sepharose column, is the same for both fluids. It is not disturbing that the overall shape of the two profiles is dissimilar since this might be expected for a protein that exists in multiple equilibrium forms.

Undoubtedly, the most convincing data so far obtained that FMP is of epididymal origin is the fact that its specific activity, whether expressed on a volume or protein concentration basis, is far higher in fluid from the cauda epididymidis than in any other body fluid (Table 3). The data in the table also clearly indicate that the forward motility activity is related in some way to the function of the male reproductive tract, since the second and third most active fluids are seminal plasma and rete testicular fluid. The exact order in which these two fluids are placed depends on the way in which specific activity is expressed, *i.e.*, on a protein concentration or fluid volume basis. Perhaps the most valuable information in the table with regard to body fluid, however, is that the maximum forward motility index obtainable reaches a value of greater than 600 only in

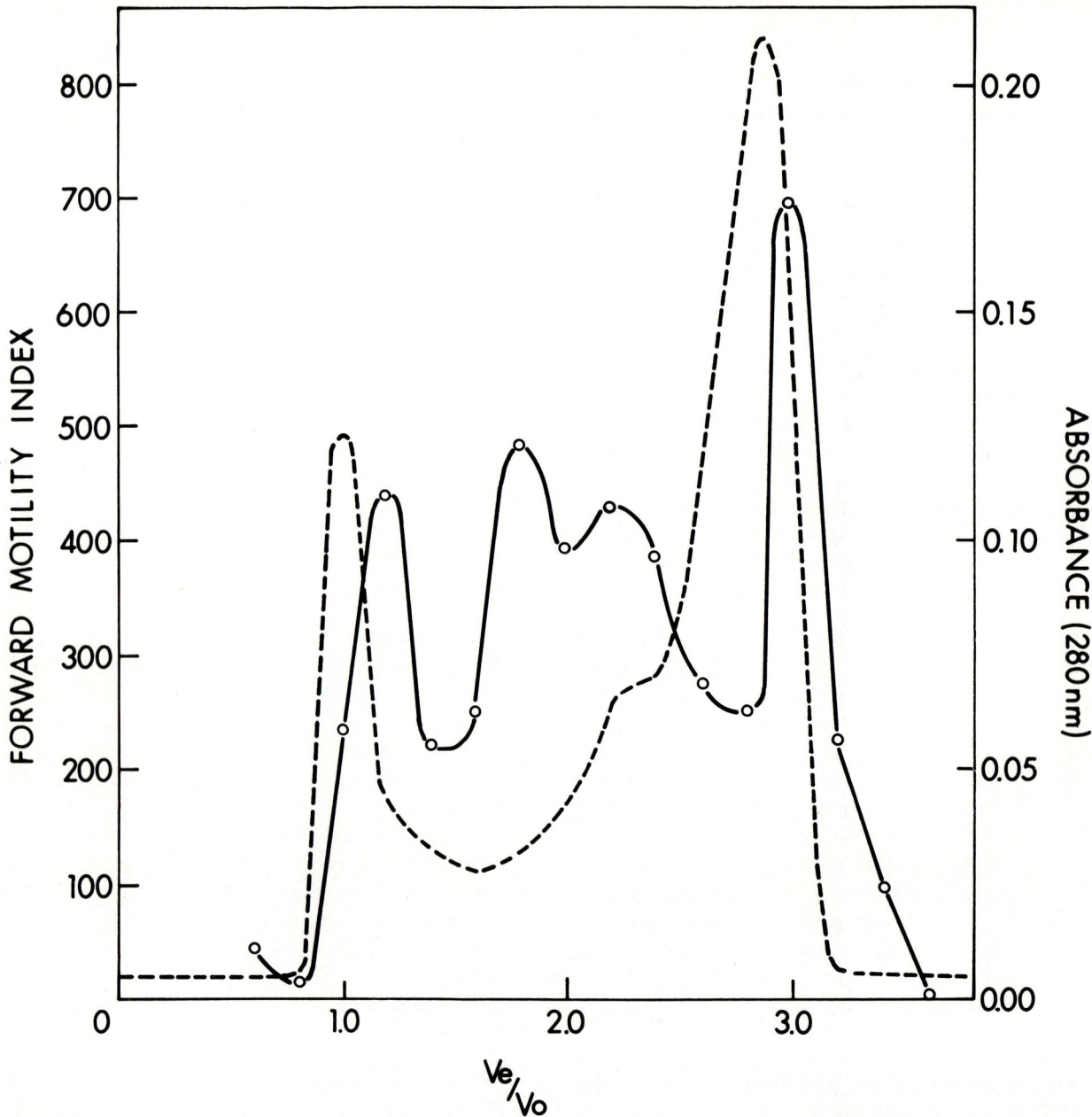

Figure 2. Fractionation of bovine seminal plasma forward motility factor on Sepharose 6B. Heat-treated seminal plasma (2 ml, 20 mg/ml) was applied to a 1.5 × 30 cm column. Fractionation was carried out at 5°C in assay buffer. FMI; (0——0), A_{280} (---), V_e/V_o, elution volume/void volume.

the case of caudal fluid and seminal plasma. All other fluids, including those from the rete testis, are only capable of attaining FMI_{max} values in the range from 200-300.

There is yet another bit of information contained in Table 3 that supports the idea that FMP is of epididymal origin. This information is contained in the second column of the table and is concerned with the relative specific activities of caudal fluid and seminal plasma when expressed on the basis of protein concentration. The consideration here is a theoretical one and is based on the fact that all of the glycerylphosphoryl choline found in seminal plasma is of epididymal origin (Mann, 1964). From this information, and from a knowledge of the average protein concentrations in these two fluids, it is possible to calculate how much the epididymal fluid protein should be diluted by the proteins derived from fluids of the other male accessory glands. From this, it

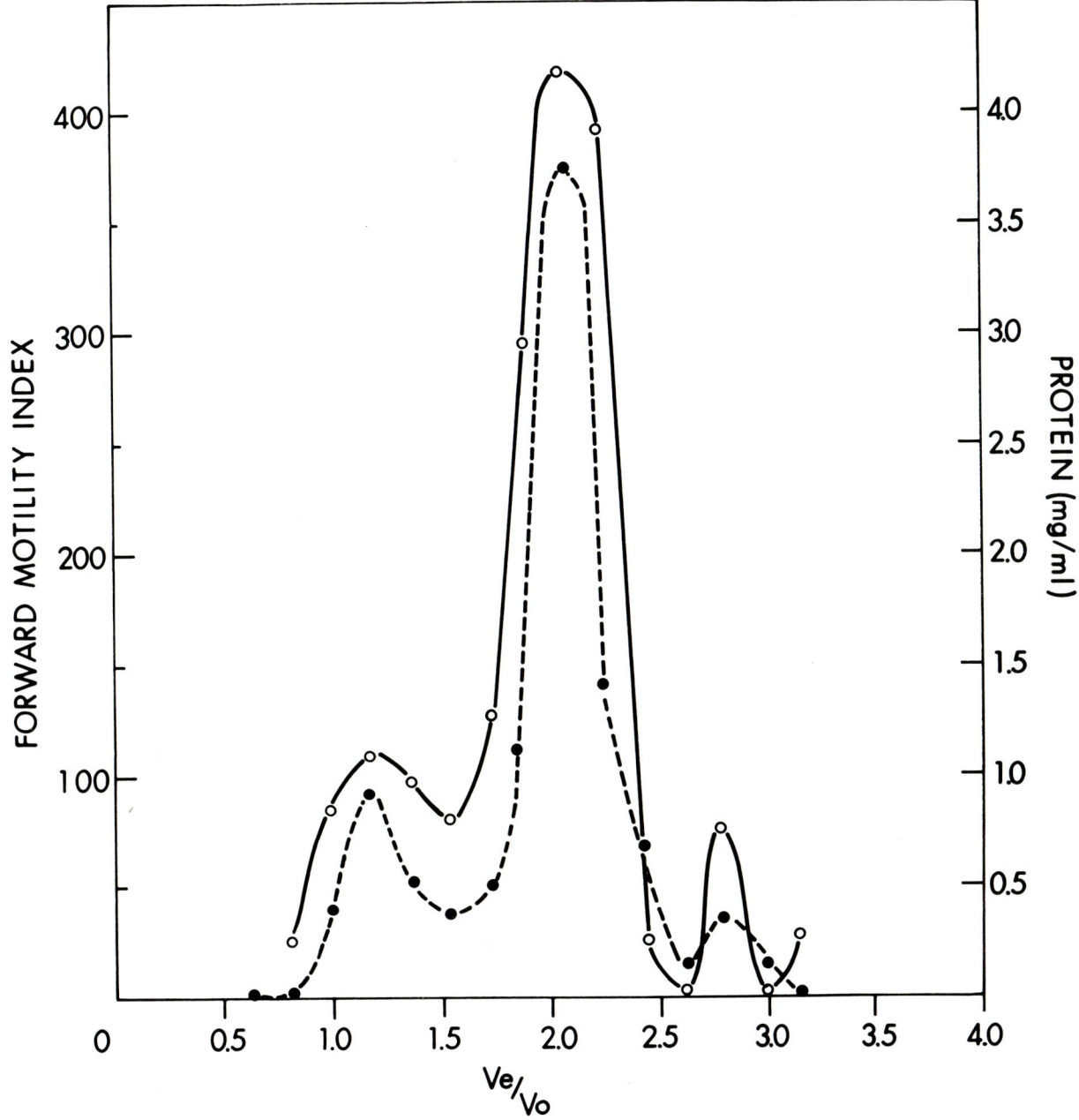

Figure 3. Fractionation of bovine seminal plasma forward motility activity on Sepharose 6B in the presence of SDS; FMI, (0——0) protein concentration (●---●). Heat-treated seminal plasma (2 ml, 15 mg/ml) was dialyzed overnight against a column of buffer containing 1% SDS, 2mM DDT (dithiothreitol), 2mM EDTA (ethylenediaminetetraacetate), and 50mM Tris-HCl, pH 7.5, before application to the column. After fractionation, the dissociating buffer was removed before assay by passage of eluates over Dowex AG 2X-10.

is possible to calculate how much less the seminal plasma-specific FMI should be than the caudal fluid-specific FMI if all of the FMP is derived from the epididymis. When these calculations are made, they show that the seminal plasma-specific activity should be one-fourth that of caudal fluid. The data in the figure show, in fact, that this activity is one-fifth that of caudal fluid. These calculations thus strongly suggest an epididymal origin for FMP.

The final evidence obtained so far to support this view derives from studies carried out with vasectomized rhesus monkeys *M. mulatta*. Here, advantage was taken of the fact that rhesus monkey seminal plasma has the ability to induce forward motion in bovine caput sperm

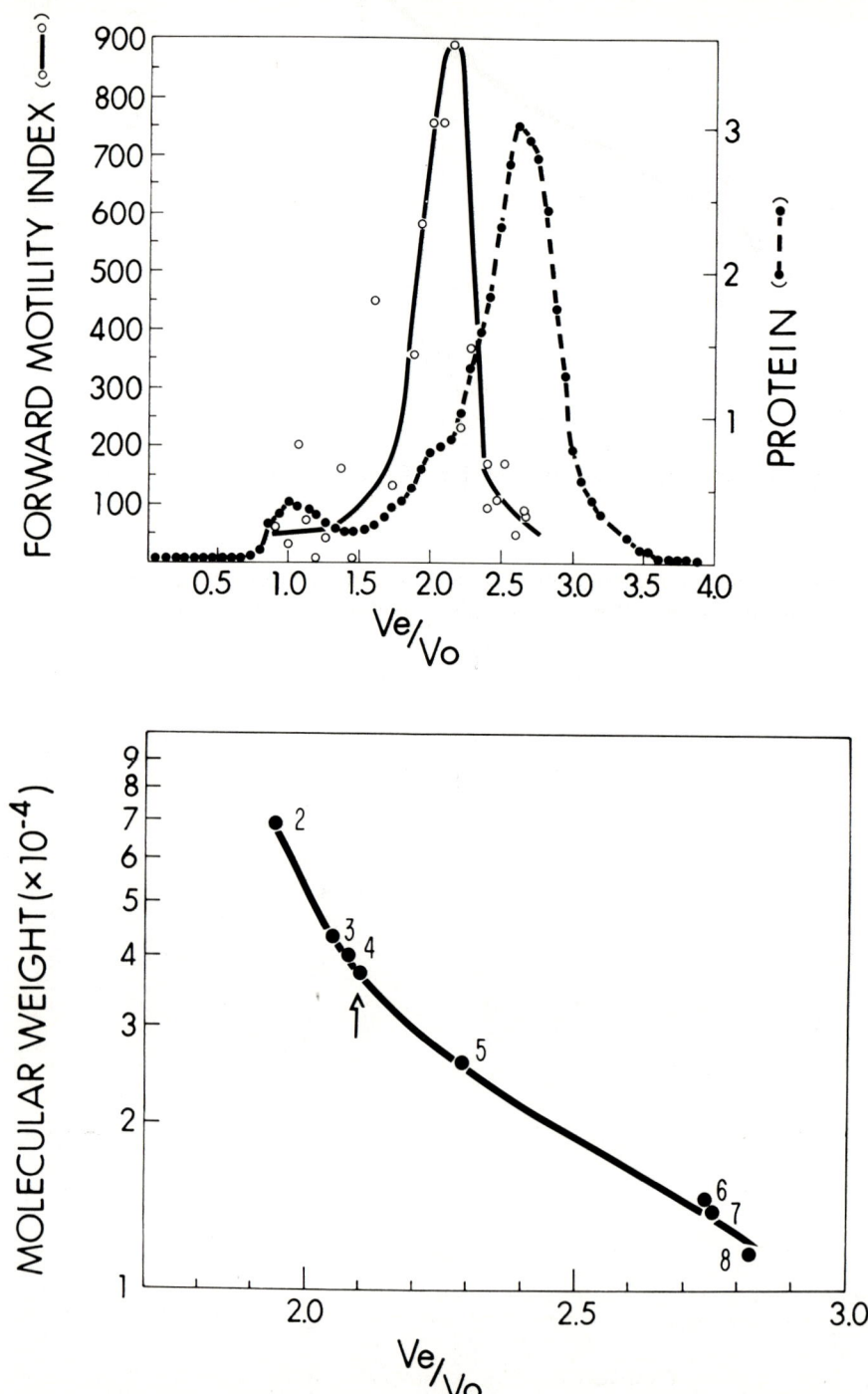

Figure 4. Molecular weight estimate of FMP by chromatography on Sepharose 6B in the presence of 6M urea. Upper: fractionation; lower: calibration curve with standard proteins (phosphorylase A, bovine serum albumin, ovalbumin, aldolase, chymotrypsinogen A, lysozyme, ribonuclease A, and cytochrome C). Arrow on lower graph indicates elution point for FMP.

in the presence of phosphodiesterase inhibitors (Table 2). Thus, if FMP is derived from the monkey epididymis, the seminal plasma of vasectomized animals should activate bovine caput sperm to a much smaller degree than the plasma of control animals. The data shown in Figure 6 indicate that this is, in fact, the case. Values taken from the linear portions of the two plots indicate that the specific activity of the seminal

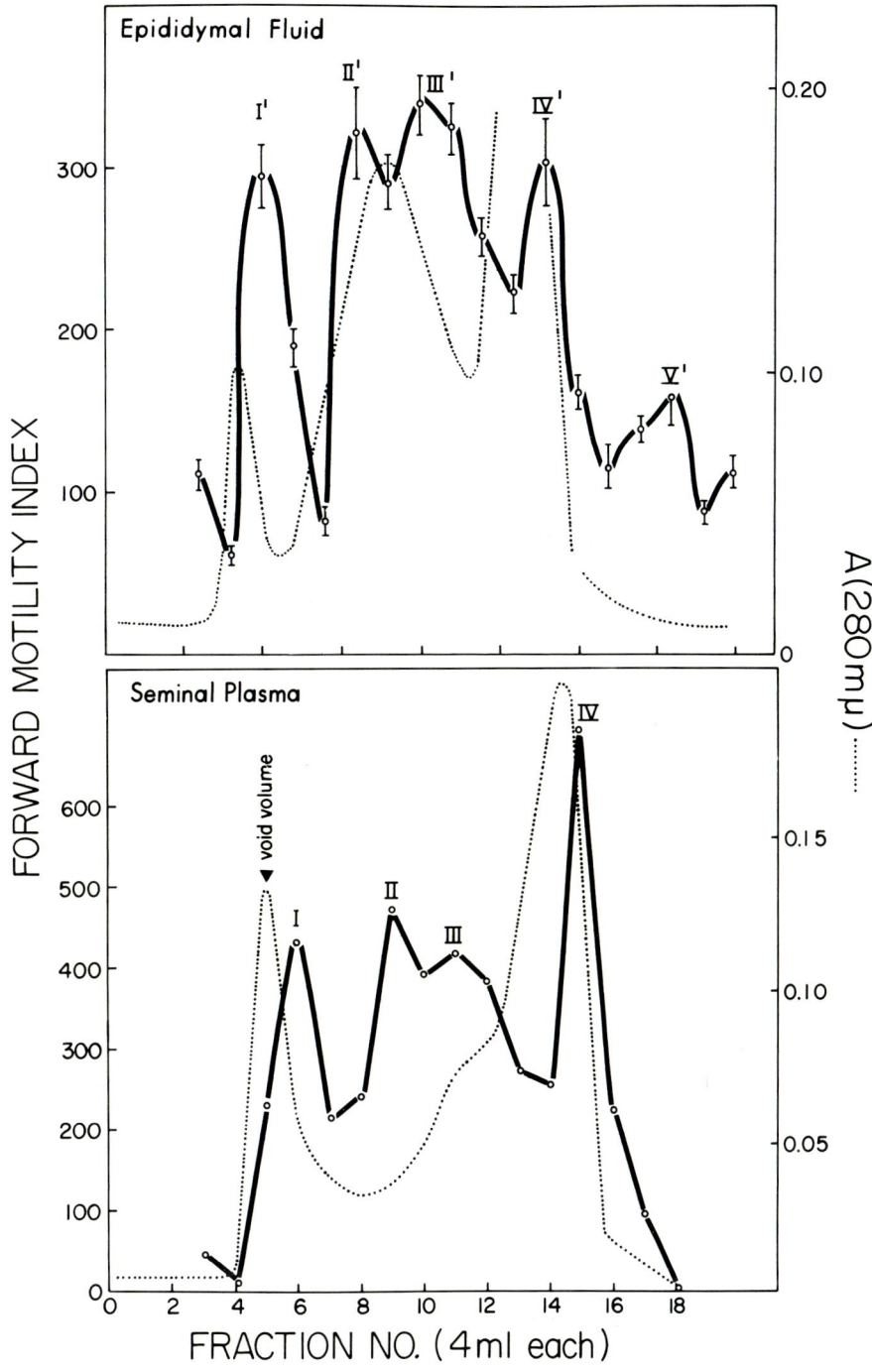

Figure 5. Chromatographic profile of epididymal fluid and seminal plasma on Sepharose 6B.

plasma of control animals is some 5-7 times higher than that of the vasectomized monkeys. Note also, in the lower curve, that the forward motility index in experimental animals never reaches a value greater than 200-300. As shown above in Table 3, this low level of activity is characteristic of many nonreproductive tract and body fluids, and thus may be nonspecific in nature.

The above evidence suggests that a forward motility protein is produced in the bovine and monkey epididymis and somehow interacts with sperm as they pass through the epididymis. Verification of these two ideas must occupy our attention in the immediate future. Of greatest importance will be the development of an assay that is less laborious and more specific than the current

Table 3. Distribution of Forward Motility Protein in Various Bovine Body Fluids

Source	Relative FMI[a]		Maximum FMI[a,b]
	Per μl of Fluid[b]	Per μg of Protein[b]	
Seminal plasma	100 ± 9.6	100 ± 9.6	630 ± 30
Caudal fluid	174 ± 17	470 ± 46	630 ± 24
Rete fluid	5.6 ± 1	105 ± 19	310 ± 34
Testis	0.35 ± 0.09	21.2 ± 5.3	350 ± 53
Vitreous humor	0.64 ± 0.19	17.9 ± 5.4	260 ± 39
Adrenal	0.86 ± 0.2	12.9 ± 3	300 ± 51
Serum	1.5 ± 0.39	0.5 ± 0.13	280 ± 22
Liver	0.52 ± 0.1	0.48 ± 0.09	300 ± 39
Heart	0.37 ± 0.19	0.24 ± 0.12	175 ± 71
Spinal cord	0.00 ± 0.04	0.00 ± 0.28	2.6 ± 26

[a] Mean ± SEM.
[b] Volumes and protein values correspond to the neat, nonheat-treated fluids or supernatants of the tissue homogenates.

photographic procedure. Thus, the forward motility protein in seminal plasma is currently being purified with the intent of developing a radioimmunoassay. Once in hand, this assay method will be used to verify the body fluid and species distribution of the factor as well as to purify the protein from epididymal fluids. The availability of purified epididymal forward motility protein is essential for carrying out meaningful studies on the interaction between FMP and developing sperm.

In summary, the data contained in this chapter indicate that the initiation of motility in the bovine epididymis involves at least two events, an elevation in the intrasperm content of cyclic AMP during epididymal transit and the production by the epididymis of a specific forward motility protein.

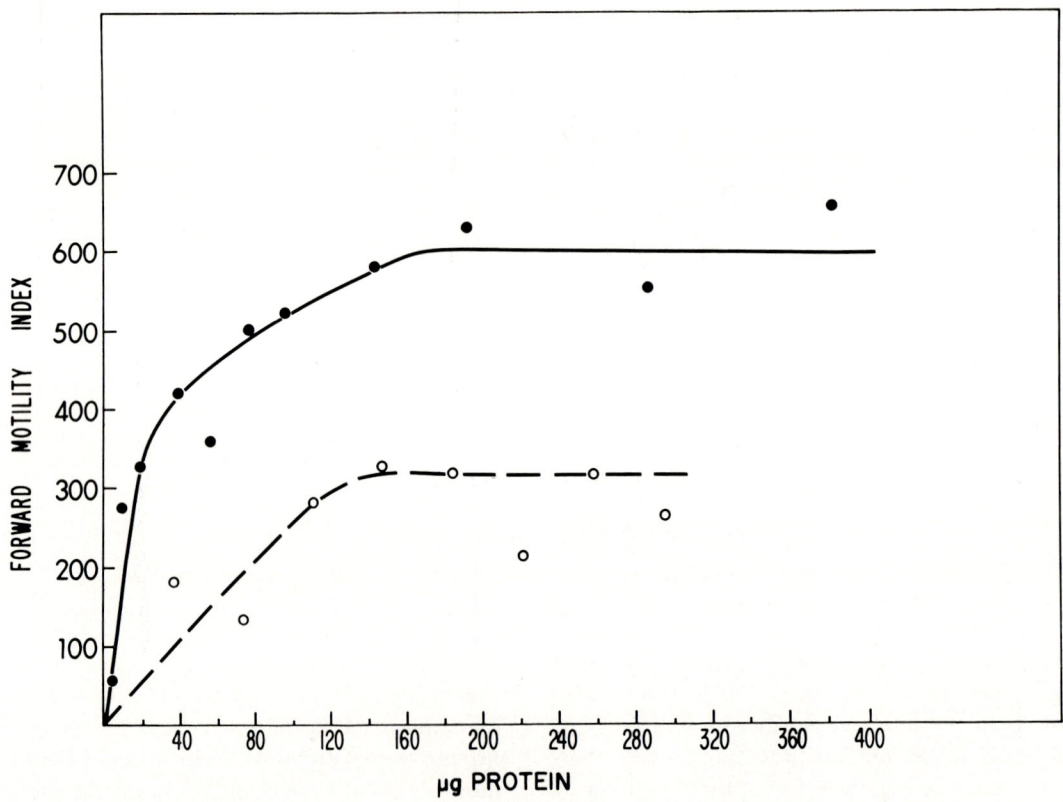

Figure 6. The relative abilities of seminal plasma protein from vasectomized (0---0) and normal (•——•) rhesus monkeys to induce forward motion in bovine caput spermatozoa.

REFERENCES

Acott, T.S.; Hoskins, D.D.: Bovine Sperm Forward Motility Protein: Partial Purification and Characterization. J Biol Chem, 253(1978)6744-6750

Bedford, J.M.: Maturation, Transport, and Fate of Spermatozoa in the Epididymis. In: Handbook of Physiology, Section on Endocrinology, pp. 303-317, ed. by E. Astwood and R.O. Greep. American Physiology Society, Washington, D.C., 1975

Bedford, J.M.: Effect of Duct Ligation on the Fertilizing Ability of Spermatozoa from Different Regions of the Epididymis. J Exp Zool 166(1967)271-282

Bedford, J.M.; Calvin, H.; Cooper, G.W.: The Maturation of Spermatozoa in the Human Epididymis. J Reprod Fertil Suppl 18(1973)199-213

Burgos, M.H.; Tovar, E.S.: Sperm Motility in the Rat Epididymis. Fertil Steril 25(1974)298-291

Calvin, H.; Bedford, J.M.: Formation of Disulfide Bonds in the Nucleus and Accessory Structures of Mammalian Spermatozoa during Maturation in the Epididymis. J Reprod Fertil Suppl 13(1971)65-75

Frenkel, G.; Peterson, R.N.; Freund, M.: The Role of Adenine Nucleotides and the Effect of Caffeine and Dibutyryl Cyclic AMP on the Metabolism of Guinea Pig Spermatozoa. Proc Soc Exp Biol Med 144(1973)420-425

Gaddum, P.; Glover, T.: Some Reactions of Rabbit Spermatozoa to Ligation of the Epididymis. J Reprod Fertil 9(1965)119-130

Glover, T.D.: The Response of Rabbit Spermatozoa to Artificial Cryptorchidism and Ligation of the Epididymis. J Endocrinol 23(1962)317-328

Horan, A.H.; Bedford, J.M.: Development of Fertilizing Ability in the Syrian Hamster. J Reprod Fertil 30(1972)417-423

Hoskins, D.D.; Casillas, E.R.: The Function of Cyclic Nucleotide in Mammalian Spermatozoa. In: Handbook of Physiology, Section on Endocrinology, pp. 453-460, ed. by E. Astwood and R.O. Greep. American Physiological Society, Washington, D.C., 1975

Hoskins, D.D.; Hall, M.L.; Munsterman, D.: Induction of Motility in Immature Bovine Spermatozoa by Cyclic AMP Phosphodiesterase Inhibitors and Seminal Plasma. Biol Reprod 13(1975)168-176

Hoskins, D.D.; Stephens, D.T.; Hall, M.L.: Cyclic Adenosine $3':5'$-Monophosphate and Protein Kinase Levels in Developing Bovine Spermatozoa. J Reprod Fertil 37(1974)131-133

Igboeli, G.; Foote, R.H.: Maturational Changes in Bull Epididymal Spermatozoa. J Dairy Sci 51(1968)1703

Janick, J.; MacLeod, J.: The Measurement of Human Sperm Motility. Fertil Steril 21(1970)140-146

Lindholmer, C.: The Importance of Seminal Plasma for Human Sperm Motility. Biol Reprod 10(1974)533-542

Mann, T.: The Biochemistry of Semen and of the Male Reproductive Tract. London, Methuen, 1964

Mooney, J.K.; Horan, A.H.; Latlimer, J.K.: Motility of Spermatozoa in the Human Epididymis. J Urol 108(1972)443-445

Nelson, L.: Spermatozoan Motility. In: Handbook of Physiology, Section on Endocrinology, pp. 421-435, ed. by E. Astwood and R.O. Greep. American Physiology Society, Washington, D.C., 1975

Orgebin-Crist, M.-C.: Maturation of Spermatozoa in the Rabbit Epididymis: Effect of Castration and Testosterone Replacement. J Exp Zool 188(1973)301-309

Stephens, D.T.; Wang, J.-L.; Hoskins, D.D.: The Cyclic AMP Phosphodiesterase of Bovine Spermatozoa: Multiple Forms, Kinetic Properties, and Changes during Development. Biol Reprod, in press

Tournade, A.: Difference de Motilite des Spermatozoides Preleves dans les Divers Segments de l'Epididyme. C R Soc Biol (Paris) 74(1913)738-739

Wyler, R.; Howards, S.S.: Micropuncture Studies of the Motility of Rete Testis and Epididymal Spermatozoa. Fertil Steril 28(1977)108-112

Young, W.C.: A Study of the Function of the Epididymis. III. Functional Changes Undergone by Spermatozoa during Their Passage through the Epididymis and Vas Deferens in the Guinea Pig. J Exp Biol 8(1931)151-163

CONTRIBUTED PAPER

SOME CHARACTERISTICS OF SALT AND WATER TRANSPORT IN THE RAT EPIDIDYMIS

P.Y.D. Wong, C.L. Au, and H.K. Ngai

Department of Physiology, Faculty of Medicine, University of Hong Kong

The rat epididymis has many characteristics of a salt-absorbing gland. The mitochondria-rich epithelial (principal) cells possess microvilli at the luminal border and the cells are held by tight junctions at the apical side (Wong et al., 1978). Enzymes involved in ion transport mechanism have been identified in the epithelium (Martan, 1969; Cohen et al., 1976). In the rat the epididymis absorbs about 90% of the testicular fluid, which process takes place along the entire length of the epididymis (Levine and Marsh, 1971).

The ionic mechanism of fluid reabsorption in the rat cauda epididymidis has been studied in the isolated epididymal duct in vitro (Wong and Yeung, 1977a) and in anesthetized rats in vivo (Wong and Yeung, 1978). It was found that the driving force of water reabsorption is an active transport of Na^+. Absorption of Na^+ is coupled to the secretion of K^+, and this process is maintained by the adrenocortical hormones (Au et al., 1978).

The mechanism of fluid reabsorption in the more proximal regions of the rat epididymis is less clear although there is evidence that these segments have a high blood flow and are likely to be engaged in active reabsorption of fluid (Setchell et al., 1964). In this work electrolyte and water transport has been measured in the caput and corpus epididymidis and compared with the cauda epididymidis. It is now evident that different regions of the epididymis do not only show morphological and ultrastructural differences (Reid and Cleland, 1957; Glover and Nicander, 1971; Hamilton, 1975), they have different sensitivity and responsiveness to different sources of androgens (Fawcett and Hoffer, 1978).

Electrolyte and water transport in the rat epididymis is highly dependent on the supply of circulating androgens (Wong and Yeung, 1977b). In this work the effect of an antiandrogen cyproterone acetate was also studied.

This work received financial support from the World Health Organization. The authors thank Schering AG, Berlin for the supply of cyproterone acetate, and the technical assistance of Mr. Raymond Wong is gratefully acknowledged.

© 1979 Urban & Schwarzenberg, Inc. Baltimore-Munich *The Spermatozoon*, edited by D.W. Fawcett and J.M. Bedford

METHODS

Microperfusion of the Rat Epididymis

Fertile male Sprague-Dawley rats weighing 350-450 g were anaesthetized with pentobarbitone (50 mg/kg body wt.). Tracheostomy was performed to ensure a clear air passage. A paramedial incision was made in the scrotum to expose the epididymis. Under a dissecting microscope, a small piece of the connective tissue sheath (about 1 mm^2) was removed at zone 5 (Reid and Cleland [1957] classification) and a small loop of the coiled epididymal duct was freed from the connective tissue (Fig. 1). The duct was cannulated by insertion of fine (Clay-Adams PE-50) polyethylene tubing pulled to a tip diameter of about 300 μm. The cannula was held in place by anchoring in plasticine. The ipsilateral vas deferens was freed from the adjacent blood vessel and was slit open using ultrafine irridectomy scissors. The cauda epididymidis was then flushed with Krebs bicarbonate solution to remove all the spermatozoa using a tuberculin syringe after which a polyethylene cannula (Clay-Adams PE-10) with tip diameter of about 300 μm was inserted into the lumen of the vas deferens and ligated in place. The clear segment of the cauda epididymidis (about 18 cm long) was then perfused in situ with Krebs bicarbonate solution using a syringe infusion pump (Harvard 970) set to deliver from a 1-ml glass syringe at constant rate of 1 μl/min (Fig. 1). The Krebs bicarbonate solution has the following composition (mM): NaCl, 118; KCl, 4.7; CaCl$_2$, 2.56; MgSO$_4$, 1.17; NaH$_2$PO$_4$, 1.13; NaHCO$_3$, 25; glucose, 11.1. This solution when bubbled with 95% O$_2$ and 5% CO$_2$ had a pH of 7.4 with osmolarity of 310 mOsm/L. Perfusate was collected into sample cups (Bel-Art) and was collected over 60 min. The effluent rate was obtained from weight of the perfusate divided by the collection time. The duct was perfused for 40 min before experimentation. The rectal temperature was monitored by a thermistor probe and was maintained at 37°C by direct illumination. At the end of the experiment, the perfused segment of the cauda epididymidis was dissected out and the length determined. In 13 experiments, the length was 17.9 ± 0.6 cm (mean ± S.E.).

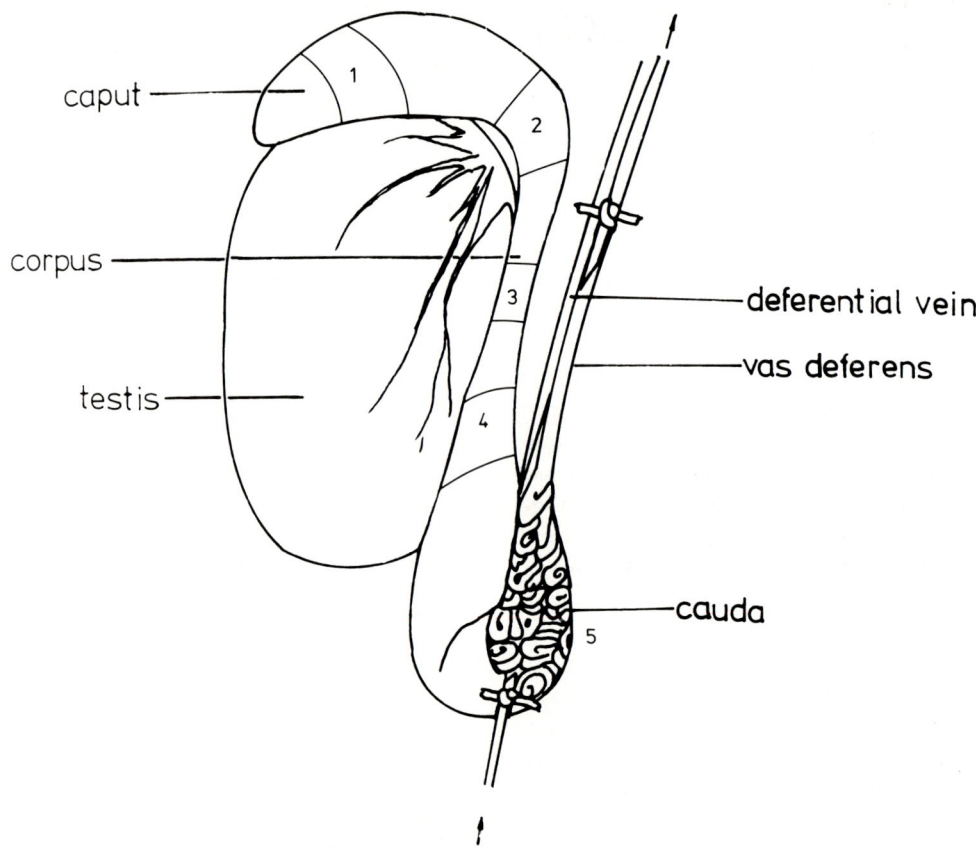

Figure 1. Schematic diagram of the rat testis. The epididymis was divided into five zones. 1, caput epididymidis; 2, proximal corpus epididymidis; 3, mid-corpus epididymidis; 4, distal corpus epididymidis, and 5, cauda epididymidis. Only the perfused cauda epididymidis is shown. The arrows show the direction of perfusion (see text for explanation).

Similar procedures were applied to the caput and the three regions of the corpus epididymidis (Fig. 1), except that the cannulae used had tip diameters of about 150 μm. For the caput epididymidis, the inflow cannula was tied at a place just distal to the incision separating the caput from the initial segment. The initial segment was therefore not included in the perfusion. The perfused lengths of the caput, proximal corpus, midcorpus and distal corpus epididymidis were 8.34 ± 0.91 cm (mean ± S.E.); 7.42 ± 0.75 cm (mean ± S.E.); 5.26 ± 0.15 cm (mean ± S.E.) and 8.01 ± 0.82 cm (mean ± S.E.) respectively. The lumens were flushed free of sperm and perfused at a rate of about 0.8 μl/min for 40 min before experimentation. Perfusates were collected over the next 2 h and analyzed for Na^+, K^+, Cl^-, inulin, and protein (see below). Histological examination of the perfused segments of the epididymis was also undertaken. The tissues were fixed in 10% formalin and stained with haemotoxylin and eosin (Fig. 1).

Analytical Procedure

The rate of water reabsorption was measured by using [^{3}H]-inulin as volume marker. The inulin ratio IR, *i.e.* [^{3}H]-inulin in perfusate over [^{3}H]-inulin in perfusion fluid was determined and the rate of water reabsorption was calculated by:

$$\text{Rate per cm duct} = \text{effluent rate } (IR - 1)/d$$

where d is the length of the perfused epididymis.

The concentration of Na^+ and K^+ in the perfusate was determined by flame photometry (Zeiss PF5) and chloride by a chloridometer (Buchler-Cotlove). The perfusate was diluted 500 times for the determination of Na^+ and K^+ and 80 times for the determination of chloride. The net electrolyte fluxes were determined from the perfusion rate and the initial and final electrolyte concentrations in the perfusion solutions. Protein concentration in the perfusate was determined by Lowry's method (Lowry et al., 1951). The rate of protein secretion was expressed as ng protein secreted/cm duct/min.

Treatment with Cyproterone Acetate

A group of sexually mature male Sprague-Dawley rats weighing approximately 400 g were given daily subcutaneous injections of 10 mg of cyproterone acetate suspended in 0.2 ml of a castor oil and benzylbenzoate mixture (4:1 v/v). Control rats were injected daily with 0.2 ml vehicle. Electrolyte and water transport was studied after 10, 25, or 50 days of injection. Another group of rats was injected for 50 days and then allowed to recover for 21 days before transport study was made. The motility of the spermatozoa collected from the cauda epididymidis was examined. The cauda fluid was diluted with physiological Ringer's solution and observed under a phase contrast microscope. The motility was expressed as the percent of motile sperm.

RESULTS

The histology of the perfused segments of the rat epididymis is shown in Figure 2. The epididymal epithelial cells were intact with stereocilia still present in the luminal border. At the level of light microscope, there

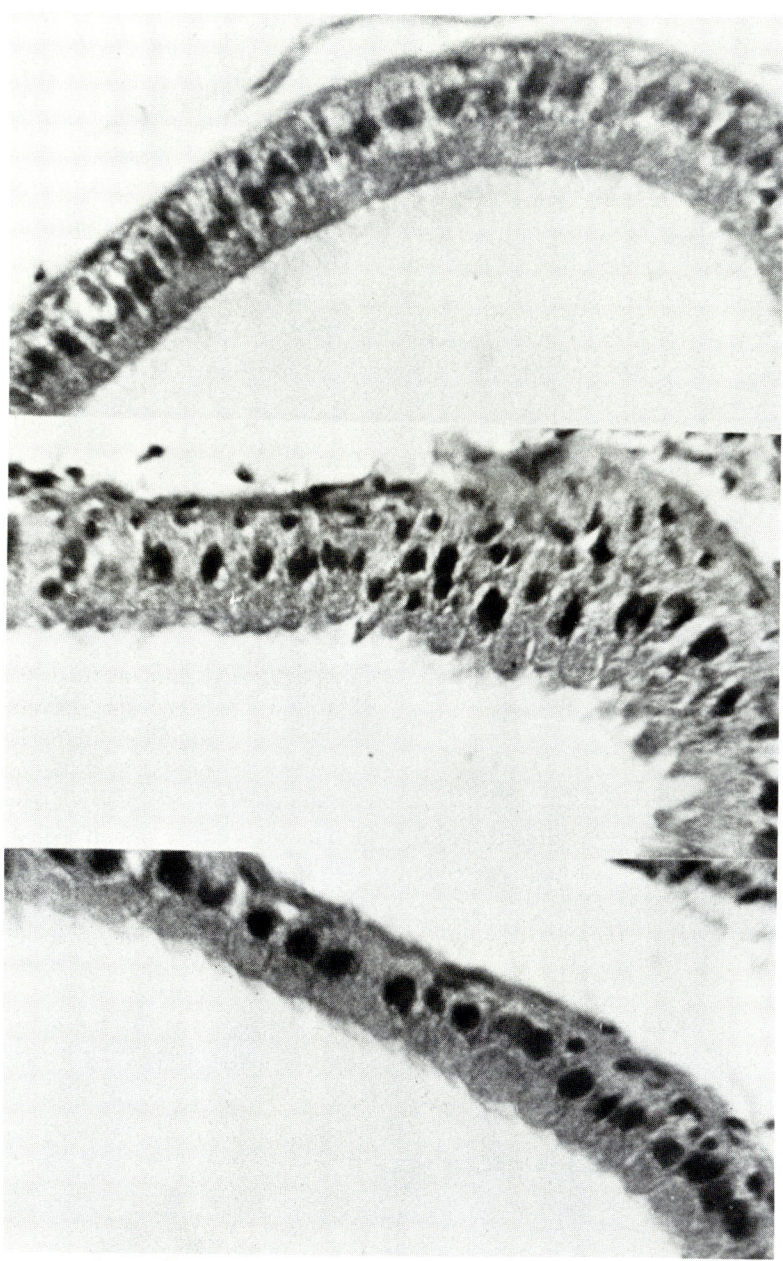

Figure 2. Photomicrograph of the cells lining the caput (upper), proximal corpus (middle), and distal corpus (lower) epididymidis which have been perfused with Krebs solution. Note the cells are intact with stereocilia present in the luminal membrane.

was no indication of cell damage by the perfusion of the lumen.

Basal Rate of Electrolyte and Water Transport in Different Regions of the Epididymis

When different segments of the rat epididymis were perfused with normal Krebs solution at rates ranging from 0.5-1 μl/min, the inulin ratio always exceeded 1. This indicated a net water reabsorption along the entire length of the duct. After correction for the net water flux, Na^+ and Cl^- were found to be reabsorbed while K^+ secreted into the ductal lumen. The rates of reabsorption of Na^+, Cl^-, and water and secretion of K^+ and protein are summarized in Figure 3. Among these five regions, the cauda epididymidis has the highest rate of electrolyte and water transport. Calculation showed that reabsorption of Na^+ was isotonic and was higher than that of the Cl^-. However, in the more proximal part of the epididymis, reabsorption of Cl was hypertonic. Na^+ and water reabsorption and K^+ secretion were carried out at much lower rates. The transport processes have the lowest activities in the mid and distal parts of the corpus epididymidis. The secretory rate of protein in the caput and cauda epididymidis was higher than that in the corpus epididymidis.

Effect of Cyproterone Acetate on Transport Functions of the Rat Cauda Epididymidis

The effect of cyproterone acetate treatment (10 mg/rat/day) is shown in Table 1. Injection of the antiandrogen for 10 days slightly diminished the rates of Na^+, Cl^-, and water reabsorption and secretion of K^+. Treatment for 25 days further reduced these rates to about 50% of the control. After 50 days, reabsorption of Na^+, Cl^-, and water and secretion of K^+ were completely abolished and the secretion of protein was significantly reduced. The effect of cyproterone acetate was partially reversible within 21 days of cessation of treatment. Concomitant with the inhibitory action on electrolyte and water transport, there was an increasing percent of nonmotile sperm in the cauda epididymidal fluid (Table 1).

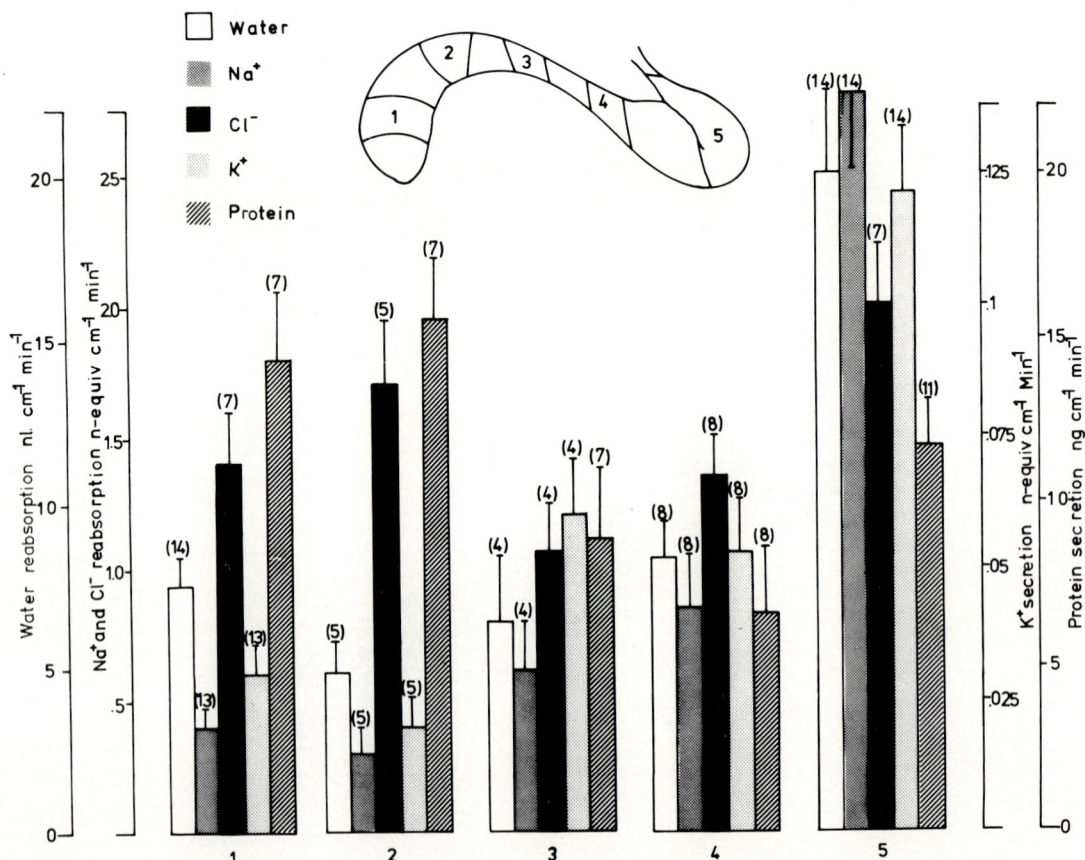

Figure 3. The rates of reabsorption of Na^+, Cl^-, and water and secretion of K^+ and protein in five different regions of the rat epididymis (see text). Each column shows the mean ± S.E. with the number of experiments shown in parentheses.

Table 1. The Effect of Cyproterone Acetate (CPA) (10 mg/rat/day) on the Rate of Transport of Electrolytes and Water in the Perfused Rat Cauda Epididymidis

Treatment	H_2O Reabsorption nl cm^{-1} min^{-1}	Na$^+$ Reabsorption nEq cm^{-1} min^{-1}	Cl$^-$ Reabsorption nEq cm^{-1} min^{-1}	K$^+$ Secretion nEq cm^{-1} min^{-1}	Protein Secretion ng cm^{-1} min^{-1}	(%) Motile Sperm
Control	13.7 ± 2.25 (n = 7)	1.75 ± 0.35 (n = 7)	1.43 ± 0.27 (n = 7)	0.097 ± 0.02 (n = 7)	22.0 ± 5.2 (n = 7)	60 ± 10.5 (n = 6)
CPA treated 10 days	11.0 ± 2.20 (n = 4)	1.40 ± 0.25 (n = 4)	0.95 ± 0.24 (n = 4)	0.030 ± 0.01* (n = 4)	22.2 ± 4.3 (n = 4)	28 ± 8.4* (n = 4)
CPA treated 25 days	6.8 ± 1.5* (n = 6)	0.75 ± 0.23* (n = 6)	0.78 ± 0.26 (n = 6)	0.038 ± 0.01* (n = 6)	13.0 ± 3.1 (n = 6)	—
CPA treated 50 days	0.19 ± 1.3*** (n = 7)	−0.54 ± 0.13*** (n = 7)	−0.78 ± 0.15*** (n = 7)	0.057 ± 0.01 (n = 7)	2.82 ± 0.51** (n = 7)	3.89 ± 1.45*** (n = 7)
CPA treated 50 days + 21 days recovery	7.2 ± 1.2** (n = 8)	0.82 ± 0.19** (n = 8)	0.84 ± 0.21** (n = 8)	0.080 ± 0.01 (n = 8)	11.0 ± 3.2* (n = 8)	14.0 ± 2.7** (n = 8)

Each value shows the mean ± S.E. All values were compared to control except for the recovery values which were compared to CPA treated 50 days.
*$P < 0.05$
**$P < 0.01$
***$P < 0.001$
— a net secretion

DISCUSSION

Absorption and secretion of fluid in many transporting glands are thought to involve an active transport of ions (Diamond and Wright, 1969). In the rat cauda epididymidis, reabsorption of water is passive and is secondary to an active transport of Na$^+$. This mechanism of water flow coupled to Na$^+$ transport conforms to the standing gradient model of Diamond and Bossert (1967). Sodium diffuses into the cell and is pumped into the intercellular spaces at its apical end by sodium pumps at the basolateral membranes. A local hypertonicity is then created at the blind end of the interspace so that water moving through the cell osmotically increases the volume and pushes the fluid out of the interspace as isotonic fluid. In this way a standing gradient is set up causing osmotic water flow (Fig. 4). The entry of Na$^+$ at the apical membrane is passive and is found to be blocked by a diuretic drug amiloride (N—amidino—3, 5—diamino—6 chloropyrazine—2—carboxamide) (Wong and Yeung, 1976). Electron microscopic studies have shown widely dilated intercellular spaces in the isolated ducts of the rat cauda epididymidis which were absorbing water at a maximal rate (Wong et al., 1978). In the cauda epididymidis, K$^+$ is found to be secreted in exchange of Na$^+$. This Na$^+$/K$^+$-coupled transport is stimulated by adrenocortical hormones (Au et al., 1978). In these respects, the cauda epididymidis has transport processes similar to those occurring in the distal kidney tubule.

The transport processes of the more proximal parts of the rat epididymis, however, are very different from those of the cauda. In the caput and proximal corpus, reabsorption of Cl$^-$ was hypertonic (Fig. 2). Na$^+$ reabsorption and K$^+$ secretion were carried out at lower rates. There was also very little reabsorption of water in these regions. One possible explanation of these results is that the proximal parts of the epididymis are characterized by an active transport of Cl$^-$ across an epithelium which is poorly permeable to Na$^+$ and water. Levine and Marsh (1971) using micropuncture on the rat epididymis found that as the seminiferous tubular fluid passed down the caput epididymidis, there was a marked reduction in the Cl$^-$ concentration while the Na$^+$ concentration remained unchanged. Presumably Cl$^-$ was reabsorbed without being accompanied by Na$^+$. Active Cl$^-$ transport has also been demonstrated in other tissues such as the loop of Henle (Burg and Green, 1973), cornea (Zadunaisky, et al., 1971), and teleost gill (Degnan et al., 1977).

The transport of electrolytes and water in the rat cauda epididymidis was found to be dependent on the supply of circulating androgens (Wong and Yeung, 1977b, 1978) and the authors' present results with the antiandrogen cyproterone acetate further support this view. There was a time dependent decrease in the electrolyte and water transport in the cauda epididymidis after treatment (10 mg/rat/day). Histological and ultrastructural studies have shown that cyproterone acetate caused an involution of the epididymal cells with depletion of secretory granules (Rajalakshmi and Prasad, 1975; Flickinger and Loving, 1976). Back et al. (1977) measured the composition of the epididymal

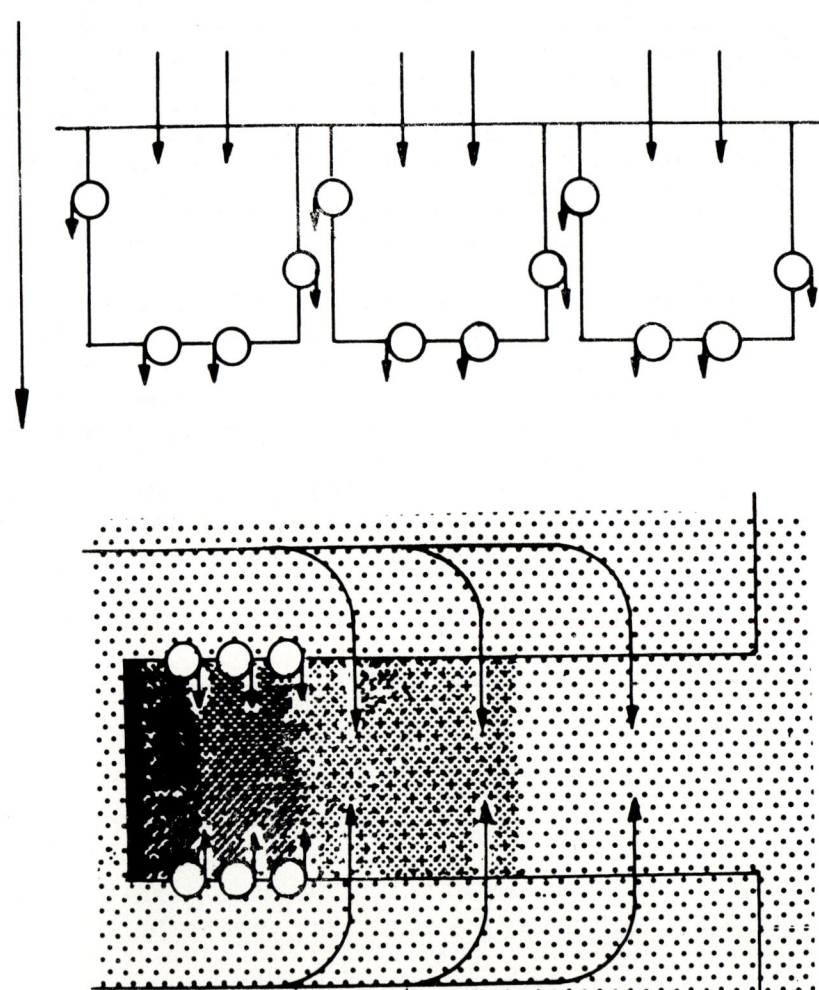

Figure 4. Models of ion and water transport in the rat cauda epididymidis. The upper model is of sodium transport through the epithelium. Na+ (short straight arrows) enters the apical side of the cells down an electrochemical gradient. Na+ pumps (circles with short arrows) in the basolateral membranes expel sodium into peritubular side Cl− (long straight arrow) move passively through the tissue down the electrical gradient created by active sodium transport. The lower model illustrates how solute and water transport may be coupled to give isotonic transport. Na+ that has entered the cells is pumped into the intercellular spaces (ICS) to give a hypertonic solution that moves water osmotically (curved arrows) into ICS. The tight junctions are impermeable and the solute pumps are confined to the apical end of ICS. The transported fluid is diluted in its passage along the ICS and is isotonic when it enters the peritubular fluid. The density of dots suggests the solute concentration.

plasma in rats and observed a slight but significant increase in Na+ concentration after cyproterone treatment. This finding is consistent with an inhibition of Na+ transport by the antiandrogen.

Although transport of electrolytes and water were markedly reduced or completely abolished after injection with cyproterone acetate, the plasma level of testosterone measured in these rats over the entire injection period remained unchanged.[1] Similar results have been obtained by Back et al. (1977) and Schenck and Neumann (1978). The effects of cyproterone acetate evidently resulted from the antiandrogenic action of the drug at the target organs (Fang and Liao, 1969). Cyproterone acetate injection was also found to inhibit the motility of the cauda epididymidal sperm. A result which is consistent with an antifertility effect of the drug (Prasad et al., 1970; Back et al., 1977).

It has previously been reported that low doses of alpha-chlorohydrin inhibited Na+ and water transport in the rat cauda epididymidis. This effect was dose dependent and reversible. The mininal effective dose was comparable to that required to induce sterility in rats. Furthermore, compounds with structure similar to alpha-chlorohydrin but devoid of an antifertility effect

---

[1] Wong, P.Y.D.; Wang, C.; Au, C.L.: in preparation

was found to have no effect on electrolyte and water transport in the rat epididymis (Wong and Yeung, 1977c; Wong *et al.*, 1977). The mechanism of action of alphachlorohydrin is unknown but it may inhibit active transport processes by inhibiting glycolysis of the epithelial cells. The effects of both alpha-chlorohydrin and cyproterone acetate may indicate a disruption of the normal epididymal transport functions as the primary cause of their antifertility action.

REFERENCES

Au, C.L.; Ngai, H.K.; Yeung, C.H.; Wong, P.Y.D.: Effect of Adrenalectomy and Hormone Replacement on Sodium and Water Transport in the Perfused Rat Cauda Epididymidis. J Endocrinol 77(1978)265-266

Back, D.J.; Glover, T.D.; Shenton, J.C.; Boyd, G.P.: Some Effects of Cyproterone Acetate on the Reproductive Physiology of the Male Rat. J Reprod Fertil 49(1977)237-243

Burg, M.; Green, N.: Function of the Thick Ascending Limb of Henle's Loop. Am J Physiol 224(1973)659-668

Cohen, J.P.; Hoffer, A.P.; Rosen, S.: Carbonic Anhydrase Localization in the Epididymis and Testis of the Rat: Histochemical and Biochemical Analysis. Biol Reprod 14(1976)339-346

Degnan, K.J.; Karnaky, K.J.; Zadunaisky, J.A.: Active Chloride Transport in the *in Vitro* Opercular Skin of a Teleost (*Fundulus heteroclitus*), a Gill-like Epithelium Rich in Chloride Cells. J Physiol (Lond) 271(1977)155-191

Diamond, J.M.; Bossert, W.H.: A Mechanism for Coupling of Water and Solute Transport in Epithelia. J Gen Physiol 50(1967)2061-2083

Diamond, J.M.; Wright, E.H.: Biological Membranes: The Physical Basis of Ion and Non-electrolyte Selectivity. Ann Rev Physiol 31(1969)581-646

Fang, S.; Liao, S.: Antagonistic Action of Anti-androgens on the Formation of a Specific Dihydrotestosterone Receptor Protein Complex in Rat Ventral Prostate. Mol Pharmacol 5(1969)420

Fawcett, D.W.; Hoffer, A.P.: Failure of Exogenous Androgen to Prevent Regression of the Initial Segments of the Rat Epididymis after Efferent Duct Ligation or Castration. Biol Reprod, in press

Flickinger, C.J.; Loving, C.K.: Fine Structure of the Testis and Epididymis of Rats Treated with Cyproterone Acetate. Am J Anat 146(1976)359-384

Glover, T.D.; Nicander, L.: Some Aspects of Structure and Function in the Mammalian Epididymis. J Reprod Fertil Suppl 13(1971)39

Hamilton, D.W.: Structure and Function of the Epithelium Lining the Ductuli Efferentes, Ductus Epididymidis, and Ductus Deferens in the Rat. In: Handbook of Physiology. Vol. V, Endocrinology, sect. 7, Male Reproductive System, pp. 259-301, ed. by D.W. Hamilton and R.O. Creep. The American Physiological Society, Washington, D.C., 1975

Levine, N.; Marsh, D.J.: Micropuncture Studies of the Electrochemical Aspects of Fluid and Electrolyte Transport in Individual Seminiferous Tubules, the Epididymis and the Vas Deferens in Rats. J Physiol (Lond) 213(1971)557-570

Lowry, O.H.; Rosebrough, N.J.; Farr, A.L.; Randall, R.J.: Protein Measurement with the Folin Phenol Reagent. J Biol Chem 193(1951)265-275

Martan, J.: Epididymal Histochemistry and Physiology. Biol Reprod Suppl 1(1969)134-154

Prasad, M.R.N.; Singh, S.P.; Rajalakshmi, M.: Fertility Control in Male Rats by Continuous Release of Microquantities of Cyproterone Acetate from Subcutaneous Silastic Capsules. Contraception 2(1970)165-170

Rajalakshmi, M.; Prasad, M.R.N.: Action of Cyproterone Acetate on the Accessory Organs of Reproduction in Prepubertal and Sexually Mature Rats. Fertil Steril 26(1975)137-143

Reid, B.L.; Cleland, K.W.: The Structure and Function of the Epididymis. I. The Histology of the Rat Epididymis. Aust J Zool 5(1957)223-246

Schenck, B.; Neumann, F.: Some Comments on the Use of Antiandrogens for Male Contraception. Int J Androl Suppl 2(1978)155-161

Setchell, B.P.; Waites, G.M.H.; Till, A.R.: Variation in Flow of Blood within the Epididymis of Sheep and Rat. Nature 203(1964)317

Wong, P.Y.D.; Yeung, C.H.: Inhibition by Amiloride of the Sodium Dependent Fluid Reabsorption in Isolated Rat Caudal Epididymis. Br J Pharmacol 58(1976)529-532

Wong, P.Y.D.; Yeung, C.H.: Fluid Reabsorption in the Isolated Duct of the Rat Cauda Epididymidis. J Reprod Fertil 49(1977a)77-81

Wong, P.Y.D.; Yeung, C.H.: Hormonal Regulation of Fluid Reabsorption in Isolated Rat Cauda Epididymidis. Endocrinology 101(1977b)1391-1397

Wong, P.Y.D.; Yeung, C.H.: Inhibition by Alpha-Chlorohydrin of Fluid Reabsorption in the Rat Cauda Epididymidis. J Reprod Fertil 51(1977c)469-471

Wong, P.Y.D.; Yeung, C.H.: Absorptive and Secretory Functions of the Perfused Rat Cauda Epididymidis. J Physiol (Lond) 275(1978)13-26

Wong, P.Y.D.; Yeung, C.H.; Ngai, H.K.: Effect of Alpha-Chlorohydrin on Transport Processes in Perfused Rat Cauda Epididymidis. Contraception 16(1977)637-642

Wong, Y.C.; Wong, P.Y.D.; Yeung, C.H.: Ultrastructural Correlation of Water Reabsorption in Isolated Rat Cauda Epididymidis. Experientia 34(1978)485-487

Zadunaisky, J.A.; Lande, M.A.; Hafner, J.: Further Studies on Chloride Transport in the Frog Cornea. Am J Physiol 221(1971)1832-1836

PART II
MOTILITY

Three hundred years have passed since Leeuwenhoek described the swimming movements of spermatozoa, and 25 since the discovery of the nearly universal occurrence of a 9+2 pattern of microtubules in the axoneme of cilia and flagella.

In the past decade methods have been developed for the isolation and biochemical characterization of several structural components of the motor apparatus of sperm tails. These studies have led to the identification of dynein, a protein with adenosine triphosphatase (ATPase) activity that forms the arms on the nine peripheral doublets. A sliding-microtubule hypothesis for the generation of waves of bending has been advanced and strongly supported by ingenious experiments. The finding of completely immotile sperm due to congenital absence of arms on the axonemal doublets in infertile men has provided clinical confirmation of the essential role of dynein in motility. Although the tempo of discovery has noticeably quickened in recent years, we are far from understanding the mechanism of sperm locomotion. Even the exact form of the tail movements remains controversial. Still to be elucidated is the function of the central pair of microtubules, the role of the radial spokes, and the mechanism of initiation of bending waves and of their propagation along the tail. The functional significance of the outer dense fibers of the mammalian spermatozoon, and the fibrous sheath of its principal piece are still unknown. The attachment of the outer fibers proximally to the head and distally to the axonemal doublets would seem to impose mechanical restraints to microtubule sliding which have yet to be explored. This section summarizes current concepts and presents new findings that help to fill important gaps in our understanding of the mechanisms of sperm motility.

SYMPOSIUM PAPERS

INTERPRETATIONS OF THE PATTERN OF SPERM TAIL MOVEMENTS

D.M. Woolley

Department of Physiology, The Medical School, University of Bristol, Bristol BS8 1TD UK

In mammals the waveform of the undulating sperm flagellum is the manifestation of the underlying displacements of the axonemal microtubules, compounded with whatever restraints or augmentations are due to the structures surrounding the axoneme. These accessory structures might be expected to complicate the shape generated by the axoneme, although their actual influence is largely unknown. On the other hand, the sperm flagellum of a mammal, because it is thicker than a simple axoneme and therefore brighter in dark-ground illumination, may be technically easier to observe in the deep chambers that are necessary if unrestrained three-dimensional flagellar movement is to occur. It remains an important technical problem to work out the three-dimensional geometry of the active flagellum. If it could be done, progress could be made toward understanding the relative activity of the nine axonemal doublets and the significance of their radial symmetry. Discussion of the sliding-filament model for flagellar motility has been confined to date to the simplified case of planar movement without axonemal torsion, except for a brief account of the principles involved in extending the idea to various three-dimensional waveforms (Schreiner, 1977). In addition to this, a definitive account of the three-dimensional movements would greatly facilitate progress in understanding hydrodynamic aspects of flagellar propulsion, since it is clear from recent discussions (Yundt et al., 1975; Keller and Rubinow, 1976) that the limitations of current theory are due mainly to the simplifications made necessary by our ignorance of the actual waveforms. Blum and Lubliner (1973) and Holwill (1977) have provided general reviews of flagellar biophysics. This chapter assesses the available observational data relating to the pattern of flagellar activity in mammalian spermatozoa and attempts to show how some of the contending interpretations may be resolved. For it is still considered reasonable to postulate that there is one basic pattern underlying flagellar undulations, in spite of the cell's versatility in responding to environmental conditions.

THE GENERAL SHAPE OF THE WAVE

As the bends travel distally along the flagellum there is an increase in their amplitude or lateral deviation from the axis of progression (Gray, 1958; Rikmenspoel, 1965; Denehy, 1975). This was the first indication that the bends must be generated actively in each successive segment of the flagellum (Machin, 1958). An increase in lateral displacement is not seen as bends are propagated in the structurally simpler sperm of invertebrates (Brokaw, 1974; Rikmenspoel, 1978). It seems probable that in mammalian spermatozoa the increasing amplitude is a result of the reduced resistance to bending as the nine dense accessory fibers taper and then terminate in the distal flagellum. This view is consistent with Phillips' (1972) observation that among mammalian species the bend angle of the proximal flagellum seems to be inversely proportional to the total cross-sectional area of the dense fibers. The precise geometry of the flagellar bends has not yet been investigated for mammalian sperm flagella. For invertebrate sperm, it is becoming accepted that the undulation is best described as having alternating arcs and straight lines (Brokaw, 1965). Such an undulation, originating in the axoneme, is presumably also a component in the mammalian waveform. The dense fibers, however, if they act as passive elastic structures would *per se* be expected to conform to a different, meander-type undulation (Holwill, 1977). The true shape therefore, is probably a result of these two tendencies and would be expected to change along the flagellum as the dense fibers become thinner.

In this discussion of bend-shapes, it is implied that the undulations are planar. This is a simplification, as there is now general agreement that the waveform in mammalian spermatozoa is not flat but three-dimensional. Interpretations of the three-dimensional geometry are still varied and conflicting. To some extent different interpretations seem to have emerged from the

---

The author gratefully acknowledges the support of the Agricultural Research Council of Great Britain (Research grant AG 15/111).

© 1979 Urban & Schwarzenberg, Inc. Baltimore-Munich *The Spermatozoon,* edited by D.W. Fawcett and J.M. Bedford

differing techniques employed, and this provides a convenient format for reviewing the available information.

Multiple-Exposure Micrography

Gray (1958) was the first to use a series of electronic flashes to record instants in the movement of bull spermatozoa. He experimented with both still and continuously moving film and made several observations relevant to the question of three-dimensionality in the form of the distal tail-wave. Some spermatozoa, which appeared to be rolling freely about the longitudinal axis, were photographed "edge on" and showed "most, if not all, elements of the tail . . . in a plane coincident with that of the median transverse axis of the head." Gray's micrograph actually shows the tail having a very slight undulation. In many other examples, however, the most distal part of the flagellum was found to be considerably deflected from this plane. Unfortunately, this deflection was not examined in cells seen with the plane-of-flattening-of-the-head parallel to the focal plane, and it remains uncertain whether the loss of clarity in the relevant parts of these micrographs was due, as one might expect, to a departure of the tail from the plane of focus.

In summary, Gray proposed that most of his observations "suggest that the tail is slightly twisted when a wave of curvature passes over its distal region." Further analysis of the distal tail-wave was based on multiple exposures of spermatozoa that were attached to the microscope slide; in fact, the four cells whose movements were plotted were attached by both the head and the midpiece. When so restrained, distal elements of the tail were seen to follow a figure-eight path. There is some difficulty in appreciating this from the published sequences and it seems doubtful, given that the relevant sections of the image must be always out of focus, that the direction taken around the figure-eight path could have been deduced. Gray's figure-eight model has been widely quoted but it should be viewed cautiously since it may represent the result of an interaction between the flagellum and the glass slide.

Cinemicrography

High-speed cinecameras provide a virtually continuous record of the changing configurations of a flagellum. There is an upper limit to the framing rate imposed by the need for sufficient illumination, especially when using dark-ground optics. Otherwise the technical problems are no worse than those that apply to any microscopical technique, the principal difficulty being that the camera records two-dimensional projections of three-dimensional forms. To gain all the geometrical information would require either simultaneous observation in more than one plane or some (as yet undeveloped) technique of stereomicroscopy applicable to objectives of large numerical aperture. Nevertheless, there have been two detailed analyses of the waveform in mammalian spermatozoa using cinefilm, and there is a measure of agreement between the two reports.

In Rikmenspoel's study (1965) bull spermatozoa were photographed in dark-ground at 200 frames per second. Sequences for 10 rotating sperm were analyzed by projecting the images and measuring the successive displacements at six standard locations along the flagellum, from the sperm's average path. These plots were interpreted as reflecting a summation of two sinusoidal waves with amplitudes of approximately 3 to 1. The records for the sixth, most distal location were incomplete on account of its large deviations from the plane of focus but, for the remaining locations, in seven of the ten cells, a given ratio between the frequencies in the two planes would account for all the displacements throughout the flagellum. Rikmenspoel used the term "helical" in a general sense to describe these waveforms. The helix is of course not regular in that its cross-section is approximately elliptical and its area increases distally. The waveform might be described as elliptically conical. It must be mentioned, however, that in an earlier paper (Rikmenspoel et al., 1960) a very clear micrograph of a rotating sperm was reproduced from a cine-sequence and its pattern in-focus and out-of-focus segments suggests a twisted-planar rather than an elliptically conical shape (as explained in Fig. 2).

Denehy et al. (1975) photographed ram spermatozoa at 300 frames per second using positive phase contrast optics. In addition, to get more resolution, they made some still pictures on 35 mm film with an electronic flash. Six rotating spermatozoa were filmed for at least one cycle of rotation; the images were projected and (as in Rikmenspoel's method) lateral displacements from an average path (or progression axis) were plotted. However, where Rikmenspoel followed six locations, Denehy et al. traced only two—the neck of the sperm and the distal end of the midpiece—arguing that more distal locations could not be identified (e.g., at successive 10 μ intervals) owing to the bending of the tail in the plane parallel to the line of sight. The displacement data for these two points were found to fit their model—an elliptically helical waveform. At the neck, the elliptical section was very flat, with a ratio between the two perpendicular components of 0.08; at the end of the midpiece the axes of the ellipse still had the same orientation with respect to the head but the ratio between them had increased to 0.17. That is, the ellipse was becoming *less* eccentric (or more nearly circular) at more distal locations. (Denehy *et al.* do not use the standard mathematical definition of *eccentricity* and their statements which include this word are open to misinterpretation.)

Thus, both Rikmenspoel and Denehy *et al.* conclude that the waveform is elliptically helical but report quite different eccentricities. Their results are not merely quantitatively different, however. In Rikmenspoel's account, the eccentricity is constant for all segments of the flagellum, whereas Denehy *et al.* have it increasing to twice its initial value within the first 14 μ of the tail. As they point out, this is exactly what would be expected if the waveform were of the planar-becoming-helical type.

Rapid Fixation

As an alternative to "arresting" moving cells by photography, one may attempt to bring about their actual arrest, either by chemical or physical treatments. If this could be achieved in a negligibly short time, the arrested flagellar configuration would represent instants in the beat cycle. The principal advantage of such preparations is that a full three-dimensional analysis is technically feasible. Such methods naturally have their limitations: the dynamics of bend propagation, or rotation, for example, cannot be studied directly in fixed cells; there are dangers in disregarding the possibility that different cells in a population may be behaving differently; and the question whether agonal or other artifactual changes are occurring is always arguable. Nevertheless any technique that actually arrests cell movement provides, in principle, material that can be further studied by electron microscopy. In this way it was first possible, by studying cilia rapidly fixed in osmium tetroxide, to establish the relationship between the overall geometry of a cilium and the internal geometry of its axonemal doublet microtubules (Satir, 1967).

In recent years the author has explored the use of a physical method, ultra-rapid freezing, as a means of approaching an instantaneous arrest of mammalian spermatozoa. Calculating from published estimates of cooling rates (*e.g.*, Costello and Corless, 1978) it appears that thick films of cells, cooled from room temperature to the frozen state by quenching them in Freon-22, are immobilized in about 50 ms. Sperm films were frozen in this way and then kept at low temperatures and infiltrated with an ethylene glycol-glutaraldehyde solution. By this "freeze-substitution" procedure a chemical fixation was superimposed on the sperm after their initial physical fixation (Woolley, 1974).

In a study of golden hamster spermatozoa, mobile cells (from the cauda epididymidis) were quench-frozen, substitution fixed, then warmed and allowed to sediment before being examined by light microscopy (Woolley, 1977). Some of the flagella had been fractured by the Freon treatment but, in the majority, it was clear that—at least in its proximal part—the flagellar waveform resembled that seen in life. Then flagella were classified and recorded photographically, often by a series of micrographs made in different focal planes. It was found that the most common waveform contained three bends. About half of these flagella were uniplanar. The remainder were three-dimensional in that the third bend (*i.e.*, the most distal) lay outside the plane containing the proximal bend cycle (Fig. 1). It appeared that, in the unbent region of the flagellum between the second and third bends, a twist in the plane of action had occurred. For 40 spermatozoa, the magnitude of the twist fell within the range 26-71°, with a mean and standard error of 46.6 ± 1.7°. In almost all the sperm, the direction of this twist was clockwise as viewed from the proximal end of the flagellum. There was some indication also in a few sperm which contained five bends, that the plane of action of the third bend cycle was further twisted in the same direction. As will be discussed later, a three-dimensional waveform consisting of twisted planes, with each bend or bend cycle being essentially planar, is geometrically quite different from helical or conical forms.

Other Published Observations

Blokhuis (1961) observed bull spermatozoa by a system of two-color dark-ground illumination, which apparently allowed him to assess displacements of the tail in the plane parallel to the line of sight. However, the color filters presumably reduced the light intensity below that required for photography. The rapidity of the movements was reduced by aging the semen samples. Blokhuis reported that in aged spermatozoa there was a "fixed screw" in the tail, over which the waves of bending travelled. This recalls the sentence quoted from Gray's paper (see above). But in less aged semen Blokhuis saw a different waveform which he described as a flat sinusoidal wave undergoing, as it travelled, a twist in its plane of vibration.

Further (Unpublished) Findings

The author has recently made still micrographs of rotating hamster spermatozoa, using a Leitz Microflash electronic flash lamp (flash duration approximately 1 ms) and Kodak Tri-X 35 mm film. The intention has been to interpret, as far as possible, the projections of the living waveforms in the light of the "twisted-plane" model derived from the analysis of frozen-substituted

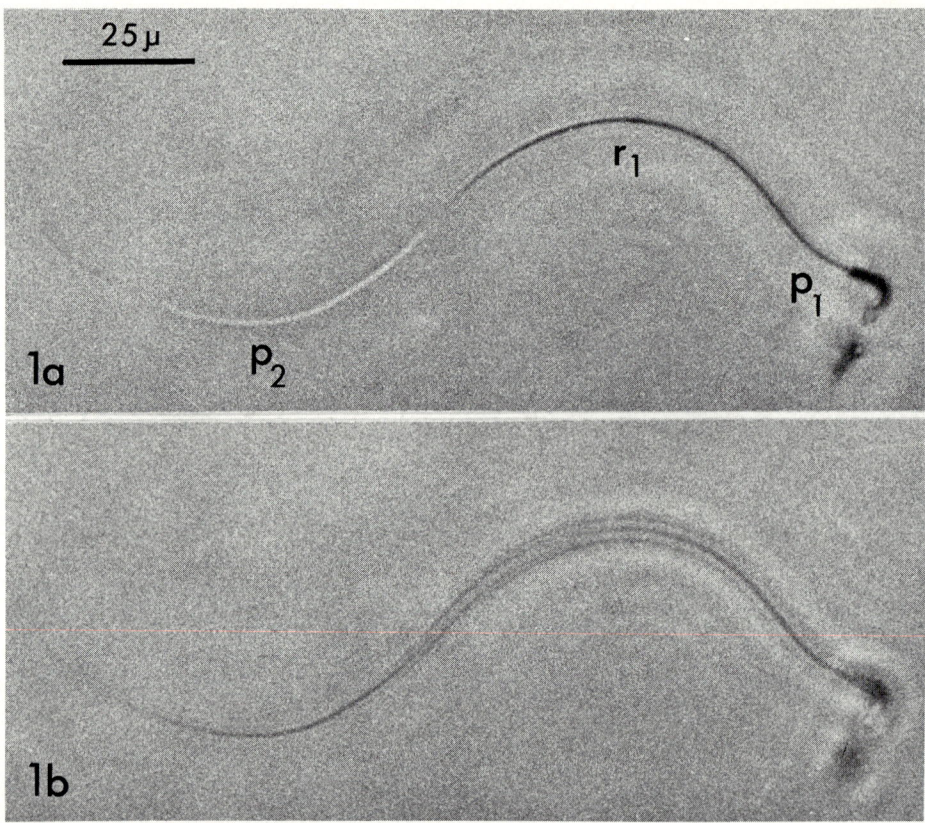

Figure 1. A spermatozoon from a golden hamster prepared by the freeze-substitution technique and allowed to settle. This cell illustrates the most common three-dimensional waveform. The most proximal principal and reverse bends (p_1, r_1) lie in the same plane as the head (a) but the plane containing the second principal bend (p_2) appears to be twisted clockwise as viewed from the sperm head, causing the center of bend p_2 to be displaced vertically (b). In this example the distance between the focal planes of Figures 1a and 1b was 12 μ. Note that the torsion appears to be restricted to the region of the flagellum *between* the bends and that the distal part of bend p_2 returns to the plane of focus again on the axis of progression. X725

cells. Spermatozoa were taken from the cauda epididymidis and allowed to suspend for 5 min in Hanks solution at room temperature as in previous work (Woolley, 1977). The dilute suspension was then placed in a sealed chamber approximately 70 μ deep and examined by dark-ground illumination at a total magnification of 400X. Focusing in the center of the chamber, micrographs were taken of sperm that swam progressively, rotating, across the center of the field. To date, interpretations have been attempted only where a flat surface of the sperm head happened to be perpendicular to the line of sight. Out-of-focus segments of the flagellum can be recognized as such but of course the magnitude of their displacements from the plane of focus cannot be measured and the direction of the displacement (whether upward or downward) is unknown. However, it is possible to determine the general character of the waveform, even though long segments are out of focus (Fig. 2). The difference between, for example, a twisted-plane sequence and an elliptically conical form emerges, in projection, in terms of whether the flagellum comes into focus on the progression axis or at its points of maximal curvature (Fig. 2b, d). Observations made to date (Fig. 3-5) are consistent with a twisted-plane undulation. It is thus unlikely that the twisted-plane waveform is an artifact of the freeze-substitution procedure. However, two discrepancies have appeared between the waveforms in the living and the frozen-substituted cells: most of the living examples showed two-bend, not three-bend, waveforms; and the torsion between bends seemed to occur between each successive bend in living spermatozoa, rather than between bends 2 and 3, as after freeze-substitution. The reason for these differences is not known with certainty but a plausible explanation is that the cells that were about to be quench-frozen became attached by their heads to the silver foil support. This might account for both discrepancies. On the other hand the two-bend, living waveforms may have resulted from the general decrease in beat frequency found to result from prolonged incubation in tissue-culture media (Bavister and Yanagimachi, 1977).

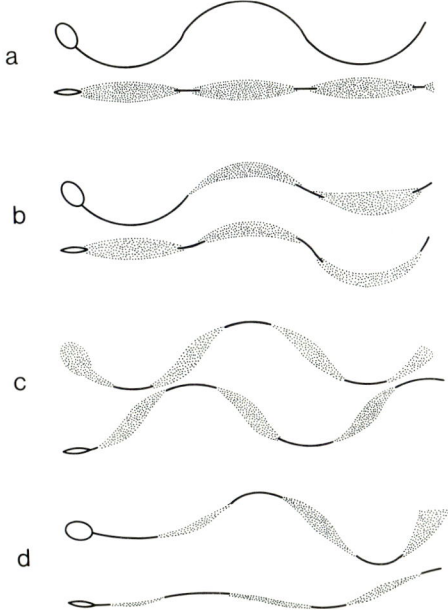

Figure 2. A diagram of some possible waveforms, showing how they may be distinguished even in partially out-of-focus two-dimensional projected images. In each case (a-d) the upper drawing shows the plane-of-flattening of the head perpendicular to the line of sight; the lower drawing shows the same form rotated through 90°. For simplicity, the undulations are drawn as arc-line series, with out-of-focus segments uniformly stippled. Figure 2a: an entirely planar waveform. Figure 2b: a twisted-plane waveform with the torsions restricted to the inter-bend segments. In this scheme, successive torsions are given equal magnitude and continue in the same direction. Notice that in such waveforms, the in-focus segments lie on the progression axis. The upper diagram should be compared with Figures 3-5. Figure 2c: a helical waveform. The flagellum is imagined to lie in the surface of a regular cylinder. Notice that the in-focus segments coincide with the points of maximum amplitude in the projection. Figure 2d: a more realistic waveform of the helical type in which the flagellum lies in the surface of a "squashed" cone (the elliptically-conical type). The pattern of in-focus and out-of-focus segments is similar to that of 2c and unlike that in 2b.

Conclusion

The different interpretations of the geometry of the three-dimensional waveform cannot yet be resolved but it is worth examining the nature and importance of these differences, particularly with respect to the required disposition of the underlying axonemal microtubules. As Gray (1962) explained, when a filament undergoes bending simultaneously in two planes normal to each other, the resultant wave is helical provided the amplitudes in the two waves are equal and the waves are one-fourth cycle out of phase. Elliptically helical waves arise either from having the amplitudes unequal or from having an altered phase difference between the cycles. When the two cycles are in phase or 180° out of phase, the wave is planar. We can therefore think of the planar-becoming-helical shape as resulting from a gradual phase shift between the two cycles; and the elliptically conical shape as resulting from gradual and proportionate increments in the two amplitudes. In any of these related three-dimensional waveforms any given segment of the flagellum would move around the circumference of a circle (or ellipse). However, it is not necessarily the case that the plane of its bending would change continuously with respect to (say) the plane bisecting the axonemal central pair. This would occur only in the absence of torsion of the axoneme. If the axoneme were appropriately twisted, it would be possible to maintain the relationship between the plane of bending and a given plane within the axoneme. These two types of helix—which are identical in *external* form—are clearly illustrated in an earlier paper by Gray (1953; see Fig. 10).

The twisted-plane types of waveform are different in character from the shapes discussed above in that here the flagellum cannot be imagined as lying always in contact with the surface of a cylinder or cone. Where a continuously twisted plane is envisaged (Gray, 1958; Blokhuis, 1961) the bending of a given segment is always in the same plane while successive elements are twisted with respect to this plane so that the whole flagellum can be thought of as lying in a screw surface. The waveform proposed by Woolley (1977) is similar except that the torsion is restricted to the region between bends, and any individual plane of bending along the flagellum is thought to depend on the number of following bends rather than on the particular flagellar segment (as might be defined by its distance from the neck). There is some similarity between this model and the current idea that sections of the axoneme are either actively sliding and bent, or straight and not rigidly cross-linked (Warner and Satir, 1974; Goldstein, 1977). It is also noteworthy that rigor waveforms in sea urchin spermatozoa do not resist torsion and that large torsions can occur within portions of the axoneme only 2-3 μ long (Gibbons and Gibbons, 1974). As with helical waves, the twisted-plane waveforms, in principle, could exist either with or without torsion of the axoneme itself. These options are best presented diagrammatically (Fig. 6).

If the discontinuously twisted waveform has general validity, it should be found in "primitive" spermatozoa and might well be more distinctly expressed there, in the absence of extra-axonemal structures. Almost all recent observations of sea urchin spermatozoa have been made on those swimming near an interface and having planar tail-waves. Yet, when allowed to swim freely they undoubtedly rotate (Gray, 1955; Brokaw,

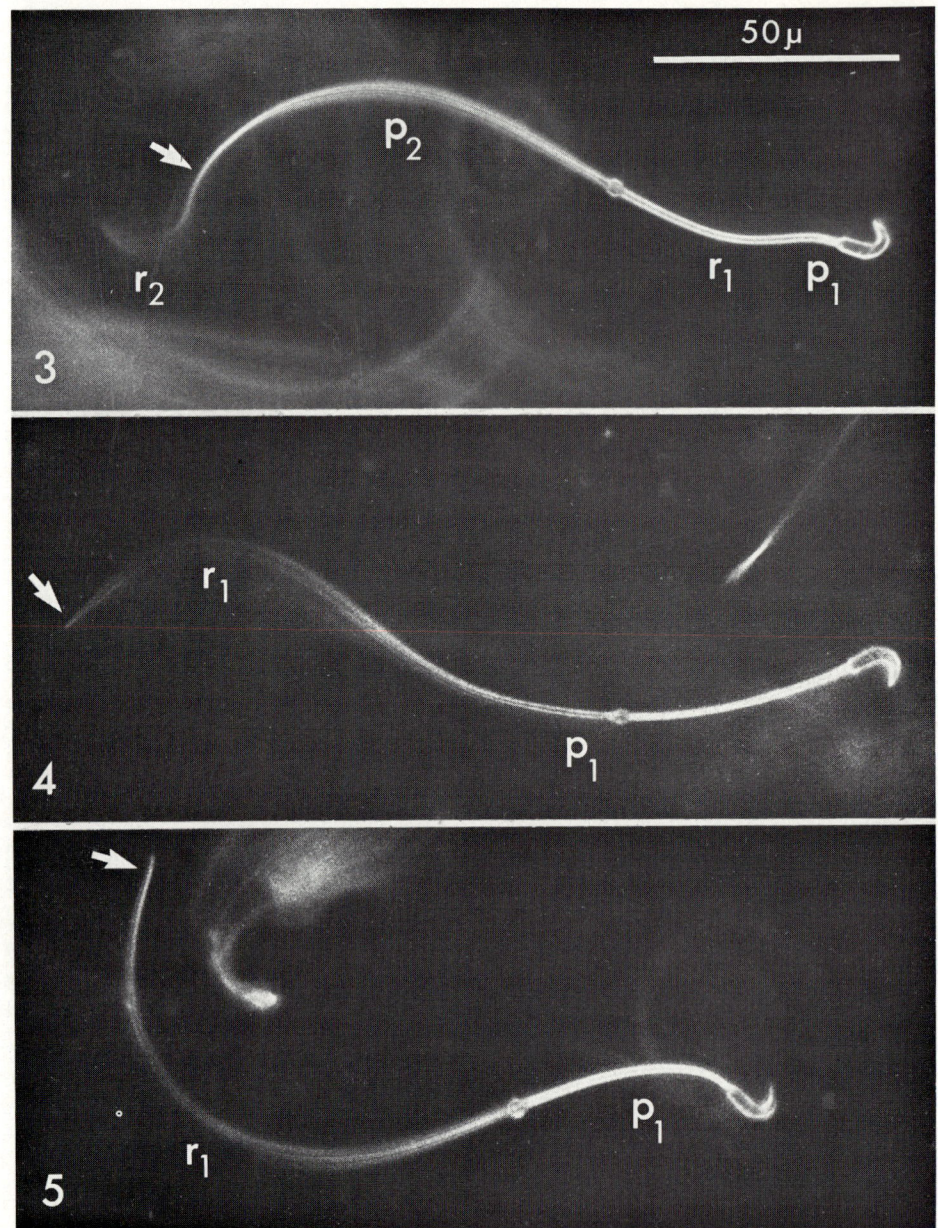

Figure 3-5. Living spermatozoa from a golden hamster, photographed by electronic flash. These cells were swimming progressively and rotating. Figure 3: This flagellum contains four bends. Bends r_1 and the incompletely developed p_1 lie in the same plane as the head; bend p_2 is twisted out of this plane, returning to it on or near the progression axis (arrow); bend r_2 is inclined at a larger angle to the plane of the micrograph. Figures 4 and 5: Examples of the more common two-bend waveforms. In each case bend r_1 leaves the plane occupied by p_1 and the sperm head, returning to this plane on or near the progression axis (arrows). X664

1974), which strongly suggests that the flagellar undulations are three-dimensional. One study does suggest that torsions occur between successive bends in *Colobocentrotus* but the true overall geometry of these rigor-waves, which appeared, surprisingly, to be planar, could not be established reliably (Gibbons, 1975).

ASYMMETRY

If we assume the most proximal bend to be planar, it is possible to define its plane of action in relation to the axonemal microtubules. The most direct evidence, from rapidly frozen rat spermatozoa, indicated that the plane of action is perpendicular to the plane that contains the

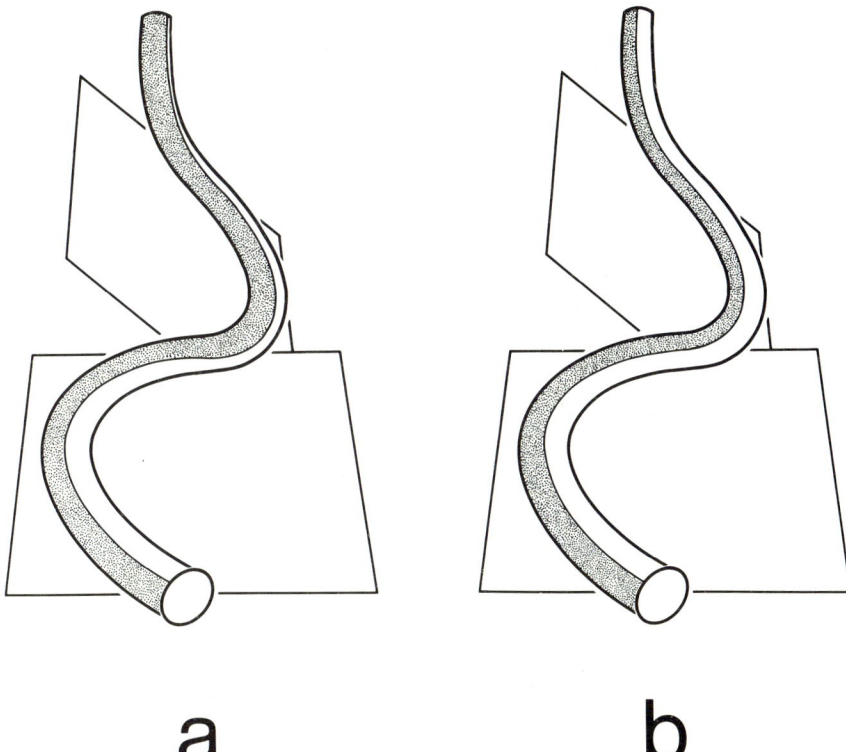

Figure 6. This illustration demonstrates how a twisted-plane waveform may or may not involve torsion of the flagellum itself. In each case two adjoining planar bends and the first portion of a third planar bend are drawn in perspective. The line drawn on the flagellum indicates a plane within the flagellum that is fixed with respect to the axonemal doublets: it might represent one of the longitudinal columns of the fibrous sheath. In Figure 6a, the plane of bending keeps its relationship to this line and the flagellum itself becomes twisted. In Figure 6b, the plane of bending is imagined to change with respect to this line, and the flagellum itself is not twisted. In each case the flagellum makes the same shape in space but the conformation of the axoneme, as emphasized by the shading, is different.

two central microtubules (Woolley, 1974). This confirmed Gibbons' conclusion, based on serial sections of conventionally fixed bull spermatozoa (Gibbons, 1963). Thus in one-half of the bending cycle, doublets No. 5 and 6 lie in the convex edge of the bend and in the other half doublet 1 does so. In all species in which the dimensions of these two bends have been compared, they have been found to be dissimilar. Asymmetry is seen in invertebrate sperm flagella without accessory fibers (Gray, 1955; Brokaw, 1974) and also in invertebrate sperm known to have accessory fibers of equal size, such as the cephalopod *Loligo* (Bishop, 1958). From this it is unlikely that the asymmetry in mammalian sperm results solely from size differences among the nine accessory (dense) fibers.

Asymmetry was first reported in bull spermatozoa by Rikmenspoel *et al.* (1960) who noted that in the absence of rotation it caused them to swim in circular paths, a behavior pattern that was later seen by Blokhuis (1961), and has since been seen in the rabbit (Branham, 1969; Phillips, 1972), in the sheep (Denehy, 1975), and in man (Phillips, 1972). But the phenomenon is best studied in those rodent species where the relationship of the bends to the hook-shaped sperm head permits the two halves of the flagellum to be distinguished. In this way the asymmetries in mouse, rat, and Chinese hamster sperm tails were all found to be the same with respect to the morphology of the sperm heads (Phillips, 1972). Phillips named the alternating bends the "effective" and "recovery" strokes, the latter having the smaller bend angle. In fact there is some doubt which of these bends exerts the greater thrust. The author has observed golden hamster and mouse spermatozoa attached to the slide by one of the flat sides of the head and turning around the point of attachment. The formation of the recovery stroke causes a greater angular movement than does the formation of the effective stroke with the result that the net movement is in a circle, always in the same direction with respect to the hook of the sperm head (Fig. 7). This indicates that a greater force is produced by the bend with the smaller angle. In an alternative terminology, the bend that takes longer to form and

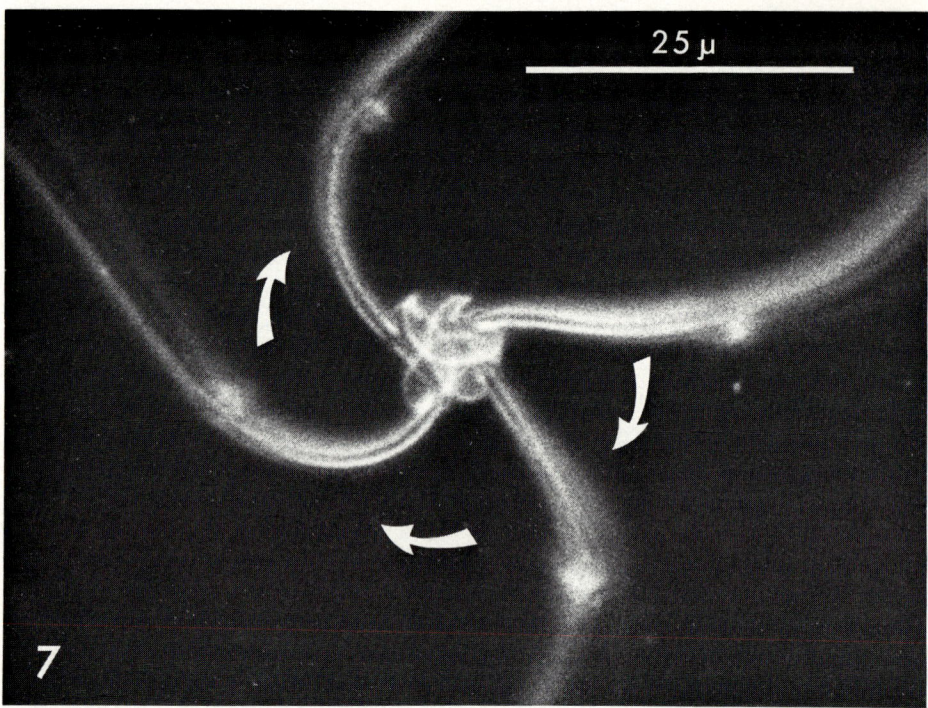

Figure 7. A mouse spermatozoon attached by its head to the coverslip and circling around its point of attachment. Four electronic flash exposures were made in the sequence indicated at intervals of 2 s (Strobex 136 Power Unit with Lamp No. 72 manufactured by Chadwick Helmuth Ltd., Monrovia, California). The direction of circling is always the same with respect to the head asymmetry, from which, it is argued, the reverse bend exerts the greater thrust (see text). X1770

develops the greater angle is called the "principal bend" as opposed to the "reverse bend"; for rat and mouse spermatozoa the principal bend has doublet 1 in its convex edge while the convex edge of the reverse bend contains doublets 5 and 6 (Woolley, 1977). In cilia, the leading edge of the effective stroke contains doublets 5 and 6 (Gibbons, 1961); therefore the reverse bend and the effective stroke of the cilium are analogous, at least structurally. In echinoderm spermatozoa the terms "principal" and "reverse" had already been applied, the former referring similarly to the bend that develops the greater angle (Gibbons and Gibbons, 1974). It is not known, however, whether the internal structure of these bends corresponds with that established for rodent spermatozoa.

ROTATION

The mammalian spermatozoon, when not swimming near an interface, gives the appearance of rolling about its longitudinal axis. The term "rotation" will be used to describe actual rolling about the longitudinal axis and should not, for the sake of clarity, be used to describe the various other angular displacements of the cell or its parts. Until recently it was possible to doubt that rotation occurs and to suggest instead that the sperm oscillate through 180° (*e.g.,* Zorgniotti *et al.,* 1958). This possibility may now be rejected in view of the following work on high-speed cine records: 1) tracing the movement of the head hook in and out of focus (mouse; Phillips, 1972); 2) tracing the movement of asymmetric cytoplasmic droplets (human; Phillips, 1972), or asymmetric head features (bull; Drake, 1974); 3) observing the color sequences under two-color darkground illumination (bull; Blokhuis, 1961 and Drake, 1974); and 4) observing accurately in dark-ground illumination, the changing shape of the light flash that is emitted from the sperm nucleus when it turns "edge-on" to the line of sight (bull; Drake, 1974).

The rotation is caused by the three-dimensional movement of the flagellum. In principle it is possible to imagine a planar waveform rotating on account of the shape of the sperm head or because of flexures between head and neck, but the matter has been settled decisively by the observation made in several species that motile flagella which have lost their heads continue to rotate as they swim (Harvey, 1953; Gray, 1958; Phillips and Olson, 1975). The unlikely possibility of rotational movement *between* the head and the tail, has been ruled out, at least in rodents (Phillips, 1972; Woolley, 1974).

Since the detailed three-dimensional geometry of the tail-wave is still disputed, it cannot yet be decided how the flagellum produces a turning couple. However, a helical wave will lead to rotation (Taylor, 1952) as will elliptically-helical, conical, or twisted-plane waveforms (Gray, 1962), and in each case the rotation of the spermatozoon will be opposite in sense to the direction of angular movement of segments of the flagellum. Therefore, a knowledge of the direction of rotation does reveal the overall sense of the three-dimensional component of the wave, whatever its precise geometry. This information, which for sperm moving at normal speed can be gained only from high-speed cinematography, has proved very elusive. The rotation is best specified as following either a left-handed or right-handed screw. (A left-handed screw motion means that a point on the edge of the cell rotates clockwise when viewed from a position in advance of the anterior extremity.) The only pictorial evidence in the literature is a sequence of frames from a film of bull spermatozoa (Drake, 1974), from which it was convincingly claimed that all six cells photographed moved as right-handed screws. However, using a different optical principle, Drake claimed to see some cells rolling in the opposite direction. But according to Blokhuis (1961) all bull spermatozoa move as left-handed screws. From the sense of the twisted-plane waveform suggested for the golden hamster, it was predicted that virtually all the sperm should rotate as right-handed screws (Woolley, 1977). Information for invertebrates sheds no light on the problem: Bishop (1958) reported predominantly right-handed motion in *Loligo*, whereas for the sea urchin *Psammechinus*, Gray (1955) claimed predominantly left-handed rotation. There is no reason, of course, to suppose *a priori* that rotation sense is the same for all species, for all sperm within a population, or for a spermatozoon under different physiological conditions.

VARIATIONS IN THE WAVEFORM

There is much evidence that physiological changes occur in the pattern of flagellar activity during the life history of the mammalian spermatozoon. The flagellum becomes capable of movement long before its development is complete. Undulatory motion is first seen in the simple axonemes of very early spermatids, before the various accessory structures develop, and it persists and may be vigorous, in all later stages of spermiogenesis (Austin and Sapsford, 1951; Clermont, 1964). It is not known, however, whether these movements occur *in vivo*. After release into the seminiferous tubule, most of the young spermatozoa are capable of weak vibratory movements (Setchell *et al.*, 1969). In the environment of the epididymal duct, sperm motility is suppressed but the flagellum continues to mature and its potential for motility changes. When sperm are released from the head of the epididymis and diluted, they generally swim with a fixed curvature of the proximal flagellum. Because this has been studied in rat spermatozoa it can be seen in the published micrographs that this fixed bend is usually in the "reverse" direction (see Fray *et al.*, 1972; Burgos and Tovar, 1974) but under some circumstances there is a fixed "principal" bend (the retroflexion seen by Blandau and Rumery, 1964). Bends originate distal to this region, propagate distally, and propel the cell around a circular path. Fray *et al.* suggested that the rigid curvature of the proximal flagellum was responsible for the circular swimming, which is a plausible idea, since the oppositely curved flagella seen by Blandau and Rumery circled in the other direction. The distal undulations, though described as planar, do have some displacement in the third dimension, as is clear from the drawings of Fray *et al.* and the cinemicrographs published by Burgos and Tovar. This is occasionally sufficient to produce rotation of these immature spermatozoa. A fixed proximal bend has also been seen in immature sperm of the rabbit (Gaddum, 1968) and may well be a general feature in mammals.

By the time the spermatozoa reach the tail of the epididymis most of them are capable, upon dilution, of the rotatory progressive motility discussed in the earlier sections of this chapter. Even though such sperm have usually been studied after dilution and in artificial media, their rotating movement is generally considered to be normal and mature in that it resembles the activity seen in the ejaculate (in those species in which the ejaculate is normally dilute). However, it is sometimes argued that in order to see a truly mature motility pattern, sperm should be examined in fluids from the female tract. In this regard, there is information on the motility of sperm in cervical mucus and descriptions of changed swimming behavior coincident with the onset of the acrosome reaction.

When swimming through cervical mucus (taken at the appropriate stage of the cycle) bovine spermatozoa swim relatively slowly, in straight parallel paths, making intermittent progress (Tampion and Gibbons, 1962a, b). Under these conditions the spermatozoa do not rotate as they swim: the flagellar bends, which develop large angles distally, appear to be exactly planar. (This behavior was demonstrated during the Woods Hole meeting in two cine films presented by Drs. P. Gaddum-Rosse, and D.F. Katz). But in the preceding section it has been argued that straight-line swimming requires a three-dimensional waveform and rotation. The relatively slow, directional movement seen in cervical mucus is in fact determined by the visco-elastic nature of the mucus and the micellar arrangement of its macromolecules. The failure of the sperm to rotate may well be due to a lateral compression of the intermicellar channels under the weight of the mucus. This explanation is suggested because the plane of bending seems to be the same for all sperm in a field and is always perpendicular to the line of vision.

The change in motility pattern which coincides with the acrosome reaction has been termed "activation." It was observed first in golden hamster, then in guinea pig spermatozoa, after they had been capacitated *in vitro* (Yanagimachi, 1970, 1972). Recently a very similar result was reported in mouse spermatozoa (Fraser, 1977). The change in the movement pattern has recently been confirmed in a quantitative study (Katz et al., 1978): it involves a reduction in the beat frequency and a large increase in amplitude of the undulations. The spermatozoa no longer swim progressively but move erratically and adopt contorted shapes. Visually this seems a more vigorous motility but the calculated power output is apparently unchanged (Katz et al., 1978). The causal relationships, if any, between the acrosome reaction and activation have not yet been worked out. In the guinea pig the two phenomena occur synchronously whereas in the mouse 64% of the activated sperm still possess their acrosomes. Yet these species are similar in that activation has been shown to be Ca^{2+} dependent (Yanagimachi and Usui, 1974; Fraser, 1977). Activated motility is interesting in that it presumably entails a sudden increase in the amount of inter-doublet sliding and perhaps a change in the plasticity of the dense fibers. Whether activation occurs *in vivo* is uncertain, though Phillips (1972) did observe an increase in bend amplitude and a serpentine "crawling" motility pattern in mouse spermatozoa recovered from the oviduct and uterus.

CONCLUSION

The idea that the mammalian sperm tail has a twisted-planar waveform has emerged from studies of rapidly frozen hamster spermatozoa. It was proposed that the plane of action twists in the straight regions between actively bending planar segments; that the torsions are progressive; and that they are clockwise in direction as viewed from the sperm head. Current work on living hamster sperm supports these proposals (except the last—for technical reasons). In light of this it is important now to re-examine the movement pattern in other species, such as the bull and ram, where the geometry has been described as elliptically conical. It would be interesting also to see whether the "immature" and "activated" motility patterns, which have been reported in rodents, are varieties of this twisted-planar model. In seeking the mechanism of the twisting, an important first step must be to overcome the technical problems and establish whether the axoneme itself becomes twisted in the inter-bend regions. Nontwisting of the axoneme would imply sequential dominance of the axoneme doublets in determining (topographically) the plane of bending. Whatever the mechanism, torsion of the *waveform* is not invariable and occurs only in the absence of surface forces. One effect of the twisted waveform, presumably, is the rotation of the cell: it should be possible therefore to make deductions concerning the magnitude and direction of the torsion from the frequency and direction of the rotation. Unfortunately, though it might seem a simple matter, no one has yet established unequivocally the direction of rotation in populations of mammalian spermatozoa.

REFERENCES

Austin, C.R.; Sapsford, C.S.: The Development of the Rat Spermatid. J R Microsc Soc 71(1951)397-406

Bavister, B.D.; Yanagimachi, R.: The Effects of Sperm Extracts and Energy Sources on the Motility and Acrosome Reaction of Hamster Spermatozoa in Vitro. Biol Reprod 16(1977)228-237

Bishop, D.W.: Motility of the Sperm Flagellum. Nature 182(1958)1638-1640

Blandau, R.J.; Rumery, R.E.: The Relationship of Swimming Movements of Epididymal Spermatozoa to their Fertilizing Capacity. Fertil Steril 15(1964)571-579

Blokhuis, E.W.M.: Optical Investigations on the Movement of Bull Spermatozoa. In: Proceedings of the Fourth International Congress on Animal Reproduction, Vol. 2, pp. 243-248. The Congress, The Hague, 1961

Blum, J.J.; Lubliner, J.: Biophysics of Flagellar Motility. Ann Rev Biophys Bioeng 4(1973)181-219

Branham, J.M.: Movements of Free-swimming Rabbit Spermatozoa. J Reprod Fertil 18(1969)97-105

Brokaw, C.J.: Non-sinusoidal Bending Waves of Sperm Flagella. J Exp Biol 43(1965)155-169

Brokaw, C.J.: Movement of the Flagellum in some Marine Invertebrate Spermatozoa. In: Cilia and Flagella, pp. 93-109, ed. by M.A. Sleigh. Academic Press, London-New York, 1974

Burgos, M.H.; Tovar, E.S.: Sperm Motility in the Rat Epididymis. Fertil Steril 25(1974)985-991

Clermont, Y.: Motility of the Flagellum and Cytoplasmic Membrane in the Rat Spermatids. Anat Rec 148(1964)271A

Costello, M.J.; Corless, J.M.: The Direct Measurement of Temperature Changes during Rapid Quenching in Liquid Coolants. J Microsc 112(1978)17-37

Denehy, M.A.: The Propulsion of Nonrotating Ram and Oyster Spermatozoa. Biol Reprod 13(1975)17-29

Denehy, M.A.; Herbison-Evans, D.; Denehy, B.V.: Rotational and Oscillatory Components of the Tailwave in Ram Spermatozoa. Biol Reprod 13(1975)289-297

Drake, A.D.: Observations on Bull Sperm Rotation. Biol Reprod 10(1974)78-84

Fraser, L.: Motility Patterns in Mouse Spermatozoa before and after Capacitation. J Exp Zool 202(1977)439-444

Fray, C.S.; Hoffer, A.P.; Fawcett, D.W.: A Re-examination of Motility Patterns of Rat Epididymal Spermatozoa. Anat Rec 173(1972)301-308

Gaddum, P.: Sperm Maturation in the Male Reproductive Tract: Development of Motility. Anat Rec 161(1968)471-482

Gibbons, B.H.; Gibbons, I.R.: Properties of Flagellar "Rigor Waves" Formed by Abrupt Removal of Adenosine Triphosphate from Actively Swimming Sea Urchin Sperm. J Cell Biol 63(1974)970-985

Gibbons, I.R.: The Relationship between the Fine Structure and Direction of Beat in Gill Cilia of a Lamellibranch Mollusc. J Biophys Biochem Cytol 11(1961)179-205

Gibbons, I.R.: A Method for Obtaining Serial Sections of Known Orientation from Single Spermatozoa. J Cell Biol 16(1963)626-629

Gibbons, I.R.: The Molecular Basis of Flagellar Motility in Sea Urchin Spermatozoa. Soc Gen Physiol Ser 30(1975)207-232

Goldstein, S.F.: Asymmetric Waveforms in Echinoderm Sperm Flagella. J Exp Biol 71(1977)157-170

Gray, J.: Undulatory Propulsion. QJ Microsc Sci 94(1953)551-578

Gray, J.: The Movement of Sea Urchin Spermatozoa. J Exp Biol 32(1955)775-801

Gray, J.: The Movement of the Spermatozoa of the Bull. J Exp Biol 35(1958)96-108

Gray, J.: Flagellar Propulsion. In: Spermatozoan Motility, pp. 1-12, ed. by D.W. Bishop. American Association for the Advancement of Science, Washington, 1962

Harvey, C.: See the published discussion in: Mammalian Germ Cells, p. 132, ed. by G.E.W. Wolstenholme. Ciba Foundation Symposium, publication No. 53. Churchill, London, 1953

Holwill, M.E.: Some Biophysical Aspects of Ciliary and Flagellar Motility. Adv Microb Physiol 16(1977)1-48

Katz, D.F.; Yanagimachi, R.; Dresdner, R.D.: Movement Characteristics and Power Output of Guinea Pig and Hamster Spermatozoa in Relation to Activation. J Reprod Fertil 52(1978)167-172

Keller, J.B.: Rubinow, S.I.: Swimming of Flagellated Microorganisms. Biophys J 16(1976)151-170

Machin, K.E.: Wave Propagation Along Flagella. J Exp Biol 35(1958)796-806

Phillips, D.M.: Comparative Analysis of Mammalian Sperm Motility. J Cell Biol 53(1972)561-573

Phillips, D.M.; Olson, G.: Mammalian Sperm Motility—Structure in Relation to Function. In: Functional Anatomy of the Spermatozoon, pp. 117-126, ed. by B.A. Afzelius. Pergammon Press, Oxford, 1975

Rikmenspoel, R.: The Tail Movement of Bull Spermatozoa. Observations and Model Calculations. Biophys J 5(1965)365-392

Rikmenspoel, R.: Movement of Sea Urchin Sperm Flagella. J Cell Biol 76(1978)310-322

Rikmenspoel, R.; Van Herpen, G.; Eijkhout, P.: Cinematographic Observations of the Movement of Bull Sperm Cells. Phys Med Biol 5(1960)167-181

Satir, P.: Morphological Aspects of Ciliary Motility. J Gen Physiol 50(1967)241-258

Setchell, B.P.; Scott, T.W.; Voglmayr, J.K.; Waites, G.M.H.: Characteristics of Testicular Spermatozoa and the Fluid which Transports them into the Epididymis. Biol Reprod 1(1969)40-66S

Schreiner, K.E.: Displacement and Sliding of Twisted Filaments in Cilia and Flagella. J Biomech 10(1977)1-4

Tampion, D.; Gibbons, R.A.: Orientation of Spermatozoa in Mucus of the Cervix Uteri. Nature 194(1962a)381

Tampion, D.; Gibbons, R.A.: The Effects of Mucus on the Swimming Rate of Sperms. Nature 196(1962b)290

Taylor, G.: The Action of Waving Cylindrical Tails in Propelling Microscopic Organisms. Proc R Soc Lond Ser A 211(1952)225-239

Warner, F.D.; Satir, P.: The Structural Basis of Ciliary Bend Formation. Radial Spoke Positional Changes Accompanying Microtubule Sliding. J Cell Biol 63(1974)35-63

Woolley, D.M.: Freeze-Substitution: A Method for the Rapid Arrest and Chemical Fixation of Spermatozoa. J Microsc 101(1974)245-260

Woolley, D.M.: Evidence for "Twisted Plane" Undulations in Golden Hamster Sperm Tails. J Cell Biol 75(1977)851-865

Yanagimachi, R.: Movement of Golden Hamster Spermatozoa before and after Capacitation. J Reprod Fertil 23(1970)193-196

Yanagimachi, R.: Fertilization of Guinea Pig Eggs in Vitro. Anat Rec 174(1972)9-20

Yanagimachi, R.; Usui, N.: Calcium Dependence of the Acrosome Reaction and Activation of Guinea Pig Spermatozoa. Exp Cell Res 89(1974)161-174

Yundt, A.P.; Shack, W.J.; Lardner, T.J.: Applicability of Hydrodynamic Analyses of Spermatozoan Motion. J Exp Biol 62(1975)27-41

Zorgniotti, A.W.; Hotchkiss, R.S.; Wall, L.C.: High-speed Cinephotomicrography of Human Spermatozoa. Med Radiogr Photogr 34(1958)44-49

BASIS OF FLAGELLAR MOTILITY IN SPERMATOZOA: CURRENT STATUS

P. Satir

Department of Anatomy, Albert Einstein College of Medicine Bronx, New York 10461 USA

In the middle of the 1950s, it became clear that at ultrastructural resolution in an extremely wide variety of species, the spermatozoan tail consisted of an axoneme composed of a 9+2 pattern of microtubules, surrounded by a portion of the cell membrane. Moreover, a similar ultrastructure also characterized motile somatic cell cilia and flagella. Within a short time, this realization led to the hypothesis that the molecular basis of movement was similar in all these organelles, which still applies today in attempts to discern the mechanism of movement. In regard to such attempts, two reports proved rather prophetic. The first is from Afzelius (1959) who realized that the microtubules

> must not necessarily be contractile in the ordinary sense of the word; the work done by them could also be the result of sliding, [each microtubule] retaining its original length and thickness.

Afzelius also suggested that the arms on each doublet microtubule, which he described for the first time, "would be active" in the mechanism of sliding. In essence, this is the understanding we now have of the mechanism which powers the motility of 9+2 sperm tails, cilia, and flagella. From the classic studies of Gibbons (1963) and his colleagues the arms are, of course, now identified with the protein dynein 1.

The second report is found in the first volume of the series of symposia "Spermatozoan Motility" of which this conference volume is the successor. It is a comment by Rothschild (1962) on technique:

> One way to gain further insight into the mode of action of the fibrils and, therefore of their *raison d'etre*, might be by trying to observe them during activity. Given that in the nineteenth and early twentieth century zoologists were apparently able to see sperm tail fibrils with the light microscope, should we not have another shot at doing the same ourselves, using dark-ground illumination?

The sliding microtubule model of the motion of cilia and flagella relies absolutely on the first of these sentences; its most exciting experimental verification relies on the second.

The author thanks Winfield Sale, Jacobo Wais, and Marika Walter for their important contributions to the data. Paulette Setzer and later, Stephen Lebduska provided photographic assistance. This work was supported by a grant from the USPHS (HL 22560).

© 1979 Urban & Schwarzenberg, Inc. Baltimore-Munich *The Spermatozoon*, edited by D.W. Fawcett and J.M. Bedford.

SLIDING AXONEMAL MICROTUBULES AS THE BASIS OF CILIARY AND FLAGELLAR MOVEMENT

In the decade 1964-1973, the basic outlines of the sliding-microtubule mechanism of ciliary and flagellar motility took form. The status of the subject was summarized at the end of that decade (Satir, 1974), a time when the model was gaining wider acceptance. The model essentially rests on two lines of experimental evidence:

1. Geometrical considerations—arising from the fact that the microtubules do not change length during sliding (Satir, 1965, 1968).
2. Work on isolated axonemes essentially begun by Hoffmann-Berling (1955) and including the direct dark-field demonstration of sliding in trypsin-treated axonemes by Summers and Gibbons (1971, 1973).

Both lines of evidence have received considerable corroboration in the intervening years. For example, Warner and Satir (1974) have been able to extend the geometric tests by making use of an intrinsic marker of distance along subfiber A of each doublet microtubule, the radial spoke periodicity. The radial spokes, which originate at subfiber A and extend toward the central complex of the axoneme occur in groups of three with uneven spacing, so that the greater spacing between successive spokes of the same group is toward the axonemal base. Warner and Satir (1974) showed that this intricate periodicity is maintained for all doublets studied along both straight and bent regions of a cilium, and conclude that this effectively makes even minimal contraction of the microtubules highly unlikely. Further, the spokes allow direct measurement of sliding displacements. The general equation of sliding, derived from geometrical studies (Satir, 1968, 1974) is:

$$\Delta l = d_n \Sigma \alpha$$

where sliding displacement (Δl) of doublet No. n is related to bend angle ($\Sigma \alpha$) by a constant indicating effective axonemal diameter (d). Such Δl displacements were originally seen at the tips of certain cilia, but Warner and Satir were able to show that the Δl displacements of the axonemal doublets predicted by the above equation occur locally in an axonemal bend as expected, and that, also as predicted, Δl is constant when the axoneme is unbent.

Sale and Satir (1976) have extended these studies to *Tetrahymena* ciliary axonemes and, by critical point methods, have obtained views of the intact spoke lattice in three-dimensions. After detergent treatment, some axonemes in these preparations may unroll and splay apart (Fig. 1). In such images, the central pair falls to the side as a unit, while the nine doublets follow one another in sequence and can be numbered. By convention, we now number the doublets: n, $n+1$, $n+2$, etc., where n is the doublet whose dynein arms extend toward subfiber B of doublet $n+1$. Doublet 5 can be identified since subfiber A of that doublet is morphogenetically the shortest of the nine. Spoke organization and tip patterns are preserved in the opened axonemes. Direct graphic demonstrations of sliding at the ciliary tip are seen by comparing one axoneme to another, and the measured tip displacements fit well with prior geometrical predictions for all nine doublets.

Geometrical predictions of the sliding hypothesis have also been fulfilled in certain recent experiments on sperm behavior. Shingyoji et al., (1977) pipetted adenosine triphosphate (ATP) onto local regions of triton-treated sea urchin sperm whose heads had been attached to a microneedle. ATP induces local equal and opposite bends without change in head or tail position, exactly conforming to the necessary constraints imposed by the geometry of sliding. Similar results have been obtained by Goldstein (1976) who has carefully analyzed angular changes accompanying bend initiation in spermatozoa.

The second evidential line involves chemical dissections of sperm tails and cilia that rely upon dissolution by detergents of the ciliary membrane. Detergent treatment apparently causes little change in the arrangements of the structural components of the axoneme proper, while the axonemal environment becomes accessible to external solutions. As the membrane dissolves, beat ceases. The critical components that are necessary to restore normal beat to the membraneless axonemes are mM concentrations of ATP and Mg^{2+}. Beat frequency can be varied by changes in ATP concentration.

Summers and Gibbons (1971) demonstrated that if isolated sea urchin sperm tail axonemes were treated briefly with trypsin before the addition of ATP, the axonemes would, instead of beating, grow longer and thinner in a manner consistent with sliding. The axonemes could elongate many times their original length, which implies that sliding occurs between nearest neighbor microtubules. In these experiments, sliding and bending, which normally occur together in the beating cilium, are uncoupled. Structural analysis indicates that trypsin, as applied to yield sliding, disrupts the radial spokes and interdoublet links (nexin?), while leaving the dynein arms and doublet microtubules functionally intact (Summers and Gibbons, 1973). This suggests that the arm-microtubule interactions are directly responsible for sliding.

These considerations have made possible direct demonstrations of microtubule sliding in a variety of species. To date, in dark-field microscopy, as well as for invertebrate sperm, sliding has been shown for a) mammalian sperm (human, Summers, 1974 and Lindemann and Gibbons, 1975; rat, Olsen and Linck, 1977); b) algal flagella (*Chlamydomonas*, Allen and Borisy, 1974 and Witman et al., 1976); c) protozoan (*Tetrahymena*, Sale and Satir, 1977); and d) metazoan somatic cilia (Walter and Satir, 1977). As indicated below, the studies with *Tetrahymena* have been carried further to show unequivocally that the movement of the doublet microtubules is responsible for the elongation of the axoneme seen with the light microscope. Significantly, individual axonemal doublets, once extruded, usually remain associated with the body of the axoneme, and, even when they do not, are not observed to move actively by themselves. Evidently, the interaction of two doublets—one (n) which contributes the active dynein arms and one ($n+1$) to which the arms intermittently attach—is always necessary for the sliding interaction and the axonemal elongation.

THE ELECTRON MICROSCOPY OF SLIDING

The thrust of recent probes is no longer simply confirmation and clarification of the broad outlines of the sliding hypothesis, but rather a more detailed examination of 1) the chemistry and morphology of events leading to microtubule displacement and 2) the regulation of sliding. Sale and Satir (1977) have contributed to the first of these studies by extending the Summers and Gibbons (1971) approach to electron microscope resolution.

Tetrahymena axonemes have been isolated, trypsin-treated, and "glued" to polylysine-coated Formvar-carbon stabilized electron microscope grids. In axonemes that do not unroll, some doublets are attached to the polylysine and subsequently do not move, while others lie above them and are held in position only by their links to other axonemal structures, most of which, except for the dynein arms, are presumably digested by trypsin. When ATP is added, these doublets are free to slide and they then may be captured by the polylysine substratum so that after fixation and prepa-

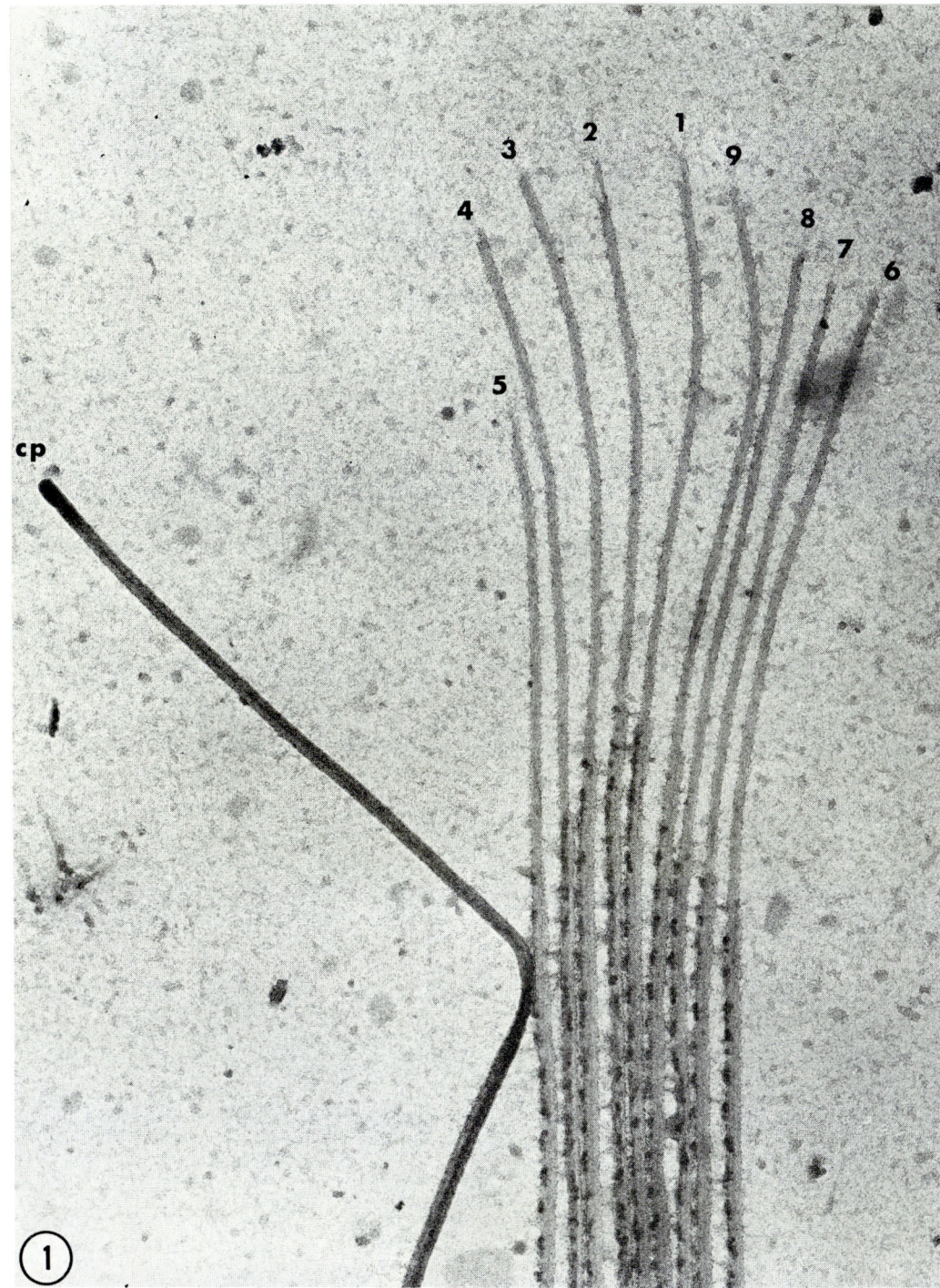

Figure 1. Splayed *Tetrahymena* axoneme. The restricted microtubule displacement correlated with bending is best seen by comparing successive points at which subfiber B ends (constrictions and simultaneous loss of dense spoke group staining). Starting at edge where n = 6 and n + 1 = 7, the doublets are displaced progressively tipward. At n = 1, this displacement reverses. From Sale and Satir (1976), (*cf.* for method of numbering the doublets). Courtesy of W.S. Sale and *J. Cell Biol.* X48,000

Table 1. Measurement of Doublet Lengths of ATP-treated, Digested Axonemes*

Cilium Number	Doublet Lengths (μm)									Mean Length (μm)	S.D. (μm)	Deviation (%)
	1	2	3	4	5	6	7	8	9			
1	5.8	5.8	5.5	5.5	5.8	6.0	5.8	5.5	—	5.7	0.17	2.9
2	5.2	5.2	5.0	5.0	5.3	5.3	5.5	5.3	—	5.2	0.17	3.2
3	4.7	4.7	4.7	4.7	5.0	—	—	—	—	4.7	0.08	1.7
4	4.9	4.5	4.6	4.6	4.5	—	—	—	—	4.5	0.09	2.0
5	6.7	6.7	6.7	6.1	—	—	—	—	—	6.4	0.26	4.0
6	5.0	5.0	4.7	4.7	—	—	—	—	—	4.8	0.13	2.8
7	3.8	3.8	4.2	4.2	4.2	4.2	—	—	—	4.0	0.21	5.3
8	5.0	5.0	5.0	5.0	5.5	6.0	5.0	5.0	—	5.2	0.36	6.9

*Reproduced from Sale (1977), courtesy W.S. Sale.

ration for electron microscopy by critical-point methods, they are preserved. Two criteria were originally rigorously used to identify axonemal configurations where sliding had occurred:

1. The sliding configuration is not seen in the absence of ATP addition.
2. Displaced and residual microtubule components of the axoneme (i.e., all doublets of the fragment) have the same length (Table 1).

These criteria were met by images such as that seen in Figure 2. Elongation by sliding of an axonemal fragment results in an extended series of doublets whose origins are displaced longitudinally while intimate lateral connections are maintained, generally for 0.8-2.0 μm. With experience, similar configurations are identifiable in preparations that are negatively stained rather than subjected to critical-point drying. In negatively stained images, the dynein arms, some of which presumably maintain the lateral associations, are visible (Fig. 3).

Although doublets can be ejected either from the tip or the base of such fragments, Sale and Satir (1977) have demonstrated that the active direction of force production always appears constant. Consider the sliding interaction between two doublets: as noted previously, the arms of doublet No. n push actively against doublet No. n+1; the arms of doublet No. n+1 do not contribute to the production of displacement. In every instance of active sliding studied, doublet n+1 was displaced relatively tipward, while doublet n moved relatively baseward. The conclusion is that the active direction of dynein-force generation must be base to tip, i.e., doublet n pushes n+1 tipward. The dynein arms of all nine doublets must act with identical polarity in the sliding preparations, but when doublets extend several times the length of the original axonemal fragment, piggybacking or asynchronous sliding may be involved.

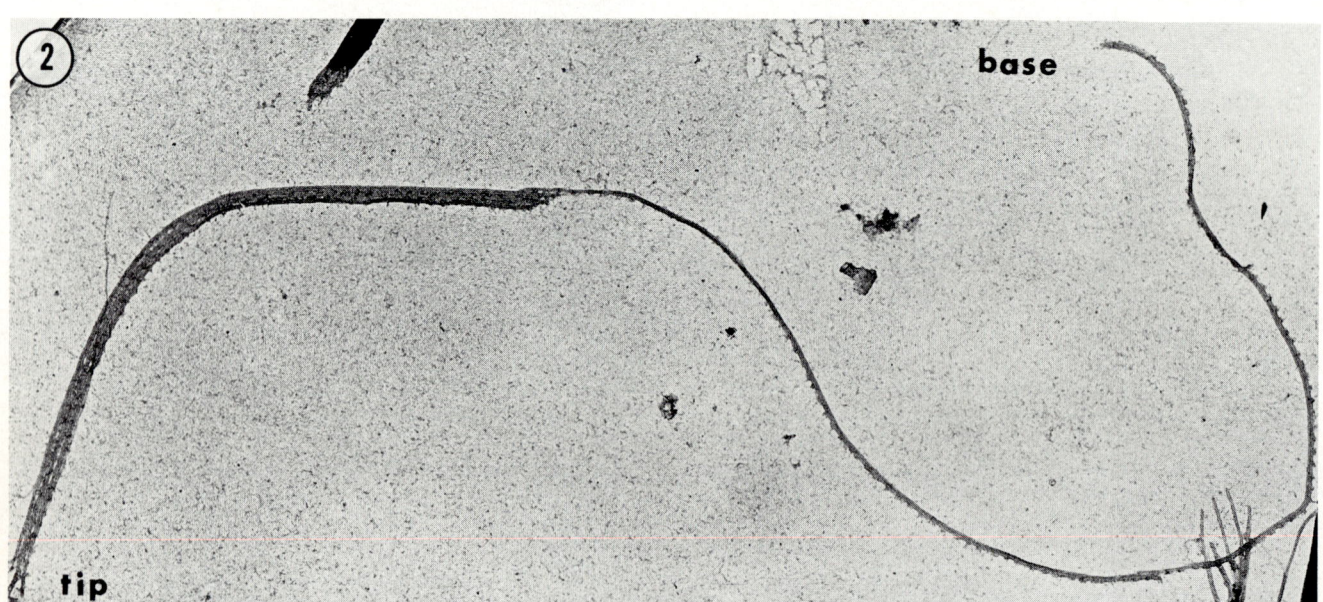

Figure 2. Critical-point dried digested axoneme after addition of ATP, showing two doublets that have been extruded, presumably by sliding. From Satir and Sale (1977). Courtesy J Protozool. X21,000

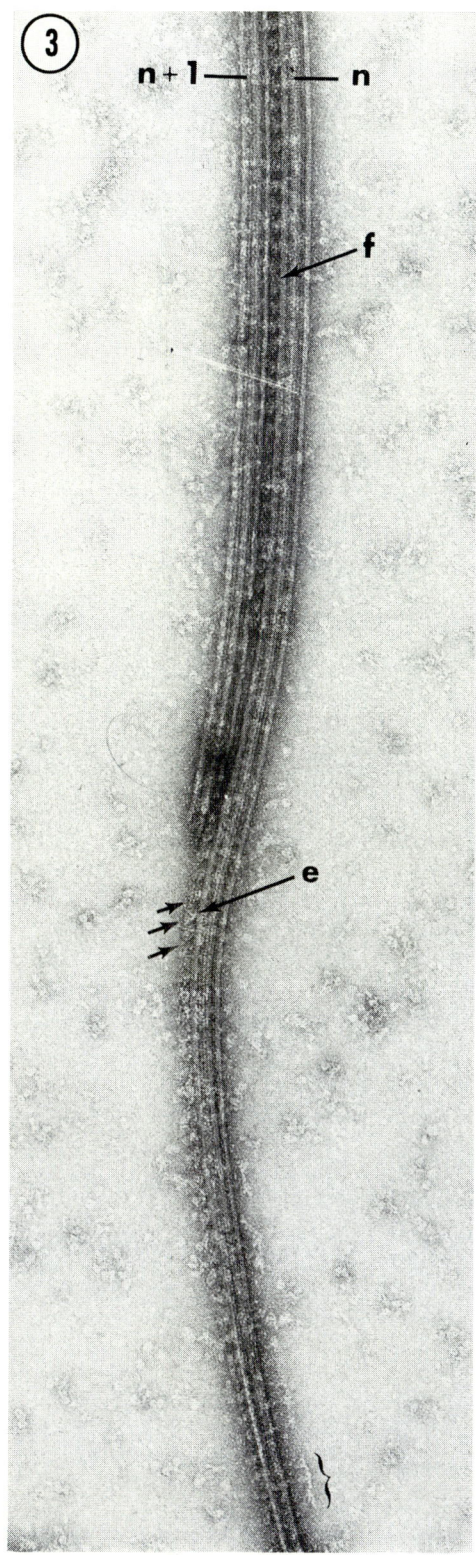

Figure 3. Negatively stained preparation of doublets in the sliding configuration. Dynein arms (arrows) and spokes (bracket) of doublet n are indicated. The arms are seen in the extended (e) and flattened (f) configurations. Doublet n + 1 is displaced tipward during the sliding interaction. From Satir and Sale (1977). Courtesy *J Protozool.* X128,000

The Dynein Arm

The term "dynein" has recently been extended to include all members of a class of divalent cation-dependent ATPase isoenzymes that occur associated with axonemal microtubules and have a very high molecular weight subunit (Gibbons *et al.,* 1976). Differential salt extraction procedures have shown that the arms can be dissociated from subfiber A in preparative amounts. In appropriate gel electrophoretic systems, more than six bands appear in the high molecular weight region (>300 kdaltons) corresponding to dynein; at least two of these components have ATPase activity. Under extraction conditions where only the outer row of dynein arms is extracted, approximately half of the major ATPase band, dynein 1, appears in the gels (Kincaid *et al.,* 1973). Such axonemes can still be reactivated but they beat with half normal frequency. Most workers conclude that dynein 1 is a major component of both arms, although it is probably not the sole component. The mechanochemical transduction event (*i.e.,* sliding) is likely to involve dynein 1 directly, since the conditions required for activity of the isolated enzyme correspond to the conditions of axonemal beat or sliding activity. Dynein 1, in a special "latent activity" form, can be re-added to axonemes whose outer arms have previously been extracted (Gibbons and Gibbons, 1976). During incubation of this mixture with ATP, outer arms reappear on the axonemes and, simultaneously, beat frequency doubles. The location of the second ATPase, dynein 2, within the axoneme is still unknown. For further recent studies of the biochemistry of dynein, see the chapter by B.H. Gibbons *et al.* in this volume.

Warner *et al.* (1977) have examined KCl-extracted, isolated dynein arms by negative-stain methods. A prevalent image in these preparations consists of approximately three subunit aggregates of a cylindrical protomer. Some substructure is also observed in the protomer itself. The arms identified by Sale and Satir (1977) at the 24-nm periodicity along axonemal microtubules in negatively stained preparations in *Tetrahymena* (Fig. 3) also have a tripartite organization, as shown dramatically after the application of linear translation re-enforcement techniques in Figure 4.

In such preparations, the arms clearly have two different appearances: extended and flattened. The characteristics of these states are summarized diagrammatically in Figure 5. In the extended form, the arms point toward the base of the cilium at an angle of approximately 40° from horizontal. The protomers are approximately 10 nm in diameter and 7-8 nm in length so that the 24 nm-long extended arm is long enough to bridge the interdoublet distance. In the flattened form, the arms are tilted further, about 70° from horizontal. The sub-

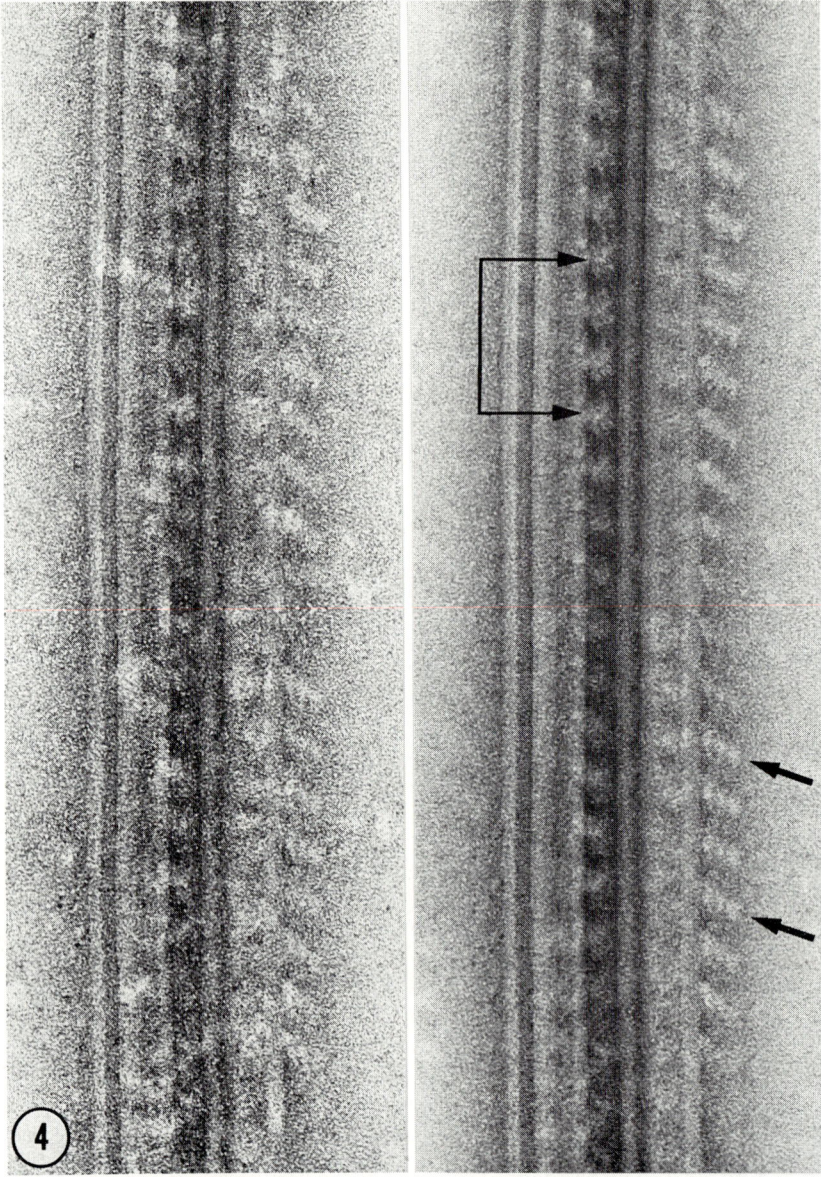

Figure 4. Negatively stained axonemal doublets. Left: original image. Right: Image translated photographically to reinforce arm structure. Free arrows delimit group of extended arms; bracket indicates group of flattened arms. Both show tripartite structure. Note that negative stain penetrates between the flattened arms and the next doublet, *i.e.*, flattened arms do not bridge the interdoublet distance. From Sale and Satir (1977, unpublished micrograph). X285,000

unit construction is still apparent, but the arms are more squat and shorter, too short to bridge the interdoublet distance. In some cases, it appears as if the attachment between subfiber A and arm is via the central subunit.

As has been indicated elsewhere (Satir, 1978), three possibilities exist as to the significance of these different appearances:

1. The two forms may represent intrinsic differences in outer versus inner arms. This explanation is the one favored by Warner and Mitchell (1978) who have obtained images similar to Figure 4.

2. The differences in form may only be apparent, caused by differences in negative-stain penetration and/or doublet (rather than arm) tilt and foreshortening upon drying.

3. The differences may be indicative of different stages in a dynein arm work-cycle related to sliding.

In the untranslated image in Figure 4 (left), the arms are not as uniform as they appear after translation (right); such images could be interpreted as indicating positional movement. However, under the conditions employed, many arms dissociate from the doublets and

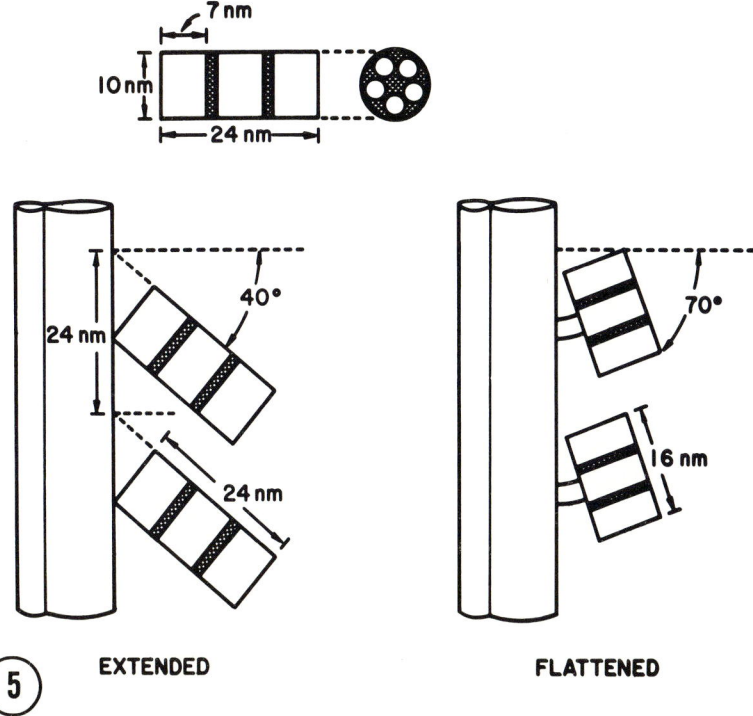

Figure 5. Diagrammatic interpretation of arm configurations of Figure 4.

it may be dissociation rather than movement that is captured in Figure 4. Nevertheless, in Figure 3, where the arms are probably inner arms, the two appearances of the arms can be seen along the same doublet. There is also the suggestion that the appearance of an arm corresponds with its position, in that most arms found between the sliding doublets have the flattened appearance, while at the point where doublet n+1 has just passed doublet n, the arms are extended.

Possibilities 1) and 2) are probably ruled out because of thin-section information. In cross-sectioned axonemes of mussel gill cilia, both inner and outer arms behave similarly. There are two appearances of arms in such sections (Fig. 6). These are the standard image, where the arm does not bridge the interdoublet distance and, the bridged or rigor image (Gibbons, 1975). Both images occur in both inner and outer arms even between different doublets of the same axoneme (as might be expected if the doublets act asynchronously). Moreover, both images can be found in longitudinal sections of axonemes, and they roughly correspond in morphology to the negative-stain images. In Figures 3 and 4, extended arms are completely free. Warner and Mitchell (1978) have observed that in negative stain, extended arms can also appear rather firmly attached to subfiber B of an adjacent doublet. In the longitudinal sections of Figure 6, showing mussel gill cilia, an additional detail is observed: the extended arms may be tilted or they may run normally to the doublets. In this case, the positional difference observed cannot be a reflection of arm dissociation, but may indicate different arm attachment stages.

A scenerio of the dynein arm cycle consistent with the electron microscopic information presented here is diagrammed in Figure 7. A corresponding enzymological sequence based on the work of Taylor and his colleagues (*cf.* Taylor, 1972) for myosin cross-bridge enzymology would also be feasible, but is largely speculative. Two aspects that are reasonably fixed are: the arm is usually unattached (standard image) when sufficient ATP is present, and the arm is usually attached (rigor image) when high Mg^{2+} and little or no ATP is present (*see also* Warner, 1978). In Figure 7 it has been assumed that the flattened form and standard image are equivalent and that in this form, the dynein arm has bound ATP. To yield the cycle, the flattened form extends when ATP is converted to $ADP-P_i$ at the enzymatic site. The extended form can now bind to the tubulin lattice of subfiber B. Positional change occurs as mechano-chemical transduction takes place. The products of ATP hydrolysis are released and the rigor image is produced. Addition of new ATP will presumably plasticize the final dynein-tubulin interaction and re-convert the attached extended arm to the standard, shortened, unattached form.

With less morphological information available, simi-

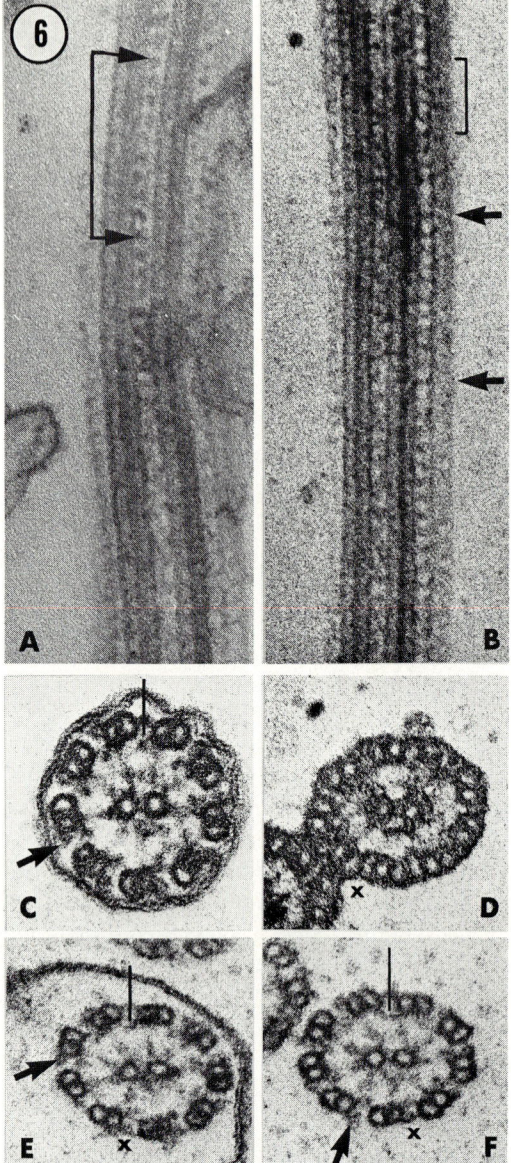

Figure 6. Arm appearances in thin-sectioned axonemes of mussel gill cilia. The standard image of arm is seen in longitudinal (A, especially at bracket) and cross (C, arrow) sections. Note that both inner and outer arms behave similarly and that neither completely spans the interdoublet space. The bridged or rigor image is seen in B and D (at x). In B, tilted (bracket) and normal (arrows) positions occur. In E and F, some arms are in the standard (arrows), some in the rigor (x) images in the same axoneme. The bridge between doublets 5-6 is always present (vertical line in C,E,F). A. X151,000 B. X113,000 C-F. X126,000

lar scenarios have been proposed by Bloodgood (1975) and Sleigh (personal communication). In the present state of affairs, most of the evidence is preliminary, and considerable controversy still exists with regard to correspondence of the structural and physiologically important states of the arms, in part because the correspondences are not yet reproducible from time to time or laboratory to laboratory. Several laboratories are now focusing more closely on these questions.

RESTRICTION AND REGULATION OF SLIDING

Although the beating sperm tail or cilium does not slide apart, as do the trypsin-treated axonemes, some actual displacement of microtubules does occur during beat (Fig. 1), but in the intact axoneme sliding is highly restricted. The limited doublet displacements of Figure 1 should be compared with displacements seen after the removal of sliding constraints in Figure 2. A major part of the system that restricts sliding is thought to involve action of the radial spokes. Mutants of *Chlamydomonas*, deficient in either the spokes themselves or the central complex against which the spokes abut, are paralyzed, despite the demonstrable presence of the intact sliding system (Witman *et al.*, 1976). The spokes apparently restrict sliding by forming local transient attachments to projections from the central microtubules in regions where bends develop (Warner and Satir, 1974). However, other components of the axoneme—perhaps even the arms themselves—may also contribute to the control system, and under certain circumstances, might substitute for or even supplant the spokes.

The most obvious feature of the components that normally constrain sliding is that they must be trypsin-sensitive. In general, the mechanisms involved in the feedback loop that limit sliding, and the coupling of these mechanisms to produce and propagate bend within the axoneme, are much less well understood than is the basic sliding event. The findings that there is constant polarity of force generation in the trypsin-treated sliding systems by themselves suggest that to produce actual bending, the doublets must slide asynchronously. One of the important actions of the trypsin-sensitive control system must be to regulate and coordinate this asynchrony. Satir and Sale (1977) reason that images such as Figure 1 actually display such regulation. Since we know that in trypsin-resistant sliding, doublet n actively pushes doublet n+1 tipward, it is possible to distinguish in intact nontrypsin-treated bending axonemes, such as in Figure 1, doublets that show this polarity from those that do not. This is a critical distinction, because the latter are never seen

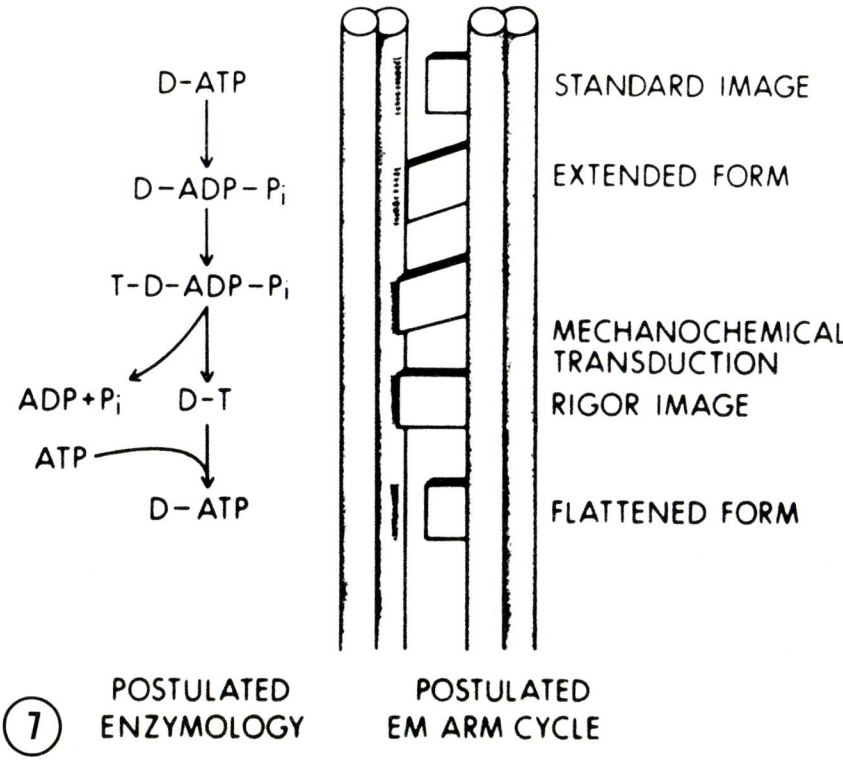

Figure 7. The presumptive dynein-arm cycle. From top to bottom successive stages of one complete cycle are shown. At each level, the postulated enzymology is correlated with the postulated arm morphology. The hatched vertical line along subfiber B of doublet n + 1 as diagrammed indicates hypothetical arm attachment site.

after trypsin treatment and must, therefore, be a product of the action of the control system. If the rule governing direction of active sliding of doublet microtubules can be extrapolated from the models to the intact axoneme, those doublets that obey the rule can be considered active, while those that do not can be considered inactive. By this reasoning, in Figure 1 doublets 6-9 must be active, while doublets 2-4 must not be. In the model constructed by Satir and Sale (1977) for ciliary motility, Figure 1 represents a recovery stroke position; during the effective stroke, doublets 1-4 would be actively sliding, while 6-9 would be inactive and only passively moved.

This analysis has one or two unexpected implications. First, the two halves of the axoneme that slide asynchronously are doublets 1-4 as opposed to 6-9 (*i.e.*, generally parallel to the plane of beat), but the doublets that move tipward are 4, 5, 6, 7 as the effective stroke progresses and 9, 1, 2 as the recovery stroke progresses (*i.e.*, groups generally perpendicular to the beat plane). Thus, not all doublets in the half axoneme moving tipward at any one time during beat have active arms. In addition, the stable plane around which doublet displacement is measured by the axoneme itself is the plane of the central pair. The morphology of certain ctenophore cilia (Afzelius, 1961) supports this conclusion. The finding of Olson and Linck (1977) that, in rat spermatozoa, sliding disintegration in the presence of ATP displays a specific pattern such that doublets 4-7 are extruded as a half-axoneme also suggests that the numerology will apply to the principal and reverse bends of flagellar motility, as does the geometry of sliding. Second, what activates the axonemal halves? For 9+2 axonemes, one speculation looks immediately promising: the sheath projections on the central microtubules are asymmetric in relation to the doublets, such that radial spokes of doublets 2-4 and 6-9 abut against different projections that are on opposite sides of the central complex. This is exactly what one might hope to find if the central complex provided the appropriate switch point for microtubule sliding activation. The existence of switch points for sliding activation may be experimentally testable by application of agents that produce ciliary arrest. Wais and Satir (in preparation) have recently obtained preliminary evidence that suggests that in some cilia, some agents (*e.g.*, high concentrations of Ca^{2+}) may act primarily at one switch point and some (*e.g.*, vanadate) at another. By extending this experimentation to indicate the structural points of action of such agents we may be able to dissect more effectively the feedback loop that governs beating in cilia and sperm.

REFERENCES

Afzelius, B.: Electron Microscopy of the Sperm Tail. Results Obtained with a New Fixative. J Biophys Biochem Cytol 5(1959)269-278

Afzelius, B.: The Fine Structure of Cilia from Ctenophore Swimming-Plates. J Biophys Biochem Cytol 9(1961)383-394

Allen, C.; Borisy, G.G.: Flagellar Motility in Chlamydomonas: Reactivation and Sliding in Vitro. J Cell Biol 63(1974)5A

Bloodgood, R.A.: Biochemical Analysis of Axostyle Motility. Cytobios 14(1975)101-120

Gibbons, B.H.; Gibbons, I.R.: Functional Recombination of Dynein-1 with Demembranated Sea Urchin Sperm Partially Extracted with KCl. Biochem Biophys Res Commun 73(1976)1-6

Gibbons, I.R.: Studies on the Protein Components of Cilia from Tetrahymena pyriformis. Proc Natl Acad Sci USA 50(1963)1002-1010

Gibbons, I.R.: The Molecular Basis of Flagellar Motility in Sea Urchin Spermatozoa. In: Molecules and Cell Movement, pp. 207-232, ed. by S. Inoue and R.E. Stephens. Raven Press, New York, 1975

Gibbons, I.R.; Fronk, E.; Gibbons, B.H.; Ogawa, K.: Multiple Forms of Dynein in Sea Urchin Sperm Flagella. In: Cell Motility, pp. 915-932, ed. by R.D. Goldman, et al. Spring Harbor Laboratory, New York, 1976

Goldstein, S.F.: Form of Developing Bends in Reactivated Sperm Flagella. J Exp Biol 64(1976)173-184

Hoffmann-Berling, H.: Geisselmodelle und Adenosintriphosphate. Biochem Biophys Acta 16(1955)146-154

Kincaid, H.L., Jr.; Gibbons, B.H.; Gibbons, I.R.: The Salt-extractable Fraction of Dynein from Sea Urchin Flagella: An Analysis by Gel Electrophoresis and Adenosine Triphosphatase Activity. J Supramol Struct 1(1973)461-470

Lindemann, C.B.; Gibbons, I.R.: Adenosine triphosphate-induced Motility and Sliding of Filaments in Sperm Extracted with Triton X-100. J Cell Biol 65(1975)147-162

Olson, G.E.; Linck, R.W.: Observations of the Structural Components of Flagellar Axonemes and Central Pair Microtubules from Rat Sperm. J Ultrastruct Res 61(1977)21-43

Rothschild, Lord: Sperm Movement—Problems of Observation. In: Spermatozoan Motility pp. 13-29, ed. by D.W. Bishop, Amer Assoc Adv Science, 1962

Sale, W.S.: Fine Structure and Direction of Active Microtubule Sliding in the Cilia of Tetrahymena. Ph.D. Thesis, University of California, Berkeley, 1977

Sale, W.S.; Satir, P.: Splayed Tetrahymena Cilia. J Cell Biol 71(1976)589-605

Sale, W.S.; Satir, P.: The Direction of Active Sliding of Microtubules in Tetrahymena Cilia. Proc Natl Acad Sci USA 74(1977)2045-2050

Satir, P.: Studies on Cilia. II. Examination of the Distal Region of the Ciliary Shaft and the Role of the Filaments in Motility. J Cell Biol 26(1965)805-834

Satir, P.: Studies on Cilia. III. Further Studies on the Cilium Tip and a "Sliding Filament" Model of Ciliary Motility. J Cell Biol 39(1968)77-94

Satir, P.: The Present Status of the Sliding Microtubule Model of Cilia. In: Cilia and Flagella, pp. 131-142, ed. by M.A. Sleigh. Academic Press, New York, 1974

Satir, P.: Regulation of Microtubule Sliding in Cilia. Acta Protozool, in press

Satir, P.: Sale, W.S.: Tails of Tetrahymena. J Protozool 24(1977)498-501

Shingyoji, C.; Murakami, A.; Takahashi, K.: Local Reactivation of Triton-extracted Flagella by Iontophoretic Application of ATP. Nature 265(1977)269-270

Summers, K.E.: ATP-induced Sliding of Microtubules in Bull Sperm Flagella. J Cell Biol 60(1974)321-324

Summers, K.E.; Gibbons, I.R.: Effect of Trypsin Digestion on Flagellar Structures and Their Relationship to Motility. J Cell Biol 58(1973)618-629

Taylor, E.W.: Chemistry of Muscle Contraction. Ann Rev Biochem 41(1972)577-616

Walter, M.F.; Satir, P.: Calcium Does Not Inhibit Sliding of Microtubules from Mussel Gill Cilia. J Cell Biol 75(1977)287A

Warner, F.D.: Cation-induced Attachment of Ciliary Dynein Cross-Bridges. J Cell Biol 77(1978)R-19-R26

Warner, F.D.; Mitchell, D.R.: Structural Conformation of Ciliary Dynein Arms and the Generation of Sliding Forces in Tetrahymena Cilia. J Cell Biol 75(1978)261-277

Warner, F.D.; Mitchell, D.R.; Perkins, C.R.: Structural Conformation of the Ciliary ATPase Dynein. J Mol Biol 114(1977)367-384

Warner, F.D.; Satir, P.: The Structural Basis of Ciliary Bend Formation. J Cell Biol 63(1974)35-63

Witman, G.B.; Fay, R.; Plummer, J.: **Chlamydomonas** Mutants: Evidence for the Roles of Specific Axonemal Components in Flagellar Movement. In: Cell Motility, ed. by R. Goldman, et al. Cold Spring Harbor Laboratory, New York, 1976.

STUDIES ON THE MECHANISM OF FLAGELLAR MOVEMENT

B.H. Gibbons

Pacific Biomedical Research Center, University of Hawaii, Honolulu, Hawaii 96822   USA

This chapter reviews four topics of recent experimental work: The first is a description of a latent activity form of dynein 1 and its properties. This enzyme preparation seems to resemble most closely the physiological form of dynein 1 *in vivo*. The second topic is the recombination of this latent dynein 1 with KCl-extracted sea urchin sperm with a concomitant restoration of functional activity. The third topic deals with the discovery of a potent, selective inhibitor of dynein and of the motility of reactivated cilia and sperm flagella. And the fourth topic, which is separate from the others, concerns a phenomenon of intermittent swimming behavior in live sea urchin sperm which may provide information about the coordination of events necessary to produce regularly propagated waves.

The involvement of the dynein arms in the sliding tubule mechanism of ciliary and flagellar movement has by now been established with great certainty by several lines of evidence (Gibbons and Gibbons, 1973, 1974, 1976). The most direct of these was the work of Summers and Gibbons (1971) which demonstrated that adenosine triphosphate (ATP) induced sliding between doublet tubules in axonemes that had been briefly digested with trypsin to remove connecting structures that normally maintain the structural integrity of the axoneme. The trypsin digestion left intact primarily the arms and the doublet tubules to which they were attached (Summers and Gibbons, 1973). Thus the hypothesis first proposed by Afzelius (1959) and supported by Satir (1968) is now widely accepted.

About six years ago the possibility of removing the membrane from sea urchin sperm flagella by treatment with Triton X-100 and then reactivating them by addition of ATP was demonstrated (Gibbons and Gibbons, 1972). Such demembranated sperm swim with movements closely resembling those of live sperm. The technique permits study of the effect of different conditions on the various parameters of movement such as beat frequency and waveform, and it has yielded much information about the mechanism of motility (Brokaw, 1975; Brokaw and Gibbons, 1973; Brokaw and Josslin, 1973; Brokaw et al., 1974; Brokaw and Simonick, 1976, 1977; Gibbons and Gibbons, 1972, 1973, 1974, 1976; B.H. Gibbons et al., 1976).

A second important use of these demembranated flagella is for the differential extraction of the proteins of the axoneme. So far, this technique has largely been applied to the group of high molecular weight proteins which include dynein. In the high molecular weight region of polyacrylamide gels on which axonemal proteins have been electrophoresed in the presence of sodium dodecyl sulfate (SDS), there are four main bands, originally called A, B, C, and D (I.R. Gibbons et al., 1976). It has been shown that two of these have ATPase activity and correspond to two isoenzymes of dynein 1 and 2. Dynein 1 accounts for 75% of the total ATPase activity of the axoneme and is found in the arms on the doublet tubules. Dynein 2, which has been isolated and described by Ogawa and Gibbons (1976), accounts for about 15% of the axonemal ATPase activity, and so far its location in the axoneme is unknown.

LATENT ATPase ACTIVITY DYNEIN 1

Gibbons and Fronk (1979) have now shown that dynein 1 can be obtained from sea urchin sperm axonemes in a latent, low activity state. This has been called latent activity dynein 1, or LAD-1, and it is extracted from sperm of the sea urchin *Tripneustes gratilla* by treatment with $0.6M$ NaCl in imidazole buffer at pH 7 in the presence of Ca^{2+} and Mg^{2+}. LAD-1 has a specific ATPase activity of approximately 0.25 μmol Pi min^{-1} mg^{-1} when assayed under standard conditions in the absence of KCl, and its activity is enhanced by several different treatments. Incubation of LAD-1 with 0.1% Triton X-100 for 10 min at 25°C causes a 10-15-fold activation of the ATPase activity. A similar activation is obtained by treating at 42°C in the absence of Triton (Fig. 1) or by reacting with 60 mol p-chloromercuribenzenesulfonate (PCMS) per 10^6 g of protein. The effects of the exposure of LAD-1 to these various treatments are not additive, but appear to cause equivalent changes in the enzyme. The ATPase activity of LAD-1 can also be partially activated, *i.e.*, about threefold,

---

The following people have contributed to the work: I.R. Gibbons, Marie Paule Cosson, John A. Evans, Earl Fronk, Becky Houck, Karl Martinson, Winfield S. Sale, and Wen-Jing Y. Tang. This work was supported by grants HD 06565 and HD 10002 from the National Institutes of Health.

© 1979 Urban & Schwarzenberg, Inc. Baltimore-Munich *The Spermatozoon*, edited by D.W. Fawcett and J.M. Bedford

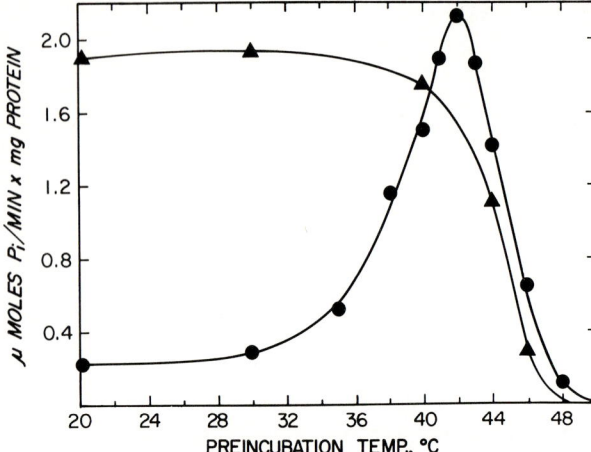

Figure 1. Specific ATPase activity of LAD-1 after preincubation for 10 min at various temperatures in the presence (—▲—) or absence (—●—) of 0.1% Triton X-100. All assays were performed at 25°C. (Gibbons and Fronk, 1979)

by dialysis for 24 h against an imidazole/ethylenediaminetetraacetate (EDTA) solution at pH 7. This partial activation can be completed by subsequent incubation with Triton X-100 as described above.

LAD-1 rebinds to axonemes from which all the dynein 1 has been extracted. Electron microscopy shows that all the outer arms are missing from such axonemes, and in most cases the inner arms appear to be missing also although they are difficult to score because of overlap with the nexin links. After adding NaCl-extracted axonemes to LAD-1 in a 1:1 ratio, based upon the relative quantities of these components obtained from intact axonemes, 41% of the outer arms could be seen in micrographs. An axoneme to LAD-1 ratio of approximately 1:2 restored 95% of the outer arms to the doublet tubules. The NaCl-extracted axonemes cause a marked activation of the ATPase activity of LAD-1 with a maximal sixfold activation occurring also at an axoneme to LAD-1 ratio of 1:2. These results suggest that the rebinding of LAD-1 is specific.

Preparations of LAD-1 consist of a monodisperse form of dynein 1, sedimenting at 21S on a 5-20% sucrose gradient (Gibbons and Fronk, 1979). Dynein 1 that has been activated by dialysis against imidazole/EDTA migrates as a single peak with a sedimentation coefficient of 10S. Electrophoretic analysis on polyacrylamide gels in the presence of SDS shows that the material in the 21S ATPase peak contains a principal component corresponding to the A electrophoretic band of dynein 1 described previously, plus three minor components that migrate at positions corresponding to molecular weights of 126,000, 95,000, and 77,000, which together account for approximately 25% of the total protein. These minor components co-purify with the ATPase peak both on sucrose density gradient centrifugation and on Sepharose 4B chromatography, suggesting that they are true components of the 21S LAD-1 particle. The minor components seem to become separated from the dynein 1 when the 21S particle breaks down to the 10S particle upon dialysis against imidazole/EDTA.

The molecular weight of LAD-1 has been determined both by sedimentation equilibrium and by sedimentation diffusion in the ultracentrifuge; the value obtained is 1,250,000. Based upon the estimated values for the molecular weights of the various polypeptides constituting the 21S particle, Gibbons and Fronk (1979) propose that it may contain three heavy A-band subunits of about 330,000 molecular weight and one each of the smaller subunits. In as much as the 10S particle obtained by dialysis against imidazole/EDTA does not rebind to salt-extracted axonemes and does not contain the medium-weight polypeptides, it is possible that these polypeptides play a role in the binding of the A-band protein to the axoneme.

FUNCTIONAL RECOMBINATION OF DYNEIN 1

For some time we have known that the dynein 1 can be partially extracted from demembranated sperm of the sea urchin *Colobocentrotus atratus* by brief treatment with $0.5M$ KCl. This treatment preferentially removes the outer arms from the doublet tubules, and the sperm remain reactivatable with ATP (Gibbons and Gibbons, 1973). In such preparations, the sperm swim with normal waveform at approximately half the normal frequency. Addition of LAD-1 to these KCl-extracted sperm causes their beat frequency to increase from about 14 Hz to 25 Hz. The beat frequency of standard reactivated sperm is approximately 30 Hz under the same conditions. Electron microscopy shows that up to 90% of the outer arms have been restored on the doublet tubules (Gibbons and Gibbons, 1976). Preparations of LAD-1 are the first in which it has been possible to demonstrate functional activity, and Gibbons and Fronk (1979) suggest that each 21S LAD-1 particle may represent a single functionally intact dynein arm unit.

With this recombination technique, it is possible to assay various preparations of dynein 1 for functional activity (Gibbons and Gibbons, 1979). LAD-1 which has been activated by treatment with Triton X-100 does not restore the beat frequency of KCl-extracted axonemes nor does it rebind to form outer arms on the doublet tubules. Likewise, heat-treated LAD-1 is not functionally active. Figure 2 shows the ATPase activity of samples of LAD-1 that had been preheated at vari-

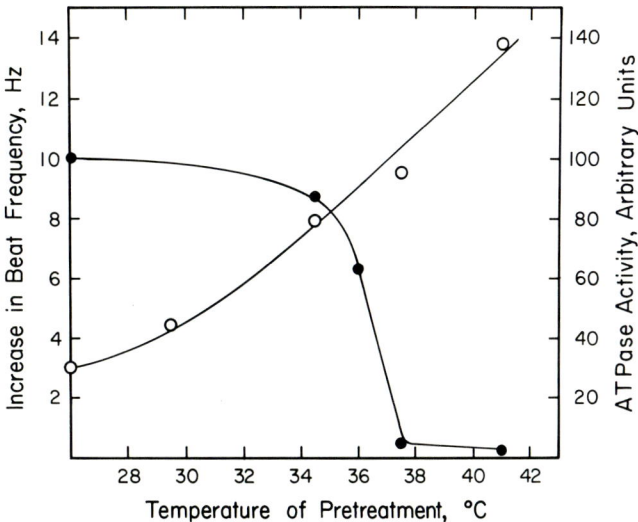

Figure 2. Effect of preincubation of LAD-1 for 10 min at the temperatures shown on its ATPase activity (−O−) and its ability to restore beat frequency to KCl-extracted sperm (−●−). (Gibbons and Gibbons, 1979)

ous temperatures with the corresponding increases in beat frequency obtained when these samples were incubated with KCl-extracted sperm. Maximal restoration of beat frequency was obtained when the specific activity of the dynein-1 ATPase was the lowest, whereas no significant increase in the beat frequency was obtained when the specific activity of the dynein 1 had risen threefold after being heated at 37.5°C. Examination by electron microscopy showed that heat-activated dynein 1 did not recombine structurally with the outer doublet tubules of KCl-extracted sperm. LAD-1 which has been maximally activated by PCMS also did not produce functional or structural recombination. Dialysis of LAD-1 against imidazole/EDTA produces only a threefold activation of the ATPase activity, but this material also lacks all ability to recombine functionally or structurally with KCl-extracted sperm. Thus the 10S particle of dynein 1 is not able to recombine. Only the latent, 21S form of dynein 1 appears able to recombine and restore the beat frequency.

INHIBITION BY VANADATE

Another approach to the investigation of the mechanism of motility that has recently become available involves the discovery that the vanadate anion (vanadium in the 5+ oxidation state) is a potent selective inhibitor of dynein ATPase and of the motility of demembranated cilia and sperm flagella (I.R. Gibbons et al., 1978; Kobayashi et al., 1978). Addition of 4 μM vanadate (NaVO$_3$) to sea urchin sperm reactivated in 0.1 mM ATP produces a complete inhibition of motility; 0.5 μM vanadate is sufficient to inhibit the movement of reactivated cilia from sea urchin embryos. In both cases the inhibition can be reversed by the addition of 2.5 mM catechol or norepinephrine (I.R. Gibbons et al., 1978), and in the case of reactivated sperm the inhibition can also be reversed by simply diluting the sperm so that the vanadate concentration falls below the critical level. Live sperm are insensitive to even 10 mM vanadate, presumably because the inhibitor cannot cross the cell membrane. Inhibition of reactivated sperm motility or of enzyme activity by vanadate was rapid, whereas the reversal by catechol was relatively slow, requiring 1-2 min to go to completion.

Kinetic studies of both the inhibition of beat frequency by a subcritical concentration of vanadate or of enzyme activity (Fig. 3) suggest that vanadate is not competitive with ATP (I.R. Gibbons et al., 1978). The results suggest that the inhibition of motility of reactivated cilia and sperm flagella is a consequence of the inhibition of dynein 1. However, the detailed response of the beat frequency to vanadate suggests that the inhibition of dynein 2 may also be involved. Experiments with isolated dynein 2 have not yet been done.

Previously Cantley et al. (1977) reported the inhibition of the (Na, K)-ATPase from porcine brain by vanadate. They also found a high affinity, and reversal by norepinephrine. This study confirms their report that actomyosin ATPase is not inhibited by vanadate under several different conditions of assay. With concentrations of vanadate up to 500 μM—1000-fold greater than is effective with dynein—no inhibition was seen of either actomyosin or myosin ATPase activity; there seems to be rather an activation in some conditions with high concentrations of vanadate. This result means that vanadate may provide an important means for distinguishing between the dynein-dependent and

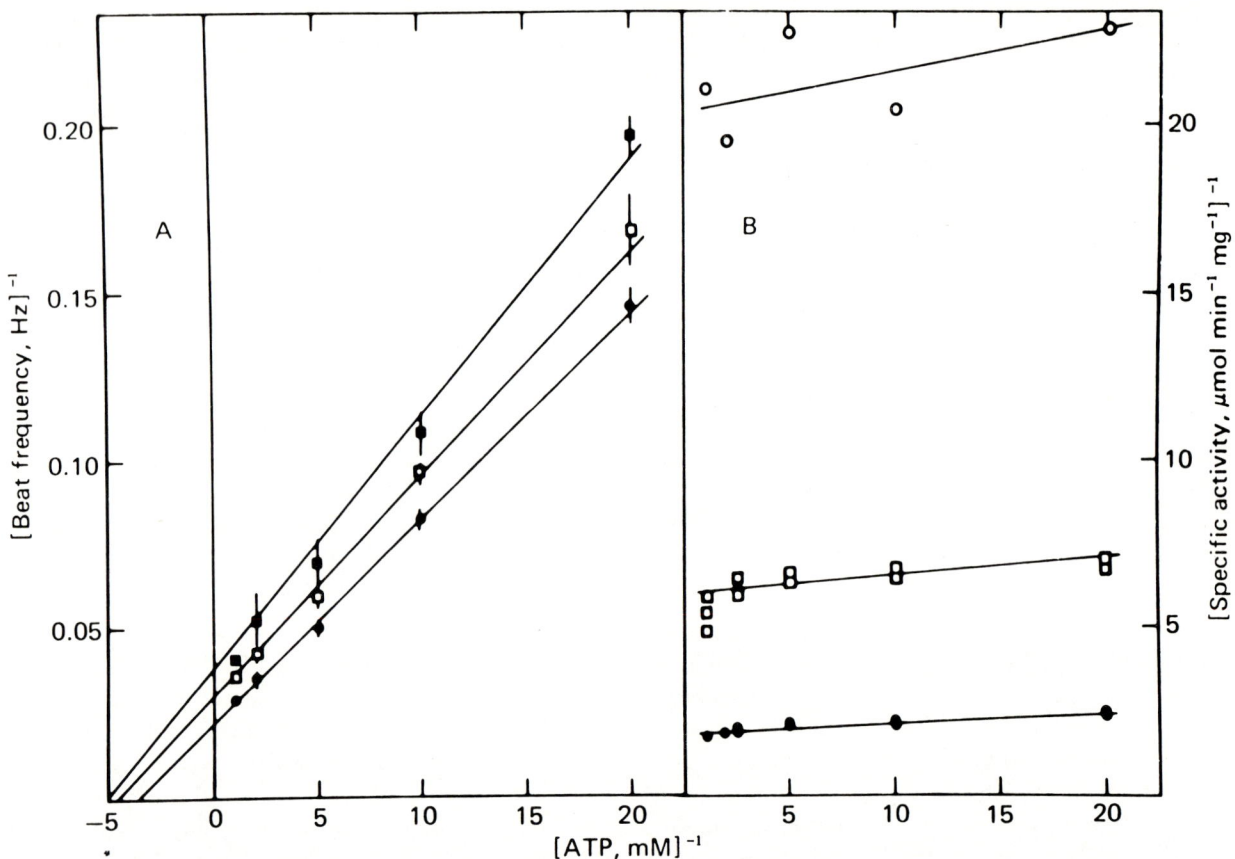

Figure 3. Double reciprocal plots of ATP dependence in presence of vanadate. Vanadate concentrations were: zero (●); 1 μM (□); 1.5 μM (■); 10 μM (○). (A) Beat frequency of reactivated sperm in 10mM Tris-HCl pH 8.0, 2mM MgSO$_4$, 0.5mM EDTA, 1mM dithiothreitol, 0.15M KCl, and ATP as shown. Bars show standard deviation for measurements of 20 sperm. (B) ATPase activity of LAD-1. The assay contained reagents for coupling ATP hydrolysis to NADH, and ATP as shown. (I.R. Gibbons et al., 1978)

actomyosin-dependent forms of cell motility (I.R. Gibbons et al., 1978; Kobayashi et al., 1978).

In preliminary experiments, vanadate was also found to inhibit the motility of human sperm reactivated following the procedure of Lindemann and Gibbons (1975). The inhibitor appears to have a high affinity, with about 0.5 μM being sufficient to block motility at pH 8 and 1mM ATP. This result strengthens the hypothesis that motility in human sperm is dependent upon a dynein ATPase rather that an actomyosin ATPase system (Lindemann and Gibbons, 1975). Little inhibition of the live sperm is discernible even at 10mM vanadate presumably as a consequence of the impermeability of the membrane.

Addition of 0.5mM vanadate to human sperm that are partially damaged by treatment with the commercial contraceptive Koromex Jelly IIA (Holland-Rantos Co., Piscataway, N.J.) in a 1000-fold dilution renders them nonmotile. At present it is unclear whether vanadate could have any usefulness in vaginal contraception. Such usefulness would depend on the development of a better method for transporting it into the sperm cell.

TRANSIENT WAVEFORMS DURING INTERMITTENT SWIMMING IN LIVE SEA URCHIN SPERM

So far the work described has dealt little with the problem of coordination in the mechanism of motility. Sliding alone will not produce bends in the axoneme, and little is known as yet about the coordination and localization of sliding movements between tubules to produce bends. The spokes and spoke heads as well as the nexin links possibly provide the elastic restraints to sliding that cause bend formation and propagation (Warner and Satir, 1974). A coordinated turning on and off of certain components may be involved in producing any given waveform. The simple 9+2 axoneme can produce either the highly asymmetric beating pattern of a cilium, or the symmetrical form of the normal sperm flagellum. In Chlamydomonas, the flagella can produce either type of bending depending on the concentration of free Ca^{2+} (Hyams and Borisy, 1975) and the existence of a Ca^{2+}-mediated regulation of symmetry in reactivated sea urchin sperm has been demonstrated by the work of Brokaw et al., (1974).

A phenomenon has recently been observed in live sea urchin sperm which involves a turning on and off of the sliding process together with localized changes in the coordination of bending (I.R. Gibbons, 1976; Gibbons and Gibbons, 1977). These sperm normally swim uninterruptedly in seawater, but when they are illuminated with blue light a proportion of them repeatedly stops and starts swimming. The phenomenon is nonperiodic and the quiescent phase is generally much shorter than the swimming phase and is of the order of 1 sec. Analysis with high-speed movies has been made of the transient waveforms that occur during stopping and starting, in terms of the changing parameters of the principal and reverse bends as they form and propagate.

The flagella of sperm that are lying in the quiescent state have a very characteristic shape that resembles a cane. There is a sharp principal bend (Gibbons and Gibbons, 1972) of about 3 rad in the flagellum near the head, while the rest is essentially straight except for a slight curve near the tip (Gibbons and Gibbons, 1977). Figure 4 is a composite of consecutive images traced from a movie film made at 214 frames per second that shows the progressive changes in waveform of a sperm starting up from the quiescent state. Movement begins spontaneously with an increase in the angle of the principal bend and simultaneous initiation of a new reverse bend close to the head. The principal bend then begins propagating, but soon decreases in angle, and dies away after passing only one-fourth to one-third of the length. The reverse bend, which achieves only a much smaller angle, dies away even sooner. Subsequent principal and reverse bends travel progressively farther down the tail until finally the flagellum is beating in the normal steady state manner.

It is apparent that the transient waveforms during starting are characterized by a high degree of asym-

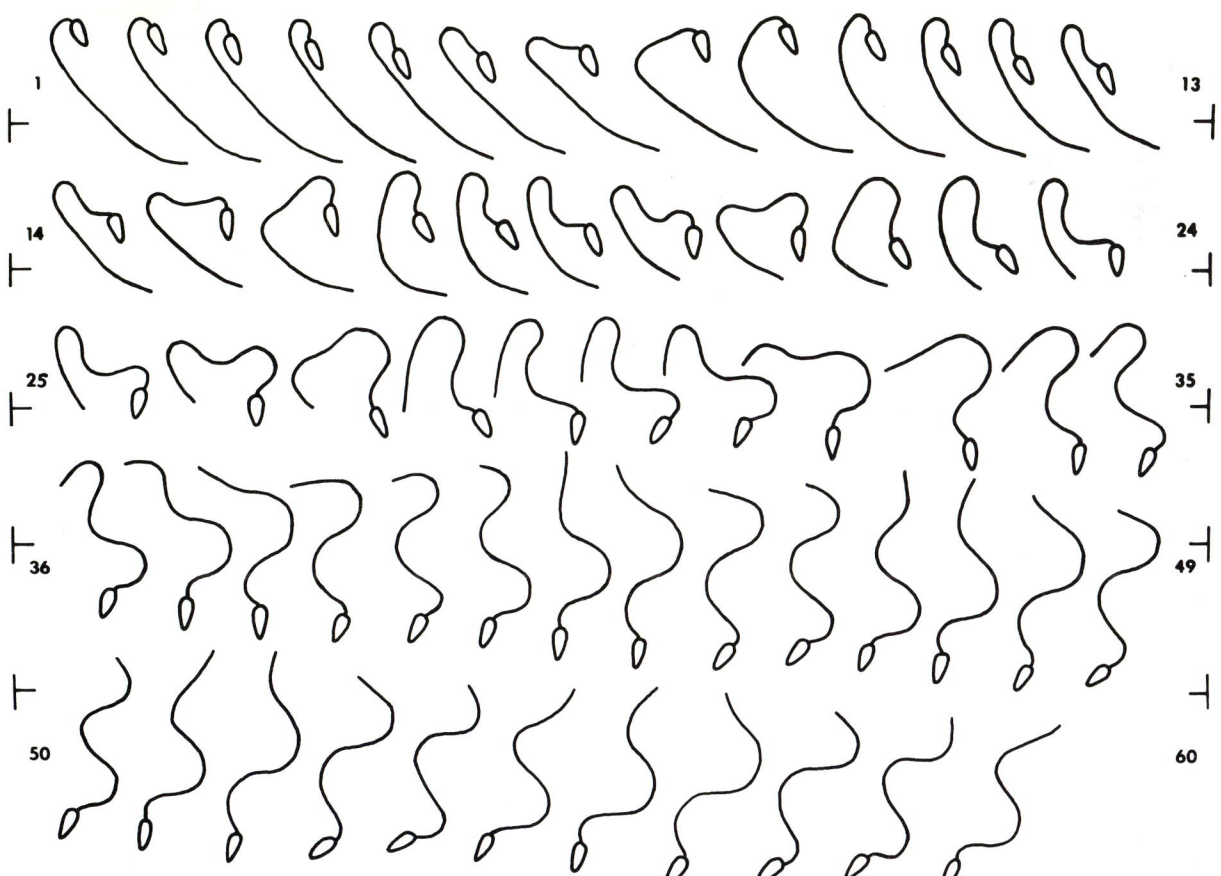

Figure 4. Tracings of consecutive frames of a movie film showing a live sperm from the sea urchin *Tripneustes gratilla* in seawater containing 0.2mM EDTA and adjusted to pH 8.3. At the beginning, the sperm is lying quiescent in a cane shape, and at the end of the series it is swimming normally. Framing rate, 214/s. Temperature, 23°C.

metry. The maximum angle of the first principal bend is much greater than that of the first reverse bend. The maximum angles of successive principal and reverse bends become more nearly equal, and the difference in curvature of the two bends decreases, so that eventually the waveform is much more symmetrical. When the sperm finally moves away from its original location, its swimming path is often quite straight along the bottom surface of the dish.

The process of stopping resembles qualitatively that of starting, except for being reversed in time. One significant quantitative difference is that stopping requires a shorter time and involves fewer beat cycles. The time period for starting is approximately 250 msec while it is 150 msec for stopping. Differences also exist in the detailed shape of the transient waveforms during starting and stopping.

A striking feature of the intermittent swimming behavior is that in the quiescent state there is a fixed bend of large angle near the head, which implies a large shear displacement between the doublet tubules in the tip region of the quiescent flagellum. This large shear displacement suggests that a sperm stops swimming as a result of an increasing degree of inhibition of sliding between the doublet tubules on the side of the flagellum responsible for generating the reverse bends, while the sliding on the other side that generates principal bends remains uninhibited, so that the axoneme rapidly accumulates increasing amounts of shear displacement on this latter side, until the last principal bend is trapped at the proximal end, unable to propagate (Gibbons and Gibbons, 1977). Re-initiation of motility would occur upon the release of sliding on the previously inhibited side of the axoneme leading to formation of a small reverse bend with propagation of the trapped principal bend. If this is correct, it would provide further confirmation for a difference between the properties of the principal and reverse bends that was suggested earlier (Gibbons and Gibbons, 1972), and that has also been reported by Goldstein (1976).

The transient, asymmetric waveforms described here resemble those seen in demembranated sperm that are reactivated in the presence of concentrations of Ca^{2+} greater than $10^{-6}M$ (Brokaw et al., 1974). Experiments with artificial seawater have shown that the intermittent swimming behavior occurs only when Ca^{2+} is present in the seawater. Calcium has been shown to play a role in the arrest response in cilia (Satir, 1975; Satir et al., 1976), and Tsuchiya (1976, 1977) has demonstrated a Ca^{2+}-induced arrest response in Triton-extracted cilia of *Mytilus* gill. The intermittent swimming behavior just described has not so far been reported in reactivated sperm, and the reason for the calcium requirement is not yet clear. It is hoped that study of this intermittent swimming phenomenon may give further information about the ionic and molecular regulation of sliding and bending in cilia and flagella.

REFERENCES

Afzelius, B.A.: Electron Microscopy of the Sperm Tail. Results Obtained with a New Fixative. J Biophys Biochem Cytol 5(1959)269-278

Brokaw, C.J.: Effects of Viscosity and ATP Concentration on the Movement of Reactivated Sea Urchin Sperm Flagella. J Exp Biol 62(1975)701-719

Brokaw, C.J.; Gibbons, I.R.: Localized Activation of Bending in Proximal, Medial and Distal Regions of Sea Urchin Sperm Flagella. J Cell Sci 13(1973)1-10

Brokaw, C.J.; Josslin, R.: Maintenance of Constant Wave Parameters by Sperm Flagella at Reduced Frequencies of Beat. J Exp Biol 59(1973)617-628

Brokaw, C.J.; Josslin, R.; Bobrow, L.: Calcium Ion Regulation of Flagellar Beat Symmetry in Reactivated Sea Urchin Spermatozoa. Biochem Biophys Res Commun 58(1974)795-800

Brokaw, C.J.; Simonick, T.F.: CO_2 Regulation of the Amplitude of Flagellar Bending. In: Cell Motility, pp. 933-940, ed. by R. Goldman, T. Pollard, and J. Rosenbaum. Cold Spring Harbor Laboratory, Cold Spring Harbor, New York, 1976

Brokaw, C.J.; Simonick, T.F.: Mechanochemical Coupling in Flagella. V. Effects of Viscosity on Movement and ATP-Dephosphorylation of Triton-demembranated Sea Urchin Spermatozoa. J Cell Sci 23(1977)227-241

Cantley, L.C., Jr.; Josephson, L.; Warner, R.; Yanagisawa, M.; Lechene, C.; Guidotti, G.: Vanadate is a Potent (Na-K)ATPase Inhibitor Found in ATP Derived from Muscle. J Biol Chem 252(1977)7421-7423

Gibbons, B.H.; Gibbons, I.R.: Flagellar Movement and Adenosine Triphosphatase Activity in Sea Urchin Sperm Extracted with Triton X-100. J Cell Biol 54(1972)75-97

Gibbons, B.H.; Gibbons, I.R.: The Effect of Partial Extraction of Dynein Arms on the Movement of Reactivated Sea Urchin Sperm. J Cell Sci 13(1973)337-357

Gibbons, B.H.; Gibbons, I.R.: Properites of Flagellar "Rigor Waves" Produced by Abrupt Removal of Adenosine Triphosphate from Actively Swimming Sea Urchin Sperm. J Cell Biol 63(1974)970-985

Gibbons, B.H.; Gibbons, I.R.: Functional Recombination of Dynein-1 with Demembranated Sea Urchin Sperm Partially Extracted with KCl. Biochem Biophys Res Commun 73(1976)1-6

Gibbons, B.H.; Gibbons, I.R.: Transient Waveforms during Intermittent Swimming in Live Sea Urchin Sperm. J Cell Biol 75(1977)276A

Gibbons, B.H.; Gibbons, I.R.: Relationship Between the Latent Adenosine Triphosphatase State of Dynein 1 and Its Ability to Recombine Functionally with KC1-extracted Sea Urchin Sperm Flagella. J. Biol Chem 254(1979) 197–201

Gibbons, B.H.; Ogawa, K.; Gibbons, I.R.: The Effect of Antidynein-1 Serum on the Movement of Reactivated Sea Urchin Sperm. J Cell Biol 71(1976)823-831

Gibbons, I.R.: Structure and Function of Flagellar Microtubules. In: International Cell Biology, pp. 348-357, ed. by B.R. Brinkley and K.R. Porter. The Rockefeller University Press, New York, 1976

Gibbons, I.R.; Cosson, M.P.; Evans, J.A.; Gibbons, B.H.; Houck, B.; Martinson, K.H.; Sale, W.S.; Tang, W-J.Y.: Potent Inhibition of Dynein Adenosine Triphosphatase and of the Motility of Cilia and Flagella by Vanadate. Proc Natl Acad Sci 75(1978)2220-2224

Gibbons, I.R.; Fronk, E.: A Latent Adenosine Triphosphatase Form of Dynein 1 from Sea Urchin Sperm Flagella. J Biol Chem 254(1979)187–196

Gibbons, I.R.; Fronk, E.; Gibbons, B.H.; Ogawa, K.: Multiple Forms of Dynein in Sea Urchin Sperm Flagella. In: Cell Motility, pp. 915-932, ed. by R. Goldman, T. Pollard, and J. Rosenbaum. Cold Spring Harbor Laboratory, Cold Spring Harbor, New York, 1976

Goldstein, S.F.: Bend Initiation in Quiescent Sperm Flagella. J Cell Biol 70(1976)71A

Hyams, J.S.; Borisy, G.G.: The Dependence of the Waveform and Direction of Beat of *Chlamydomonas* Flagella upon Calcium Ions. J Cell Biol 67(1975)186A

Kobayashi, T.; Martensen, T.; Nath, J.; Flavin, M.: Inhibition of Dynein ATPase by Vanadate and Its Possible Use as a Probe for the Role of Dynein in Cytoplasmic Motility. Biochem Biophys Res Commun 81(1978)1313-1318

Lindemann, C.B.; Gibbons, I.R.: Adenosine Triphosphate-induced Motility and Sliding of Filaments in Mammalian Sperm Extracted with Triton X-100. J Cell Biol 65(1975)147-162

Ogawa, K.; Gibbons, I.R.: Dynein-2: A New Adenosine Triphosphatase from Sea Urchin Sperm Flagella. J Biol Chem 251(1976)5793-5801

Satir, P.: Studies on Cilia. III. Further Studies on the Cilium Tip and a "Sliding Filament" Model of Ciliary Motility. J Cell Biol 39(1968)77-94

Satir, P.: Ionophore-mediated Calcium Entry Induces Mussel Gill Ciliary Arrest. Science 190(1975)586-587

Satir, P.; Reed, W.; Wolf, D.I.: Ca^{++}-Dependent Arrest of Cilia without Uncoupling Epithelial Cells. Nature 263(1976)520-521

Summers, K.E.; Gibbons, I.R.: Adenosine Triphosphate-induced Sliding of Tubules in Trypsin-treated Flagella of Sea Urchin Sperm. Proc Natl Acad Sci 68(1971)3092-3096

Summers, K.E.; Gibbons, I.R.: Effects of Trypsin Digestion on Flagellar Structures and Their Relationship to Motility. J Cell Biol 58(1973)618-629

Tsuchiya, T.: Ca^{++}-Induced Arrest Response in Triton-extracted Lateral Cilia of *Mytilus* Gill. Experientia 32(1976)1439-1440

Tsuchiya, T.: Effects of Calcium Ion on Triton-extracted Lamellibranch Gill Cilia: Ciliary Arrest Response in a Model System. Comp Biochem Physiol 56A(1977)353-361

Warner, F.D.; Satir, P.: The Structural Basis of Ciliary Bend Formation. Radial Spoke Positional Changes Accompanying Microtubule Sliding. J Cell Biol 63(1974)35-63

ADVANCES IN THE ULTRASTRUCTURAL ANALYSIS OF THE SPERM FLAGELLAR AXONEME

R.W. Linck

Department of Anatomy, Harvard Medical School, Boston, Massachusetts 02115 USA.

The sperm flagellar axoneme is a chemically and structurally complex organelle, capable of generating bending waves from energy derived from the hydrolysis of adenosine triphosphate (ATP). The axoneme is composed of two principal proteins, the dynein ATPase enzymes and the microtubule protein tubulin, and as many as 100 minor component proteins. These macromolecules are arranged in the familiar 9+2 cross-sectional pattern (Fig. 1), characteristic of cilia as well as flagella. Two lines of research have previously indicated the importance in motility of the dynein arm-doublet microtubule interactions and the radial spoke-central pair interactions. First, Gibbons and colleagues (Gibbons, 1963; Gibbons and Gibbons, 1976; Summers and Gibbons, 1971) and Satir and colleagues (Sale and Satir, 1977; Satir, 1968) demonstrated that the principal motive force for flagellar bending derives from sliding movements between doublet microtubules, generated by the interaction of the dynein ATPase arms of one doublet microtubule with the adjacent doublet microtubule. Second, Warner and Satir (1974) and Witman and colleagues (Witman et al., 1976; Witman et al., 1978) showed that some form of interaction between the central-pair microtubules and the radial spokes provides a regulatory function in the conversion of doublet-tubule sliding to bending waves.

Before the molecular mechanism of ciliary and flagellar motility can be understood, several gaps must be filled in our knowledge of the axoneme. First, the three-dimensional arrangement of the various structural elements associated with doublet microtubules, *e.g.*, dynein arms, radial spokes, and nexin fibers, should be determined, since the interactions of these structures must be crucial to the development of bending waves. Second, the high-resolution fine structure of the central-pair microtubule apparatus must be analyzed as well as its interactions with the radial spokes. Ultimately, the various minor component proteins must be analyzed as to their loci in the axoneme and their biochemical function in the propagation and regulation of flagellar bending waves.

The aim of this chapter is to review the ultrastructure of the doublet microtubule and central-pair microtubule apparatuses in relation to ciliary and flagellar motility. Considerable progress has recently been made on analyzing the structure of the central-pair apparatus, and somewhat more attention is given this subject. Although of obvious overall importance to sperm motility, the ultrastructure of the sperm flagellar membrane, mitochondria, fibrous sheath, and dense fibers and the biochemistry of the axoneme proteins are not discussed, and the reader is referred to the other chapters in this volume and to several excellent reviews on these subjects (Fawcett, 1977; Gibbons, 1977; Linck, 1976; Piperno, Huang and Luck, 1977; Stephens and Edds, 1976).

THE THREE-DIMENSIONAL STRUCTURE OF THE DOUBLET-MICROTUBULE COMPLEX

Radial Spokes and Nexin Filaments

As shown in Figure 1, cilia and flagella are typified by a cylindrical arrangement of nine doublet microtubules, each bearing two rows of arms that project toward the adjacent doublet tubule and one row of radial spokes that radiate inward toward the central pair of microtubules. Note that mammalian and cephalopod spermatozoa have additional "dense fibers" associated with the doublet microtubules (Baccetti *et al.*, 1976; Fawcett, 1975).

The radial spokes (Fig. 2) were first observed in thin section by Afzelius (1959) and Gibbons and Grimstone (1960) and subsequently more thoroughly described in negative stain by Hopkins (1970) and in thin section by Warner (1970). Hopkins described the radial spokes of *Chlamydomonas* flagella as consisting of hammer-shaped structures attached perpendicularly to the A-tubule of the doublet microtubule, each spoke with a shaft 5 x 33 nm and a head 5 x 15 nm; the spokes were found to be arranged in pairs with alternate spacings of 30 nm between members of a pair and 70 nm between adjacent pairs. Warner showed similarly paired spoke struc-

---

The author is particularly grateful to Drs. Linda Amos and Gary Olson whose stimulating ideas and efforts contributed greatly to this paper. The work was supported principally by Research Grant No. GM 21527 from the National Institute of General Medical Sciences and by a Postdoctoral Fellowship from the American Cancer Society, both to the author.

© 1979 Urban & Schwarzenberg, Inc. Baltimore-Munich *The Spermatozoon*, edited by D.W. Fawcett and J.M. Bedford

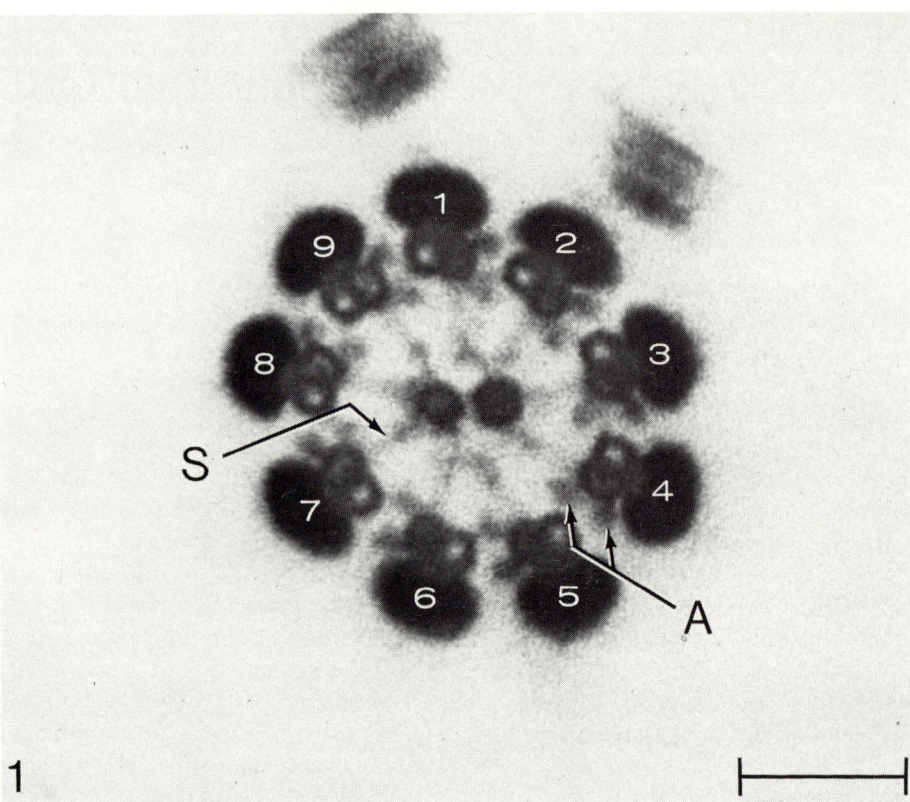

Figure 1. Cross section of demembranated squid (*Loligo pealei*) spermatozoon near the midpiece region and viewed from base to tip. Dense fibers (numbered) are attached to their respective doublet microtubules; the numbering system is that of Afzelius (1959). Pairs of dynein arms (A) are attached to each A-tubule and point in a clockwise direction toward the B-tubule of the adjacent doublet microtubule. Radial spokes (S) emanate from the doublet tubules and point inward where they abut against the central-pair apparatus. Of the central-pair microtubules, the somewhat hollow one nearest doublet tubule No. 8 is believed to be the C_1-tubule possessing the "barbs"; the more solid central tubule nearest doublet No. 3 corresponds to the C_2-tubule containing the projections (see Fig. 11). Scale bar = 0.1 μ.

tures in insect spermatozoa, but reported an alternate spacing of 32 and 56 nm. Subsequently, Warner and Satir (1974) observed radial spokes in molluscan gill cilia to be grouped in triplets, but with complex spacings of 22 and 29 nm between alternate members of a triplet and 36 nm between adjacent triplets. Furthermore, Warner and Satir demonstrated the polarity of the spoke triplets along the axis of the microtubule: the spoke triplets are arranged with the longer 29-nm repeat oriented toward the proximal (basal) end of the axoneme and the shorter 22-nm repeat oriented toward the distal end. In Figure 2 a triplet arrangement of radial spokes is shown as they occur in scallop (*Pecten maximus*) sperm. Several other arrangements of radial spoke pairs and triplets have been reported for various species (Benke and Forer, 1967; Burton, 1967; Chasey, 1972; Olson and Linck, 1977; Perotti, 1969; Witman *et al.*, 1978). From these reports, however, there seems to be no consistent pattern to the arrangement or spacings of radial spokes. Some of the inconsistencies may be real and some may be artifactitious; for example, the processes of fixation, dehydration, and embedment frequently cause specimen shrinkage. Furthermore, some published measurements may result from investigators rounding off their estimates or using noncalibrated electron microscopes. Even with calibrated microscopes, however, the actual magnification may vary by 5-10% owing to hysteresis in the lenses unless precautions are taken (Agar *et al.*, 1974).

Figure 2. Negatively stained preparation of scallop (*Pecten maximus*) sperm flagellar axonemes. Doublet microtubules are displayed on carbon film showing profiles of radial spoke triplets (numbered) and arms (A). The spokes are arranged with the same polarity determined from gill cilia by Warner and Satir (1974); *i.e.*, spoke 1 is located toward the flagellar base and spoke 3 toward the tip. The set of arms remaining on the one tubule is more stable than those on the other tubules and is believed to correspond to the 5-6 bridge arms. These arms appear to be composed of a globular head and a thin tail portion connecting the head to the tubule and pointing distally. See Table 1 for axial spacings. Scale bar = 100 nm.

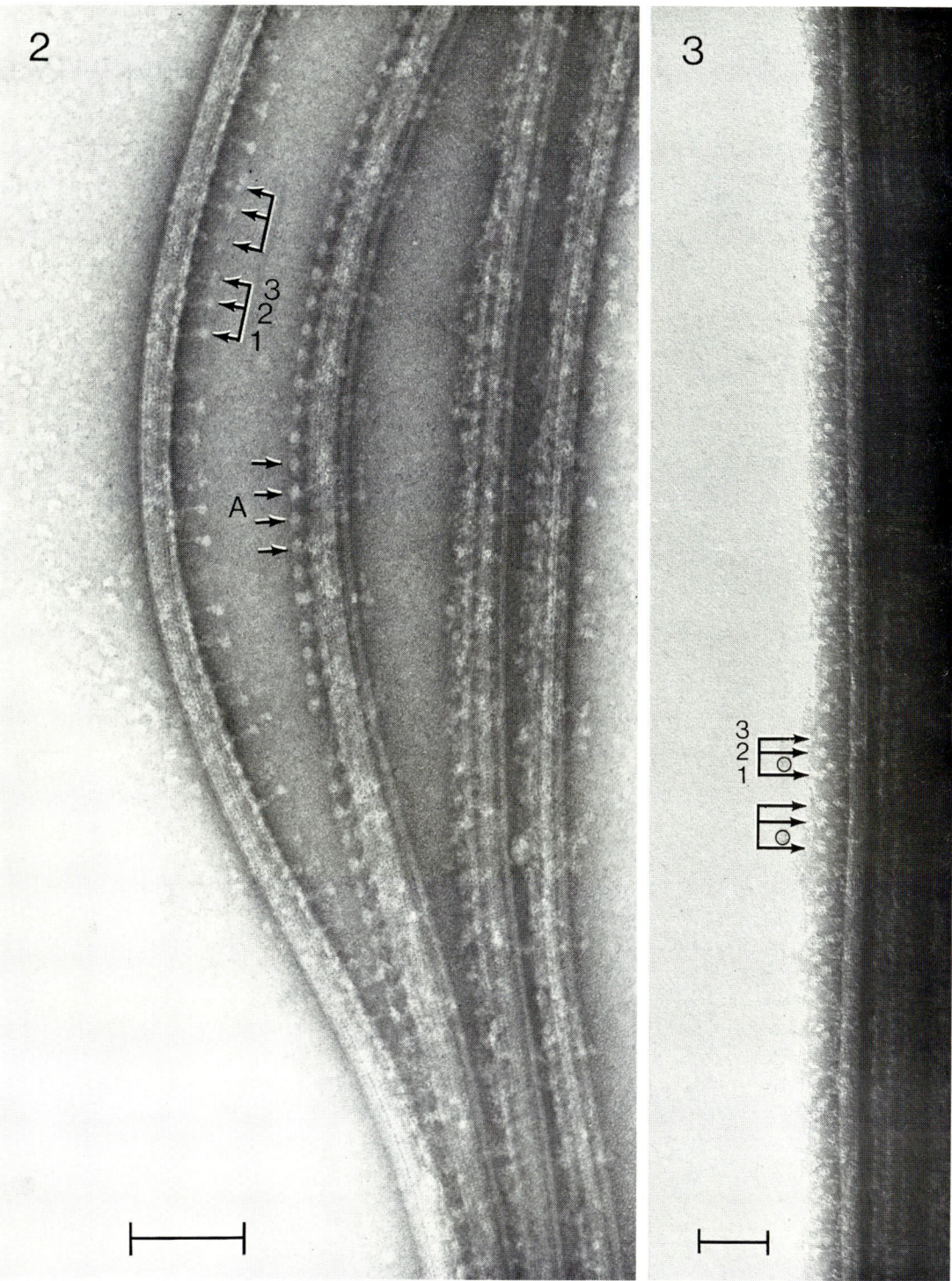

Figure 3. Negatively stained preparation of demembranated rat sperm flagella, showing the radial spoke triplets (numbered). The spokes are arranged with the same polarity as determined from gill cilia by Warner and Satir (1974): spoke 1 toward the flagellar base, spoke 3 toward the flagellar tip. In rat sperm an additional structure a round globule (circles), is seen between spokes 1 and 2 and appears attached to the distal side of spoke 1; its axial repeat along the doublet tubule is therefore 96 nm. See Table 1 for axial spacings of spokes. Reprinted with permission from Olson and Linck (1977). Scale bar = 100 nm.

The author and colleagues have investigated the morphology and axial spacings of the various accessory structures associated with sperm flagella of sea urchins, scallops, and rats, using negative-stain electron microscopy coupled with optical diffraction analysis (Amos et al., 1976; Olson and Linck, 1977). Optical diffraction analysis enables one to calculate periodic spacings independent of any specimen shrinkage or expansion, calibration standards or hysteresis in the microscope. The axial period of the microtubule monomeric subunit is 4.0 nm as determined by X-ray diffraction of native, hydrated microtubule preparations (Cohen et al., 1971; Mandelkow et al., 1977); thus the microtubule subunit represents an internal standard against which the spacings of accessory structures can be measured in optical transforms of images of negatively stained axonemes. Figures 2 and 3 show radial spokes from scallop and rat sperm respectively; Table 1 gives their axial spacings. The spokes are lollipop-shaped structures with shafts measuring 5 x 28 nm attached to the A-tubule and possessing globular spoke heads approximately 17 nm in diameter. The spokes are grouped in triplets with alternate spacings of 24 and 32 nm with 40 nm between adjacent triplets, the overall axial repeat of the spoke triplets being 96 nm. All axial spacings of the spoke triplets, and furthermore the axial spacings of all axoneme components, are exact multiples of the 4-nm tubulin monomer (8-nm tubulin dimer) repeat (Table 1); thus these structures must be arranged in some precise way on the surface lattice of the microtubule (Amos et al., 1976; Amos and Klug, 1974; Linck and Amos, 1974). The polarity of the spokes in rat spermatozoa is also the same as that determined by Warner and Satir (1974) for the gill cilia of fresh water molluscs, namely, the longer 32-nm spoke repeat is located toward the sperm head and the shorter 24-nm spacing toward the flagellar tip (Fig. 3 and 4). Therefore, according to the numbering system of Warner and Satir, radial spoke 1 is located proximally and spoke 3 distally. The arrangement and polarity of the radial spokes on the doublet microtubule is depicted in Figure 5.

Rat spermatozoa possess two additional structural elements associated with the axoneme. First, a globular component is positioned between radial spokes 1 and 2 (Fig. 3 and 4). The diameter of the globule is approximately 17 nm, and successive structures along a given tubule have a center-to-center spacing of 96 nm. The globule appears most likely to represent a hitherto unresolved structural component of the radial spoke triplet; however, whether it is specific to rat spermatozoa or is a universal structure of the flagellar axoneme remains to be determined.

A second type of structural element is seen as a system of long, thin filaments traversing between adjacent doublet tubule-dense fiber complexes (Fig. 4). These filaments are attached to the tubule axis at 96-nm intervals, and although their precise point of attachment is not certain, they appear to join in register either with the globules just mentioned or with the radial spoke proximal to the globule (i.e., radial spoke 1). These thin filaments probably correspond to the so-called nexin fibers described in other species. In partially fractionated axonemes of *Tetrahymena* cilia, Gibbons (1965) showed adjacent A-tubules to be connected by thin filaments, for which Stephens (1970) suggested the term "nexin" fibers. Subsequent workers provided further evidence that the nexin fibers were attached at 96-nm intervals along the doublet tubules (Dallai et al., 1973; Linck, 1973; Warner, 1976; Witman et al., 1978). A controversy exists as to whether the nexin filaments directly interconnect the A-tubules of adjacent doublet tubules (Gibbons, 1965; Linck, 1973; Stephens, 1970), or whether they connect the A-tubule of one doublet to the B-tubule of the adjacent doublet (Warner, 1976; Witman et al, 1978). Although the reasoning is good on both sides of the argument, the fact is that the exact structural attachments of the nexin fibers are still unclear. Furthermore, the possibility must be considered that a single nexin fiber may run continuously from one doublet to the next with structural contacts to both A- and B-tubules of each doublet tubule.

Nexin fibers are considered to play two roles in the axoneme: 1) a purely structural role to maintain the ninefold symmetric cylinder of doublet microtubules in the "resting" state of the axoneme, and 2) an active role as elastic elements to regulate the amount of shear displacement between adjacent doublet tubules during active sliding (Brokaw and Simonick, 1977; Dallai et al., 1973; Olson and Linck, 1977; Stephens, 1970; Warner, 1976; Witman et al., 1978). The highly stretched appearance of the nexin fibers in Figure 4 attests to these hypotheses.

Dynein Arms

The pairs of arms attached to each A-tubule and projecting toward the neighboring B-tubules were first described in thin section by Afzelius (1959). Gibbons (1961) and Gibbons and Grimstone (1960) showed that these arms exist as two rows of periodic projections attached along the surface of the microtubule; and Gibbons (1963, 1965) subsequently demonstrated that these arms are composed of the ATPase protein dynein. The inner and outer row of dynein arms are now known to differ both in their morphology (Allen, 1968) and in their chemical composition (Gibbons & Gibbons, 1973;

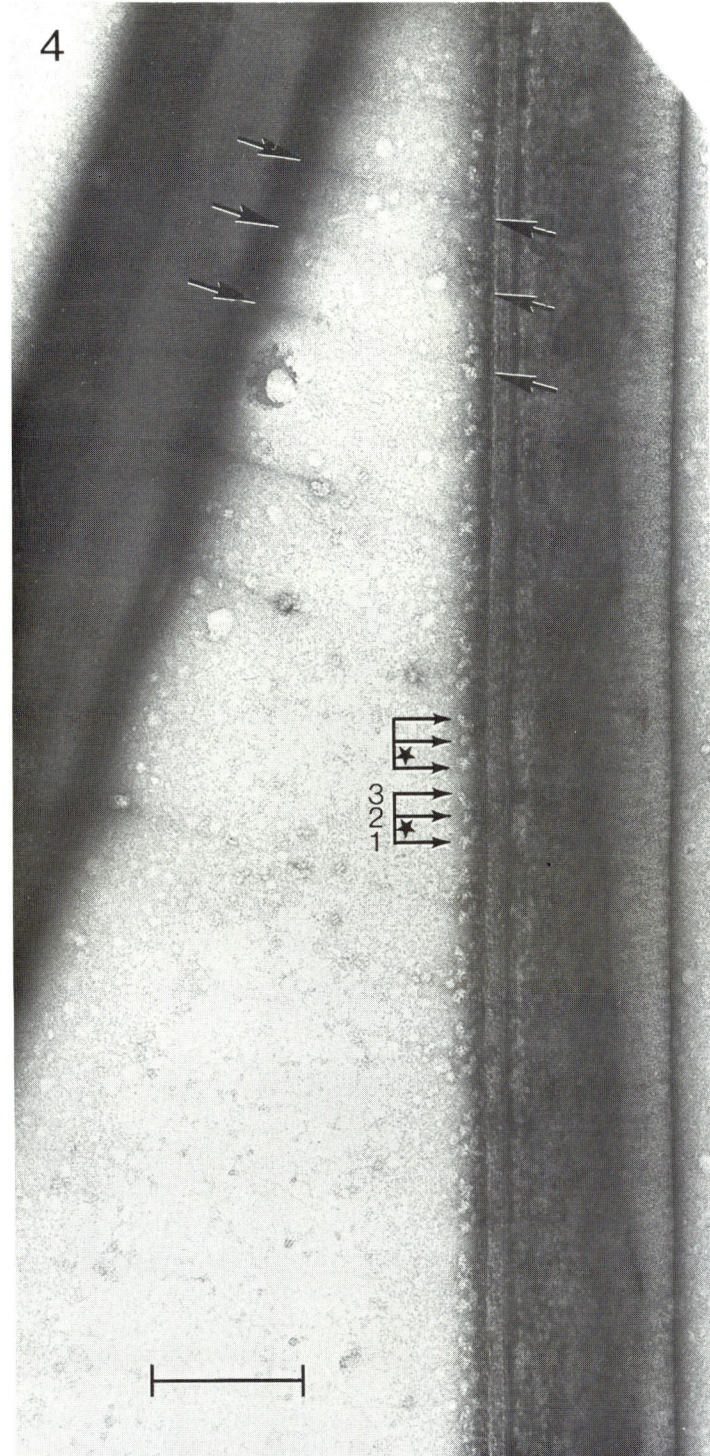

Figure 4. Negatively stained preparation of demembranated rat sperm flagella. The radial spoke triplets (numbered) and the associated globules (stars) are arranged along a doublet microtubule and associated dense fiber. Thin, filamentous strands (large arrows), apparently elastic in nature, interconnect two adjacent doublet tubules; these strands appear to attach to the doublet tubule in register with radial spoke 1 or its associated globule. The axial repeat of these fibers is therefore 96 nm. These filaments probably correspond to the so-called nexin fibers. Reprinted with permission from Olson and Linck (1977). Scale bar = 200 nm.

Table 1. Axial Spacings and Relative Numbers of Axoneme Components

Axoneme Component:	Axial Spacing* (nm)	Number of Components per 96 nm of Axoneme
Doublet microtubule complex:		
Doublet microtubules	4 (monomer)[a]	
	8 (dimer)[b]	2484 tubulin dimers[c]
Inner dynein arms[d]	24	32
Outer dynein arms[d]	24	32
5-6 bridge arms (inner & outer)	24[e]	8
Radial spokes[f,g]		27 radial spokes
S_1-S_2	32	9 (S_1)
S_2-S_3	24	9 (S_2)
S_3-S_1	40	9 (S_3)
S_1-S_1	96	
Nexin fibers	96[h]	?
Central-pair apparatus:		
Microtubules	4 (monomer)[a]	
	8 (dimers)[b]	312 tubulin dimers[c]
Central bridges	16[i]	6 (one row?)
Sheath projections	16	6 (one row)
		24 (four rows)
C_1-barbs	32	3 (one row?)

*Values were obtained by optical diffraction analysis of scallop sperm (Amos, et al., 1976) and rat sperm (Olson and Linck, 1977), except as noted.

[a]From X-ray diffraction of native microtubules (Cohen et al., 1971; Mandelkow et al., 1977).

[b]From optical diffraction of negatively stained microtubules (Amos and Klug, 1974).

[c]Based on 23 protofilaments/doublet tubule, 13 protofilaments/singlet tubule (Tilney et. al., 1973).

[d]Does not include 5-6 bridge.

[e]See text; corrected from original measurements of Warner and Satir (1974).

[f]Nomenclature of spokes is that of Warner and Satir (1974) who obtained slightly smaller repeat values from thin sections of gill cilia.

[g]The only known exception to this pattern of spacings is in Chlamydomonas (Witman et al., 1978).

[h]Dallai et al., 1973; Linck, 1973; Olson and Linck, 1977; Stephens, 1970; Warner, 1976; Witman et al., 1978.

[i]See text; corrected from original measurements of Warner (1976).

Gibbons et al., 1976; Kincaid et al., 1973; Linck, 1973); the chemistry of the dyneins, however, will not be dealt with here, and the reader is referred to the recent review by Gibbons (1977). Numerous values for the axial periodicity of the dynein arms have been reported, the inconsistencies apparently due to specimen shrinkage and to the superimposition of the two rows of dynein arms in the plane of viewing. Chasey (1972) and Allen and Borisy (1974) obtained what is now considered to be the correct value for the axial spacing of the dynein arms, i.e. 24 nm; however, considering that the inner and outer dynein arms differ chemically and morphologically, it was not clear whether the 24-nm repeat applied to only one or to both sets of arms. Amos et al. (1976) and Warner (1976) correctly determined that the axial spacing of both rows of arms is 24 nm. In addition, these investigators found that the two rows of dynein arms are not in register, but that the outer row of arms is shifted by approximately 4 nm (Warner) or approximately 9 nm (Amos et al.) toward the flagellar tip relative to the inner arm; thus a pair of arms are arranged in a left-handed manner on the A-tubule surface lattice (Fig. 5). Finally, Warner and colleagues (Warner and Mitchell, 1978; Warner et al., 1977) have recently shown that in negatively stained preparations the dynein arm appears to be composed of three morphological subunits with molecular weights of approximately 350,000 daltons. These findings are also in agreement with biochemical data from Gibbons' laboratory (Gibbons, 1977; Gibbons et al., 1976).

Details concerning the arrangement of the dynein arms and radial spokes are summarized in Table 1 and diagrammed in Figure 5.

The 5-6 Bridge

Afzelius (1959) and Gibbons and Fronk (1972) noted that in sea urchin sperm the inner and outer arms of doublet tubule No. 5 are connected to doublet tubule

No. 6, forming what is now commonly referred to as the 5-6 bridge. The 5-6 bridge has also been observed in the gill cilia of the fresh water molluscs *Anodonta cataracta* (Gibbons, 1961) and *Elliptio complanatus* (Satir, 1965; Warner, 1974). The structural and chemical composition of the "arms" comprising the 5-6 bridge cannot be assumed to be the same as that of the other eight sets of dynein arms. Gibbons (1961) and Warner and Satir (1974) reported values of 22.5 nm and 21.9 nm respectively for the axial spacing of the arms of the 5-6 bridge; however, these values are subject to the errors of specimen shrinkage discussed earlier and furthermore the values given do not distinguish between the inner and outer arms of the bridge. Regardless, Warner and Satir (1974) state that the axial repeat of the 5-6 bridge (21.9 nm, uncorrected) is identical to that of the dynein arms; thus assuming the correct values of 24 nm for the dynein arm spacing (Amos *et al.*, 1976), the axial repeat of the 5-6 bridge must also be 24 nm. Preliminary observations by Linck (Fig. 2) suggest that the axial periodicity of the 5-6 bridge is in fact 24 nm, but that the structural conformation of the bridge is different from that of the other dynein arms (*cf.* Fig. 2 with those of Warner and Mitchell, 1978).

The 5-6 bridge is apparently not always well preserved and has not been observed in many species. Olson and Linck (1977), however, made the following observation which demonstrates that a specialization must exist between doublets 5 and 6 in rat spermatozoa. When rat spermatozoa are demembranated with Triton X-100 in the presence of Mg^{2+}-adenosine triphosphate (ATP), the flagella undergo a disintegrating process wherein doublet tubules 4, 5, 6, and 7 (and their accompanying dense fibers) slide out of the fibrous sheath in a proximal direction, leaving doublet tubule-dense fiber complexes 8, 9, 1, 2, and 3 and the central pair in their unaltered conformation within the fibrous sheath (Fig. 6). Of doublet tubule-dense fiber complexes 4, 5, 6, and 7, numbers 4 and 7 are always left as individual members, whereas doublet tubule-dense fibers 5 and 6 are always paired. A 5-6 bridge is not observed in thin sections or negative stain of normal or disintegrated rat sperm; thus either a 5-6 bridge exists in rat spermatozoa but is not preserved by conventional fixation conditions, or some other structural specialization besides the "arms" is responsible for the connection between doublets 5 and 6. (For a more detailed analysis of the ATP-dependent sliding phenomena of rat sperm flagella, see Olson and Linck, 1977).

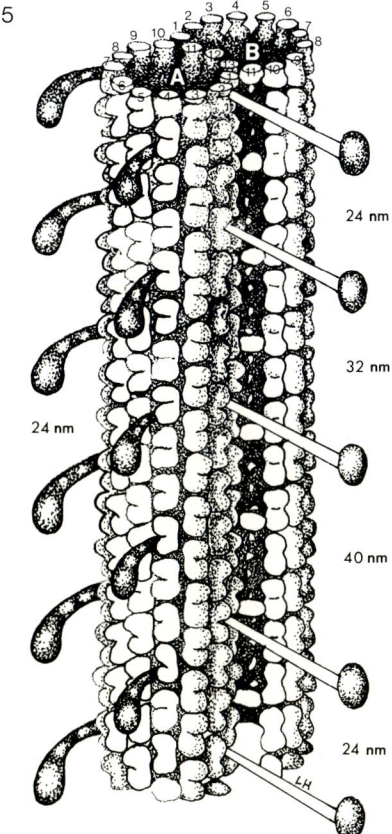

Figure 5. A 3-dimensional model of the doublet microtubule complex based on data from electron microscope images, optical diffraction analysis and computer reconstruction of flagellar axonemes (Amos, Linck & Klug, 1976; Olson & Linck, 1977). The doublet tubule is oriented with the proximal or basal end down. Certain structural features of the model have been established: (1) The two rows of dynein arms are arranged each with axial repeats of 24 nm, and the arms are slightly staggered such that the outer arms are approximately 9 nm nearer the flagellar tip relative to the inner arms. The dynein arms appear to be composed of three morphological subunits as demonstrated by Warner & Mitchell (1978). (2) Members of the radial spoke triplets have alternate spacings of 24 and 32 nm with 40 nm separating adjacent triplets. (3) The polarity of the spoke triplets is that determined by Olson & Linck (1977) and Warner & Satir (1974); i.e., the 32 nm spacing is proximal to the 24 nm spacing. Other details of the model are shown for the sake of illustration only: the exact attachment sites of the arms and spokes on the surface lattice of the tubule are not known, nor is the axial position (i.e., phase relationship) of the spokes relative to the inner dynein arms; periodic subunits (asterisk) are shown connecting the inner wall of the B-tubule to the A-tubule (Linck, 1976).

ULTRASTRUCTURE OF THE CENTRAL-PAIR MICROTUBULE COMPLEX

Cilia and flagella of most species possess a pair of singlet microtubules in the center of the axoneme (Fig. 1). Flagella of some species lack their central pair (*i.e.*, 9+0

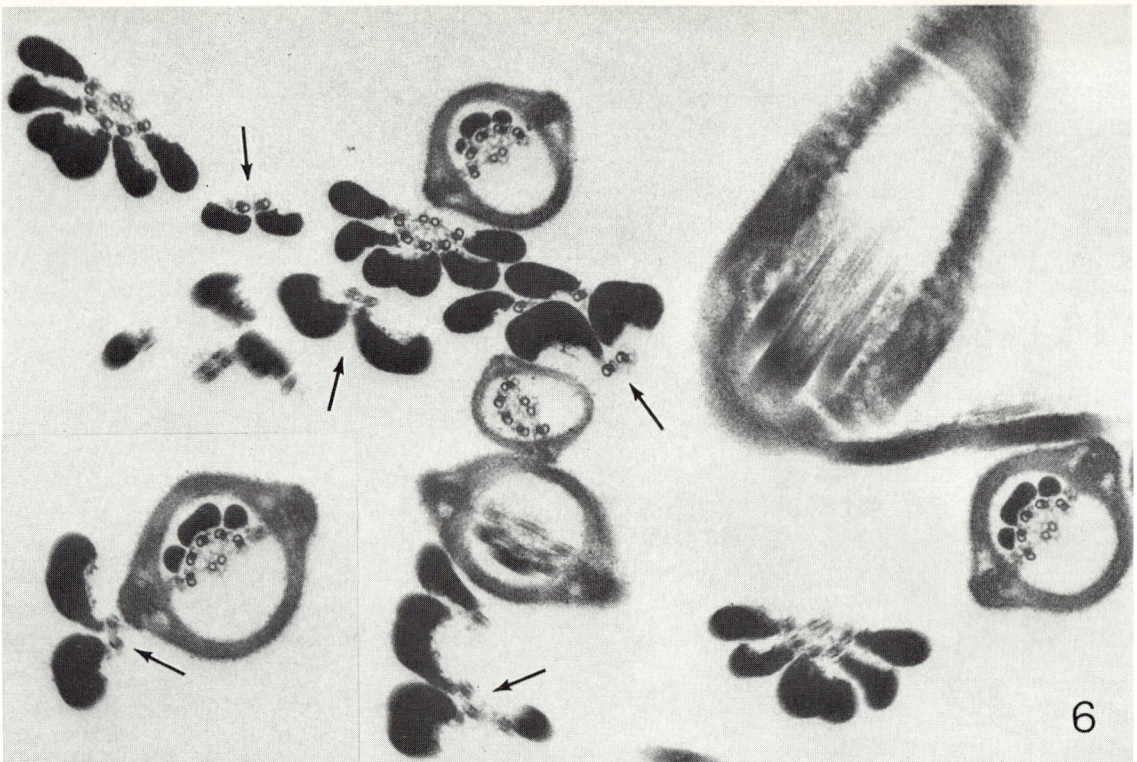

Figure 6. ATP-dependent disintegration of demembranated rat sperm. Cross sections show that doublet microtubules 4, 5, 6, and 7 and their associated dense fibers specifically slide out of the fibrous sheath; doublet tubule-dense fibers No. 8, 9, 1, 2, and 3 and the central-pair apparatus are retained within the fibrous sheath. Of the disintegrated fibers, No. 4 and 7 remain free, while 5 and 6 almost always remain paired (arrows), suggesting the presence of a 5-6 bridge or some other structure preventing these fibers from sliding apart. See Olson and Linck (1977); reprinted with permission.

axonemes), yet are motile (Baccetti et al., 1978); in other cases the central microtubules are replaced by a single dense core of material (Burton, 1967; Henley et al., 1969; Phillips, 1969; Silveira, 1960). In species whose flagella naturally possess a central pair, however, it has been elegantly demonstrated by Witman et al. (1976, 1978) that genetic removal of the central pair results in the loss of motility; furthermore, these investigators have shown that interactions between the radial spokes and the central pair regulate the dynein-mediated sliding between outer doublet tubules. The work of Warner and Satir (1974) had previously demonstrated that a cycle of spoke detachment-reattachment to the central "sheath" occurs in bent regions of ciliary axonemes, and postulated that this mechanism is responsible for converting outer doublet microtubule sliding into bending waves. With the above as an introduction to the role of the central pair in axoneme motility, the fine structure of the central-pair microtubule apparatus will now be considered.

In cross section, the two central-pair tubules are connected at their closest points by short bridges (6 nm long) corresponding to the rungs of a ladder (Gibbons, 1961; Olson and Linck, 1977; Warner, 1976; Witman et al., 1978). Occasionally in cross section (Fig. 7a) the bridge appears to be divided, and it is not yet clear whether one or two rows of bridges join the two central tubules. Warner (1976) reported an axial repeat of 14.5 nm for the central bridge in negatively stained gill cilia; this value, however, should probably be corrected to 16 nm because of the measuring errors discussed above and because the bridge is reported to be the same

Figure 7. A montage showing the appearance of the central-pair microtubule apparatus in rat sperm flagella. a: In cross section a central-pair apparatus remains attached to a doublet tubule-dense fiber complex by means of a connection between the radial spoke (S) and one of the central sheath projections (P). Four rows of sheath projections are found in rat sperm, although all rows may not be chemically and structurally equivalent. A central bridge (CB) joins the two tubules of the central pair. Scale bar = 50 nm. b: In negative stain a central-pair apparatus is seen twisting along its length and out of the plane of the carbon film; as the central pair twists, the sheath projections (P) seen in profile in the bottom section of the specimen appear as globules superimposed over the tubules (top section of specimen). c: Usually in negative stain the two central tubules differ in appearance; the C_1-tubule appears coated with extra material while the C_2-tubule is clean and more evenly stained. Scale bar = 100 nm for b and c. Reprinted with permission from Olson and Linck (1977).

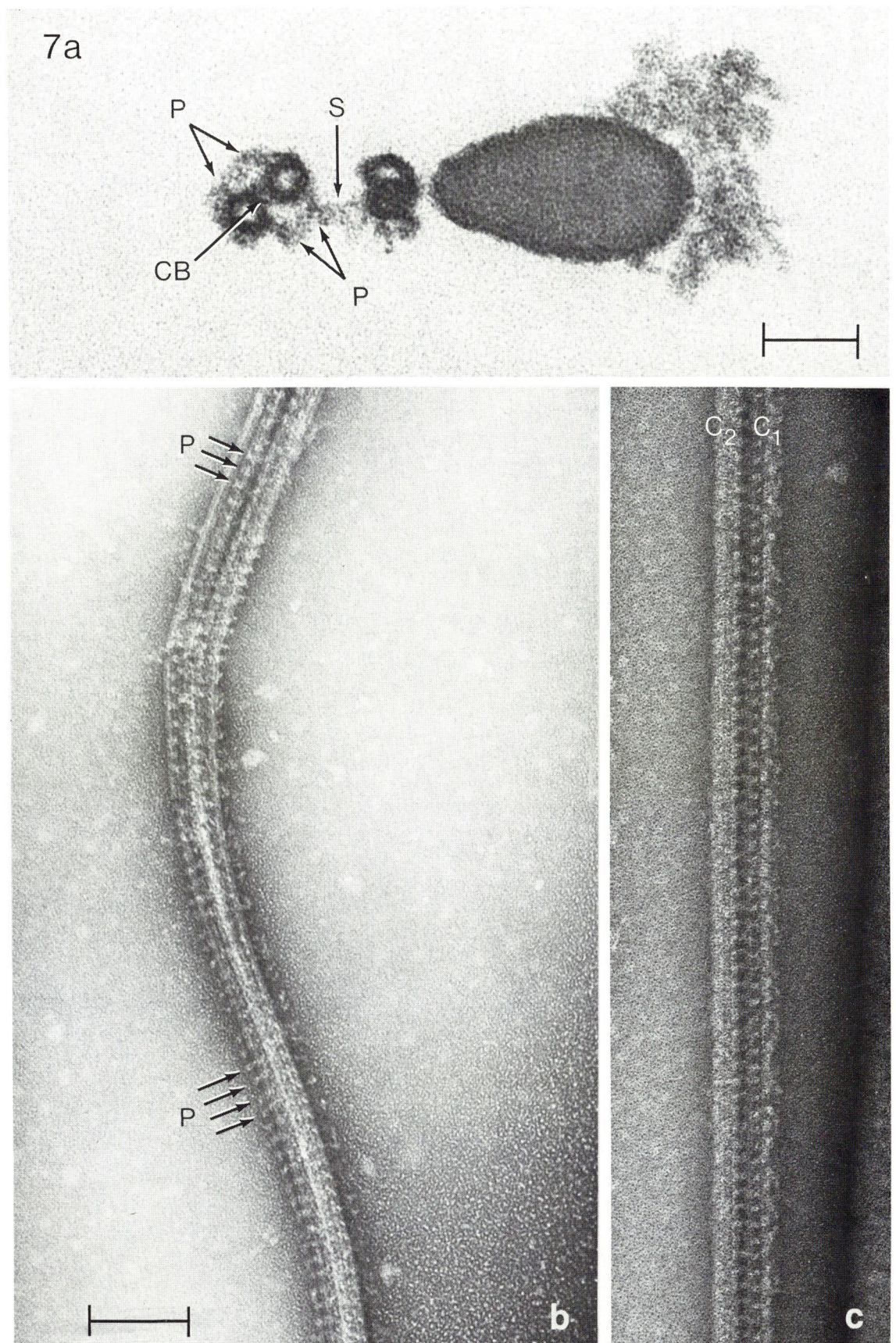

as the 16-nm repeating sheath projections (Olson and Linck, 1977; Warner, 1976).

Early studies described a helical filament or sheath wrapped about the central tubules (Gibbons and Grimstone, 1960; Gibbons, 1961). Later investigations by Chasey (1969), Hopkins (1970) and Warner and Satir (1974) indicate, however, that the "sheath" is more likely composed of rows of projections attached to each central-pair tubule. The projections measure 18 nm long and are attached at 16 nm intervals along the tubule axis (Fig. 7b). With certain exceptions noted below, each microtubule of the central pair possesses two rows of projections which subtend an angle of 120° (Fig. 7a). The tips of the projections in each row are in close apposition to the tips of the projections emanating from the neighboring tubule, however, whether the tips of one row of projections are in structural contact with the projections on the adjacent tubule is unclear. This description is characteristic of gill cilia of molluscs (Warner and Satir, 1974), rat spermatozoa (Olson and Linck, 1977), and *Chlamydomonas* flagella (Witman et al., 1978). The flagella of some species appear to lack one or more rows of the central sheath projections: for example, in squid spermatozoa one central-pair tubule possesses a single row of projections and the other tubule possesses none (Fig. 11); this is discussed in more detail below. In *Tetrahymena* cilia, one central tubule bears two rows of projections while the other tubule bears none (Chasey, 1969). Perhaps in some species certain rows of projections are more labile than others and are missed in observation, but it may be that these differences are real and consequently that a flagellum need not possess a full complement of projections to be functionally motile. Also, it is not known whether the different rows of projections are chemically and/or functionally equivalent.

Recently several new observations have been made regarding the high resolution ultrastructure of the central-pair microtubule complex (Olson and Linck, 1977; Linck and Olson, 1976,[1]). These observations were made by optical diffraction analysis of negatively stained rat spermatozoa and from direct electron microscopic analysis of isolated squid sperm central pair. Because of some differences in these species, they are discussed separately. The results are summarized in Table 1.

Rat Sperm Central Pair

Rat sperm central pair as discussed above possess four sets of sheath projections with axial repeats of 16 nm (Fig. 7); however, in negative stain the two microtubules usually appear to be different (Fig. 7c). Invariably the C_2-tubule is relatively smooth and evenly stained, while the C_1-tubule is coated with extra material. In order to analyze the possible periodic nature of this material, negatively stained specimens were analyzed by optical diffraction techniques. Diffraction patterns (Fig. 8) indicated a strong 16-nm^{-1} layer line, as expected from the 16-nm repeat of the projections. In addition, however, a 32-nm layer line and its harmonics were also present. Such images were optically analyzed by layer-line filtering to average periodic information and to eliminate "noise" according to the technique of Klug and DeRosier (1966) (Fig. 9). The prominent 16-nm axial repeats are superimposed over both tubules and correspond to the sheath projections. The most notable feature, however, is a row of barb-shaped structures attached along the outer edge of the C_1-tubule, repeating at 32-nm intervals. Details of the barb-shaped structure are best seen in the filtered image, but their presence is also apparent in the original image. The barbs are straight, approximately 24 nm long and are set at an angle of about 30° from the axis of the tubule; in nearly all specimens the barbs possess globular tips and larger globular bases. The tips of the barbs are oriented toward the proximal (or basal) end of the flagellum. This polarity was determined by relating their orientation to other polarity markers along the flagellum, such as the fibrous sheath or the radial spokes of adjacent doublet tubules (Fig. 10).

The barb-shaped components are not trivial structures specific to rat spermatozoa. They have been observed in the flagella of sea urchin, scallop, and squid sperm (Linck and Olson, 1976) and evidence for them has been seen in other published micrographs of cilia as well (Chasey, 1972; Warner and Satir, 1974). The function of these components is unclear, but there is some evidence to suggest that a row of barbs may interact with the radial spokes of one (or more) doublet tubule. In Figure 10 for example, a central-pair apparatus and a doublet tubule are attached to one another in a negative stain preparation, presumably by means of radial spoke-central sheath interactions. Optical filtering of this image reveals a number of features regarding the structural organization preserved in this specimen but not readily apparent in the original image. First, the radial spokes appear in their usual triplet form, spoke triplets being spaced at 96 nm axially, center to center, and individual members of the triplets spaced at 24 and 32 nm. As described earlier, the polarity of the spoke triplet is such that the 32-nm spacing is located proximally. Located between spokes 1 and 2 is an electron density corresponding in shape and position to the

---

[1] Linck, R.W.; Olson, G.E.: in preparation

96-nm globule described in Figure 3. These globules are faintly visible between spokes 1 and 2 in the original, unfiltered image. A most interesting result of the filtering is that a system of barbs arising from the C_1-tubule can be seen projecting toward and apparently contacting the radial spoke heads. The barbs are set at an angle of approximately 65° to the tubule axis, and they display the same polarity as described above on free central pairs, *i.e.*, the tip of the barb is oriented toward the base of the flagellum. The angle of the barb is greater in the case of the doublet-central pair complex (65°) than in the case of individual dissociated central pairs (*i.e.*, 30°; Fig. 9). Furthermore, every third barb, *i.e.*, those adjacent to radial spoke 3, are set at a somewhat more shallow angle of 45°. The significance of the changes observed in the barb angle is unclear; however, these changes could reflect structurally altered states of barb components in their interaction with the radial spokes.

Squid Sperm Central Pair

In order to study further the interaction between radial spokes and central pairs, it is desirable to obtain quantities of pure central pairs sufficient for biochemical and further structural analysis. Methods have recently been developed for the isolation of milligram amounts of pure central-pair apparatuses from squid, *Loligo pealei*, sperm (Linck and Olson, 1976, in preparation). The method involves first a demembranation of the sperm with Triton X-100, followed by extraction with 0.5M KCl. The method relies on the fact that the cen-

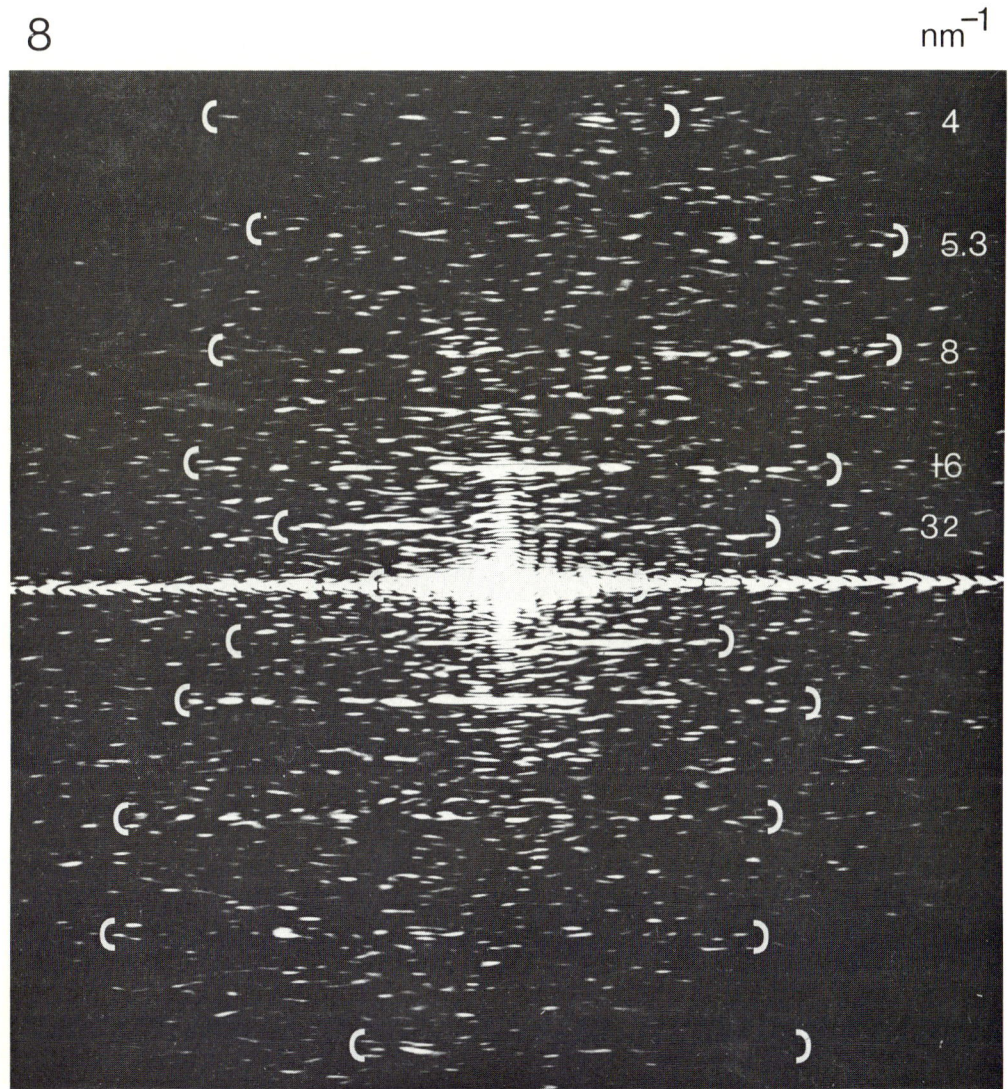

Figure 8. Optical diffraction pattern of the central-pair apparatus shown in Figure 9a. Layer lines indexing on a fundamental 32-nm repeat can be seen. Only the even orders are labelled; however, odd order layer lines can also be seen at 10.7, 6.5, and 4.6 nm^{-1}. Parentheses designate the length and width of each layer line and equatorial reflections used in the optical reconstruction of Figure 9b. Reprinted with permission from Olson and Linck (1977).

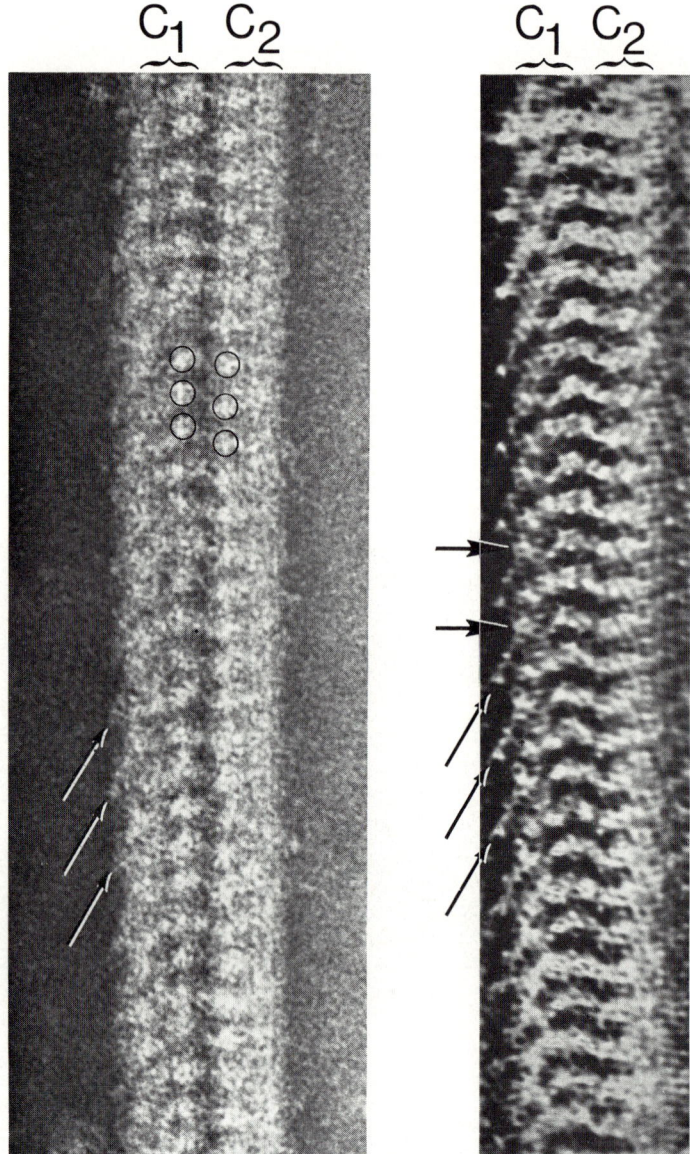

Figure 9. a: Original image of a negatively stained central-pair apparatus from rat sperm showing the C_1- and C_2-tubules and the projections (circles) superimposed over the tubules. b: Filtered image reconstructed from a mask prepared from the optical transform shown in Figure 8. Note the prominent "barb-shaped" elements (oblique arrows) repeating at 32 nm axially along the left lateral edge of the C_1-tubule. The "barbs" are set at an angle of approximately 30° to the tubule axis and have globular tips and larger globular bases (large arrows) where they attach to the tubule surface. The barbs can be faintly seen in the original image. Details of the projections in the filtered image are obscured by the superimposition of the front and back sides of the central pair.

Figure 10. Image analysis of a doublet microtubule-central pair complex from rat sperm. a: Original image of a negatively stained specimen wherein a doublet microtubule (D) remains attached to the central-pair apparatus (C_1C_2) by means of a connection between the radial spokes (numbered) and the central sheath components. b: filtered image and c: tracing made directly from Figure b, reveal the structural details between the doublet tubule (D) and the C_1-tubule of the central pair. (All images are oriented with the base of the flagellum toward the bottom of the page, and a segment of the filtered image is shown below Figure a to clarify the spatial relationship of the doublet and central-pair tubules in the two images.) The radial spoke heads are evident as large electron-dense structures (white globules designated by numbered arrows in Figure b, black dots in Figure c). The 96-nm repeating globules (open circles) is located on the distal side of spoke 1. The polarity of the spoke triplets is shown in Figures

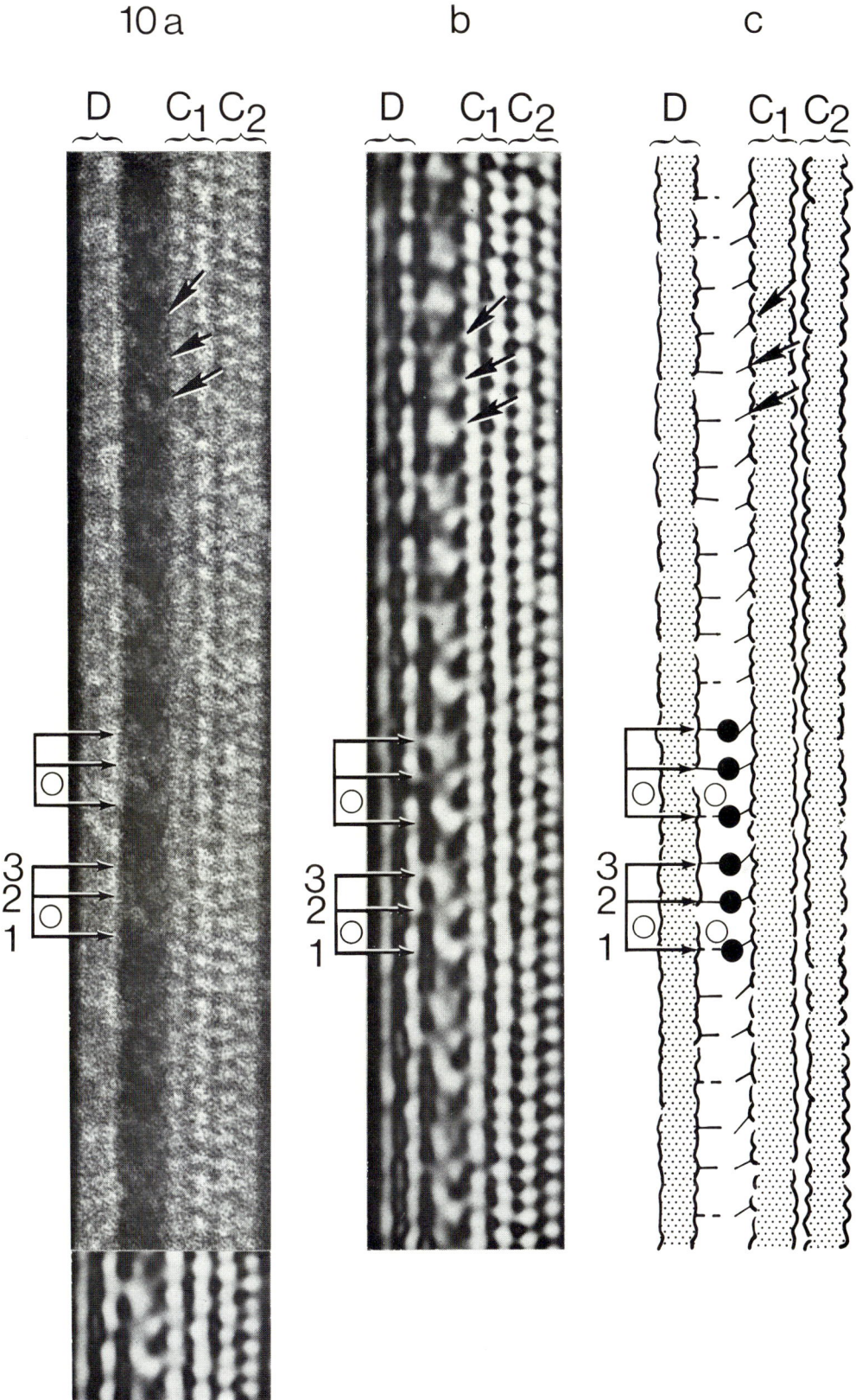

2 and 3. Barb-shaped elements (diagonal arrows) are attached to the left lateral edge of the C_1-tubule. The tips of the barbs point toward the proximal end of the flagellum and are in register with the radial spoke heads. The barbs associated with spoke heads 1 and 2 are tilted at an angle of 65° to the tubule axis (compare with the 30° angle of barbs in Figure 9). Barbs associated with spoke head 3 appear to be tilted somewhat less, i.e., 45°. The significance of these changes in barb angle is unclear but would be expected if all barbs in Figure 10 are attached to their respective spoke heads. Some of the details of the filtering are faintly visible in the original image.

tral-pair tubules are released by such treatment whereas the doublet tubules and their associated dense fibers remain firmly associated with the sperm heads. The central pair can thus be easily purified and recovered by differential centrifugation. A preparation of isolated central pairs is shown in cross section in Figure 11a. Examination of cross sections and negatively stained preparations have revealed a number of interesting findings.

As with rat sperm the two members of the central-pair microtubules from squid sperm appear to be different. First, in negative stain one tubule, the C_1-tubule, possesses the barb-shaped elements along its outer edge (Fig. 11b, c); these components have the same structure and axial repeat (32 nm) as in rat sperm. The C_2-tubule appears to have but a single row of 15-17 nm long projections repeating at 16 nm axially (Fig. 11b, c) in contrast to rat sperm which have four rows. In hundreds of particles examined by negative stain the C_1-tubules have never been observed to possess the 16-nm repeating projections, and the C_2-tubules have never been seen to possess the 32-nm periodic barbs. Although only one row of projections seems to exist in the squid central pair, it is of course possible that certain rows of projections might be selectively solubilized by the isolation or staining procedures, in which case we are describing here a subset of stable structures. The number of rows of barbs is less certain: since they lie at a shallow angle to the tubule axis, additional rows could be superimposed over the tubule surface in negative stain; cross sections in fact indicate as many as three tufts of material associated with the surface of the C_1-tubule (Fig. 11a, inset).

A second feature of the squid central pair is that the two tubules appear to be fundamentally different. In negative stain the outer surface of the C_2-tubule with its 16-nm repeating projections appears smooth and evenly contrasted by uranyl acetate, while the lumen of this tubule is rarely filled with stain (Fig. 11b, c). Correlated with this observation is the fact that in cross section (Fig. 11a) the C_2-tubule, which can be identified as having a single prominent projection, appears solid. The negative stain and cross-sectional views would, therefore, suggest that some additional material (*i.e.*, protein) is continuously organized along the lumen of the C_2-tubule. The C_1-tubule on the other hand appears periodically mottled in negative stain (Fig. 11c) and in cross section appears either hollow or solid with about equal frequency, indicating that material is also arranged within the lumen of the C_1-tubule but with a definite periodic repeat.

On the basis of the details discussed above, it is possible to define the asymmetry of the central pair within the axoneme. Comparison of cross sections of demembranated squid spermatozoa (Fig. 1) and cross sections of isolated central pairs (Fig. 11a), indicates that the C_2-tubule (solid with projection) is positioned near outer doublet tubule No. 3, while the C_1-tubule (hollow) is nearest doublet No. 8. Although there is no direct proof, this same asymmetric pattern has been deduced to apply to rat spermatozoa (Olson and Linck, 1977).

A third and final observation regarding the central-pair microtubules isolated from squid sperm is that they can be induced to form paracrystalline sheets. Isolated central-pair apparatuses tend to hybridize with one another and in negatively stained preparations they can be seen lying side by side along their coaxial plane (Fig. 12). The way in which this pairing occurs is highly regular. The C_2'-tubule of one central-pair apparatus always hybridizes with its homologous tubule, the C_2''-tubule of another central-pair apparatus. This homologous pairing always takes place in an antiparallel fashion, such that the barbs of the adjoining C_1'-tubule point in one direction while those of the C_1''-tubule point in the opposite direction. The exact mechanism by which such pairing takes place between homologous C_2-tubules is not known at this time, but presumably it involves the interactions of the C_2-projections or the surfaces of the two C_2-tubules. Optical diffraction analysis of central-pair apparatuses is now underway, and hopefully this technique will reveal answers to the three-dimensional structure, the unique differences, and this unusual pairing phenomenon of central-pair microtubules.

Figure 11. Montage showing the structural details of central-pair microtubules isolated from squid sperm. a: Thin section showing a field of isolated central pair; inset, one central-pair apparatus displays the frequently hollow appearance of the C_1-tubule, the always solid appearance of the C_2-tubule, a single prominent projection (P) on the C_2-tubule, and three tufts of material attached to the outer surface of the C_1-tubule (cf. Fig. 1). b and c: Specimens negatively stained with uranyl acetate showing the 32nm-repeating barbs (B) on the C_1-tubule and the 16nm-repeating projections (P) on the C_2-tubule. Note the inherent differences in the C_1- and C_2-tubules: The C_2-tubule is smooth and evenly stained in uranyl acetate and appears solid in cross section (Fig. a, inset), indicating that the lumen is filled with stain-excluding material. On the other hand, the lumen of the C_1-tubule is regularly mottled in negative stain and is frequently hollow in cross section, suggesting a periodic arrangement of material in the lumen.

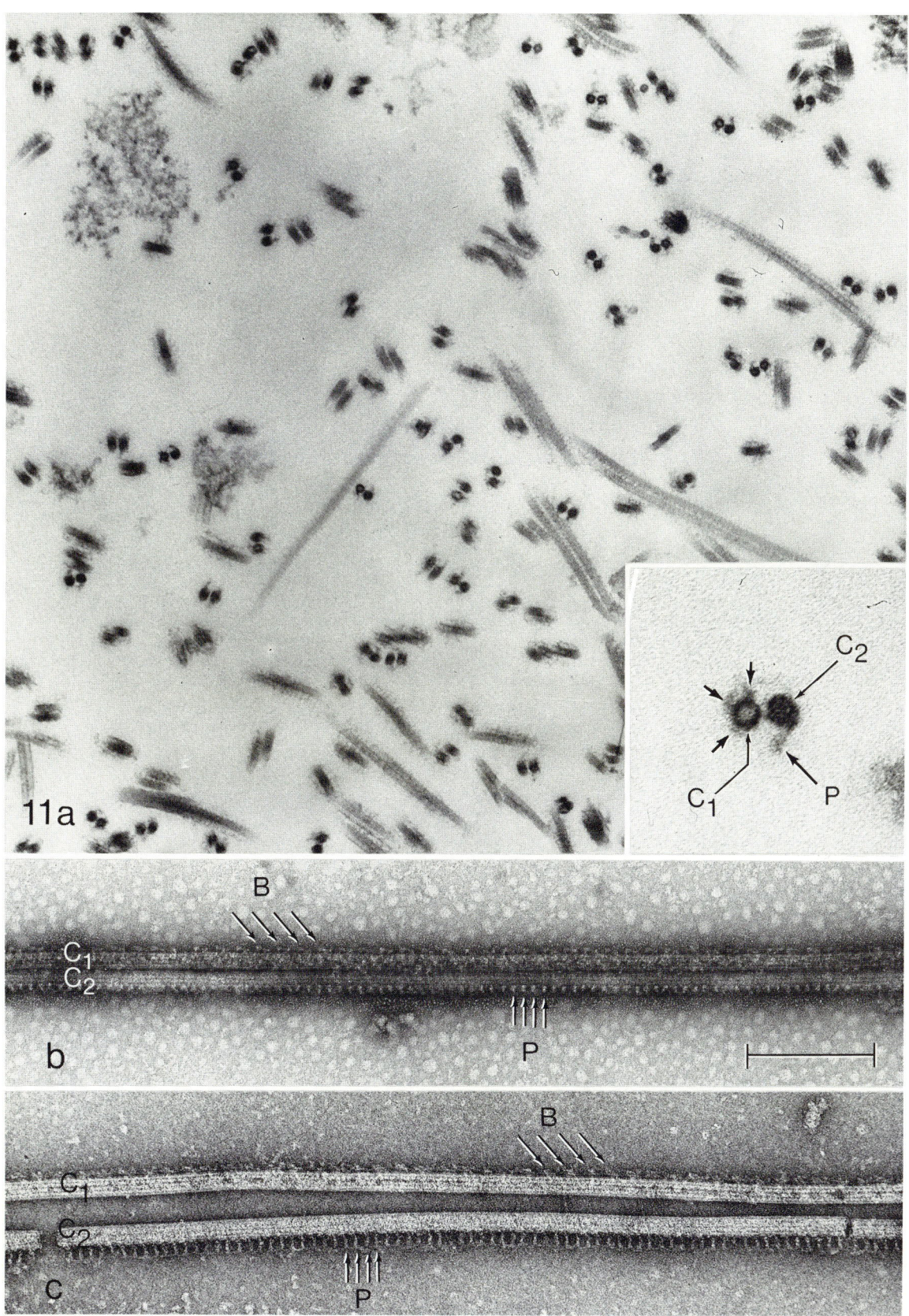

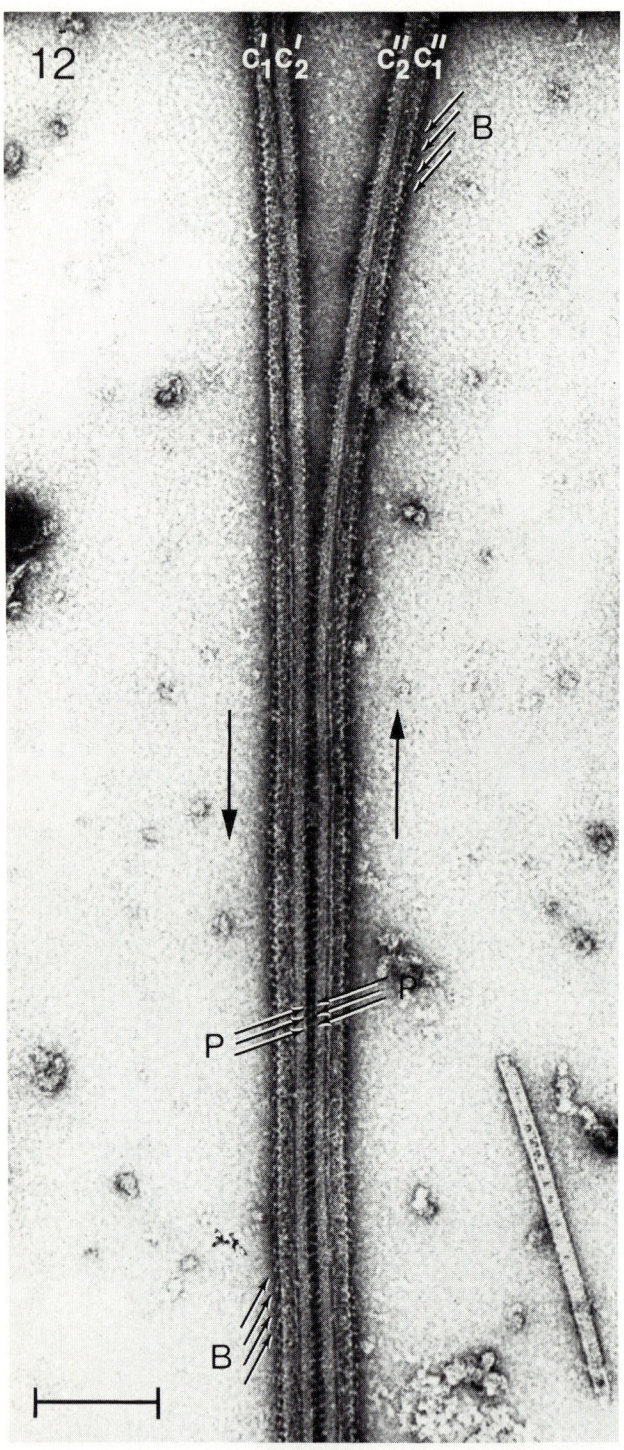

Figure 12. A negatively stained specimen showing a central-pair duplex obtained from isolated squid sperm. The duplex is formed by the pairing of homologous C_2-tubules in an antiparallel fashion. Barbs (B) on the left central pair ($C_1'C_2'$) point down, while the barbs on the right central pair ($C_1''C_2''$) point up; the large arrows indicate the polarity of their respective central pair and point toward the basal end. A regular interaction of the rows of projections (P) can be seen in the region between the C_2-tubules in contact. The pairing of the C_2-tubules in an antiparallel manner commonly occurs in preparations of isolated central pairs and thus is not merely a coincidental stacking phenomenon. Scale bar = 200 nm.

REFERENCES

Afzelius, B.: Electron Microscopy of the Sperm Tail. Results Obtained with a New Fixative. J Biophys Biochem Cytol 5(1959)269-278

Agar, A.W.; Alderson, R.H.; Chescoe, D.: Principles and Practice of Electron Microscope Operation. In: Practical Methods in Electron Microscopy, ed. by A.M. Glauert. North-Holland/American Elsevier, New York, 1974

Allen, C.; Borisy, G.G.: Structural Polarity and Directional Growth of Microtubules of *Chlamydomonas* Flagella. J Mol Biol 90(1974)381-402

Allen, R.D.: A Reinvestigation of Cross Sections of Cilia. J Cell Biol 37(1968)825-831

Amos, L.A.; Klug, A.: Arrangement of Subunits in Flagellar Microtubules. J Cell Sci 14(1974)523-549

Amos, L.A.; Linck, R.W.; Klug, A.: Molecular Structure of Flagellar Microtubules. In: Cell Motility, Book C, pp. 847-867, ed. by R.D. Goldman, T.D. Pollard and J.L. Rosenbaum. Cold Spring Harbor Laboratory, Cold Spring Harbor, New York, 1976

Baccetti, B.; Burrini, A.G.; Dallai, R.; Pallini, V.: The Dynein Electrophoretic Bands in Axonemes Naturally Lacking the Inner or the Outer Arm. J Cell Biol, 80(1979)334-340

Baccetti, B.; Pallini, V.; Burrini, A.G.: The Accessory Fibers of the Sperm Tail. III. High Sulfur and Low Sulfur Components in Mammals and Cephalopods. J Ultrastruct Res 57(1976)289-308

Behnke, O.; Forer, A.: Evidence for Four Classes of Microtubules in Individual Cells. J Cell Sci 2(1967)169-192

Brokaw, C.J.; Simonick, T.F.: Motility of Triton-demembranated Sea Urchin Sperm Flagella during Digestion by Trypsin. J Cell Biol 75(1977)650-665

Burton, P.R.: Fine Structure of the Unique Central Region of the Axial Unit of Lung Fluke Spermatozoa. J Ultrastruct Res 19(1967)166-172

Chasey, D.: Observations on the Central Pair of Microtubules from the Cilia of *Tetrahymena pyriformis*. J Cell Sci 5(1969)453-458

Chasey, D.: Further Observations on the Ultrastructure of Cilia from *Tetrahymena pyriformis*. Exp. Cell Res 74(1972)471-479

Cohen, C.; Harrison, S.C.; Stephens, R.E.: X-ray Diffraction from Microtubules. J Mol Biol 59(1971)375-380

Dallai, R.; Bernini, F.; Giusti, F.: Interdoublet Connections in the Sperm Flagellar Complex of *Sciara*. J Submicrosc Cytol 5(1973)137-145

Fawcett, D.W.: The Mammalian Spermatozoon. Dev Biol 44(1975)394-436

Fawcett, D.W.: Unsolved Problems in Morphogenesis of the Mammalian Spermatozoon. International Cell Biology, pp. 588-601, ed. by B.R. Brinkley and K.R. Porter. Rockefeller University Press, 1977

Gibbons, B.H.; Gibbons, I.R.: The Effect of Partial Extraction of Dynein Arms on the Movement of Reactivated Sea Urchin Sperm. J Cell Sci 13(1973)337-357

Gibbons, B.H.; Gibbons, I.R.: Functional Recombination of Dynein 1 with Demembranated Sea Urchin Sperm Partially Extracted with KCl. Biochem Biophys Res Comm 73(1976)1-6

Gibbons, I.R.: The Relationship between the Fine Structure and Direction of Beat in Gill Cilia of a Lamellibranch Mollusc. J Biophys Biochem Cytol 11(1961)179-205

Gibbons, I.R.: Studies on the Protein Components of Cilia from *Tetrahymena pyriformis*. Proc Natl Acad Sci USA 50(1963)1002-1010

Gibbons, I.R.: Chemical Dissection of Cilia. Arch Biol (Liège) 76(1965)317-352

Gibbons, I.R.: Structure and Function of Flagellar Microtubules. In: International Cell Biology, pp. 348-357, ed. by B.R. Brinkley and K.R. Porter. Rockefeller University Press, 1977

Gibbons, I.R.; Fronk, E.: Some Properties of Bound and Soluble Dynein from Sea Urchin Sperm Flagella. J Cell Biol 54(1972)365-381

Gibbons, I.R.; Fronk, E.; Gibbons, B.H.; Ogawa, K.: Multiple Forms of Dynein in Flagellar Axonemes of Sea Urchin Sperm. In: Cell Motility, Book C, pp. 915-932, ed. by R.D. Goldman, T.D. Pollard, J.L. Rosenbaum. Cold Spring Harbor Laboratory, Cold Spring Harbor, New York, 1976

Gibbons, I.R.; Grimstone, A.V.: On Flagellar Structure in Certain Flagellates. J Biophys Biochem Cytol 7(1960)697-716

Henley, C.; Costello, D.P.; Thomas, M.B.; Newton, W.D.: The "9+1" Pattern of Microtubules in Spermatozoa of *Mesostoma* (Platyhelminthes, Turbellaria). Proc Natl Acad Sci USA 64(1969)849-856

Hopkins, J.M.: Subsidiary Components of the Flagella of *Chlamydomonas reinhardii*. J Cell Sci 7(1970)823-839

Kincaid, H.L.; Gibbons, B.H.; Gibbons, I.R.: The Salt-extractable Fraction of Dynein from Sea Urchin Sperm Flagella: An Analysis by Gel Electrophoresis and by Adenosine Triphosphate Activity. J Supramol Struct 1(1973)461-470

Klug, A.; DeRosier, D.J.: Optical Filtering of Electron Micrographs: Reconstruction of One-sided Images. Nature 212(1966)29-32

Linck, R.W.: Chemical and Structural Differences between Cilia and Flagella from the Lamellibranch Mollusc, *Aequipecten irradians*. J Cell Sci 12(1973)951-981

Linck, R.W.: Flagellar Doublet Microtubules: Fractionation of Minor Components and α-Tubulin from Specific Regions of the A-Tubule. J Cell Sci 20(1976)405-439

Linck, R.W.; Amos, L.A.: The Hands of Helical Lattices in Flagellar Doublet Microtubules. J Cell Sci 14(1974)551-559

Linck, R.W.; Olson, G.E.: Structural Chemistry of Sperm Flagellar Central and Outer Doublet Microtubules. In: Contractile Systems in Non-Muscle Tissues, pp. 229-240, ed. by S.V. Perry, A. Margreth, R.S. Adelstein. Elsevier/North Holland, Amsterdam, 1976

Linck, R.W.; Olson, G.E.: in preparation.

Mandelkow, E.; Thomas, J.; Cohen, C.: Microtubule Structure at Low Resolution by X-ray Diffraction. Proc Natl Acad Sci USA 74(1977)3370-3374

Olson, G.E.; Linck, R.W.: Observations of the Structural Components of Flagellar Axonemes and Central Pair Microtubules from Rat Sperm. J Ultrastruct Res 61(1977)21-43

Perotti, M.E.: Ultrastructure of the Mature Sperm of *Drosophila melanogaster* Meig. J Submicrosc Cytol 1(1969)171-195

Phillips, D.M.: Exceptions to the Prevailing Pattern of Tubules (9 + 9 + 2) in the Sperm Flagella of Certain Insect Species. J Cell Biol 40(1969)28-43

Piperno, G.; Huang, B.; Luck, D.J.L.: Two-dimensional Analysis of Flagellar Proteins from Wild-type and Paralyzed Mutants of *Chlamydomonas reinhardtii*. Proc Natl Acad Sci Usa 74(1977)1600-1604

Sale, W.S.; Satir, P.: The Direction of Active Sliding in *Tetrahymena* Cilia. Proc Natl Acad Sci USA 74(1977)2045-2049

Satir, P.: Studies on Cilia. II. Examination of the Distal Region of the Ciliary Shaft and the Role of the Filaments in Motility. J Cell Biol 26(1965)805-834

Satir, P.: Studies on Cilia. III. Further Studies on the Cilium Tip and a "Sliding Filament" Model of Ciliary Motility. J Cell Biol 39(1968)77-94

Silveira, M.: Ultrastructure Studies on a "Nine Plus One" Flagellum 1. J Ultrastruct Res 26(1969)274-288

Stephens, R.E.: Isolation of Nexin—The Linkage Protein Responsible for the Maintenance of the Nine-fold Configuration of Flagellar Axonemes. Biol Bull 139(1970)438a

Stephens, R.E.; Edds, K.T.: Microtubules: Structure, Chemistry and Function. Physiol Rev 56(1976)709-777

Summers, K.E.; Gibbons, I.R.: Adenosine Triphosphate-induced Sliding of Tubules in Trypsin-treated Flagella of Sea Urchin Sperm. Proc Natl Acad Sci USA 68(1971)3092-3096

Tilney, L.G.; Bryan, J.; Bush, D.J.; Fujiwara, K.; Mooseker, M.S.; Murphy, D.B.; Snyder, D.H.: Microtubules: Evidence for 13 Protofilaments. J Cell Biol 59(1973)267-275

Warner, F.D.: New Observations on Flagellar Fine Structure. The Relationship between Matrix Structure and the Microtubule Component of the Axoneme. J Cell Biol 47(1970)159-182

Warner, F.D.: Crossbridge Mechanisms in Ciliary Motility. In: Cell Motility, Book C, pp. 891-914, ed. by R.D. Goldman, T.D. Pollard and J.L. Rosenbaum. Cold Spring Harbor Laboratory, Cold Spring Harbor, New York, 1976

Warner, F.D.; Mitchell, D.R.: Structural Conformation of Ciliary Dynein Arms and the Generation of Sliding Forces in *Tetrahymena* Cilia. J Cell Biol 76(1978)261-277

Warner, F.D.; Mitchell, D.R.; Perkins, C.R.: Structural Conformation of the Ciliary ATPase Dynein. J Mol Biol 114(1977)367-384

Warner, F.D.; Satir, P.: The Structural Basis of Ciliary Bend Formation. Radial Spoke Positional Changes Accompanying Microtubule Sliding. J Cell Biol 63(1974)35-63

Witman, G.B.; Fay, R.; Plummer, J.: *Chlamydomonas Mutants*: Evidence for the Roles of Specific Axonemal Components in Flagellar Movement. In: Cell Motility, Book C, pp. 969-986, ed. by R.D. Goldman, T.D. Pollard and J.L. Rosenbaum. Cold Spring Harbor Laboratory, Cold Spring Harbor, New York, 1976

Witman, G.B.; Plummer, J.; Sander, G.: *Chlamydomonas* Flagellar Mutants Lacking Radial Spokes and Central Tubules. Structure, Composition, and Function of Specific Axonemal Components. J Cell Biol 76(1978)729-747

CONTRIBUTED PAPERS

LOCALIZATION OF DYNEIN IN SEA URCHIN SPERM FLAGELLA

H. Mohri, K. Ogawa, and T. Miki-Noumura

Department of Biology, University of Tokyo, Komaba, Meguro-Ku, Tokyo 153, Japan; Department of Cell Biology, National Institute for Basic Biology, Okazaki 444, Japan; Department of Biology, Ochanomizu University, Tokyo 112, Japan

Since Gibbons (1963) succeeded in solubilizing the adenosine triphosphatase (ATPase) protein dynein from *Tetrahymena* cilia and in recombining dynein with the outer doublet microtubules—with concomitant disappearance and reappearance of the arms attaching along A-tubule of the outer doublets—the dynein molecule has been believed to correspond to the arms that are considered to be responsible for the sliding-microtubule mechanism of ciliary and flagellar movement (Satir, 1968; Summers and Gibbons, 1971; Brokaw, 1972). Such solubilization and recombination of dynein have also been observed in sea urchin, starfish, and fish sperm flagella (Gibbons, 1965; Mohri et al., 1969; Ogawa and Mohri, 1972; Hayashi and Higashi-Fujime, 1972; Mabuchi et al., 1976). Electron micrographs of the solubilized dynein fractions showed globular units of approximately 100Å, which appear to be a monomeric form of dynein (Gibbons and Rowe, 1965; Mohri et al., 1969; Warner et al., 1977). The evidence, however, does not appear to be sufficient for identification of dynein ATPase as the arms. There are several polypeptide bands in the high molecular weight region of sodium dodecyl sulfate (SDS)-polyacrylamide gel after electrophoresis of ciliary and flagellar axonemes or as crude dynein preparations; of these only two, designated as dynein 1 and dynein 2 in sea urchin sperm flagella, have been identified as dyneins possessing ATPase activity (Ogawa and Mohri, 1975; Ogawa and Gibbons, 1976; I.R. Gibbons et al., 1976). Furthermore, a recent electron microscopic examination of arms and solubilized dynein has suggested that each arm consists of three to four subunits, the sizes of which correspond to monomeric dynein (Warner et al., 1977).

Both the outer and inner arm have been considered to be equivalent, consisting of the same dynein molecule. However, they differ from each other in structural configuration as observed in the cross sections or negatively stained images of cilia and flagella (Allen, 1968; Warner and Mitchell, 1978). In addition, brief extraction of the axonemes with $0.5M$ KCl or NaCl solubilizes only the outer arms, preferentially extracting dynein 1 or A-band polypeptide on SDS-polyacrylamide gel and leaving the inner arms intact (Kincaid et al., 1973; Gibbons and Gibbons, 1973, 1976; Mabuchi et al., 1976; I.R. Gibbons et al., 1976; Warner et al., 1977). The experiments with Triton X-100-treated spermatozoa of the sea urchin *Colobocentrotus atratus*—which showed a reduction of beat frequency to about half that of the control after the KCl extraction and restoration of the beat frequency by adding the dynein-1 fraction to the KCl-extracted spermatozoa (Gibbons and Gibbons, 1973, 1976)—appear to prove functional equivalency between the outer and inner arm. Such a type of reduction in the beat frequency, however, has not been obtained with other species of sea urchins (Brokaw, personal communication; Okuno, personal communication).

In order to clarify the above-mentioned points, the authors have examined identification of dynein as the arms, using an antiserum prepared against a tryptic fragment of dynein 1 retaining the original ATPase activity (Fragment 1A) purified from sperm flagella of the sea urchin *Anthocidaris crassispina* (Ogawa and Mohri, 1975). Furthermore, some trials have been made to differentiate the roles played by the outer and inner arms. In this chapter, the results so far obtained on structure and function of the arms in flagellar movement are summarized.

MATERIALS AND METHODS

Anti-Fragment 1A serum was prepared in a rabbit as described by Ogawa and Mohri (1975). Fragment 1A was purified from sperm flagella of *Anthocidaris crassispina*. Details for indirect immunofluorescence microscopy (Nikon FK) and immunoelectron microscopy (Hitachi HS9) with ferritin, using the antiserum, are described elsewhere (Ogawa et al., 1977a). For the experiments, spermatozoa of the sea urchins *A. crassispina*, *Hemicentrotus pulcherrimus*, and *Pseudocentrotus depressus*

The authors are grateful to Dr. M. Okuno, Ms. H. Masuda, Ms. H. Hata, Ms. Y. Yano, and Ms. T. Mohri for their contributions to several facets of the present research. This work was supported by grants-in-aid from the Ministry of Education, Science, and Culture, Japan and a grant from the Ford Foundation.

© 1979 Urban & Schwarzenberg, Inc. Baltimore-Munich *The Spermatozoon*, edited by D.W. Fawcett and J.M. Bedford

were demembranated by extraction with 20 volumes of 0.025% (vol/vol) Triton X-100 in 0.15M KCl, 4mM MgSO$_4$, 1mM CaCl$_2$, 2mM ethylenediamine tetraacetate (EDTA), 5mM 2-mercaptoethanol, and 2mM Tris-HCl buffer, pH 8.2, for 1 min at room temperature, followed by several washings with the above medium without Triton X-100. In some cases, the demembranated flagella (axonemes) were isolated from the heads by homogenization and centrifugation.

Motility of Triton-treated spermatozoa, demembranation of spermatozoa with Triton X-100, and reactivation by ATP in the presence of either anti-Fragment 1A serum or preimmune serum have been observed as described by Okuno et al. (1976).

The ATP-driven tubule extrusion was observed by the method developed by Brokaw and Simonick (1976) with some modification (Masuda et al., 1978). One hundred μl of the demembranated spermatozoa was treated for 90 s at room temperature with 0.5 ml of ATP-free reactivation medium (0.15M KCl, 2.2mM MgSO$_4$, 2mM dithiothreitol, 2mM EGTA, 0.5mM CaCl$_2$, 2% polyethylene glycol [M$_r$ 20,000], 20mM Tris-HCl buffer, pH 8.4) containing 2 μg trypsin (Sigma Chemical Co., T 8003). For terminating the digestion, 4 μg of soybean trypsin inhibitor was added. The trypsin-treated axonemes were then broken into fragments of about 10-20 μm with a pipette and the suspension of the fragmented axonemes was diluted tenfold with the ATP-free reactivation medium. When necessary, the suspension was mixed with the ATP-free reactivation medium containing anti-Fragment 1A serum and kept for 30 min at 0°C before the addition of 0.5mM ATP. In another series of experiments, both trypsin and ATP were added at once to the fragmented axonemes without prior digestion by trypsin. Dark-field illumination was used for observation of tubule extrusion as described previously (Miki-Noumura and Kamiya, 1976). The extrusion process was recorded with a CTC-9000 Night Vision Camera System including a video tape recorder (Ikegami Tsushinki Co.).

For the removal of the outer arms, the spermatozoa were first suspended in 0.04% Triton X-100, 0.15M NaCl, 4mM MgSO$_4$, 0.5mM EDTA, 1mM dithiothreitol, 2mM Tris-HCl buffer, pH 8.0, and homogenized. The axonemes were isolated by centrifugation (12,000 rpm for 10 min at 4°C) of the supernatant produced when they were freed from the heads by a prior centrifugation at 4000 rpm for 10 min. The sedimented axonemes were treated with 0.5M NaCl, 4mM MgSO$_4$, 1mM dithiothreitol, 2mM Tris-HCl, pH 8.0, for various periods of time at room temperature, and then centrifuged at 12,000 rpm for 10 min at 4°C. The extent of extraction of the outer arms was checked by electron microscopy. The specimens were prefixed with 2.5% glutaraldehyde, postfixed with 1% osmium tetroxide, embedded in Epon 812, and thin-sectioned.

RESULTS AND DISCUSSION

Observation by Immunoelectron Microscopy

By indirect immunofluorescence microscopy, either the flagella of demembranated spermatozoa or the isolated axonemes were brightly stained with antiserum against Fragment 1A, indicating the presence of dynein 1 in the axonemes (cf. Fig. 1 in Ogawa et al., 1977a). The sperm heads, especially apical and basal regions, were also fluorescent. This latter point is discussed below.

On thin cross sections of the axonemes treated with the anti-Fragment 1A serum and the ferritin-conjugated IgG fraction of goat anti-rabbit IgG (Fig. 1a), ferritin particles were found only in the vicinity of the distal end of each outer arm, but not near the other structures (including the inner arms) within the axoneme. When either the antiserum absorbed with Fragment 1A (Fig. 1b) or the preimmune serum (Fig. 1c) was used, no ferritin particles were detected. Figure 2 shows the longitudinal thin sections of the axonemes treated with the anti-Fragment 1A serum. Again, the ferritin labels were found along the one side of outer doublet microtubules and outside the axonemes, but not inside the axonemes. When the labelling was not so heavy, the average minimum interval between the adjacent ferritin particles was approximately 20 nm, thus probably corresponding to the reported 24-nm value of the periodicity of the arms on the A-tubule, (Amos et al., 1976). The rather unexpected result of nonlabelling of the inner arms could be caused by the presence of the outer arms, which prevents the antiserum and the ferritin-conjugated IgG from reaching the inside of the axonemes. The removal of the outer arms by the extraction with 0.5M NaCl, however, did not bring about any labelling of the inner arms and other structures inside of the axonemes (Fig. 1d). Still, it is possible that the interdoublet links and other components are obstacles against the labelling of the inner arms. We have not observed any ferritin particles near the inner arms even when the 9 + 2 structures appeared as opened or fragmented arrays, or when the trypsin-treated axonemes were examined; although the outer arms were always labelled with ferritin.

Examination of electron micrographs of about 400 axonemes revealed that the outer arms from the No. 5 outer doublets were rarely labelled with ferritin particles, in contrast to almost 100% labelling of the outer

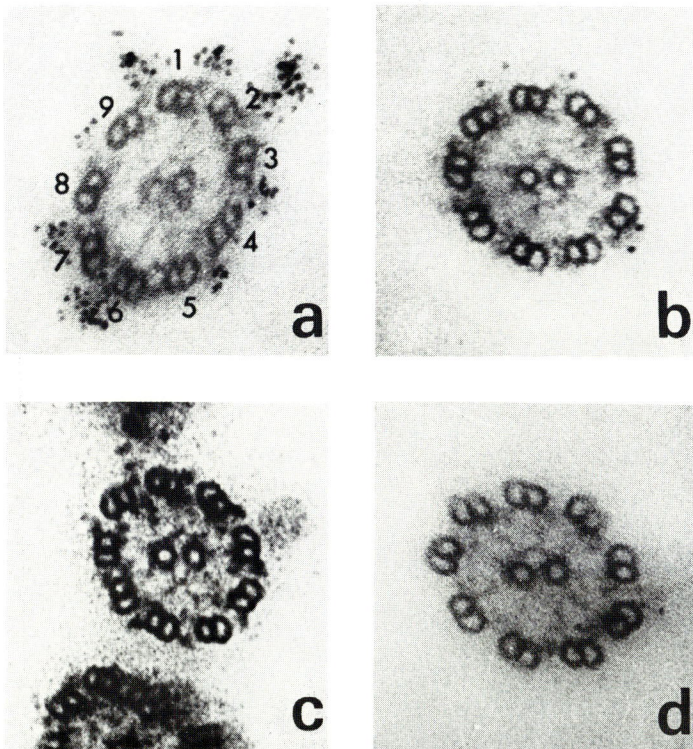

Figure 1. Immunoelectron microscopy of sea urchin (*Anthocidaris crassispina*) sperm axonemes treated with anti-Fragment 1A serum and ferritin-conjugated IgG of goat anti-rabbit IgG. Thin cross sections: (a) with antiserum; (b) with antiserum absorbed with Fragment 1A; (c) with preimmune serum; (d) with antiserum, after removal of outer arms. X125,000. Reproduced, with permission, from Ogawa et al. (1977).

arms on other doublets. It has been observed that there is a cross bridge between the No. 5 and the No. 6 doublet owing to the presence of extra projections from the No. 6 doublet in sea urchin sperm flagella (Afzelius, 1959). This cross bridge is so tight that the binding of the antibody against Fragment 1A to the distal part of the outer arm on the No. 5 doublet appears to be prevented.

From these observations, it can be concluded that at least the outer arms consist of dynein 1 and the Fragment-1A portion, *i.e.*, the active site of dynein-1 ATPase is located at the distal end of the outer arms. In regard to the mechanism by which the arms walk along the B-tubule of the adjacent outer doublet, this is consistent with the formation of cross bridges with the arms during flagellar movement (Gibbons and Gibbons, 1974); and with the specific activation of ATPase of Fragment 1A by the tubulin originated from the B-tubule (Ogawa, 1973). Among the three to four subunits of each arm recently observed (Warner *et al.*, 1977; Warner and Mitchell, 1978), the distal one would consist of (or correspond to a part of) Fragment 1A, the ATPase-active subunit of dynein 1. The firm cross bridge between the No. 5 and the No. 6 outer doublet does not seem to allow these two doublets to slide with each other. It is possible that the ATPase activity of the arms on the No. 5 doublet is also inhibited, although attempts to confirm this using electron microscopy of cytochemical detection of ATPase activity with lead nitrate were not successful, owing to the limitation of this technique. The presence of the cross bridge would be important, if the flagellar bending occurred in one direction by active sliding from the No. 1 to the No. 5 doublet, and in another direction from the No. 6 to the No. 1 doublet.

As mentioned above, some parts of the sperm heads as well as the whole axonemes were stained with the anti-Fragment 1A serum by indirect immunofluorescence microscopy. Figure 3 shows a thin section of Triton-treated sperm heads processed for immunoelectron microscopy with the anti-Fragment 1A serum. The plasma membrane (and the acrosomal membrane) remaining around the acrosomal region and at the basal region of the head was found to be labelled with ferritin particles, but not the nuclear membrane. Such a labelling was observed with neither the antiserum absorbed with Fragment 1A nor the preimmune serum. The cortical layer of sea urchin eggs was brightly stained with the anti-Fragment 1A serum by indirect immunofluorescence microscopy (Mohri *et al.*, 1976). Further

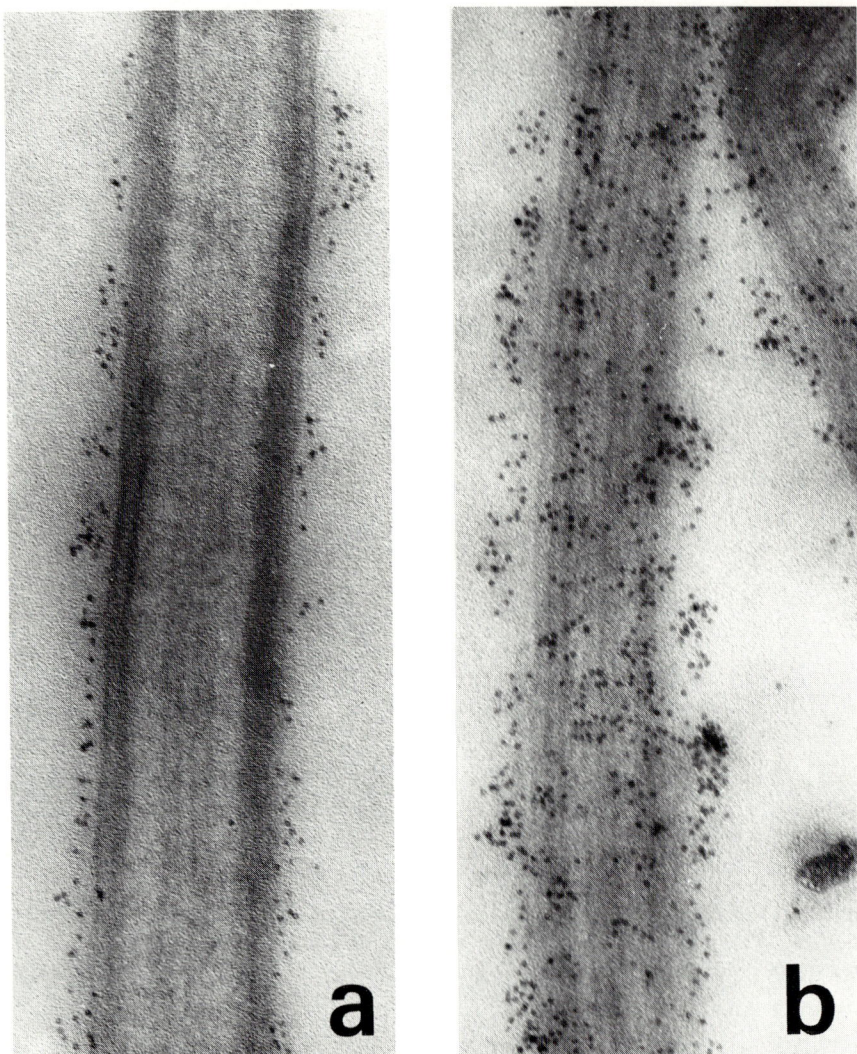

Figure 2. Same as Figure 1. Longitudinal thin sections: (a) a section through the central pair; (b) a tangential section. X125,000.

biochemical studies revealed that there is a Mg^{2+}-, Ca^{2+}-activated ATPase in the isolated cortices, exhibiting similar characteristics to those of flagellar dynein (Kobayashi et al., 1978). The ATPase activity was reduced by 60-80% with the anti-Fragment 1A serum, and a polypeptide band corresponding to dynein 1 was detected in the antigen-antibody complex precipitated from the KCl-extract of the cortices with the antiserum on the SDS-polyacrylamide gel electrophoresis. Therefore, it is conceivable that dynein 1 or a related molecule is also present in or on the sperm plasma membrane. In Figure 3a, the content of the acrosomal granule appears also to be labelled with ferritin. The presence of Mg^{2+}-, Ca^{2+}-ATPase in the acrosomal granule has been reported in starfish and bivalve spermatozoa (Mabuchi and Mabuchi, 1973).

Inhibition of Movement of Triton-demembranated Spermatozoa and of Tubule Extrusion with Anti-Fragment 1A Serum

The effects of anti-Fragment 1A serum on the ATP-induced motility of Triton-treated sea urchin spermatozoa are summarized in Figure 4 (*cf.* Okuno et al., 1976). With homologous species *A. crassispina* the majority of the spermatozoa reactivated with ATP progressed along a straight path with a beat frequency of approximately 30 Hz in both the presence (200 µl) and absence of the preimmune serum. The addition of 5 µl of the antiserum to the spermatozoa suspended in 0.95 ml of reactivation medium completely stopped the progressive movement, with only a small number of spermatozoa oscillating their heads by bending only the proximal

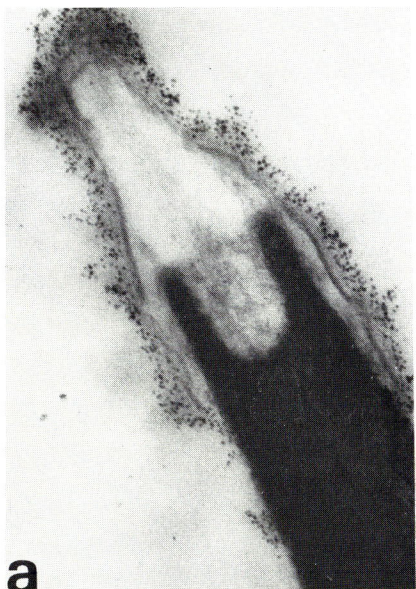 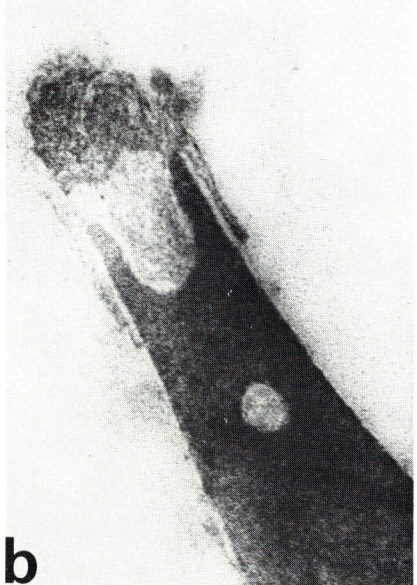

Figure 3. Immunoelectron microscopy of Triton-extracted sea urchin (*Anthocidaris crassispina*) sperm heads treated with anti-Fragment 1A serum and ferritin-conjugated IgG of goat anti-rabbit IgG: (a) with antiserum; (b) with preimmune serum. X85,000.

part of their flagella. With 10 μl of the antiserum, even the head-oscillation was completely arrested. In the case of heterologous species *H. pulcherrimus*, on the other hand, 35% of the Triton-treated spermatozoa still exhibited the head oscillation with 100 μl of the antiserum, although the progressive motion was completely inhibited with 5 μl of the antiserum. Similar results with the same antiserum have been obtained with other heterologous spermatozoa (I.R. Gibbons et al., 1976; B.H. Gibbons et al., 1976; Ogawa et al., 1977b). In *Colobocentrotus atratus*, a rapid fall in the beat frequency of the reactivated spermatozoa was observed immediately after the addition of the antiserum with little change in the waveform, except the larger bend angle in the proximal portion of the flagellum. In *Strongylocentrotus purpuratus*, however, the antiserum reduced both the bend angle and the beat frequency of the reactivated spermatozoa. The anti-Fragment 1A serum also inhibited the movement-coupled ATPase activity of the sperm models. In the case of glycerinated homologous spermatozoa, the inhibition of the ATPase activity remained at 45% even after a prolonged incubation with the antiserum under a certain condition (Okuno et al., 1976); this was, however, highly dependent on the KCl and ATP concentrations, and reached 80% with 0.33mM ATP at zero KCl (Ogawa et al., 1977a).

The ATP-driven tubule extrusion from the trypsin-treated axonemes was observed with *A. crassispina* and *H. pulcherrimus* (cf. Masuda et al., 1978). As shown in Figure 5a and b, when a small volume of 0.5mM ATP was introduced to the suspension of the axoneme fragments, almost 100% of the axonemes showed a slight undulatory movement and then extruded doublet tubules within a few seconds, sometimes reaching a total length four or five times that of the original fragments. The extruded tubules took a coiled form owing to an inherent property of the outer doublets (Miki-Noumura and Kamiya, 1976). When the trypsin-treated axonemes were pre-incubated with sufficient amounts of the anti-Fragment 1A serum, no tubule extrusion occurred even in the presence of ATP, as shown in Figure 5c. The minimum amount causing 100% inhibition was about 2 μl/ml of the mixed suspension. The preimmune serum had no inhibitory effect on the tubule extrusion.

Several interpretations can be drawn from the above results: First, since the anti-Fragment 1A serum, which reacts with dynein 1 and inhibits its ATPase activity, does not precipitate dynein 2 nor reduce the ATPase activity of dynein 2 (Ogawa and Gibbons, 1976), it is clear that dynein 1, but not dynein 2, is responsible for the sliding-tubule mechanism. The residual ATPase activity of demembranated spermatozoa in the presence of the antiserum may be due to dynein 2, the localization and function of which are as yet unknown. Second, when the above-mentioned labelling of only the outer arms by the antiserum is considered together with the complete inhibition by the antiserum of motility of Triton-treated spermatozoa and of ATP-driven tubule extrusion, the question arises as to whether the outer arms are sufficient to produce the motive force for the sliding of outer doublets. Then the inner arms would play only some supplementary role or even if not con-

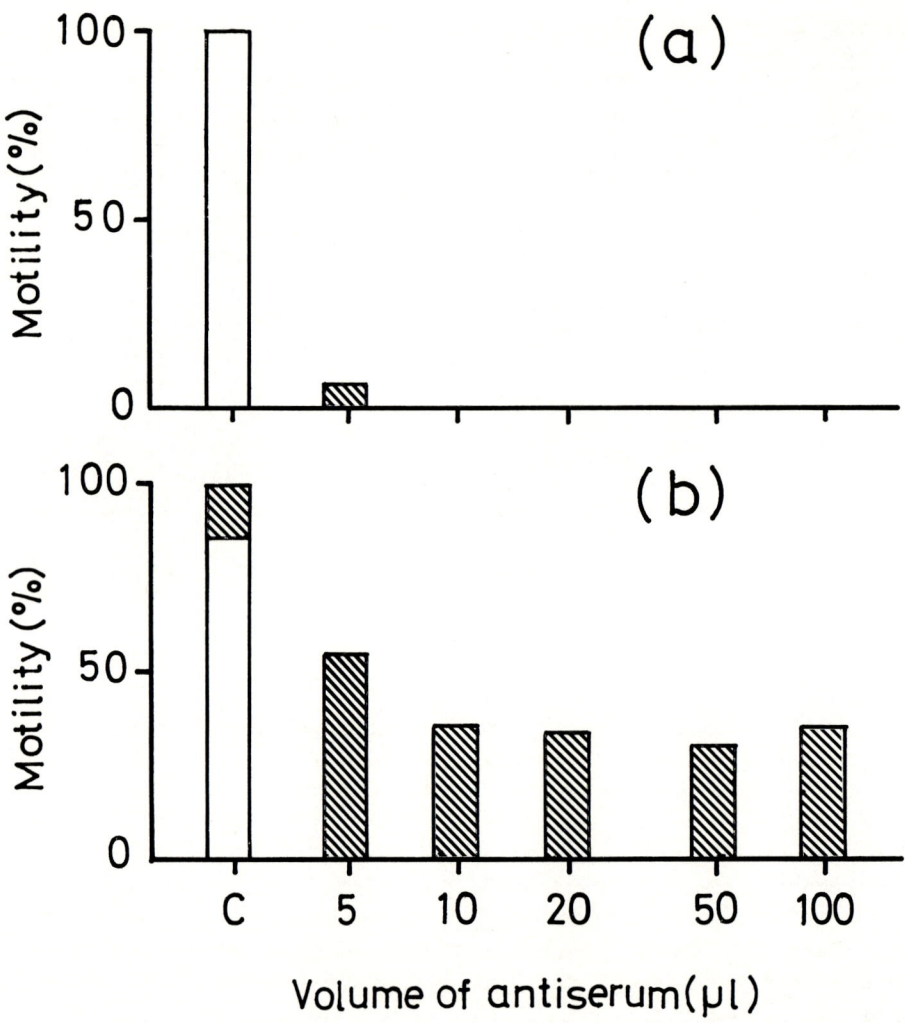

Figure 4. Effects of anti-Fragment 1A serum on reactivation of Triton-treated sea urchin spermatozoa with ATP: (a) *Anthocidaris crassispina;* (b) *Hemicentrotus pulcherrimus.* In the control (c), 200 μl of preimmune serum was added. Open portion represents percentage of spermatozoa showing progressive movement, and hatched portion that of spermatozoa showing head oscillation.

sisting of dynein ATPase, at least dynein 1. This is inconsistent with the results obtained with the Triton-treated *C. atratus* spermatozoa, which showed a reduction of the beat frequency to half that of the control after the extraction of the outer arms with 0.5M KCl (Gibbons and Gibbons, 1973, 1976). Third—because the bending of this portion persisted in the presence of large amounts of the antiserum, especially in heterologous spermatozoa—it appears that the movement of the proximal portion of the flagellum depends on a somewhat different mechanism from that of the remaining portion of the flagellum. It is possible that dynein 2 localizes at the proximal portion and is responsible for the initiation of flagellar wave. Fourth, there is some species difference in respect to the effects of the antiserum.

Tubule Extrusion in the Presence and Absence of the Outer Arms

If only the outer arms are responsible for the sliding between adjacent outer doublets, the removal of the outer arms by 0.5M NaCl extraction has to result in complete inhibition of the ATP-driven tubule extrusion. Figure 6 shows the time course of the disappearance of the outer arms by the NaCl extraction of the axonemes, obtained by inspecting hundreds of extracted axonemes. Around 60% of the ATPase activity originally found in the axonemes was solubilized by the extraction as previously reported (Kincaid *et al.,* 1973; Gibbons and Gibbons, 1973). When the fragmented axonemes of *P. depressus* were first digested with trypsin and then extracted with NaCl, tubule extrusion with ATP rap-

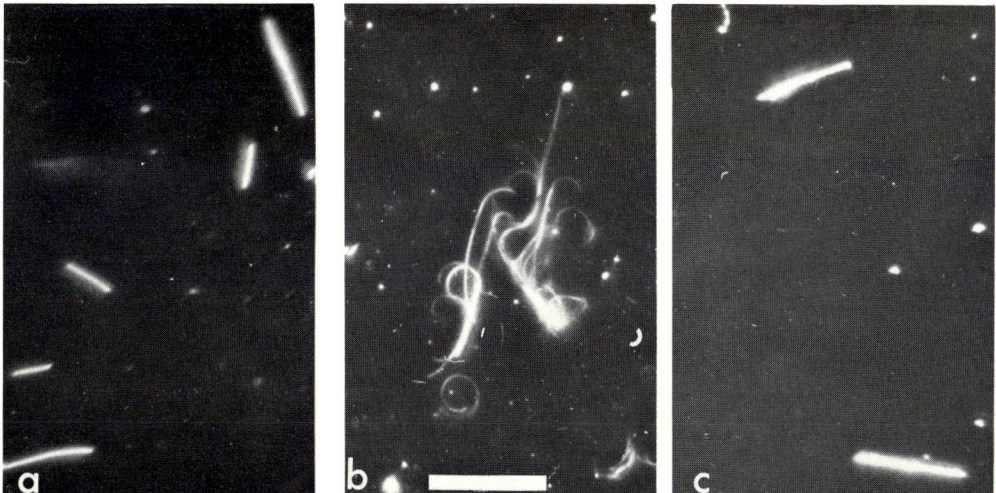

Figure 5. Effect of anti-Fragment 1A serum of ATP-driven tubule extrusion of trypsin-treated axonemal fragments (*Anthocidaris crassispina*): (a) before addition of ATP; (b) tubule extrusion from control axonemes after addition of ATP; (c) axonemes pre-treated with anti-Fragment 1A serum, after addition of ATP. Scale bar 10 μm.

idly dropped with increase in the extraction time and was completely lost after the almost complete disappearance of the outer arms. In a similar experiment with *A. crassispina*, however, some 30% of the trypsin-treated axonemes showed the tubule extrusion or were disintegrated on the addition of ATP even after a 10-min extraction with NaCl. Furthermore, when the fragmented axonemes of *P. depressus* were first extracted with NaCl and then exposed to trypsin and ATP at the same time, about 85% of the axonemes exhibited tubule extrusion, as compared with almost 100% tubule extrusion in the non-extracted axonemes. In the former case, however, the velocity of extrusion was much smaller than that of the control. More quantitative analysis is now in progress on the extrusion velocity. The axonemal structure of *A. crassispina* appears to be more resistant to NaCl treatment than that of *P. depressus*.

The last result appears to indicate the participation of the inner arms as well as the outer arms in the sliding-tubule mechanism, although the complete equivalency in function and properties between both kinds of arms has not yet been established. Nonlabelling

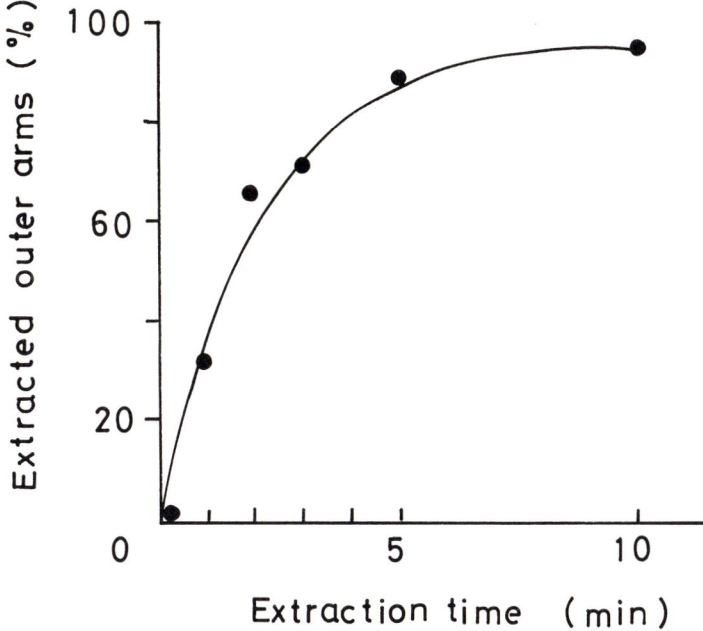

Figure 6. Removal of outer arms from axonemes of sea urchin (*Pseudocentrotus depressus*) by extraction with 0.5M NaCl.

of the inner arms with Fragment-1A serum is then somewhat difficult to understand. One possibility is that the outer and inner arms consist of similar but antigenically different dynein, such as A_1 and A_2 postulated by Kincaid *et al.* (1973), the reason being such that the A-band polypeptide still remains after the extraction of the axonemes with $0.5M$ KCl or NaCl, which preferentially solubilizes the A-band polypeptide and the outer arms. The fact that the ATPase activity of dynein preparation obtained by the extraction with a low ionic strength solution (Tris-EDTA)—which solubilizes both kinds of arms, and was almost completely inhibited by the antiserum (Ogawa and Mohri, 1975)—is not consistent with such a view. Furthermore, a new antiserum prepared against dynein 1 itself also inhibited the ATPase activity remaining in the axonemes after the KCl extraction (Ogawa, unpublished). Difference in the structural configuration between the outer and inner arms would be responsible for the nonlabelling of the inner arms. Even if the anti-Fragment 1A serum was bound to only the outer arms, the complete inhibition of motility of the Triton-treated spermatozoa and of the tubule extrusion could be obtained, provided the binding of the antiserum also gave a structural resistance to "walking" of the inner arms. In the experiments with trypsin-treated axonemes, the antiserum inhibited not only the tubule extrusion but also any disintegration of the axonemes. The above-mentioned result with *C. atratus* spermatozoa (Gibbons and Gibbons, 1973, 1976), namely, that the removal of the outer arms brought about a reduction of beat frequency to half that of the control, but no change in the waveform, is not easily interpreted. Such a result is not common among other sea urchins[1,2] (Ogawa *et al.*, 1977b) where the beat frequency was reduced to much less than that of the control and the bend angle was also reduced. Further experiments with different materials are necessary for complete understanding of the mechanism of flagellar movement.

REFERENCES

Afzelius, B.A.: Electron Microscopy of the Sperm Tail. Results Obtained with a New Fixative. J Biophys Biochem Cytol 5(1959)269-278

Allen, R.D.: A Reinvestigation of Cross Sections of Cilia. J Cell Biol 37(1968)825-831

Amos, L.A.; Linck, R.W.; Klug, A.: Molecular Structure of Flagellar Microtubules. In: Cell Motility, pp. 847-867, ed. by R. Goldman, T. Pollard and J. Rosenbaum. Cold Spring Harbor Laboratory, Cold Spring Harbor, New York, 1976

[1]Brokaw, C.J.: personal communication
[2]Okuno, M.: personal communication

Brokaw, C.J.: Flagellar Movement: A Sliding Filament Model. Science 178(1972)455-462

Brokaw, C.J.; Simonick, T.F.: CO_2 Regulation of the Amplitude of Flagellar Bending. In: Cell Motility, pp. 933-940, ed. by R. Goldman, T. Pollard and J. Rosenbaum. Cold Spring Harbor Laboratory, Cold Spring Harbor, New York, 1976

Gibbons, B.H.; Gibbons, I.R.: The Effect of Partial Extraction of Dynein Arms on the Movement of Reactivated Sea Urchin Sperm. J Cell Sci 13(1973)337-357

Gibbons, B.H.; Gibbons, I.R.: Properties of Flagellar "Rigor Waves" Formed by Abrupt Removal of Adenosine Triphosphate from Actively Swimming Sea Urchin Sperm. J Cell Biol 63(1974)970-985

Gibbons, B.H.; Gibbons, I.R.: Functional Recombination of Dynein 1 with Demembranated Sea Urchin Sperm Partially Extracted with KCl. Biochem Biophys Res Commun 73(1976)1-6

Gibbons, B.H.; Ogawa, K.; Gibbons, I.R.: The Effect of Antidynein 1 Serum on the Movement of Reactivated Sea Urchin Sperm. J Cell Biol 71(1976)823-831

Gibbons, I.R.: Studies on the Protein Components of Cilia from *Tetrahymena pyriformis*. Proc Natl Acad Sci USA 50(1963)1002-1010

Gibbons, I.R.: Chemical Dissection of Cilia. Arch Biol (Liège) 76(1965)317-352

Gibbons, I.R.; Rowe, A.J.: Dynein: A Protein with Adenosine Triphosphatase Activity from Cilia. Science 149(1965)424-426

Gibbons, I.R.; Fronk, E.; Gibbons, B.H.; Ogawa, K.: Multiple Forms of Dynein in Sea Urchin Sperm Flagella. In: Cell Motility, pp. 915-932, ed. by R. Goldman, T. Pollard and J. Rosenbaum. Cold Spring Harbor Laboratory, Cold Spring Harbor, New York, 1976

Hayashi, M.; Higashi-Fujime, S.: Binding and Adenosine Triphosphatase of Flagellar Proteins from Sea Urchin Sperm. Biochemistry 11(1972)2977-2982

Kincaid, H.L.; Gibbons, B.H.; Gibbons, I.R.: The Salt-extractable Fraction of Dynein from Sea Urchin Sperm Flagella: An Analysis by Gel Electrophoresis and by Adenosine Triphosphatase Activity. J Supramol Struct 1(1973)461-470

Kobayashi, Y.; Ogawa, K.; Mohri, H.: Evidence that the Mg-ATPase in the Cortical Layer of Sea Urchin Egg is Dynein. Exp Cell Res 114(1978)285-292

Mabuchi, I.; Shimizu, T.; Mabuchi, Y.: A Biochemical Study of Flagellar Dynein from Starfish Spermatozoa: Protein Components of the Arm Structure. Arch Biochem Biophys 176(1976)564-576

Mabuchi, Y.; Mabuchi, I.: Acrosomal ATPase in Starfish and Bivalve Mollusc Spermatozoa. Exp Cell Res 82(1973)271-279

Masuda, H.; Ogawa, K.; Miki-Noumura, T.: Inhibition of ATP-driven Tubule Extrusion of Trypsin-treated Axonemes. Exp Cell Res 115(1978)435-439

Miki-Noumura, T.; Kamiya, R.: Shape of Microtubules in Solutions. Exp Cell Res 97(1976)451-453

Mohri, H.; Hasegawa, S.; Yamamoto, M.; Murakami, S.: Flagellar Adenosine Triphosphatase (Dynein) from Sea Urchin Spermatozoa. Sci Pap Coll Gen Educ Univ Tokyo 19(1969)195-217

Mohri, H.; Mohri, T.; Mabuchi, I.; Yazaki, I.; Sakai, H.; Ogawa, K.: Localization of Dynein in Sea Urchin Eggs during Cleavage. Dev Growth Diff 18(1976)391-398

Ogawa, K.: Studies on Flagellar ATPase from Sea Urchin Spermatozoa. II. Effect of Trypsin Digestion on the Enzyme. Biochim Biophys Acta 293(1973)514-525

Ogawa, K.; Mohri, H.: Studies on Flagellar ATPase from Sea Urchin Spermatozoa. I. Purification and Some Properties of the Enzyme. Biochim Biophys Acta 256(1972)142-155

Ogawa, K.; Mohri, H.: Preparation of Antiserum Against a Tryptic Fragment (Fragment A) of Dynein and an Immunological Approach to the Subunit Composition of Dynein. J Biol Chem 250(1975)6476-6483

Ogawa, K.; Gibbons, I.R.: Dynein 2. A New Adenosine Triphosphatase from Sea Urchin Sperm Flagella. J Biol Chem 251(1976)5793-5801

Ogawa, K.; Mohri, T.; Mohri, H.: Identification of Dynein in the Outer Arms of Sea Urchin Sperm Axonemes. Proc Natl Acad Sci USA 74(1977a)5006-5010

Ogawa, K.; Asai, D.J.; Brokaw, C.J.: Properties of an Antiserum Against Native Dynein 1 from Sea Urchin Sperm Flagella. J Cell Biol 73(1977b)182-192

Okuno, M; Ogawa, K.; Mohri, H.: Inhibition of Movement and ATPase Activity of Demembranated Sea Urchin Spermatozoa by Antidynein Antiserum. Biochem Biophys Res Commun 68(1976)901-906

Satir, P.: Studies on Cilia. III. Further Studies on the Cilium Tip and a "Sliding Filament" Model of Ciliary Motility. J Cell Biol 39(1968)77-94

Summers, K.E.; Gibbons, I.R.: Adenosine Triphosphate-induced Sliding of Tubules in Trypsin-treated Flagella of Sea Urchin Sperm. Proc Natl Acad Sci USA 68(1971)3092-3096

Warner, F.D.; Mitchell, D.R.; Perkins, C.R.: Structural Conformation of the Ciliary ATPase Dynein. J Mol Biol 114(1977)367-384

Warner, F.D.; Mitchell, D.R.: Structural Conformation of Ciliary Dynein Arms and the Generation of Sliding Forces in *Tetrahymena* cilia. J Cell Biol 76(1978)261-277

PHOSPHORYLATION OF MICROTUBULES OF RAT SPERMATOZOA DURING EPIDIDYMAL MATURATION

D. Tongkao and M. Chulavatnatol

Department of Biochemistry, Faculty of Science, Mahidol University, Bangkok, Thailand

Spermatozoa of different species are known to possess both cyclic 3′,5′-adenosine monophosphate-dependent and independent protein kinases (Hoskins et al., 1972; Garbers et al., 1973; Hoskins et al., 1974; Lee and Iverson, 1976). Although the enzyme preparation from the spermatozoa can catalyze the phosphorylation of histones, protamin, and casein, the nature of their physiological substrate(s) is still unknown (Harrison, 1975). To approach this problem, the authors have selected the epididymal maturation of spermatozoa as a physiological event to be studied. Since spermatozoa in the caput region of the epididymis move circularly and those in the cauda region move with forward progressive pattern (Mooney et al., 1972; Fray, et al., 1972; Burgos and Tovar, 1974), certain components of the contractile system (Summers, 1975) may be modified during sperm maturation, leading to the change in the pattern of motility. One of the modifications may be phosphorylation of 9+2 axonemes. Therefore, phosphorylation of intact caput spermatozoa has been studied in comparison with that of the cells from the cauda epididymis. The experiment has been designed according to the previous observation by Babcock et al. (1973, 1975) that [^{32}P]-orthophosphate taken up by intact spermatozoa will appear in the sperm nucleotides and proteins.

METHODS AND MATERIALS

Assay of [^{32}P]-Orthophosphate Uptake

Spermatozoa from rat cauda epididymidis were freshly extruded into Hank's balanced salt solution containing 70 μM phosphate and 4% bovine serum albumin, pH 5.9, at room temperature by the method described previously (Chulavatnatol et al., 1977). The cells from the caput portion were similarly prepared. They were then separately incubated with 1 mCi/ml[^{32}P]-orthophosphate (Amersham) at 37°C. The final sperm concentration was 2×10^8 cells/ml. At a specified time interval, an aliquot (10 μl) was removed, diluted fivefold, and immediately applied to a millipore filter paper (Millipore Corporation). The content was carefully sucked to dryness with an air-pump and washed with five 3.0-ml portions of Hank's balanced salt solution under suction. The radioactivity retained on the paper was determined by counting Cerenkov radiation in an aqueous system. This represented the total [^{32}P]-orthophosphate uptake by the cells.

Assay of Total Protein Phosphorylation

To determine the total labelling of sperm proteins, an aliquot (0.45 ml) was removed from the incubation mixture and immediately mixed with 50 μl of 0.5N HCl. The mixture was washed three times with the acid, and then sonicated by using a Branson sonifier (setting at 60 watts) for 5 min. A portion (50 μl) of the sonicated acid-extract was applied to a Whatman 31 ET paper chromatogram which was later developed in 5% trichloroacetic acid (TCA) for 1.5 h according to the method of Li and Felmly (1973). The protein spot was cut out and the radioactivity determined as described above.

Assay of [γ-^{32}P]-ATP

Another portion (0.3 ml) of the acid-extract was treated with 5% perchloric acid and then neutralized with saturated KHCO$_3$. The amount of [γ-^{32}P]-adenosine triphosphate (ATP) was determined by incubating the neutralized extract (0.1 ml) with 20 μg of beef heart protein kinase (Sigma) and excess amount of salmon protamine (Sigma) in 80mM Tris-HCl buffer, pH 7.4, in a final volume of 0.15 ml (England and Walsh, 1976). The incubation was carried out at 30°C for 30 min which was adequate to reach the equilibrium of the transfer of label from synthetic [γ-^{32}P]-ATP, prepared according to the method of Glynn and Chappell (1964), to protamine. The radioactivity of the phosphoprotamine was determined using the TCA-chromatogram described above.

Preparation of Sperm Microtubules

To prepare microtubular protein from the spermatozoa, the cells incubated with [^{32}P]-orthophosphate for 30 min as described above were mixed with 1% sodium dodecyl sulphate (SDS) containing 50mM dithiothreitol and then washed three times with Hank's balanced salt solution. After a second treatment with 0.06% SDS containing 10mM dithiothreitol in 50mM Tris-HCl buffer, pH 8.0, the cells were dialyzed against 1mM Tris containing 0.1mM ethylenediamine tetraacetic acid and 0.1mM dithiothreitol, pH 8.0. The soluble fraction of the dialyzed cells was used for SDS-polyacrylamide gel electrophoresis. After staining for protein with Coomassie brilliant blue, the gels were cut and then the radioactivity was determined in a Triton-xylene scintillation cocktail (Anderson and McClure, 1973). The protein band corresponding to that of the microtubular protein, tubulin, prepared from rat brain, according to the method of Shelansky et al. (1973), was identified as the sperm tubulin. Furthermore, a similar preparation of sperm tubulin carried out in the absence of SDS also showed strong binding to colchicine, which was a general property of tubulin from various tissues (Wilson et al., 1974).

RESULTS

Uptake of [^{32}P]-orthophosphate

As observed previously in bovine spermatozoa (Babcock et al., 1975), the uptake of phosphate by the rat epididymal spermatozoa is rapid, reaching a maximum in 10-20 min (Fig. 1). However, it was noted that the amount of the labelled phosphate declined slowly thereafter, suggesting a gradual release of the label back into the incubation medium. This may reflect some damage of the cells during prolonged incubation. The amount of the label accumulated by the caput epididymidal spermatozoa after 10 min was slightly more than that of the cells from the caudal portion. Throughout the 1 h incubation, the spermatozoa from the caudal epididymis were motile, while those from the caput portion stopped moving after a few minutes.

Formation of [γ-^{32}P]-ATP

The labelled orthophosphate taken up was very rapidly incorporated into ATP in the γ-phosphoryl position (Fig. 2). Within the first few minutes, the level of

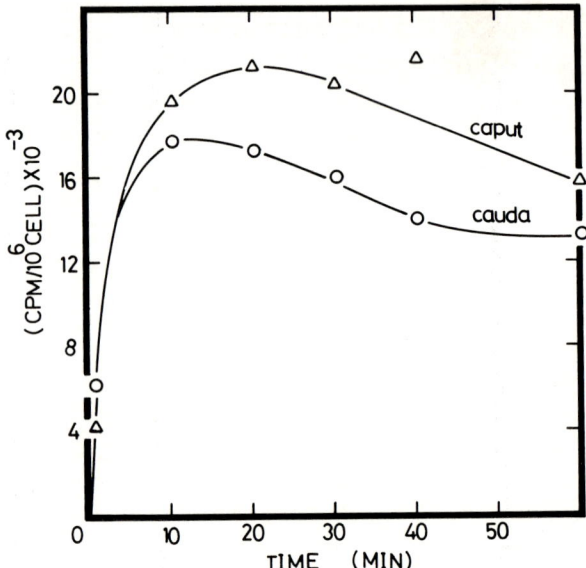

Figure 1. Uptake of [^{32}P]-orthophosphate by spermatozoa from the cauda (O) and the caput (△) epididymides.

[γ-^{32}P]-ATP was maximum, with the level in the spermatozoa from the caudal epididymis higher than that of the cells from the caput portion, suggesting a better ability to synthesize ATP by the former cell type. This interpretation would be consistent with one previous finding of a higher ATP content in the caudal epididymal spermatozoa (Chulavatnatol et al., 1977).

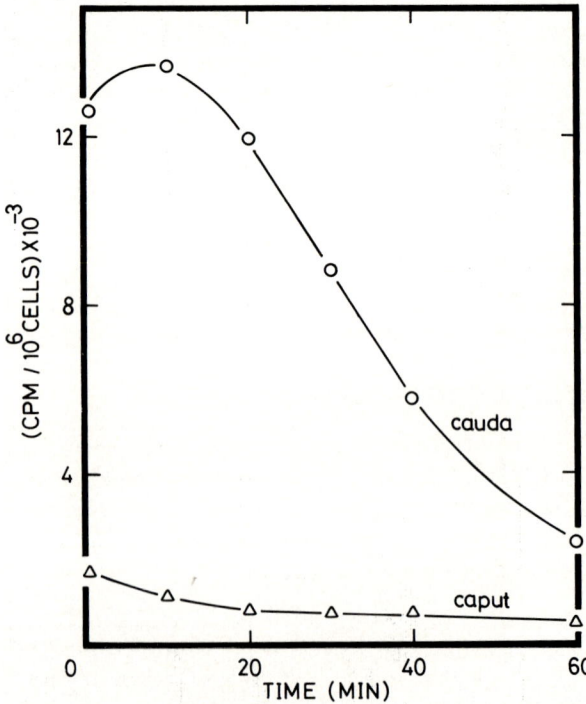

Figure 2. Incorporation of ^{32}P into γ-phosphoryl moiety of ATP by spermatozoa from the cauda (O) and the caput (△) epididymides.

Formation of [^{32}P]-phosphoproteins

Upon further incubation, the level of [γ-^{32}P]-ATP dropped slowly, suggesting the transfer of the γ-phosphoryl moiety to various acceptors, including proteins, in phosphorylation reactions. The incorporation kinetics of the labelling or phosphorylation of the proteins in the sperm appeared biphasic with a fast initial rate followed by a slower linear rate (Fig. 3). Quite distinctly, the mature sperm seemed to exhibit a faster rate of incorporation than that of the immature sperm.

Phosphorylation of Microtubules

The tubulin preparations from spermatozoa of both caput and cauda regions of the epididymis showed similar protein bands in SDS-polyacrylamide gel electrophoresis, with one intense band having electrophoretic mobility corresponding to that of purified rat brain tubulin (Fig. 4). This indicated that the tubulin was equally extractable from both types of cells even though the structure of mature spermatozoa were usually considered tougher than that of the immature cells. Further analysis showed that the tubulin band from the mature spermatozoa was most heavily labelled (Fig. 5). The protein that migrated just behind the tubulin was also labelled. No label was confidently detected on other protein bands. The most striking result was that none of the protein bands from the immature sperma-

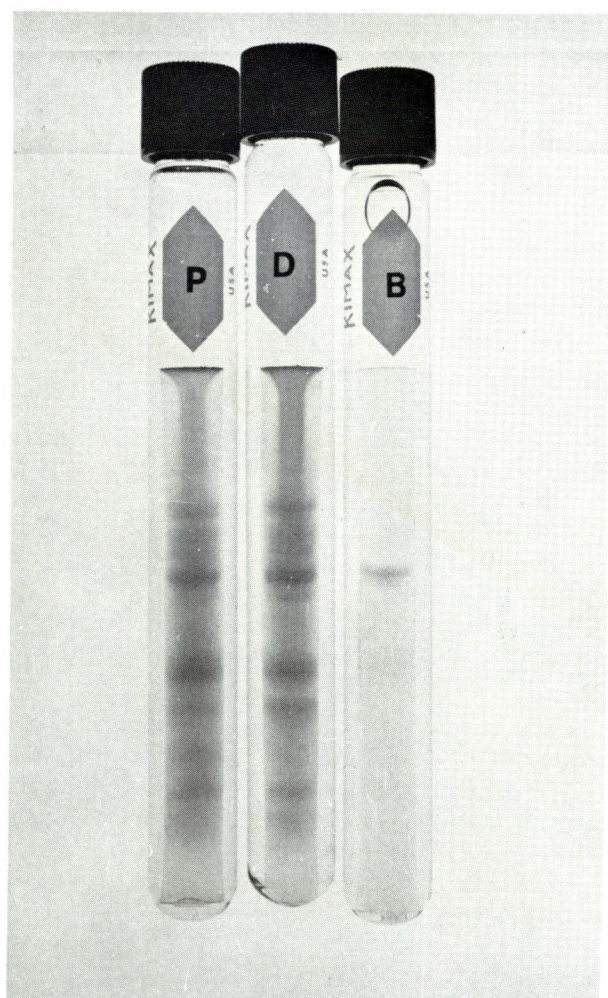

Figure 4. SDS-polyacrylamide gel electrophoretic patterns of tubulin preparations from spermatozoa of the cauda (D) and the caput (P) epididymides in comparison with that of brain tubulin (B).

tozoa contained any label (Fig. 5). Assuming that the extracted tubulins came primarily from the sperm tails, the finding implied that phosphorylation of this component in the motile apparatus was probably one of the events occurring during the epididymal sperm maturation that contributed to the change in motility pattern. The nature of the second labelled band was not identified.

DISCUSSION

The metabolic fate of the labelled orthophosphate taken up by the spermatozoa can be summarized as shown in Figure 6. The first step seems to be the rapid incorporation into the γ-phosphoryl position of ATP (Fig. 2), similar to that observed by Babcock *et al*. (1975). This is likely to be due to mitochondrial oxida-

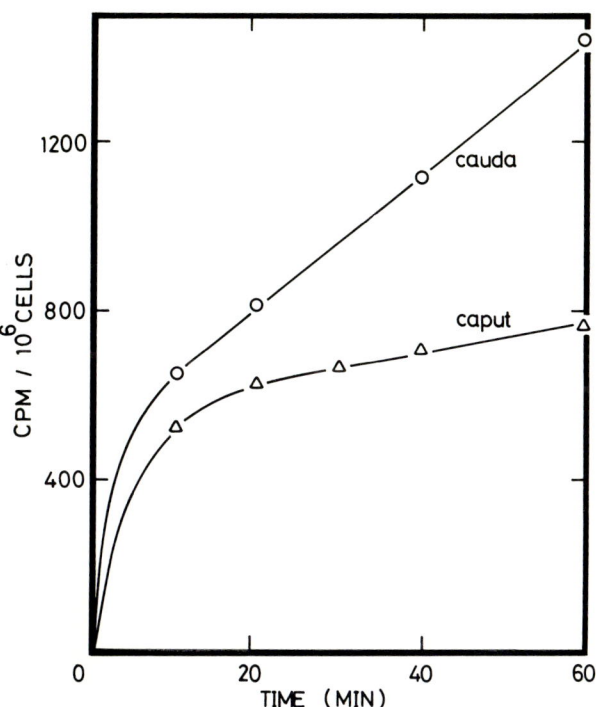

Figure 3. Incorporation of ^{32}P into phosphoproteins by spermatozoa from the cauda (○) and the caput (△) epididymides.

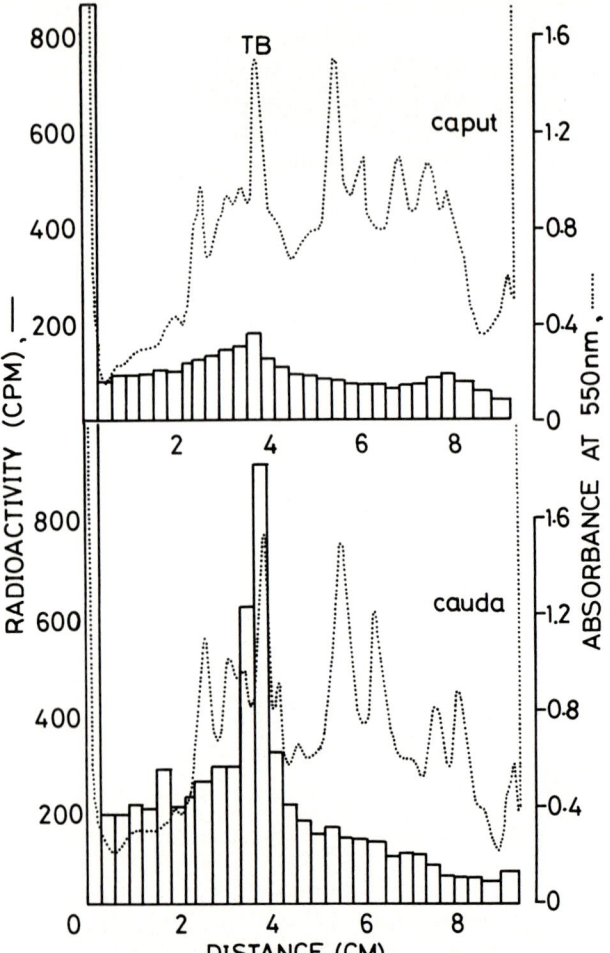

Figure 5. SDS-polyacrylamide gel electrophoretic patterns of tubulin preparations from spermatozoa from the cauda (lower panel) and the caput (upper panel) epididymides. Histograms represent radioactivity of ^{32}P. Dotted lines are protein profiles. "TB" designates band that corresponds to the position of brain tubulin.

tive phosphorylation which should be highly active under the aerobic condition of the experiment. The level of $[\gamma\text{-}^{32}P]$-ATP is expected to fall (Fig. 2) when the breakdown or utilization exceeds the synthesis. Three main types of the reactions that degrade or utilize ATP will likely be occurring in motile spermatozoa: the ATPases, especially that of dynein during active motility; the phosphorylation of proteins catalyzed by protein kinases; and phosphotransferase reactions that transfer the γ-phosphoryl group of ATP to acceptors of small molecular weight, e.g., guanine nucleotides (Babcock et al., 1973, 1975), or glucose and fructose 6-phosphate.

Likewise, the level of $[^{32}P]$-phosphoproteins will be determined by the synthesis, catalyzed by the protein kinases, and the degradation, catalyzed by the phosphatases (Tang and Hoskins, 1975). Thus, the change in the rate of increase in the level as shown in Figure 3 suggests some kinetic alteration of one or both of these processes. Similarly, the difference in the net formation of the phosphoproteins between the mature and immature spermatozoa (Fig. 3) reflects the difference in either the kinase and/or the phosphatase between these cell types. In contrast to $[\gamma\text{-}^{32}P]$-ATP, the level of $[^{32}P]$-phosphoproteins does not decline, suggesting that the degradation never exceeds the synthesis within the duration of the experiment.

Although spermatozoa from both caput and cauda portions of the epididymis possess protein kinases (Hoskins et al., 1974) and can form phosphoproteins (Fig. 3), it is rather surprising to observe that tubulin of the cells from the caput epididymis is not phosphorylated while that of the cauda is. This implies that the tubulin becomes accessible and can serve as substrate for the protein kinases during sperm maturation. Such a change may play an important role in altering the sperm motility pattern associated with maturation. The mechanism of the process is unknown and deserves further study.

Admittedly, identification of sperm tubulin by comparing it with the brain tubulin under the same electrophoretic condition is preliminary and not very precise. In this chapter, no attempt is made to remove tubulin-associated proteins (Sandoval and Cuatrecasas, 1976; Rappaport et al., 1976; Sloboda et al., 1975), if they exist in the spermatozoa. These associated proteins from brain, rather than tubulin, have been shown to be phosphorylated (Rappaport et al., 1976; Sloboda et al., 1975). Whether the situation in spermatozoa is different from that in brain remains to be investigated.

Besides tubulin, another protein has been shown to be phosphorylated in mature spermatozoa (Fig. 5). In fact, Huacuja et al. (1977) have recently demonstrated that three membrane proteins of human spermatozoa can be phosphorylated. Thus, one is tempted to suggest that several proteins in spermatozoa can be phosphorylated but the phosphorylation must at least be associable with some physiological event to be meaningful.

REFERENCES

Anderson, L.E.; McClure, W.O.: An Improved Scintillation Cocktail of High-solubilizing Power. Anal Biochem 51(1973)173-179

Babcock, D.F.; First, N.L.; Lardy, H.A.: Phosphodiesterase

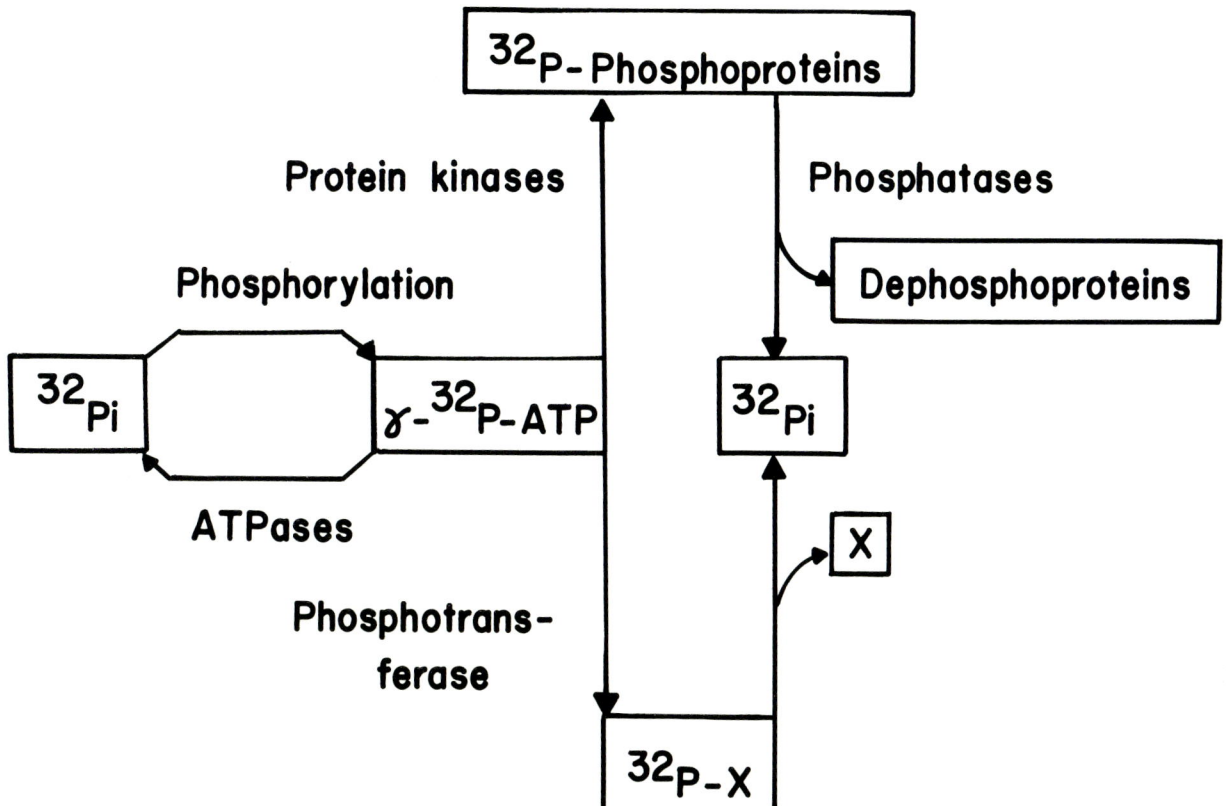

Figure 6. Simplified biochemical reactions involved in the incorporation of ^{32}P into proteins and metabolites (x) and their degradation.

Inhibitors Alter Labelling of Sperm Nucleotides and Proteins. Biol Reprod 9(1973)99-100A

Babcock, D.F.; First, N.L.; Lardy, H.A.: Transport Mechanism for Succinate and Phosphate Localized in the Plasma Membrane of Bovine Spermatozoa. J Biol Chem 250(1975)6488-6495

Burgos, M.H.; Tovar, E.S.: Sperm Motility in the Rat Epididymis. Fertil Steril 25(1974)985-991

Chulavatnatol, M.; Hasibuan, I.; Yindepit, S.; Eksittikul, T.: Lack of Effect of 2-Chlorohydrin on the ATP Content of Rat, Mouse and Human Spermatozoa. J Reprod Fertil 50(1977) 137-139

England, A.J.; Walsh, D.A.: A Rapid Method for the Measurement of [γ-^{32}P]ATP-specific Radioactivity in Tissue Extracts and its Application to the Study of $^{32}P_i$ Uptake into Perfused Rat Heart. Anal Biochem 75(1976)301-308

Fray, C.S.; Hoffer, A.P.; Fawcett, D.W.: A Reexamination of Motility Patterns of Rat Epididymal Spermatozoa. Anat Rec 173(1972) 301-308

Garbers, D.L.; First, N.L.; Lardy, H.A.: Properties of Adenosine 3':5'-Monophosphate-dependent Protein Kinases Isolated from Bovine Epididymal Spermatozoa. J Biol Chem 248(1973)875-879

Glynn, I.M.; Chappell, J.B.: A Simple Method for the Preparation of ^{32}P-labelled Adenosine Triphosphate of High Specific Activity. Biochem J 90(1964)147-149

Harrison, R.A.P.: Aspects of the Enzymology of Mammalian Spermatozoa. In: The Biology of the Male Gamete (Supplement 1 to the Biological Journal of the Linnean Society, Vol. 7), pp. 301-316, ed. by J.G. Duckette and P.A. Racey. Academic Press, New York, 1975.

Hoskins, D.D.; Casillas, E.R.; Stephens, D.T.: Cyclic AMP-dependent Protein Kinases of Bovine Epididymal Spermatozoa. Biochem Biophys Res Commun 48(1972)1331-1337

Hoskins, D.D.; Stephens, D.T.; Hall, M.L.: Cyclic Adenosine 3':5'-Monophosphate and Protein Kinase Levels in Developing Bovine Spermatozoa. J Reprod Fertil 37(1974)131-133

Huacuja, L.; Delgada, N.M.; Merchant, H.; Pancardo, R.M.; Rosado, A.: Cyclic AMP-induced Incorporation of $^{32}P_i$ into Human Spermatozoa Membrane Components. Biol Reprod 17(1977)89-96

Lee, M.Y.W.; Iverson, R.M.: An Adenosine 3':5'-Monophosphate-dependent Protein Kinase from Sea Urchin Spermatozoa. Biochim Biophys Acta 429(1976)123-126

Li, H.C.; Felmly, D.A.: A Rapid Paper Chromatographic Assay for Protein Kinase. Anal Biochem 52(1973)300-304

Mooney, J.K.; Horan, A.H.; Lattimer, J.K.: Motility of Spermatozoa in the Human Epididymis. J Urol 108(1972)443-445

Rappaport, L.; Leterrier, J.F.; Virion, A.; Nunez, J.: Phosphorylation of Microtubule-associated Proteins. Eur J Biochem 62(1976)539-549

Sandoval, J.V.; Cuatrecasas, P.: Proteins Associated with Tubulin. Biochem Biophys Res Commun 68(1976)169-177

Shelansky, M.L.; Gaskin, F.; Cantor, C.A.: Microtubule Assembly in the Absence of Added Nucleotides. Proc Natl Acad Sci USA 70(1973)765-768

Sloboda, R.D.; Rudolph, S.A.; Rosenbaum, J.L.; Greengard, P.: Cyclic AMP-dependent Endogenous Phosphorylation of a Microtubule-associated Protein. Proc Natl Acad Sci USA 72(1975)177-181

Summers, K.: The Role of Flagellar Structures in Motility. Biochim Biophys Acta 416(1975)153-168

Tang, F.Y.; Hoskins, D.D.: Phosphoprotein Phosphatase of Bovine Epididymal Spermatozoa. Biochem Biophys Res Commun 62(1975)328-335

Wilson, L.; Bamburg, J.R.; Mizel, S.B.; Grisham, L.M.; Creswell, K.M.: Interaction of Drugs with Microtubule Proteins. Fed Proc 33(1974)158-166

A SPECIFIC SELENOPOLYPEPTIDE ASSOCIATED WITH THE OUTER MEMBRANE OF RAT SPERM MITOCHONDRIA

H.I. Calvin and G.W. Cooper

Department of Human Genetics and Development and Center for Reproductive Sciences, Columbia University, New York, New York 10032 USA; Department of Obstetrics and Gynecology, Cornell University Medical College, New York, New York 10021 USA

In addition to its role in protecting against cadmium toxicity to the testis (Gunn and Gould, 1970), selenium is required for normal spermatogenesis in the rat. When rats are deprived of this trace element and supplemented with Vitamin E for two generations, the resulting male offspring display reduced spermatogenesis and produce abnormal, immotile spermatozoa, characterized by breaks within the tails (Wu et al., 1973). The substantial incorporation of subcutaneously administered ^{75}Se into testes of mice and rats (Gunn, et al., 1967; Gunn and Gould, 1970) and its retention by spermatozoa during their subsequent transit through the epididymis suggest that selenium is intrinsic to the spermatozoon and may be associated with one or more proteins required for normal spermiogenesis. Autoradiography reveals that ^{75}Se incorporated into the spermatozoon is concentrated within the midpiece (Brown and Burk (1973), a finding which may be correlated with the tail defects observed in Se-deficient spermatozoa.

The major Se-containing polypeptide in the rat spermatozoon has recently been identified and localized within a keratinous fraction of the sperm tail (Calvin, 1978). In this chapter these earlier findings are summarized and extended. Additional information is presented supporting the association of a selenopolypeptide with the keratinous outer membrane of sperm mitochondria. Its possible similarity to or identity with one of the major protein components present in these structures is considered.

MATERIALS AND METHODS

Sodium [^{75}Se]-selenite (New England Nuclear Corp.) was administered at doses of 100 µCi per testis to 350-500 g rats and spermatozoa were harvested from cauda epididymides essentially as described previously (Calvin, 1978). The sperm were expressed into 0.15M NaCl and aliquots were collected by centrifugation, either for resuspension in 20mM sodium phosphate (pH 6.0), sonication, and separation of heads and tails (Calvin, 1976) or for incubation of intact spermatozoa in various media.

Either intact spermatozoa or purified, sonicated sperm tails were employed for the procedures listed in Table 1. Sodium dodecyl sulfate (SDS) extraction was performed by incubation for at least 15 min in 1% SDS, 50mM Tris HCl, pH 7.5. Trypsin treatment was carried out by incubation for 20-30 min in 0.2 mg/ml trypsin (Grade TRL, Worthington Biochemicals), dissolved in 50mM Tris HCl (pH 8.0), followed by a 2-min sonication. The samples were sonicated in volumes not exceeding 5 ml, with a Bronwill Model II-A sonifier, fitted with a 3/16 in. titanium microtip, at a power setting of 65%. Incubation in 1% SDS, 0.20mM dithiothreitol (DTT), 50mM Tris HCl was carried out at pH 7.5 for 16-20 h or at pH 8.5 for 2-3 h. These samples were sonicated for 2 min at a power setting of 45%, in order to disrupt the mitochondrial and fibrous sheaths and release dense fibers. Incubation in 10mM DTT, 50mM Tris HCl (pH 8.5), was conducted for 2-3 h followed by sonication for 2 min at the 65% power setting. After the above treatments, samples were centrifuged at 15,000 g for 15 min, and where indicated, the supernatants were then recentrifuged at 100,000 g for 60 min to obtain a second pellet. The first pellet was washed once by resuspension in 0.1% SDS and recentrifuged at 15,000 g. The combined supernatants were then used to obtain the succeeding 100,000 g x 60 min pellet.

SDS-polyacrylamide gel electrophoresis was performed as described previously (Calvin, 1978). Samples

SDS-polyacrylamide gel electrophoresis was performed as described previously (Calvin, 1978). Samples were boiled for 2 min in 1% SDS, 40mM DTT, 10mM Tris (pH 8.5) prior to electrophoresis. Radioactivity in 1-mm gel slices was determined with a Nuclear Chicago Model 1185 gamma counter at approximately 50%

The authors gratefully acknowledge the expert technical assistance of Mr. R. Jurasinski, Ms. Chin-Yueh Hsu, and Ms. Miu-Ying Fong and the support of grants HD-05316 and HD-09215 from the National Institutes of Health.

© 1979 Urban & Schwarzenberg, Inc. Baltimore-Munich *The Spermatozoon*, edited by D.W. Fawcett and J.M. Bedford

Table 1. Retention of Labelled Se by Fractions Prepared from Intact Spermatozoa (S) or Purified Sperm Tails (T)

Treatment	Fraction	Tail Structures	Se Retained %
SDS	15,000 g × 15 min pellet (S, T)	Connecting piece, dense fibers, fibrous sheath, mitochondrial vesicles	95-98
Trypsin, sonication	15,000 g × 15 min pellet (S)	Most internal structures, except: annulus, fibrous sheath, radial spokes	95-98
1% SDS– 0.2mM DTT, sonication	15,000 g × 15 min pellet, washed (S, T)	Dense fibers, connecting piece	5-15
	100,000 g × 60 min pellet (S, T)	Mitochondrial vesicles, dense fiber fragments	50-70
10mM DTT, sonication	15,000 g × 15 min pellet (S)	Most internal structures	15-20
	100,000 g × 60 min pellet (S)	Damaged mitochondria, membrane fragments, dense fiber fragments, axial fibers	20-40

efficiency. All other measurements of radioactivity were performed either with this counter or by liquid scintillation spectrometry. For the latter, 1 ml of aqueous sample was mixed with 10 ml of Hydrofluor (National Diagnostics, Parsipanny, New Jersey) and counted in the ^{3}H window of a Packard Tri-Carb Model 3225 liquid scintillation spectrometer at 45% efficiency. Glutathione peroxidase was determined with H_2O_2 as substrate, by the method of Paglia and Valentine (1967). Protein concentration of extracts was determined by the method of Bradford (1976), with a kit furnished by Bio-Rad Laboratories (Richmond, California).

Samples were prepared for electron microscopy by refrigeration of pellets overnight in 2.5% glutaraldehyde, 20mM sodium phosphate (pH 6.0). These were postfixed at room temperature for 1 h in 1% OsO_4, 0.1M phosphate (pH 7.4), dehydrated in a graded series of ethanols and propylene oxide, and embedded in Epon 812. Thin sections for transmission microscopy were stained with lead citrate (Reynolds, 1963) and 3% uranyl acetate in 50% ethanol and were viewed with a JOEL 100B electron microscope at 80 kV.

RESULTS

Following intratesticular administration of ^{75}Se to rats, more than 1% of the counts can be recovered in association with cauda epididymidal spermatozoa. The radioactivity is not appreciably released by sonication, and sperm heads isolated from sonicates by sucrose density gradient centrifugation (yield ∼ 80%) retain less than 3% of the total sperm label. By contrast, more than 70% of the total sperm ^{75}Se is recovered from tails isolated in similar yield from sucrose gradients. Further observations, which indicate the distribution of ^{75}Se among sperm tail structures, are summarized in Table 1.

As noted previously (Calvin, 1978), ^{75}Se is recovered almost quantitatively in the 15,000 g × 15 min pellet following extraction of intact spermatozoa or sperm tails with SDS. It is thus associated with a fibrous fraction of the sperm tail stabilized by disulfide bonds, which includes four major structures: connecting piece, dense outer fibers, fibrous sheath, and vesicles derived from the outer membranes of mitochondria (Bedford and Calvin, 1974).

Additional observations suggest that of these four elements, only the mitochondrial ghosts accumulate substantial amounts of ^{75}Se. The failure of trypsin to solubilize a significant fraction of the Se, even when combined with sonication (Table 1), eliminates the fibrous sheath as a significant locus of ^{75}Se, since the latter structure is substantially eroded by trypsin, in contrast to mitochondria and dense fibers (Fig. 1); ^{75}Se does not appear to concentrate within the connecting piece or the outer dense fibers. A large particulate fraction (15,000 g × 15 min pellet) which consists almost entirely of these structures (Calvin et al., 1975), obtained after incubation of sperm tails in 1% SDS, 0.20mM dithiothreitol (DTT), sonication, and one wash with 0.1% SDS, retains only 5-15% of the label (Table 1). Conversely, the combined washes of this dense fiber-connecting piece fraction account for more than 85% of the ^{75}Se in the sperm tail (Calvin, 1978). It has subsequently been found that the ^{75}Se in these washes is largely sedimentable by centrifugation at 100,000 g for 1 h (Table 1). The labelled residue is composed essentially of mitochondrial vesicles and fine fragments of dense fibers (Fig. 2). Since the dense fibers isolated in

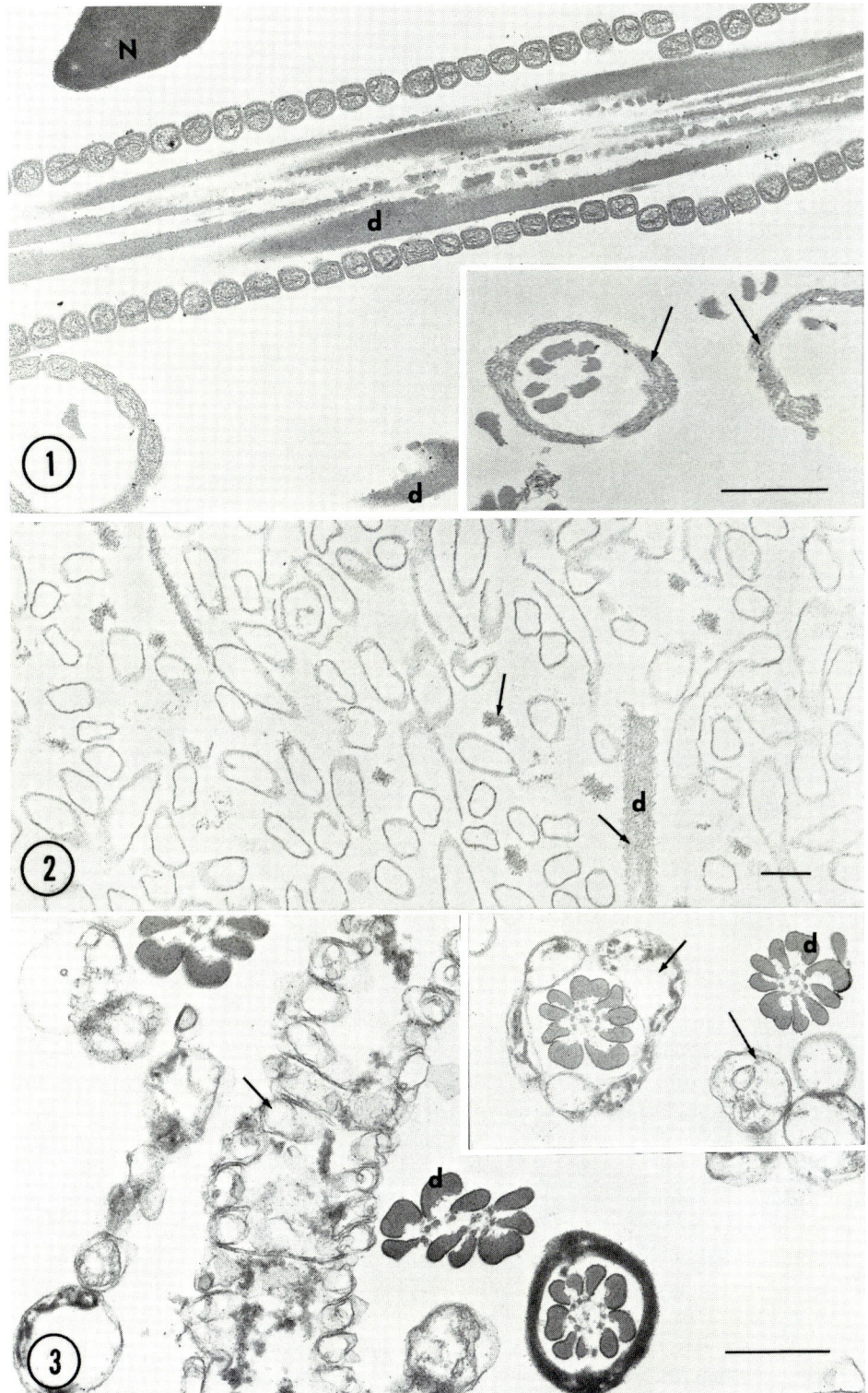

Figure 1. Rat spermatozoa treated for 30 min with trypsin, 0.20 mg/ml. The plasma membrane, annulus, axonemal complex, and fibrous sheath (arrows, inset) are extensively degraded by trypsin, while the dense fibers (d), nucleus (N), and mitochondrial sheath show little or no change in ultrastructural appearance. 15,000 g x 15 min pellet. Bar = 0.5 μm. X31,500.

Figure 2. 100,000-g pellet consisting of mitochondrial vesicles and dense fiber fragments (d, arrows) from a sperm tail supernatant produced by incubation in 1% SDS-0.20mM DTT, sonication, and one wash in 0.1% SDS. Bar = 0.2 μm. X36,000.

Figure 3. Rat spermatozoa incubated 2 h in 10mM DTT (pH 8.5), vortexed 30 s 15,000 g x 15 min pellet. Mitochondria (arrows and inset) are swollen and vesiculated by DTT treatment, while dense fibers (d) and fibrous sheath show minimal change in ultrastructure. Bar = 0.5 μm. X31,500.

The insets in Figures 1 and 3 are of the same magnification as the respective figures.

the preceding 15,000 g x 15 min pellet were sparsely labelled, it may be inferred by elimination that the ^{75}Se in the 100,000-g pellet is associated with mitochondrial vesicles.

The association of selenium with mitochondrial elements has been suggested by Brown and Burk (1973), who localized silver grains primarily over the midpiece of the spermatozoon, following administration of ^{75}Se to rats, and autoradiography. In further support of their conclusions, we find that trypsin, which leaves the mitochondrial sheath comparatively intact (Fig. 1), also releases very little ^{75}Se (Table 1). By contrast, incubation in 10mM DTT (pH 8.5) selectively degrades mitochondria (Fig. 3) and allows the release of more than 80% of the label from the sperm upon sonication and centrifugation at 15,000 g for 15 min (Table 1). A variable proportion of the ^{75}Se released into this supernatant sediments at 100,000 g within 1 h (Table 1). The remainder (40-60%) appears to have been solubilized in the presence of 10mM DTT.

Complete solubilization of ^{75}Se-labelled protein may be effected by incubation in 1% SDS, 40mM DTT at pH 8.5. The crude supernatant obtained by sonication in 1% SDS, 0.20mM DTT, and centrifugation at 15,000 g for 15 min has been solubilized in this way and examined for ^{75}Se-labelled polypeptides by SDS-polyacrylamide gel electrophoresis (Calvin, 1978). Only one radioactive component was detected on the gels. Its mobility, which was not altered by carboxymethylation, suggests a molecular weight of 17,000 daltons. The labeled material was rendered dialyzable with Pronase, confirming that it is a polypeptide (Calvin, 1978).

In more recent experiments, the crude supernatant in which the ^{75}Se-labelled polypeptide was first identified has been fractionated by centrifugation at 100,000 g for 1 h. The pellet, consisting mainly of mitochondrial vesicles and small dense-fiber fragments, retains most of the ^{75}Se in the parent supernatant fraction (Table 1). SDS-polyacrylamide gel electrophoresis reveals one peak of radioactivity (Fig. 4). The banding pattern of the 100,000-g pellet fraction is shown in Figure 5, tube 2. By comparison with the total proteins in tail keratin (tube 1), this fraction is enriched in two bands, designated bands I and II. Their apparent molecular weights are 26,000 and 21,000 daltons, respectively. The more rapidly migrating, 21,000-dalton component may coincide with the ^{75}Se peak, although identical mobility has not yet been established. Little or no label is associated with band I. Both bands I and II appear to be of slightly lower mobility than two prominent bands in the dense fiber-connecting piece protein extract (tube 3), which are designated as bands A and B, respectively.

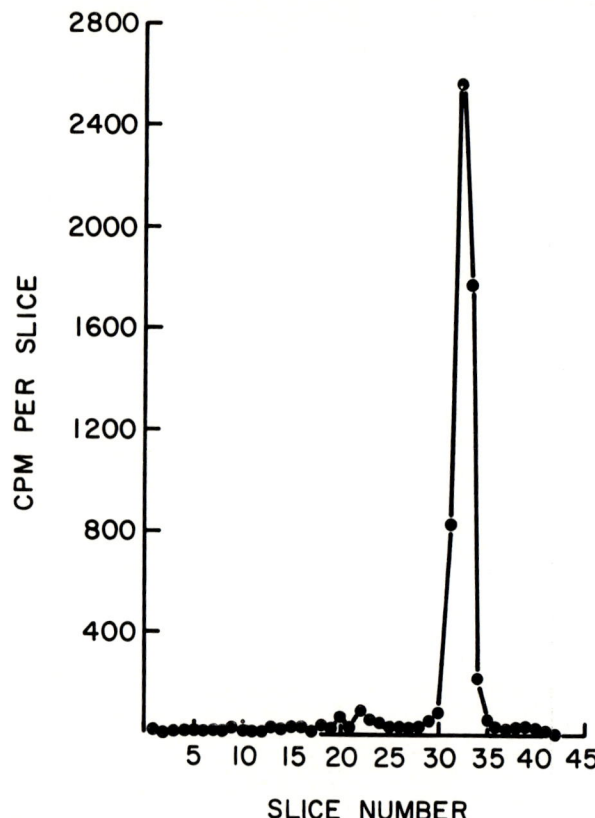

Figure 4. Radioactivity recovered in successive 1-mm gel slices following SDS-polyacrylamide gel electrophoresis of a 100,000 g x 60 min pellet composed of mitochondrial vesicles and dense fiber fragments.

The selenoenzyme glutathione peroxidase, a tetramer of 75,000-100,000 daltons (Flohé et al., 1976), has been detected in extracts of goat, human, and dog spermatozoa (Li, 1975), but is relatively deficient in spermatozoa of the rabbit, ram, and bull (Li, 1975; Brown et al., 1977). Since the molecular weight of the subunit of glutathione peroxidase is similar to that of the labelled rat sperm selenopolypeptide, attempts were made to establish whether the distribution of ^{75}Se in rat sperm fractions was correlated with glutathione peroxidase activity. Following sonication of rat spermatozoa in 20mM sodium phosphate (pH 6.0), significant enzyme activity was detected in the 1,500 g x 5 min supernatant, although, as noted previously (Calvin, 1978), such supernatants contain less than 5% of the total sperm ^{75}Se. The level of activity was of the order of 1 μmole/h/mg protein, and therefore, appeared to be comparable to that reported for goat epididymal spermatozoa (Li, 1975). Treatment of sonicated residues with 10mM DTT and further sonication, under conditions that

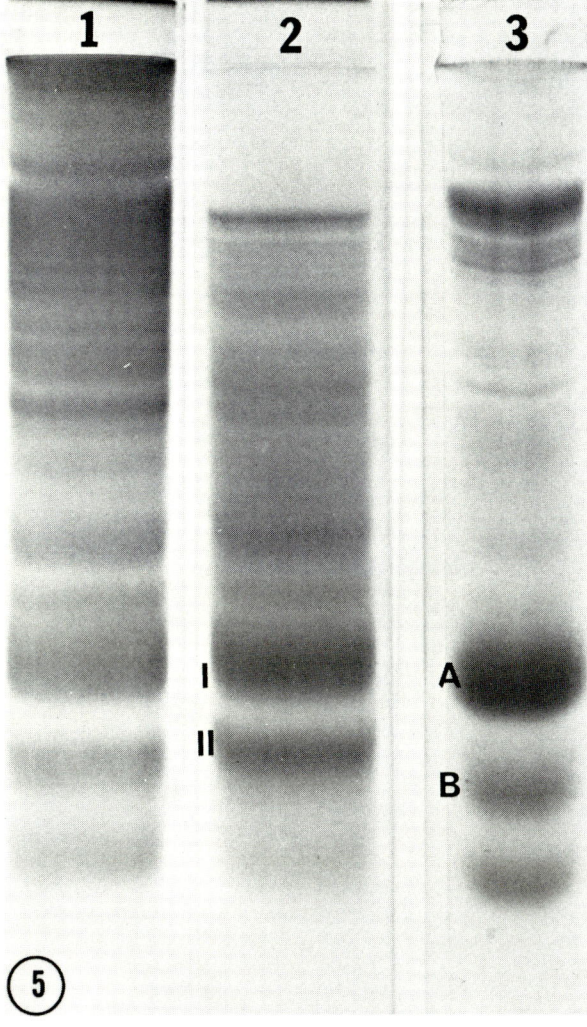

Figure 5. Staining patterns observed following SDS-polyacrylamide gel electrophoresis of (1) total tail keratin, (2) mitochondrial vesicle-dense fiber fraction, and (3) dense fiber-connecting piece fraction. Gels stained with Coomassie blue G and destained by diffusion, as described previously (Calvin et al., 1975).

release most of the ^{75}Se into a 15,000 g × 15 min supernatant fraction (Table 1), did not release further detectable enzyme activity into this supernatant. Although it is possible that the enzyme activity was inhibited by DTT in the latter extracts, this does not seem likely, since human seminal plasma glutathione peroxidase is not inhibited by DTT (Calvin, 1978)

DISCUSSION

This chapter presents evidence for highly selective labelling of a single selenopolypeptide in the rat spermatozoon. Although its molecular weight is similar to that of the subunit of glutathione peroxidase, it appears unlikely that the ^{75}Se-labelled rat sperm polypeptide is a catalytically active subunit of this peroxidase for the following reasons: 1) glutathione peroxidase activity cannot be detected in ^{75}Se-labelled sperm extracts under conditions in which activity is normally measurable; 2) unlike glutathione peroxidase, which has been found in the cytosol or the mitochondrial matrix (Flohé and Günzler, 1976), the sperm selenopolypeptide is firmly bound to fibrous material; 3) the progressive accumulation of ^{75}Se by the testis and epididymis over a period of several weeks appears to be organ-specific (Brown and Burk, 1973), whereas, by contrast, glutathione peroxidase is widely distributed throughout the body and its concentration in the testis is comparatively modest (Flohé and Günzler, 1976); and 4) the ^{75}Se in testicular cytosol is, in the main, not associated with glutathione peroxidase activity, and includes a glutathione peroxidase-negative component whose molecular weight has been estimated as 16,000 daltons (Prohaska et al., 1977).

It is proposed that the ^{75}Se-labelled sperm polypeptide is in some way essential for the assembly of the mitochondrial sheath. Subcellular fractionation suggests its association with the outer membrane of mitochondria, a conclusion consistent with the autoradiographic studies of Brown and Burk (1973), showing localization of ^{75}Se over the midpiece of rat spermatozoa. The sperm tail defects observed in Se-deficient rats by Wu et al. (1973) may well reflect a deficiency of this labelled polypeptide.

Recently, the protein composition of SDS-insoluble mitochondrial vesicles derived from bull spermatozoa has been described (Pallini et al., 1979). Among the polypeptides identified was a 20,000-dalton, cysteine-rich molecule, which may correspond to the component designated as band II in Figure 5. This cysteine-rich molecule is believed to be intrinsic to these vesicles, and its intermolecular disulfide cross-linking is probably responsible for their stability in SDS. It remains to be established whether the rat sperm selenopolypeptide is identical with or closely related to the cysteine-rich bull sperm mitochondrial protein.

Selenium is an analogue of sulfur and can substitute for the latter to form selenocysteine, the analogue of cysteine (Forstrom et al., 1978). Nevertheless, the selenium in rat spermatozoa is not randomly distributed among cysteine-rich proteins, since it is apparently absent from dense fibers, which contain high concentrations of cysteine (Baccetti et al., 1973; Calvin et al., 1975). If present as selenocysteine, it is intriguing that selenium is specifically located in one sperm polypeptide and may well be limited to one position within the molecule. The mechanism by which selenium is incorporated as a single selenocysteine residue in each of the four catalytic sites of glutathione peroxidase is unknown, but is believed to be a posttranslational event (Forstrom *et al.*, 1978).

The total amount of selenium in the rat spermatozoon has never been reported, to the authors' knowledge. This information would be necessary to establish the maximum number of selenium-containing molecules in these cells and determine whether the labelled selenopolypeptide is a sufficiently substantial constituent of the rat spermatozoon to act as a structural protein.

REFERENCES

Baccetti, B.; Pallini, V.; Burrini, A.G.: The Accessory Fibers of the Sperm Tail. I. Structure and Chemical Composition of the Bull "Coarse Fibers." J Submicros Cytol 5(1973)237-256

Bedford, J.M.; Calvin, H.I.: Changes in —S—S—linked Structures of the Sperm Tail during Epididymal Maturation, with Comparative Observations in Sub-mammalian Species. J Exp Zool 187(1974)181-204

Bradford, M.M.: A Rapid and Sensitive Method for the Quantitation of Microgram Quantities of Protein Utilizing the Principle of Protein-Dye Binding. Anal Biochem 72(1976)248-254

Brown, D.G.; Burk, R.F.: Selenium Retention in Tissues and Sperm of Rats Fed a Torula Yeast Diet. J Nutr 103(1973)102-108

Brown, D.V.; Senger, P.L.; Stone, S.L.; Froseth, J.A.; Becker, W.C.: Glutathione Peroxidase in Bovine Semen. J Reprod Fertil 50(1977)117-118

Calvin, H.I.: Isolation and Subfractionation of Mammalian Sperm Heads and Tails. Methods Cell Biol 13(1976)85-104

Calvin, H.I.: Selective Incorporation of Selenium-75 into a Polypeptide of the Rat Sperm Tail. J Exp Zool 204(1978)445-452

Calvin, H.I.; Hwang, F.H.F.; Wohlrab, H.: Localization of Zinc in a Dense Fiber-Connecting Piece Fraction of Rat Sperm Tails Analogous Chemically to Hair Keratin. Biol Reprod 13(1975)228-239

Flohé, L.; Günzler, W.A.: Glutathione-dependent Enzymatic Oxidoreduction Reactions. In: Glutathione: Metabolism and Function, pp. 17-34, ed. by I.M. Arias and W.B. Jakoby. Raven Press, New York, 1976

Flohé, L.; Günzler, W.A.; Ladenstein, R.: Glutathione Peroxidase. In: Glutathione: Metabolism and Function, pp. 115-138, ed. by I.M. Arias and W.B. Jakoby. Raven Press, New York, 1976

Forstrom, J.W.; Zakowski, J.J.; Tappel, A.L.: Identification of the Catalytic Site of Rat Liver Glutathione Peroxidase as Selenocysteine. Biochemistry 17(1978)2639-2644

Gunn, S.A.; Gould, T.C.: Cadmium and Other Mineral Elements. In: The Testis, Vol. 3, pp. 377-481, ed. by A.D. Johnson, W.R. Gomes and N.L. Vandemark. Academic Press, New York-London, 1970

Gunn, S.A.; Gould, T.C.; Anderson, W.A.D.: Incorporation of Selenium into Spermatogenic Pathway in Mice. Proc Soc Exp Biol Med 124(1967)1260-1263

Li, T.K.: The Glutathione and Thiol Content of Mammalian Spermatozoa and Seminal Plasma. Biol Reprod 12(1975)641-646

Paglia, D.E.; Valentine, W.N.: Studies on the Quantitative and Qualitative Characterization of Erythrocyte Glutathione Peroxidase. J Lab Clin Med 70(1967)158-169

Pallini, V.; Baccetti, B.; Burrini, A.G.: A Peculiar Cysteine-Rich Polypeptide as Related to Some Unusual Properties of Mammalian Sperm Mitochondria. In: The Spermatozoon, pp. 141–51, ed. by D.W. Fawcett and J.M. Bedford. Urban and Schwarzenberg, Baltimore, 1979

Prohaska, J.R.; Mowafy, M.; Ganther, H.E.: Interactions between Cadmium, Selenium and Glutathione Peroxidase in Rat Testis. Chem Biol Interact 18(1977)253-265

Reynolds, E.S.: The Use of Lead Citrate at High pH as an Electron-opaque Stain in Electron Microscopy. J Cell Biol 17(1963)210-213

Wu, S.H.; Oldfield, J.E.; Whanger, P.D.; Weswig, P.H.: Effects of Selenium, Vitamin E, and Antioxidants on Testicular Function in Rats. Biol Reprod 8(1973)625-629

A PECULIAR CYSTEINE-RICH POLYPEPTIDE RELATED TO SOME UNUSUAL PROPERTIES OF MAMMALIAN SPERM MITOCHONDRIA

V. Pallini, B. Baccetti, and A.G. Burrini

Institute of Zoology, University of Siena, 53100 Siena, Italy

Sperm mitochondria have structural and functional characteristics which are not shared by mitochondria of other mammalian cells, *i.e.* a crescentic shape and helical arrangement (Fawcett, 1970; Phillips, 1977); a multilaminar outer membrane (Elfvin, 1968) stabilized by disulfide cross-links and resistant to extraction with sodium dodecyl sulfate (SDS) (Bedford and Calvin, 1974); unusually shaped and arranged *cristae* (Fawcett, 1970); resistance to hypotonic conditions (Keyhani and Storey, 1973); a comparatively inefficient uptake of Ca^{2+} (Storey and Keyhani, 1973); and a peculiar metabolism of pyruvate (Van Dop *et al.*, 1977) connected with an intramitochondrial localization of lactate dehydrogenase isozyme X (Montamat and Blanco, 1976; Baccetti *et al.*, 1975).

Using purified preparations of bull sperm mitochondria the authors have studied the polypeptide composition of the disulfide-hardened, SDS-resistant fraction of the mitochondrial outer membrane. A peculiar cysteine- and proline-rich polypeptide was isolated from this structure which appeared to be related to the stability of the unusual shape of these mitochondria and to their resistance to swelling.

METHODS

Preparation of Sperm Subcellular Structures

Bovine epididymal sperm mitochondria were detached by sonication and isolated by isopycnic centrifugation as described elsewhere (Pallini, 1979). An SDS-insoluble fraction was prepared by suspending mitochondria in about 50 volumes of 4% SDS in $0.0125M$ Tris-HCl at pH 6.8; the residue was sedimented at $30,000\,g$ for 15 min and washed twice with $0.12M$ NaCl, $0.01M$ Tris-HCl, pH 7.5. In order to prevent sulfhydryl oxidation or rearrangement with disulfide groups, 4%-solutions of SDS in $0.02M$ EDTA (pH 5.0) were used under nitrogen (Sedlak and Lindsay, 1968). When necessary, preparations were stored at $-30\,°C$ in the presence of 0.2 mg/ml of phenylmethylsulfonyl fluoride. Bovine epididymal sperm accessory fibers were prepared as previously described (Baccetti *et al.*, 1976a).

Swelling Experiments

Swelling studies were performed by monitoring at 520 nm the turbidity of suspensions of freshly prepared mitochondria containing 0.1-0.2 mg protein/ml. Dimethylsulfoxide (1% v/v), $CaCl_2$ ($2.5\,mM$) (Lehninger, 1962) and mercaptoethanol were added to mitochondrial suspensions in $0.12M$ NaCl, $0.01M$ Tris-HCl (pH 7.5). Suspensions in $0.12M$ ammonium phosphate or acetate at pH 7.5, $10^{-4}M$ Rotenone, $10^{-3}M$ ethyleneglycol,-bis(amino-ethyl ether)-N,N tetraacetic acid (Crompton *et al.*, 1974) were also studied.

Reduction and Carboxamidomethylation

Sedimented and lyophylized structures were dissolved (4-6 mg dry weight/ml) in $7M$ guanidine-HCl, $0.5M$ Tris-HCl at pH 8.5, $0.1M$ dithiothreitol and incubated at $37\,°C$ for 2 h under nitrogen. Carboxamidomethylation of sulfhydryl groups was achieved by adding iodoacetamide to $0.25M$ final concentration. In radioactive labelling experiments, ^{14}C-iodoacetamide was mixed with the cold reagent in order to obtain a specific activity of about 50 μCi/mmol. Proteins were quantitatively recovered from the reaction mixtures by precipitation with 5 volumes of absolute ethanol at $-30\,°C$ and by centrifugation at $5,000\,g$ at $2\,°C$, or by dialyzing reaction mixtures against distilled water at $2\,°C$.

Ion-exchange Chromatography

Reduced alkylated proteins were precipitated by dialysis against distilled water, lyophilized, dissolved in $7M$ urea, $0.01M$ Tris-HCl at pH 7.5, and loaded on a dieth-

---

This investigation was supported by the C.N.R. (Centro Nazionale delle Ricerche), project "Biology of Reproduction."

© 1979 Urban & Schwarzenberg, Inc. Baltimore-Munich *The Spermatozoon*, edited by D.W. Fawcett and J.M. Bedford

ylaminoethyl (DEAE) Sephadex (A 50) column, 0.8 x 10 cm. The column was eluted with a 200 ml linear gradient of NaCl (0.2M) in 7M urea, 0.01M Tris-HCl at pH 7.5; 2-ml fractions were collected at a flow rate of 1 ml/10 min; the absorbancy at 280 nm of each fraction was determined. Fractions in the peaks were pooled, dialyzed against distilled water and lyophylized.

Aminoacid Analysis

Carboxamidomethylated proteins were hydrolyzed for 24 h at 110°C. The hydrolysates were dried *in vacuo* over P_2O_5 and NaOH and analyzed as previously described (Baccetti *et al.*, 1976b) using the M82 single column of a Beckman Multichrom B liquid column chromatograph.

SDS-polyacrylamide Gel Electrophoresis

The high-pH discontinous system described by Laemmli (1970) was used, with 5.5 x 55 mm cylindrical separation gels of 12% polyacrylamide. Proteins were dissolved by heating at 100°C for 2 min in 2% SDS, 5% mercaptoethanol, 0.06M Tris-HCl at pH 6.8, 10% glycerol, and 0.001% bromphenol blue. Mercaptoethanol was omitted when dissolving alkylated proteins. Electrophoresis was performed at 1 mA per gel. Bands were stained with 0.2% Coomassie blue in 50% methanol, 7% acetic acid and destained with 20% methanol and 7% acetic acid, followed by 7% acetic acid. The following reference proteins were used in order to estimate molecular weights: cytochrome C (M_r 11,700), carboxamidomethylated papain (M_r 23,000), tropomyosin (M_r 36,000), actin (M_r 45,000), and bovine serum albumin (M_r 68,000). In order to estimate the protein content, stained bands were cut out, rinsed with distilled water, the dye eluted with 25% aqueous pyridine, and measured at 605 nm (Fenner *et al.*, 1975). For radioactivity determinations, the stained bands were counted by the method of Senior (1975).

Chemical Determinations

Total protein was determined by the method of Lowry *et al.* (1951). Phospholipids were extracted according to Folch *et al.* (1957) and total phosphorus determined on the washed extracts by the method described by Ames (1966).

Electron Microscopy

Purified mitochondria were fixed in Karnovsky's fixative, containing 2% tannic acid, for 1 h at 4°C; washed in cacodylate buffer 0.1M pH 7.2 overnight; postfixed in 1% OsO_4 in the same buffer for 30 min at 4°C; and dehydrated and embedded in Epon. Sections were stained with uranyl acetate and lead citrate. Negative staining was performed with 1% PTA (phosphotungstic acid) in 0.4% sucrose at pH 7. The samples were examined with a Philips EM 301 electron microscope.

RESULTS

Swelling of Sperm Mitochondria

Isolated sperm mitochondria were essentially unaffected by a variety of treatments known to produce swelling in heart and liver mitochondria: the organelle ultrastructure and the turbidity of the suspension did not change over prolonged incubation (as long as 6 h) in 2mM Tris-HCl buffer of pH 7.5; only minor decreases in turbidity were noted using dimethylsulfoxide or calcium and ammonium salts as swelling agents (*cf.* "Methods").

On the other hand, after addition of mercaptoethanol the turbidity dropped at a rate roughly related to the concentration of this reagent (Fig. 1) and reached a minimum at about 70% of the initial value. Mitochondria sedimented after mercaptoethanol-induced swelling appeared in the electron microscope as markedly swollen, empty round vesicles (Fig. 2). These structures contained the whole spectrum of native mitochondrial polypeptides (Fig. 3) except for one specific polypeptide of 20,000 daltons which was extracted by mercaptoethanol and recovered in the supernatant fraction in quite pure form: it proved to account for about 15% of total

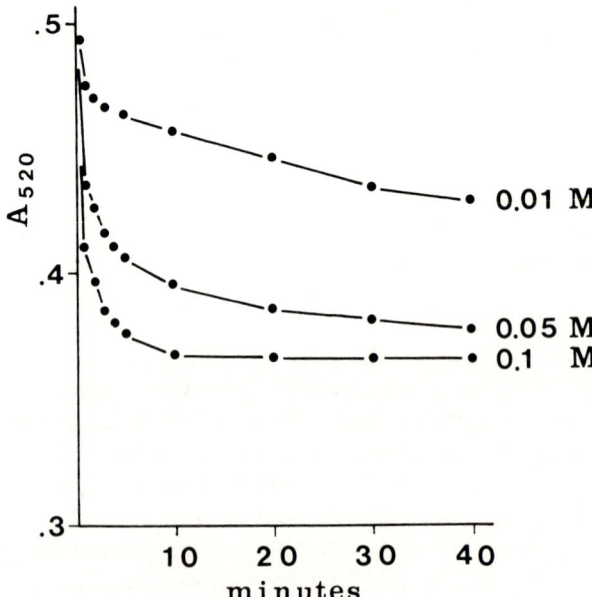

Figure 1. Time course of the turbidity decrease of sperm mitochondrial suspensions in the presence of mercaptoethanol. Mercaptoethanol (0.01, 0.05, and 0.1M) was added at the 0 time.

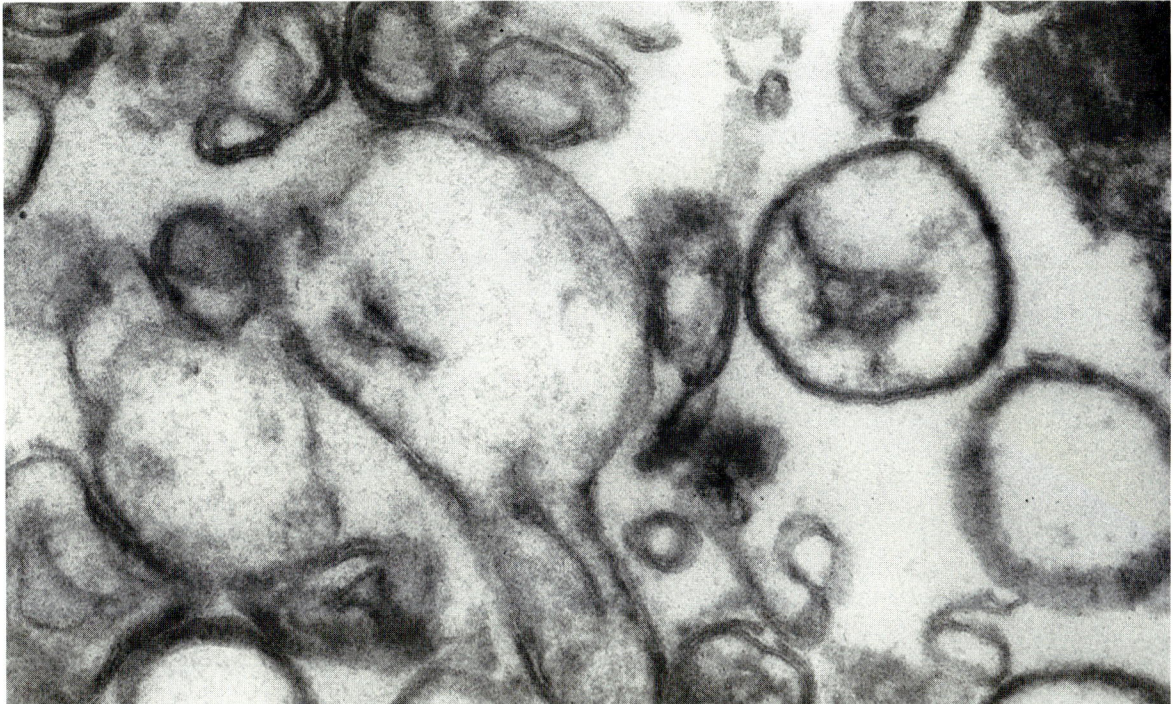

Figure 2. Electron microscopic appearance of sperm mitochondria after swelling induced by 0.05M mercaptoethanol. Tannic acid impregnation. X112,000

mitochondrial protein. Control experiments showed that not even traces of this polypeptide are released from mitochondria incubated in the absence of mercaptoethanol (Fig. 3). Preliminary experiments performed with increasing concentrations of mercaptoethanol (5-50mM) demonstrate that the turbidity decrease and the extent of release of the 20,000-dalton polypeptide are roughly proportional.

At the ultrastructural level mitochondria, after mercaptoethanol-induced swelling, show the cytoplasmic surface of the outer membrane completely smooth, even after tannic-acid treatment (Fig. 4). In the control specimens the same surface after tannic-acid treatment reveals a granular component covering its whole area (Fig. 5).

Nature of the SDS-resistent Outer Membrane

Upon extraction of isolated sperm mitochondria with excess SDS (*cf.* "Methods"), an insoluble residue is formed which can be sedimented as a tightly packed, glass-transparent pellet; in the electron microscope it appears to consist of empty mitochondrial outer membranes that preserve their crescent shape (Fig. 6, 7). These structures are stabilized by disulfide cross-links since they dissolve rapidly upon addition of mercaptoethanol (0.01-0.1M final concentration) to suspension in SDS or in saline. The SDS-resistent structure does not result from an artefactual disulfide cross-linking since it is also obtained by extraction with SDS under conditions to prevent any sulfhydryl oxidation or rearrangement with disulfides (*cf.* "Methods").

The SDS-resistent residue accounts for 30-40% of total mitochondrial protein and contains less than 0.2 μg of lipid phosphorus per mg protein, *i.e.*, less than 3% of the lipid phosphorus content of native sperm mitochondria.

As demonstrated by gel electrophoresis (Fig. 8), the SDS-resistent fraction essentially consists of three polypeptide chains having molecular weights of 31,000, 29,000 and 20,000. The 31,000-dalton chain is present also in the SDS-soluble fraction, whereas the two other components are found only in the SDS-resistent residue. It should be noted that the 20,000-dalton polypeptide is released from mitochondria by treatment with mercaptoethanol. The quantitative ratios among the 31,000-, 29,000-, and 20,000-dalton components were found very reproducibly to be 1:1:2 in several different preparations.

As a first step toward separation on a preparative scale, the polypeptides of the SDS-resistent residue were fully reduced and alkylated (*cf.* "Methods"); upon dialysis against distilled water a precipitate was formed in which the three polypeptides were present; the supernatant, however, also contained a considerable amount of

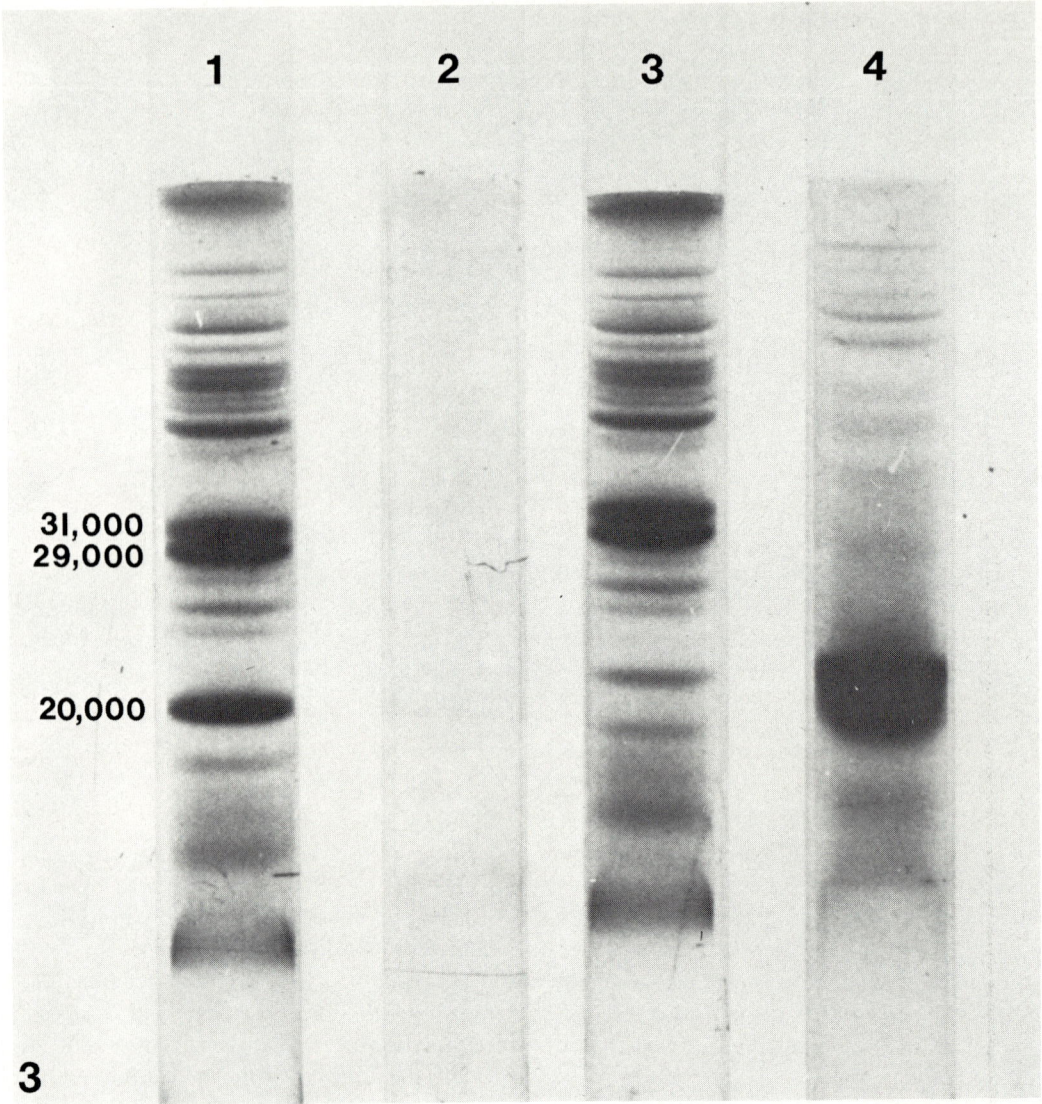

Figure 3. Extractability of sperm mitochondrial polypeptides with mercaptoethanol. Mitochondria were suspended (0.3 mg protein/ml) in 0.12M NaCl, 0.01M Tris-HCl at pH 7.5 containing 0.05M mercaptoethanol. The latter reagent was omitted in control experiments. Swelling was monitored at 520 nm for 30 min at room temperature; suspensions were then centrifuged at 20,000 rpm for 10 min; the sediment and the supernatant were analyzed by SDS-polyacrylamide gel electrophoresis. Gel 1: sediment of control experiment, corresponding to 30 μl of incubation mixture. Gel 2: supernatant of control experiment, corresponding to 300 μl of incubation mixture. Gel 3: sediment from swelling experiment, corresponding to 30 μl of incubation mixture. Gel 4: supernatant of swelling experiment, corresponding to 300 μl of incubation mixture.

the 20,000-dalton chain in very pure form (gel 1, Fig. 10). A DEAE Sephadex column chromatography of the precipitate (Fig. 9) yielded essentially two A_{280} peaks: in the first mostly the 29,000-dalton polypeptide was detected (gel 2, Fig. 10), while the second contained the 31,000-dalton polypeptide and traces of lower molecular weight components, including the 20,000-dalton chain (gel 3, Fig. 10).

The amino acid composition of the three polypeptides in the described degree of purification is reported in Table 1. The 29,000- and 31,000-dalton components do not possess any predominant amino-acid that might suggest some specialized roles. On the other hand, the very high cysteine and proline content of the 20,000-dalton polypeptide is quite unusual for a membrane protein and may be compared with those of high sulfur components of keratins and mammalian sperm accessory fibers (Baccetti et al., 1976b).

Electrophoretic Demonstration that Sperm Mitochondria and Accessory Fibers Contain Different Sulfur-rich Polypeptides

Cysteine-rich polypeptides were specifically labelled by fully reducing and alkylating with ^{14}C-iodoacetamide (cf. "Methods") the mitochondrial SDS-insoluble fraction and the accessory fibers from bull sperm; ethanol-precipitated proteins were separated by SDS-polyacrylamide gel electrophoresis (Fig. 11); due to the high load on the gel (gel 1, Fig. 11) the 29,000- and 31,000-dalton polypeptides are not well separated and several minor bands are visible; the electrophoretic pattern of sperm accessory fibers (gel 2, Fig. 11) shows a predominant band at about 30,000 daltons as previously described (Baccetti et al., 1976b). The ratio between radioactivity and dye content of a band (cf. "Methods") represents an indirect measure of the cysteine content of the polypeptide and is found to be highest in the 20,000-dalton band from mitochondria and in the 30,000-dalton band from accessory fibers (Table 2). Therefore, these molecules are rather similar as to content of cysteine, yet are easily distinguishable on the basis of their electrophoretic mobility.

DISCUSSION

Bedford and Calvin (1974) first observed by electron microscopy that the mitochondrial outer membrane of rat spermatozoa can be dissolved in SDS only after reduction of disulfide bonds with dithiothreitol. This chapter reports that extraction with SDS of purified bull sperm mitochondria results in the formation of insoluble empty structures that maintain the typical crescent shape of sperm mitochondrial outer membranes, do not contain phospholipids, and consist of three polypeptide chains (20,000, 29,000, and 31,000 daltons) cross-linked by disulfide bridges. The authors propose to call these structures mitochondrial "shells"

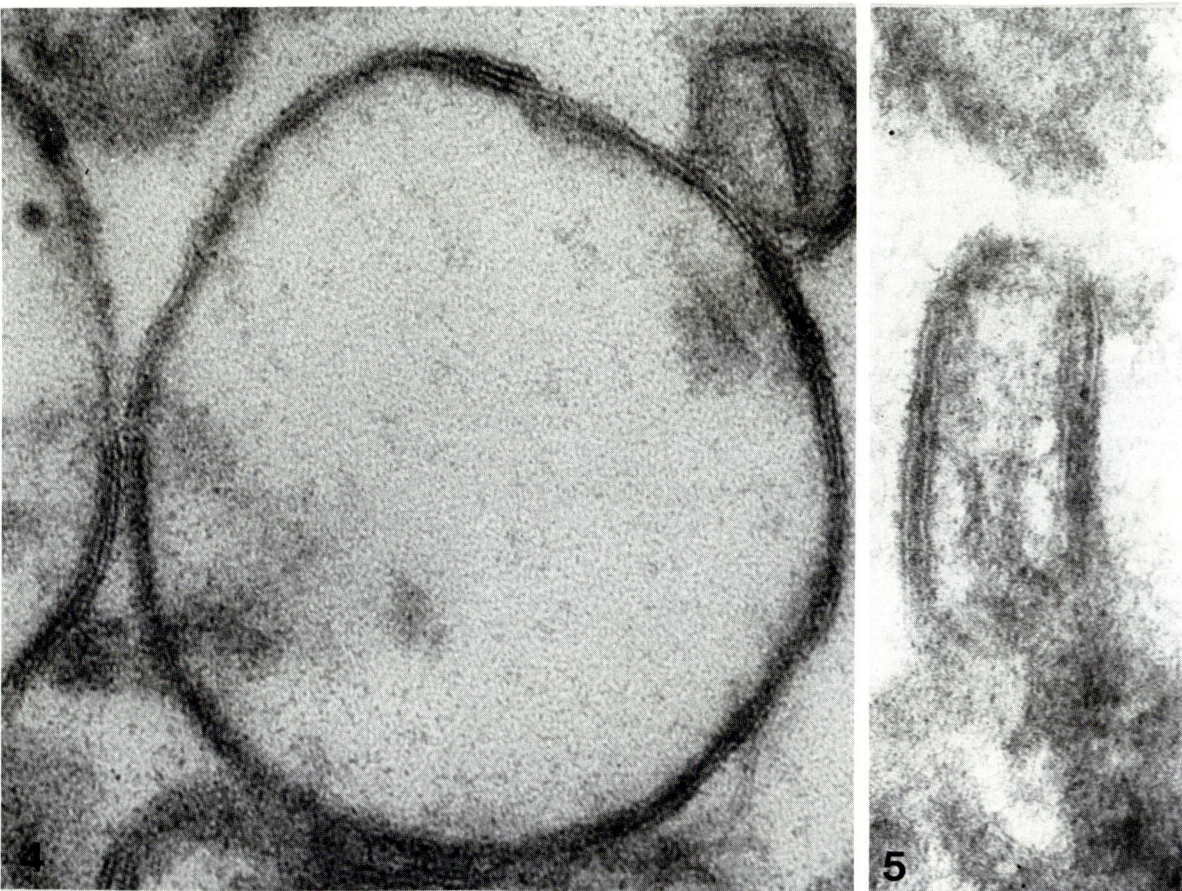

Figure 4. Thin section of a sperm mitochondrial preparation after mercaptoethanol-induced swelling. The cytoplasmic surface of the mitochondrial outer membrane is completely smooth. Tannic acid impregnation. X224,000

Figure 5. Thin section of a native sperm mitochondria preparation (control for Fig. 4). The cytoplasmic surface of the mitochondrial outer membrane in covered by a granular layer. Tannic acid impregnation. X224,000

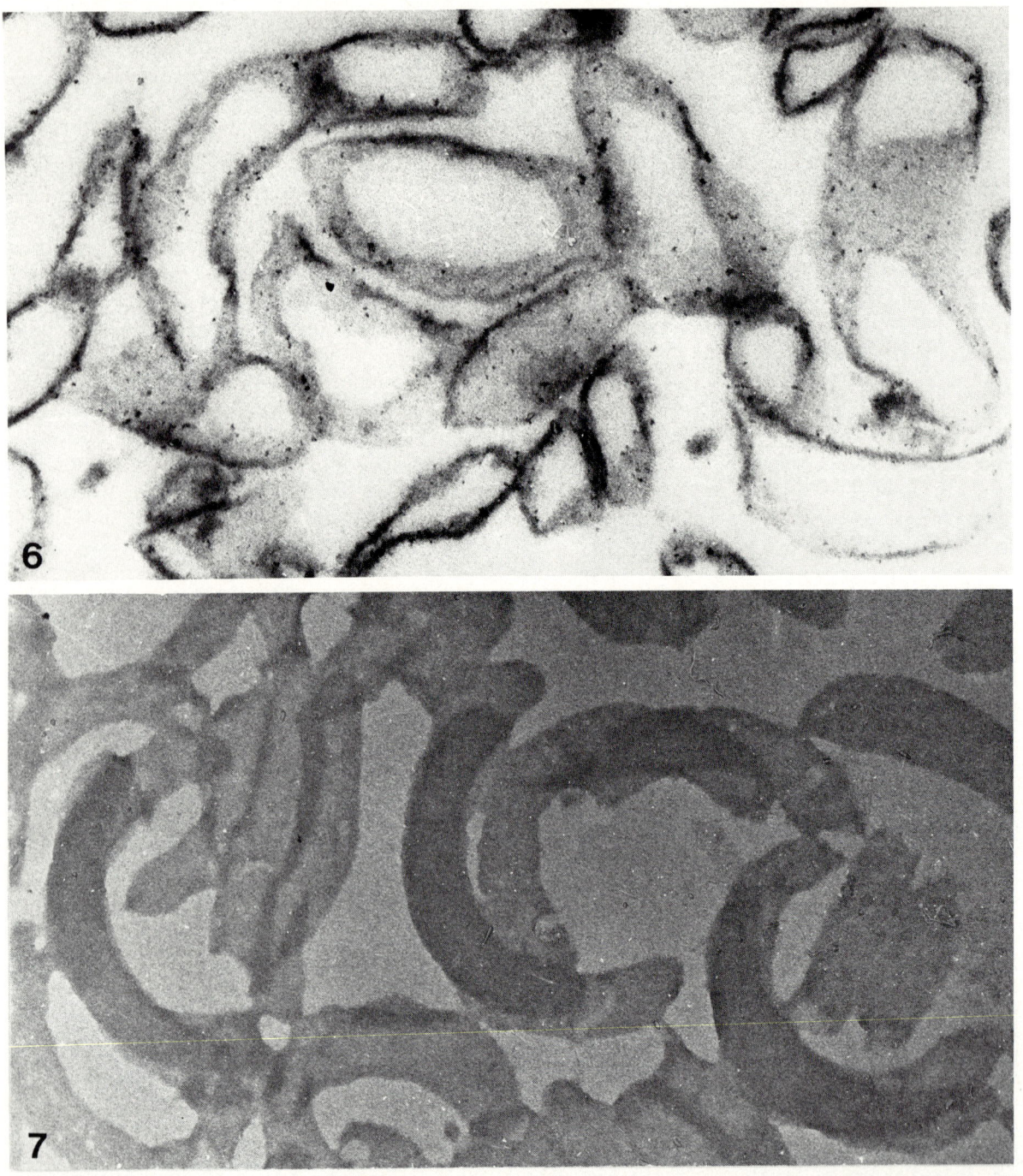

Figure 6. Electron microscopic appearance of the SDS-resistant structures from bull sperm mitochondria. Thin section. X120,000

Figure 7. Electron microscopic appearance of the SDS-resistant structures from bull sperm mitochondria. Negative staining. X30,000

rather than "ghosts" since they consist of lipid-depleted membrane structural proteins and have certainly lost all phospholipid-dependent membrane properties, which, on the contrary, are preserved in structures usually designated as ghosts.

The cross-linked polypeptides correspond to bands 8, 9, and 12 in high resolution electropherograms of sperm mitochondrial proteins (Pallini, 1979) and are absent or negligible in bull heart and liver mitochondria. The 20,000-dalton polypeptide (band No. 12 in the cited paper) may connect into a network the other two components by forming disulfide bonds with them, as is suggested by its high content of cysteine; in addition, its high content of proline may correspond to structural and functional properties quite unusual in membrane proteins. This polypeptide certainly recalls the high sulfur components of bull sperm accessory fibers (Baccetti et al., 1976b), from which, however, it is easily distinguished on the basis of its electrophoretic migration and relatively high solubility in water.

The data reported in this chapter and in the accompanying paper (Pallini, 1979) demonstrate that the crescent shape of bull sperm mitochondria is stable enough to undergo without modification the strains of the isolation procedure, i.e., sonication and exposure to hypertonic sucrose solutions; moreover, isolated bull sperm mitochondria prove resistant to hypotonic shock, in agreement with the observation of Keyhani and Storey (1973) on whole rabbit spermatozoa; in addition, it is particularly interesting that they are not affected by ammonium salts which induce a swelling based on the anion-active transport by the organelle conceivably operating in all kinds of mitochondria (Crompton et al., 1974). Until now, we have been able to induce swelling, i.e., loss of crescent shape and enlargement, only by treating sperm mitochondria with mercaptoethanol, a well known disulfide-reducing reagent; the concentrations of mercaptoethanol used to

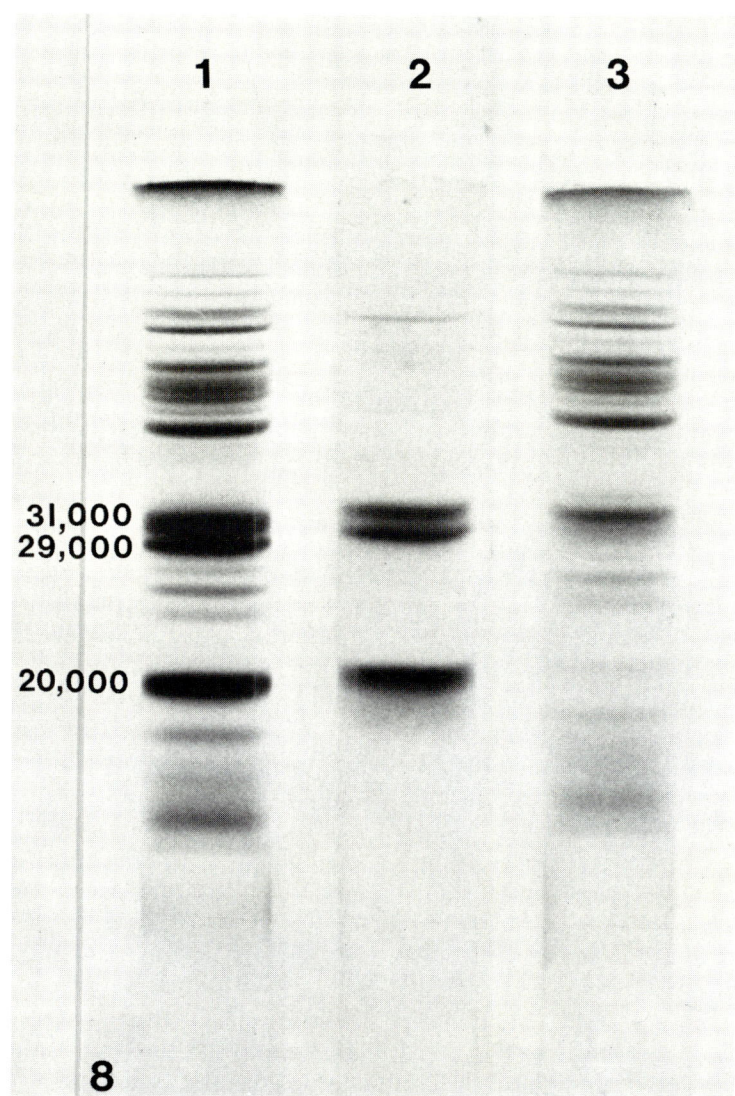

Figure 8. Extractability of sperm mitochondrial polypeptides with SDS. Gel 1: polypeptides of native mitochondria, 30 μg of total protein. Gel 2: polypeptides of the SDS-insoluble fraction from 30 μg of total mitochondrial protein. Gel 3: polypeptides of the SDS-soluble fraction from 30 μg of total mitochondrial protein.

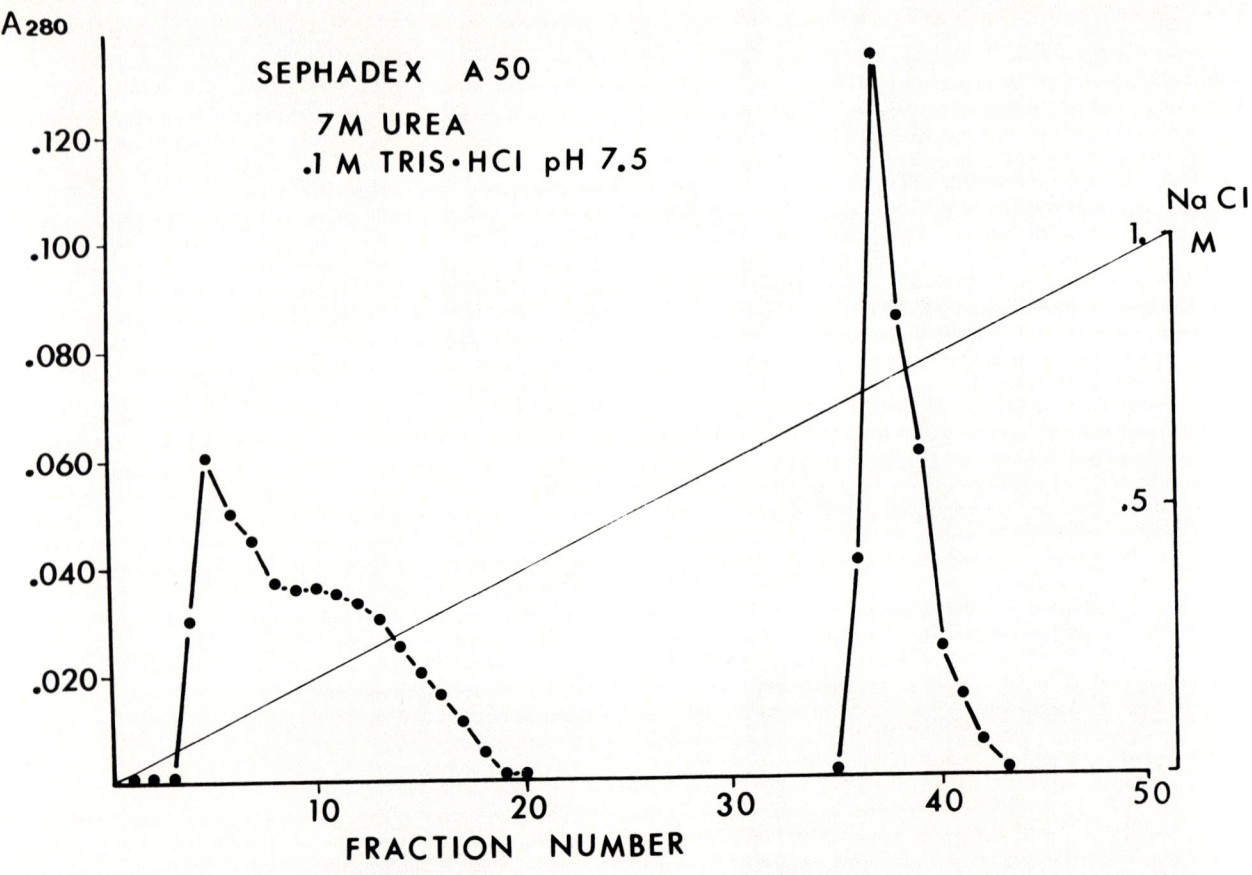

Figure 9. Ion-exchange chromatography of alkylated polypeptides from the SDS-resistant fraction of bull sperm mitochondria. The shape of the NaCl gradient is also reported (straight line and the scale on the right side of the graph).

promote swelling were also sufficient to solubilize the SDS-resistant shell and the swelling itself was concomitant with the specific release of the 20,000-dalton cysteine-rich polypeptide. These observations lead us to conclude that surface and osmotic forces are strongly opposed by the disulfide-stabilized shell as long as the disulfide cross-links are intact. This situation is quite unusual in metazoan membranes; however it is interesting to note that the abnormal shape of spheroechinocytes is stabilized by covalent cross-links, including disulfide bonds, among spectrin polypeptides (Palek et al., 1978) and that the osmotic resistance of camel erythrocytes is determined by a tight interaction between the membrane and a spectrin network (Ralston, 1975).

The present data do not allow conclusions as to the functional role of a covalently cross-linked shell in sperm mitochondria of higher mammals. Even though its significance is not yet understood, an artefactual nature of this structure may be ruled out since it may be obtained by extraction with SDS under conditions that prevent sulfhydryl-disulfide rearrangements. This conclusion is further supported by the reproducible stoichiometric ratios among its polypeptide components.

The crescent shape itself suggests that the shells consist of proteins originally localized in the mitochondrial outer membrane; their interaction with other membrane components is as yet unclear. The authors have observed (unpublished data) that the shells easily recombine with phospholipids; probably the 29,000- and 31,000-dalton components are capable of interacting with the lipid bilayer; however, the tendency of the 20,000-dalton polypeptide to stay in water solution suggests a localization extrinsic to the membrane.

The probable external localization of this polypeptide and its absence from mitochondria detached with mercaptoethanol from the spermatozoon (Pallini, 1979) may indicate that it represents at least a component of the mitochondrial cement (André, 1962; Clérot et al., 1977; Toury et al., 1977) supposed to connect mitochondria with one another during sperm development. In addition, the molecular weight and the extractability of this polypeptide seem quite similar to those of selenoflagellin, a selenium-binding protein recently detected by Calvin (1978) in rat spermatozoa.

SUMMARY

Isolated bull sperm mitochondria possess an SDS-insoluble shell which maintains the crescent shape of the outer membrane and consists of three polypeptide chains (M_r 20,000, 29,000, and 31,000) cross-linked by disulfide bridges. The 20,000-dalton polypeptide contains more than 20 prolines and about 18 cysteines per 100 residues and is selectively released when these mitochondria are induced to swell by treatment with mercaptoethanol, a disulfide-reducing reagent. Bull sperm mitochondria are otherwise resistant to all other tested swelling reagents active on heart and liver mitochondria. It is concluded that the well-documented unusual shape and resistence to swelling of mammalian sperm mitochondria are due to the stabilizing effect of disulfide-hardened structural proteins probably localized in the outer membrane.

REFERENCES

Ames, B.N.: Assay of Inorganic Phosphate, Total Phosphate and Phosphatases. In: Methods in Enzymology. Vol. VII, pp. 115-118, ed. by E.F. Neufeld and V. Ginsburg. Academic Press, New York-London, 1966

Andrè, J.: Contribution à La Connaissance du Chondriome. Etude de ses Modifications Ultrastructurales pendant La Spermatogenèse. J Ultrastruct Res 3(1962)1-185S

Baccetti, B.; Pallini, V.; Burrini, A.G.: Localization and

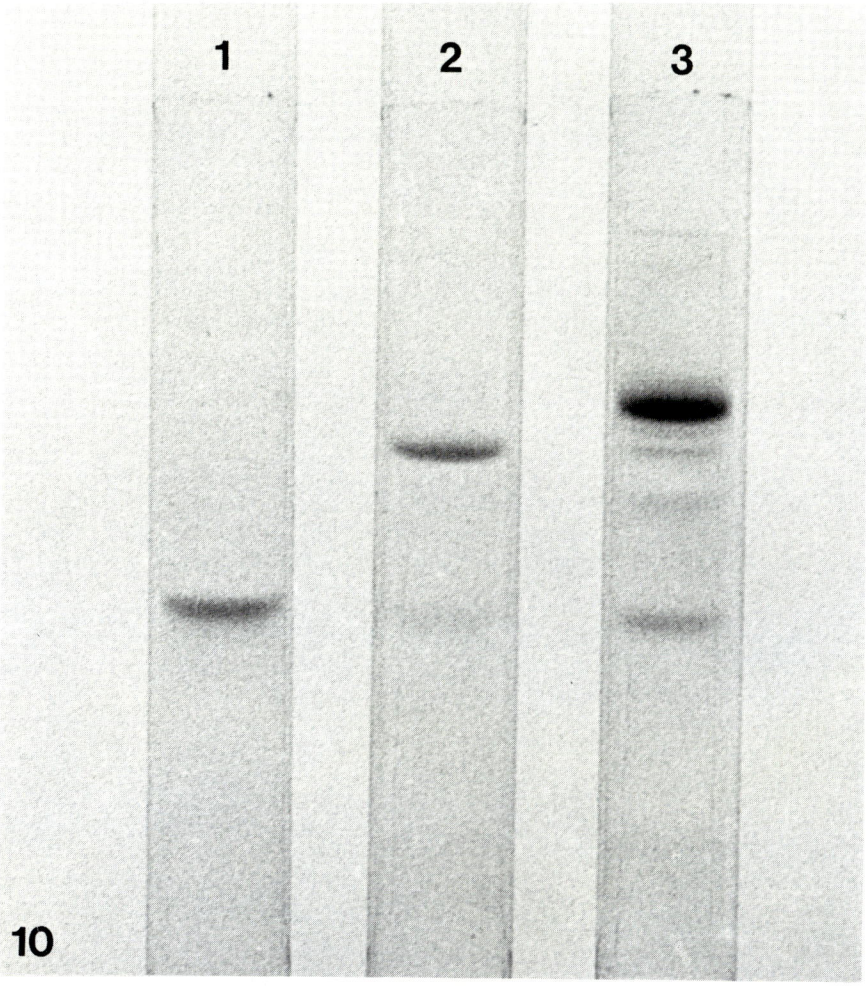

Figure 10. Purity assessment of the polypeptides isolated from the SDS-resistant fraction of bull sperm mitochondria. Gel 1: water-soluble fraction of alkylated proteins (cf. "Methods"), 0.025 A_{280} units. Gel 2: fractions 4-18 (cf. Fig. 9), 0.025 A_{280} units. Gel 3: fractions 36-44 (cf. Fig. 9), 0.05 A_{280} units.

Table 1. Amino Acid Composition of the Polypeptides Present in SDS-resistent Fraction of Bull Sperm Mitochondria (residues/100 residues)

	31,000-Dalton Polypeptide	29,000-Dalton Polypeptide	20,000-Dalton Polypeptide
SCM Cysteine*	2.1	0.4	17.9
Aspartic acid	11.3	9.9	7.0
Threonine	7.8	6.8	3.4
Serine	9.6	11.3	8.8
Glutamic acid	12.1	9.6	13.6
Proline	5.1	2.2	26.5
Glycine	10.5	13.8	3.5
Alanine	6.7	7.2	1.8
Valine	4.1	3.6	0.8
Methionine	1.2	0.7	0.2
Isoleucine	3.4	2.9	0.3
Leucine	7.7	7.0	2.7
Tyrosine	3.2	3.1	0.3
Phenylalanine	3.9	4.1	0.3
Histidine	1.1	6.7	0.0
Lysine	7.1	8.6	11.3
Argine	2.9	1.8	1.5

*S-carboxymethyl cysteine

Catalytic Properties of Lactate Dehydrogenase in Different Sperm Models. Exp Cell Res 90(1975)183-190

Baccetti, B.; Pallini, V.; Burrini, A.G.: The Accessory Fibers of the Sperm Tail. II. Their Role in Binding Zinc in Mammals and Cephalopods. J Ultrastruct Res 54(1967a)261-275

Baccetti, B.; Pallini, V.; Burrini, A.G.: The Accessory Fibers of the Sperm Tail. III. High-Sulfur and Low-Sulfur Components in Mammals and Cephalopods. J Ultrastruct Res 57(1976b)289-308

Bedford, J.M.; Calvin, H.I.: Changes in —S—S-linked Structures of the Sperm Tail during Epididymal Maturation, with Comparative Observations in Sub-mammalian Species. J Exp Zool 187(1974)181-204

Calvin, H.I.: Selective Incorporation of Selenium-75 into a Polypeptide of the Rat Sperm Tail. J Exp Zool 204(1978)445-452

Clérot, J.C.; Toury, R.; Andrè, J.: Les Groupements Mitochondriaux des Cellules Germinales des Poissons Téléostéens Cyprinidés. III. Méthode d'Isolament du Ciment Intermitochondrial. Biol Cell 30(1977)217-224

Crompton, H.; Palmieri, F.; Capano, M.; Quagliarello, E.: The Transport of Sulfate and Sulfite in Rat Liver Mitochondria. Biochem J 142(1974)127-137

Elfvin, L.G.: An Ultrastructural Difference between the Outer and Inner Membrane of the Middle Piece Mitochondria in Rat Spermatozoa. J Ultrastruct Res 24(1968)259-268

Fawcett, D.W.: A Comparative View of Sperm Ultrastructure. Biol Reprod 2(1970)90-127S2

Fenner, C.; Traut, R.R.; Mason, D.T.; Wikman-Coffelt, J.: Quantification of Coomassie Blue-stained Proteins in Polyacrylamide Gels Based on Analyses of Eluted Dye. Anal Biochem 63(1975)595-602

Folch, J.; Less, M.; Sloane Stanley, G.H.: A Simple Method for the Isolation and Purification of Total Lipids from Animal Tissues. J Biol Chem 226(1957)497-509

Keyhani, E.; Storey, B.T.: Energy Conservation Capacity and Morphological Integrity of Mitochondria in Hypotonically Treated Rabbit Epididymal Spermatozoa. Biochim Biophys Acta 305(1973)557-569

Laemmli, U.K.: Change of Structural Proteins during the Assembly of the Head of Bacteriophage T_4. Nature 227(1970)680-685

Lehninger, A.L.: Water Uptake and Extrusion by Mitochondria in Relation to Oxidative Phosphorylation. Physiol Rev 42(1962)467-517

Lowry, O.H.; Rosebrough, N.J.; Farr, A.L.; Randall, R.J.: Protein Measurement with the Folin Phenol Reagent. J Biol Chem 193(1951)265-275

Montamat, E.E.; Blanco, A.: Subcellular Distribution of the Lactate Dehydrogenase Isozyme Specific for Testis and Sperm. Exp Cell Res 103(1976)241-245

Palek, J.; Liu, P.A.; Liu, S.C.: Polymerization of Cell Membrane Protein Contributes to Spheroechinocyte-shaped Irreversibility. Nature 274(1978)505-507

Pallini, V.: Isolation of Mitochondria from Bull Epididymal Spermatozoa. In: The Spermatozoon, ed. by D.W. Fawcett and J.M. Bedford. Urban & Schwarzenberg, Baltimore-Munich, 1979

Phillips, D.M.: Mitochondrial Disposition in Mammalian Spermatozoa. J Ultrastruct Res 58(1977)144-154

Ralston, G.B.: Proteins of the Camel Erythrocyte Membrane. Biochim Biophys Acta 401(1975)83-94

Sedlak, J.; Lindsay, R.H.: Estimation of Total, Protein-bound, and Non-Protein Sulfhydryl Groups in Tissue with Ellman's Reagent. Anal Biochem 25(1968)192-205

Senior, A.E.: Mitochondrial Adenosine Triphosphatase. Location of Sulfhydryl Groups and Disulfide Bonds in the Soluble Enzyme from Beef Heart. Biochemistry 14(1975)660-664

Storey, B.T.; Keyhani, E.: Interaction of Calcium Ion with the Mitochondria of Rabbit Spermatozoa. FEBS Lett 37(1973)33-36

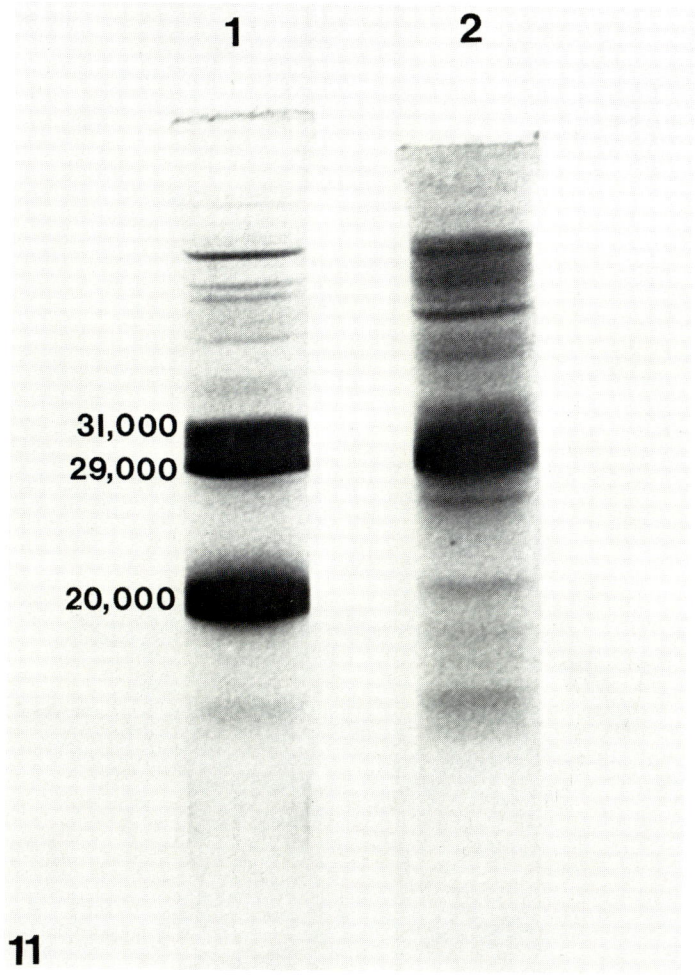

Figure 11. SDS-polyacrylamide gel electrophoresis of the mitochondrial SDS-resistant fraction and of the accessory fibers from bull epididymal spermatozoa. Gel 1: reduced ^{14}C-carboxamidomethylated mitochondrial proteins, 0.2 A_{280} units. Gel 2: reduced ^{14}C-carboxamidomethylated accessory fiber proteins, 0.2 A_{280} units.

Toury, R.; Clérot, J.C.; André, J.: Les Groupements Mitochondriaux des Cellules Germinales des Poissons Téléostéens Cyprinidés. IV. Analyse Biochimique des Constituants du "Ciment" Intermitochondrial Isolé. Biol Cell 30(1977)225-232

Van Dop, C.; Hutson, S.M.; Lardy, H.A.: Pyruvate Metabolism in Bovine Epididymal Spermatozoa. J Biol Chem 252(1977)1303-1308

Table 2. Distribution of ^{14}C-iodoacetamide in Polypeptide Chains from Bull Sperm Accessory Fibers and SDS-resistent Fraction of Mitochondria (cf. Methods and Fig. 11)

Polypeptide	Degree of Labelling* (counts/min/A_{605})
Accessory fibers	
approximately 30,000 dalton	750
Mitochondria	
31,000 dalton	78
29,000 dalton	32
20,000 dalton	807

*Expressed as the ratio between counts per minute and absorbance of dye eluted from the electrophoretic band.

ASYMMETRICAL OSCILLATION OF SEA URCHIN SPERM FLAGELLA INDUCED BY CALCIUM

C.J. Brokaw and S.F. Goldstein

Division of Biology, California Institute of Technology, Pasadena, California 91125 USA; Department of Genetics and Cell Biology, University of Minnesota, St. Paul, Minnesota 55108 USA

Modulation of beating by Ca^{2+} concentration has been demonstrated in demembranated sea urchin sperm flagella (Brokaw et al., 1974) and in several other types of cilia and flagella (Naitoh and Kaneko, 1972; Holwill and McGregor, 1975; Tsuchiya, 1976; etc.). In the case of sea urchin sperm flagella, symmetrical flagellar waveforms and nearly straight swimming paths are observed following Triton-demembranation in the presence of millimolar concentrations of Ca^{2+}, if the Ca^{2+} concentration in the reactivation solution is maintained at a low level (approximately $10^{-9}M$) with EGTA. If the Ca^{2+} concentration in the reactivation solution is increased, the flagellar waveforms become asymmetrical and the spermatozoa swim in circular paths when they are observed close to a surface. This Ca^{2+} control mechanism may be involved in generating the asymmetrical beat patterns seen when spermatozoa of other species respond chemotactically to egg extracts (Miller and Brokaw, 1970; Miller, 1976) but it has no known function in sea urchin spermatozoa.

Analysis of the changes in flagellar bending which occur when the beat pattern becomes asymmetrical may facilitate understanding of the mechanisms that control sliding between the microtubules of sperm flagella, to produce normal oscillation and bend propagation. Sea urchin spermatozoa are particularly suitable for this analysis because high-quality photographs of their planar waveforms can be readily obtained, and methods for Triton-demembranation and reactivation under controlled conditions have become routine.

This chapter is a preliminary report on a portion of the results of this analysis. A detailed report will be published (Brokaw, 1979).

EXPERIMENTAL

Spermatozoa were obtained from the sea urchin *Strongylocentrotus purpuratus* and demembranated with Triton X-100 by standard procedures (Brokaw, 1975a). The reactivation solutions for these experiments contained $0.25M$ KCl, $3mM$ Mg^{2+}, $0.10mM$ $MgATP^{2-}$, $2mM$ dithiothreitol, 2% polyethylene glycol, 0.2% methyl cellulose, and $20mM$ Tris buffer, with the pH adjusted to 8.2. In addition, $2.0mM$ ethylenediaminetetraacetate (EDTA) or EGTA and appropriate amounts of $MgSO_4$ and $CaCl_2$ were added to control the Ca^{2+} concentration. All observations were carried out at 18°C. Photographs were taken of spermatozoa swimming freely at the lower glass surface of a covered well slide (Brokaw, 1977). This surface was coated with Siliclad to reduce the tendency of the spermatozoa to adhere to the surface.

Moving-film flash photomicrographs were obtained with a Robot Star II 35 mm camera, which was modified so that the spring motor advanced the film during the time the shutter was open. This camera provided higher film transport rates and consequently allowed the use of higher flash rates than the Zeiss C35M motor-driven camera used previously for this type of photography (Goldstein, 1976, 1977). The films were analyzed on a microfilm reader by measuring angles between the central axis of the sperm head and the straight regions between flagellar bends.

Portions of typical photographic records of spermatozoa beating with symmetrical and asymmetrical waveforms are shown in Figures 1A and 1B. The results of bend-angle analysis on these photographs are shown in Figures 2 and 3. Each of these figures shows the time course of the bend angles of principal and reverse bends (Gibbons and Gibbons, 1972) as they develop and propagate along the flagellum. The data for each flagellum represent an average over four consecutive beat cycles.

Figure 1C illustrates the behavior of a "short" flagellum found in the reactivation solution containing $10^{-4}M$ Ca^{2+}.

INTERPRETATION

Analysis of the time-course of bend angle, similar to that shown in Figures 2 and 3, has been carried out previously using photographs of live and demem-

---

The authors are indebted to Tom Simonick for diligent assistance with the experiments and measurements. This work has been supported by NIH grant GM-18711 to CJB and by NSF grant BMS73-06710-A01 to SFG.

© 1979 Urban & Schwarzenberg, Inc. Baltimore-Munich *The Spermatozoon*, edited by D.W. Fawcett and J.M. Bedford

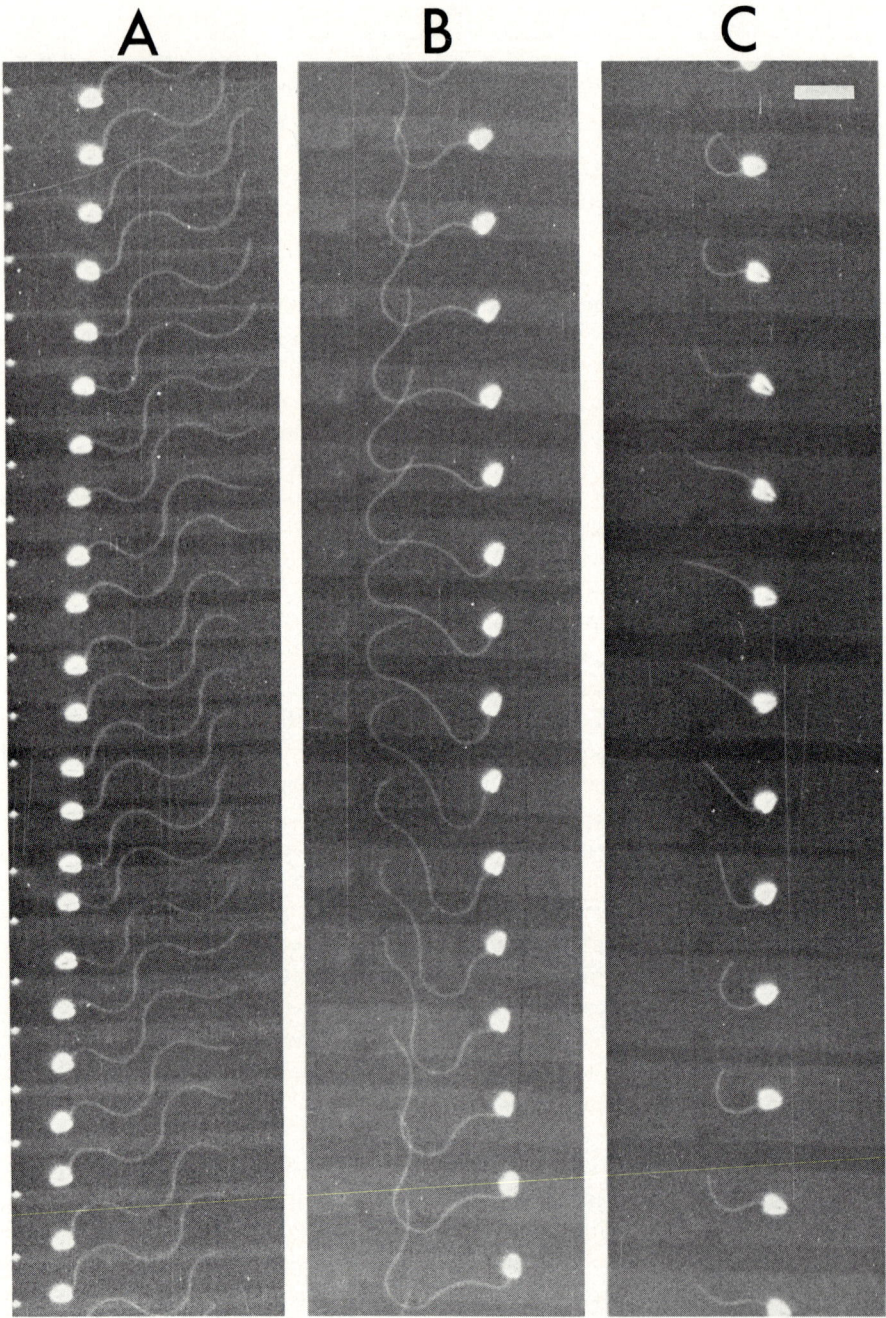

Figure 1. Moving-film flash photomicrographs of Triton-demembranated sea urchin spermatozoa swimming next to a glass surface. In A, the Ca^{2+} concentration in the reactivation solution was $10^{-9}M$, and the flash rate was 100 Hz, equivalent to 11 flashes per flagellar beat cycle. In B, the Ca^{2+} concentration was $10^{-4}M$ and the flash rate was 100 Hz, equivalent to 10 flashes per flagellar beat cycle. In C, the Ca^{2+} concentration was $10^{-4}M$ and the flash rate was 80 Hz, equivalent to approximately eight flashes per flagellar beat cycle. The scale bar indicates a length of 10 μm.

branated sea urchin sperm flagella (Brokaw, 1970; Goldstein, 1976, 1977), but the new photographs contain more data for each flagellum and reduce the "noise level." The analysis of Brokaw (1970) suggested that bend angles developed at a nearly constant rate for about one beat cycle, and then leveled off to a constant value which was maintained as the bends propagated along the flagellum. Goldstein (1976) found that in flagella with symmetrical waveforms, the two developing bends nearest the base of the flagellum tended to increase in angle at the same rate (in opposite directions). Consequently, the development of bends near

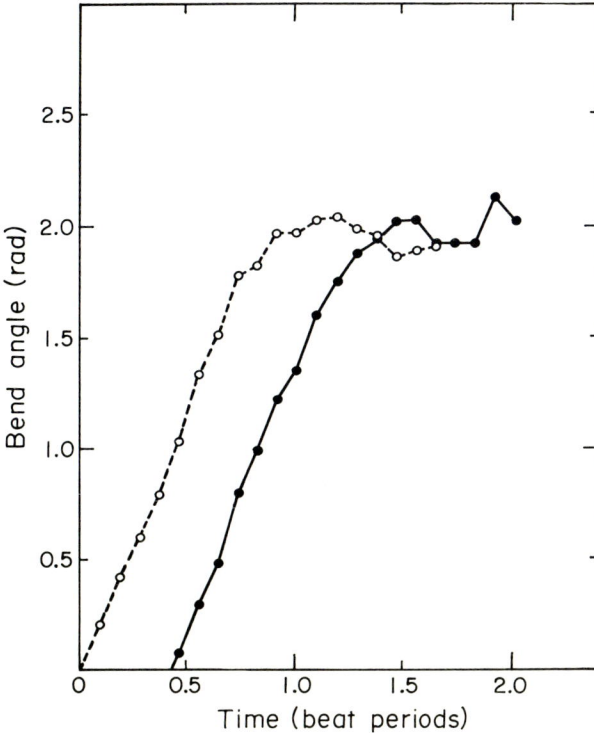

Figure 2. Time course of bend angles measured on the symmetrically beating flagellum shown in Figure 1A.

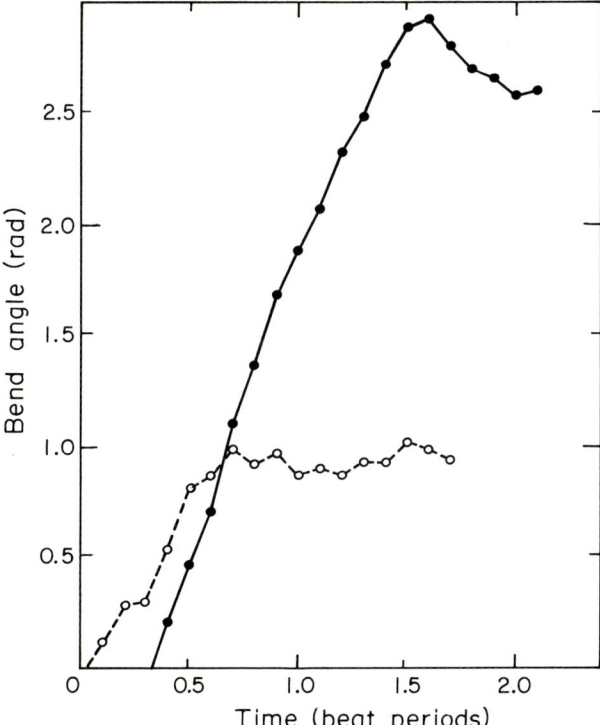

Figure 3. Time course of bend angles measured on the asymmetrically beating flagellum shown in Figure 1B.

the base of the flagellum is associated with little or no microtubular sliding in regions of the flagellum distal to these two developing bends. These features are exemplified by the symmetrical flagellum shown in Figures 1A and 2.

Goldstein (1977) studied asymmetrical bending in flagella of live spermatozoa. The angles of developing bends in asymmetrically beating flagella do not neutralize each other, and a significant amount of sliding between microtubules must occur in distal regions of the flagellum, in addition to the microtubular sliding associated with propagation of bends on the distal portion of the flagellum. This does not occur uniformly during the beat cycle. The reverse bend, which has the lower bend angle, develops for about three-fourths of a beat cycle, at a somewhat lower rate than the principal bend. It then abruptly stops growing and maintains a constant or slowly decreasing bend angle. During the remaining one-fourth of the beat cycle, before a new reverse bend is initiated at the base of the flagellum, only the principal bend closest to the base is increasing in bend angle. The development of this principal bend closest to the base must be associated with sliding between microtubules throughout the more distal portion of the flagellum. This sliding can be termed "synchronous" sliding to distinguish it from the "metachronous" sliding associated with the propagation of bends (Brokaw and Gibbons, 1975). Bends in the distal region of the flagellum propagate at a uniform rate and show no alteration during the period of synchronous sliding (*cf.* Fig. 9 of Goldstein, 1977).

Similar behavior is shown by asymmetrical Triton-demembranated flagella. In the example shown in Figures 1B and 3, the growth of the reverse bend terminates after 0.7 beat cycle, while the growth of the principal bend continues for about 1.3 beat cycles. Consequently, there is a period of approximately 0.6 beat cycle in which the growth of the principal bend is not associated with growth of a reverse bend in the opposite direction, and must be compensated by synchronous sliding between microtubules in more distal regions of the flagellum.

The difference in durations of the growth periods of principal and reverse bends is the major factor responsible for the asymmetrical bending pattern. The example shown here is an extreme one; more commonly the duration of growth of the principal bend is close to 1.0 beat cycle. In some cases, particularly at higher Ca^{2+} concentrations where the degree of asymmetry is more extreme, there may also be a difference in the rates of growth of principal and reverse bends, as shown in Figure 3. In the most extreme cases of asymmetry, there is also a decrease in angle of the reverse bend as it propagates along the flagellum. A single perturbation of microtubular sliding that can be responsible for all three of these perturbations in the time course of bend angle associated with asymmetrical bending patterns has not yet been identified.

As shown in Figure 1C, short flagella can also beat asymmetrically. Their bending patterns are similar to the bending seen in the basal region of an intact flagellum, which shows a large difference between the rates of growth of principal and reverse bends. These flagella are not long enough to display the modifications in bending pattern associated with early termination of growth of the reverse bend and synchronous sliding in distal regions of the flagellum.

The termination of growth of the reverse bend corresponds to a rather abrupt initiation of synchronous sliding in distal regions of the flagellum. Synchronous sliding in flagella is also seen when the bending of quiescent sperm flagella is initiated by formation of a principal bend at the base of the flagellum (Goldstein, 1979). Synchronous sliding must also be initiated abruptly at the beginning of the effective stroke in cilia (Rikmenspoel and Sleigh, 1970). Synchronous sliding appears to be an important capability of the mechanisms that control sliding between flagellar microtubules.

Simple models for the control of metachronous sliding in symmetrically beating flagella have been proposed, and computer stimulation methods have been used to demonstrate that these simple models can give spontaneous oscillation and bend propagation (Brokaw 1971, 1972, 1975b; Hines and Blum, 1978). However, these models are at best incomplete, since they do not explain the control of synchronous sliding in asymmetrically beating flagella and cilia.

REFERENCES

Brokaw, C.J.: Bending Moments in Free-swimming Flagella. J Exp Biol 53(1970)445-464

Brokaw, C.J.: Bend Propagation by a Sliding Filament Model for Flagella. J Exp Biol 55(1971)289-304

Brokaw, C.J.: Computer Simulation of Flagellar Movement. I. Demonstration of Stable Bend Propagation and Bend Initiation by the Sliding Filament Model. Biophys J 12(1972)564-586

Brokaw, C.J.: Effects of Viscosity and ATP Concentration on the Movement of Reactivated Sea Urchin Sperm Flagella. J Exp Biol 62(1975a)701-719

Brokaw, C.J.: Molecular Mechanism for Oscillation in Flagella and Muscle. Proc Natl Acad Sci USA 72(1975b)3102-3106

Brokaw, C.J.: CO_2-Inhibition of the Amplitude of Bending of Triton-demembranated Sea Urchin Sperm Flagella. J Exp Biol 71(1977)229-240

Brokaw, C.J.: Calcium-induced Asymmetrical Beating of Triton-demembranated Sea Urchin Sperm Flagella. J Cell Biol, in press

Brokaw, C.J.; Gibbons, I.R.: Mechanisms of Movement in Flagella and Cilia. In: Swimming and Flying in Nature, pp. 89-125, ed. by T.Y.-T. Wu, C.J. Brokaw and C. Brennan. Plenum Publishing Corp., New York, 1975

Brokaw, C.J.; Josslin, R.; Bobrow, L.: Calcium Ion Regulation of Flagellar Beat Symmetry in Reactivated Sea Urchin Sperm Flagella. Biochem Biophys Res Comm 58(1974)795-800

Gibbons, B.H.; Gibbons, I.R.: Flagellar Movement and Adenosine Triphosphatase Activity in Sea Urchin Sperm Extracted with Triton X-100. J Cell Biol 54(1972)75-97

Goldstein, S.F.: Form of Developing Bends in Reactivated Sperm Flagella. J Exp Biol 64(1976)173-184

Goldstein, S.F.: Asymmetric Waveforms in Echinoderm Sperm Flagella. J Exp Biol 71(1977)157-170

Goldstein, S.F.: Starting Transients in Sea Urchin Sperm Flagella. J Cell Biol, 80(1979)61-68

Hines, M.; Blum, J.J.: Bend Propagation in Flagella I. Derivation of Equations of Motion and Their Simulation. Biophys J 23(1978)41-57

Holwill, M.E.J.; McGregor, J.L.: Control of Flagellar Wave Movement in *Crithidia oncopelti*. Nature 255(1975)157-158

Naitoh, Y.; Kaneko, H.: ATP-Mg-reactivated Triton-extracted Models of *Paramecium:* Modification of Ciliary Movement by Calcium Ions. Science 176(1972)523-524

Miller, R.L.: Flagellar Wave Morphology during Animal Sperm Chemotaxis. J Cell Biol 70(1976)341a

Miller, R.L.; Brokaw, C.J.: Chemotactic turning Behavior of *Tubularia* Spermatozoa. J Exp Biol 52(1970)699-706

Rikmenspoel, R.; Sleigh, M.A.: Bending Moments and Elastic Constants in Cilia. J Theor Biol 28(1970)81-100

Tsuchiya, T.: Ca-Induced Arrest Response in Triton-extracted Lateral Cilia of *Mytilus* Gill. Experientia 32(1976)1439-1440

DISASSEMBLY OF THE GUINEA PIG SPERM TAIL

D.S. Friend, P.M. Elias, and I. Rudolf

Departments of Pathology and Dermatology, University of California, San Francisco, California 94143 USA

The sperm plasma membrane is a mosaic of functionally and morphologically distinct domains (Fawcett, 1975; Friend and Fawcett, 1974; Friend, 1977; Koehler, 1973). This study advances a technique for isolating two of these singular areas—the zipper and the annulus—and paves the way for their further characterization by biochemical assays.

Examined by the freeze-fracture technique, which exposes the hydrophobic interior of the membrane (Branton, 1966; Bullivant, 1974; McNutt, 1977), individual areas are most readily recognized by the differing patterns of particles in the cytoplasmic part of the plasmalemma. In guinea pig sperm, for example, the particles in the portion that overlies the acrosomal cap form a quilted design, whereas those over the major part of the postacrosomal segment are disordered. In front of the striated ring, demarcating the boundary between the sperm head and tail, particles can be observed in flower-like clusters; and covering the mitochondria of the midpiece, they appear as aggregations of circumferential beaded strings. Separating the mid- and principal-piece of the tail, the annulus exhibits rows of particles in the outer part of the membrane. Adorning the principal piece are two staggered rows of particles, commonly referred to as the "zipper," adjacent to outer dense fiber No. 1 (Fawcett, 1975; Friend, 1974; Friend, 1977).

Species other than the guinea pig possess comparable sperm membrane differentiations. Many, such as those of man, mouse, rat, rabbit, bull, boar, and hamster are simpler (Fawcett, 1975; Flechon, 1974; Olson and Linck, 1977); while others, such as those of the opossum, may have still more elaborate patterns of intramembrane particles (Olson et al., 1977). Among these distinctive regional specializations of the membrane, the particulate pattern of the annulus and zipper may be the most consistent, perhaps even universal, among species that reproduce by internal fertilization.

It is now quite generally agreed that the particles seen in freeze-fracture replicas contain proteins (McNutt, 1977; Vail et al., 1974). In the membrane of the *Halobacterium*, erythrocyte and epithelial cells with gap-junctions, proof of this generalization is quite clear (Fisher, 1974; Goodenough and Stoeckenius, 1972; Marchesi et al., 1976 Steck, 1974), and it can be assumed that the same is true of sperm. Membrane proteins function as enzymes, ion pumps, receptors, attachment sites, or parts of an integral structural framework. Methods for isolating proteins from individual regions of the spermatozoon have the potential to reveal more about the composition of the membrane, more about the specialized functions of the specific regions of membrane, and more about membrane organization and regulation in general (Nicolson, 1976).

It has very recently been recognized that in guinea pig sperm, some parts of the plasma membrane are rich in sterols (primarily non-esterified cholesterol), while other parts contain little (Friend and Elias, 1978). Like proteins, sterols are inhomogeneous in distribution. These two factors have served as a theoretical basis for isolating particles from specific regions of sperm. Using the saponins, digitonin and tomatin (Elias et al., 1978b), or the polyene antibiotic, filipin (Elias et al., 1978b; Norman et al., 1976; Verkleij et al., 1973), it was found that the plasma membrane where it blankets the acrosomal cap contains five times more sterol than the postacrosomal segment, and that the striated ring, annulus, and zipper are virtually free of such sterols (Friend and Elias, 1978). Since digitonin, particularly, acts as a membrane-disrupting detergent, it could be used to dissociate the sterol-rich portions of the membrane, sparing the sterol-poor areas (Elias et al., 1978a). The membrane-penetrating proteins of the zipper and annulus could then be detached from their underlying anchorage. Other proteins not morphologically identifiable may also be extracted.

This brief chapter describes an initial methodological approach for dissociating these two plasma-membrane components from the remainder of the tail and for disassembling the tail piece-by-piece, with major emphasis on the morphological appearance of the preparations (what is lost may not always be recognizable by electron microscopy). Workers using the myriad techniques of biochemistry will probably conceive of better ways to retrieve and purify the proteins and other

---

This study was supported by United States Public Health Service (NIH) Grants HD 10445 and AM 19098. The authors warmly thank Rosamond Michael for her superior editorial help.

© 1979 Urban & Schwarzenberg, Inc. Baltimore-Munich *The Spermatozoon*, edited by D.W. Fawcett and J.M. Bedford

structural components. The following results are only as a starting point.

In the course of disassembling the plasma membrane of the tail, selective dissolution of the microtubules, dense fibers, and satellite filaments was also achieved, and serendipitously a simple method for conserving the bulk of the dense fibers was found. To the authors' knowledge, specific degradation of the colchicine-resistant axonemal microtubules has not been heretofore reported.

The use of thin sections, freeze-fractures, and surface replicas confirmed the step-by-step dissociation of the tail.

MATERIALS AND METHODS

For each experiment, spermatozoa were removed from the tails of the epididymides and vasa deferentia of ether-anesthetized, mature, male guinea pigs. The pooled sperm were mixed with several milliliters of calcium-free Tyrode's solution (Yanagimachi, 1978), modified for specific steps in the disassembling process as follows:

Digitonin Procedure for Disrupting the Cholesterol-containing[1] Plasma Membrane

Sperm were treated with 0.2% digitonin in calcium-free Tyrode's solution, pH 7.8, at 20°C for 10 min. If the sperm were to be used for morphologic studies alone, they were mixed with 0.2% digitonin in 1.5% glutaraldehyde in $0.1M$ sodium cacodylate buffer, pH 7.4, for 30 min.

Separation of Heads and Tails

When desired, after digitonin disruption of the plasma membranes of unfixed sperm, some tails could be concentrated by differential centrifugation in discontinuous gradient solutions as described by Gall *et al.*, (1974) and Millette *et al.*, (1973) (5 ml 65% sucrose, 15 ml 60% sucrose, and 5 ml 55% sucrose). After centrifugation for 30 min at 600 g, tails are recoverable at the top interface of the 55%-sucrose layer. No attempt was made to separate the head and tail for the morphological studies.

---

[1]*Filipin procedure for determining the topographic distribution of non-esterfied cholesterol* (Elias *et al.*, 1978b): Filipin (Upjohn Co., Kalamazoo, Mich.) was purified by thin-layer chromatography in chloroform: methanol: water: acetic acid (60:35:4.5:0.5 by volume). The agent was dissolved in a drop of dimethylsulfoxide (DMSO) and added to $0.1M$ sodium cacodylate-glutaraldehyde fixative, pH 7.4, to a final concentration of 300 μmal filipin in the fixative. The solution also contained 4% sucrose and 0.05% calcium chloride.

Triton X-100 Treatment for Removal of the Zipper and Annulus

Following digitonin treatment of unfixed sperm, spermatozoa were pelleted in microfuge tubes and then resuspended in Triton X-100, as a 0.1% solution in calcium-free Tyrode's solution at pH 7.9 for 1 min. (The supernatant may be used for isolation of the dissolved membrane components.) The cells were then fixed as outlined under "Processing for Electron Microscopy, Thin Sections."

N-butylamine Treatment for Dissociation of Axonemal Microtubules

Starting with freshly removed sperm (preferable), sperm after digitonin treatment, or sperm after both digitonin and Triton treatment, spermatozoa were pelleted in microfuge tubes in Tyrode's solution, resuspended in n-butylamine (Cooper and Young, 1977) (0.01 ml/ml calcium-free Tyrode's solution), pH 8-11, and vortexed for 30 s.

The suspension may then be pelleted and the supernatant used for standard gel electrophoresis. The packed sperm were resuspended in Tyrode's solution before fixation.

SDS Treatment for Dissolving all but the Outer Dense Fibers

Whole sperm or sperm at any of the above stages of treatment may be dissolved in a 2.3% solution of sodium dodecyl sulfate (SDS) (O'Farrell, 1975). They may be pelleted in microfuge tubes. The fibers are usually heavily contaminated with partially disaggregated chromatin.

Processing for Electron Microscopy

Thin Sections The resultant pellets of all the above preparations were fixed in 1.5% glutaraldehyde in $0.1M$ sodium cacodylate buffer, pH 7.4, for ~1 h at room temperature. Standard procedures were used for subsequent processing (Friend and Fawcett, 1974; Friend, 1977), including postfixation in OsO_4, staining *en bloc* with aqueous uranyl acetate for 45 min, *en bloc* mordanting with tannic acid (Simionescu and Simionescu, 1976) for 45 min, dehydration in a series of graded alcohols and propylene oxide, and embedding in Epon. Sections were then stained with uranyl acetate and alkaline lead.

Freeze-fractures The resultant pellets of the above preparations were fixed as for thin-sectioning (but only for 30 min), immersed for 3-4 h in $0.1M$ sodium cacodylate-buffered glycerol (25%), frozen at liquid-nitrogen temperature, and fractured in a Balzers freeze-fracture apparatus at a stage temperature of −115°C.

RESULTS AND DISCUSSION

The presentation of the authors' data is oriented toward the morphological effects of digitonin, Triton X-100, n-butylamine, and SDS on the guinea pig sperm tail principal piece, annulus, and midpiece (Fig. 1).

The Principal Piece

The structural hallmark of the principal piece is the zipper, which appears opposite fiber No. 1 as a thickening of the membrane and increase in its density in cross-section (Fig. 2a); as an interrupted periodic density in grazing longitudinal sections (Fig. 2d); as a double row of intramembrane particles in freeze-fracture preparations (Fig. 2c); and as a continuous, striated strand in surface replicas (Fig. 2b). Treatment of the cell with filipin reveals that this transmembrane protein differentiation—that is, the zipper—is flanked, but not impinged upon, by an abundance of free cholesterol (Fig. 2e). The assumption that the zipper is composed of transmembrane proteins is based on the fact that its particles are morphologically represented on both fracture-faces and the outer side of the membrane. In addition, it displays a filamentous attachment to the underlying fibrous sheath.

Treatment with the detergent digitonin—which interacts with cholesterol-rich plasma membrane (Elias *et al.*, 1978a), scalloping and disrupting it—leaves the ribs of the fibrous sheath and the attached zipper exposed (Fig. 3 and 4), as would be anticipated from observations with filipin labelling. Surface replicas, as well as examination of thin sections, confirm the retention of this structure (Fig. 4).

The zipper particles are then removed with Triton X-100 (Fig. 3c and 4d). Pilot studies with lactoperoxidase-catalyzed ^{125}I-iodination of whole plasma membrane, followed by sequential digitonin membrane disruption and then Triton extraction of the sperm, indicate that the labelled surface protein may be recoverable by gel electrophoresis (Glabe, Vacquier, and Friend, unpublished results). Presumably, the residual activity is derived from those surface elements not removed by digitonin—the zipper and the plasma membrane at the site of the annulus.

The isolation of zipper particles is significant for several reasons: First, there are few retrievable transmembrane proteins available for study. Glycophorin (Marchesi *et al.*, 1976; Steck, 1974), bacteriorhodopsin (Fisher and Stoeckenius, 1977), and gap-junction parti-

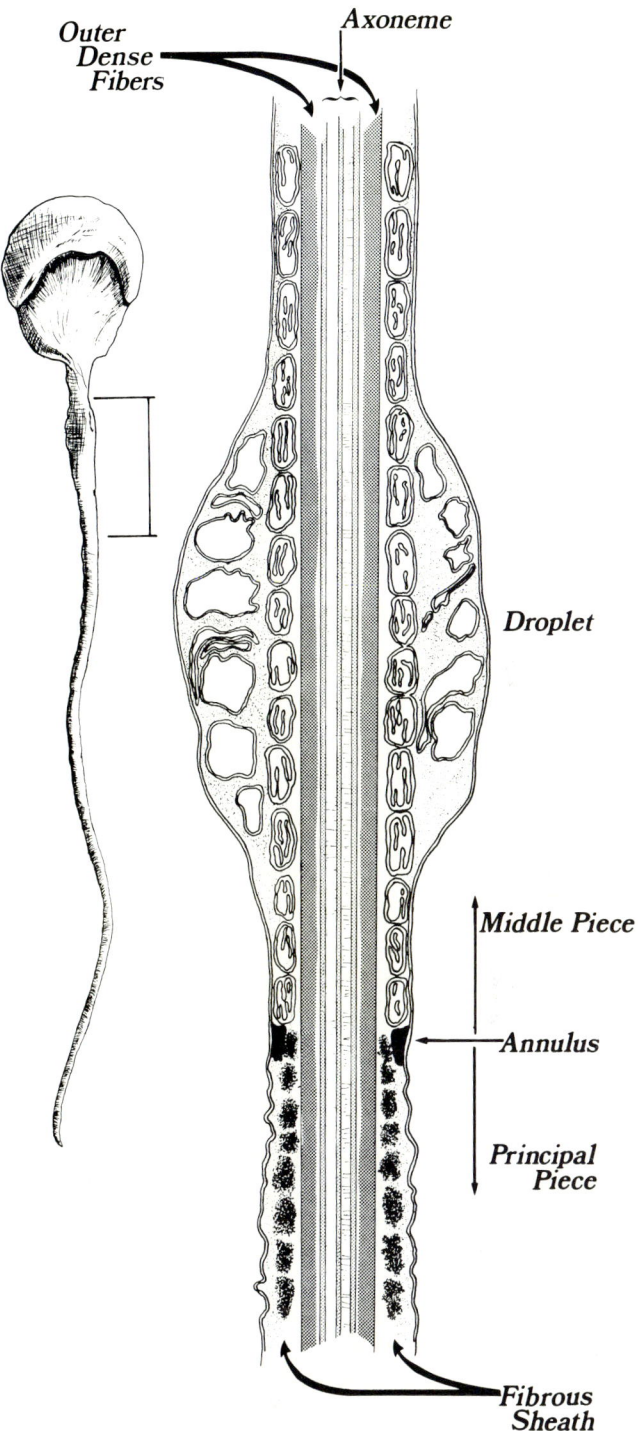

Figure 1. Diagram of the portion of the guinea pig sperm tail shown within brackets in the outline of the entire cell. The structures relevant to this chapter are the plasma membrane as a whole, the part of the membrane overlying the annulus, the axonemal microtubules, the outer dense fibers, and the fibrous sheath. The zipper and satellite filaments will be illustrated in subsequent micrographs.

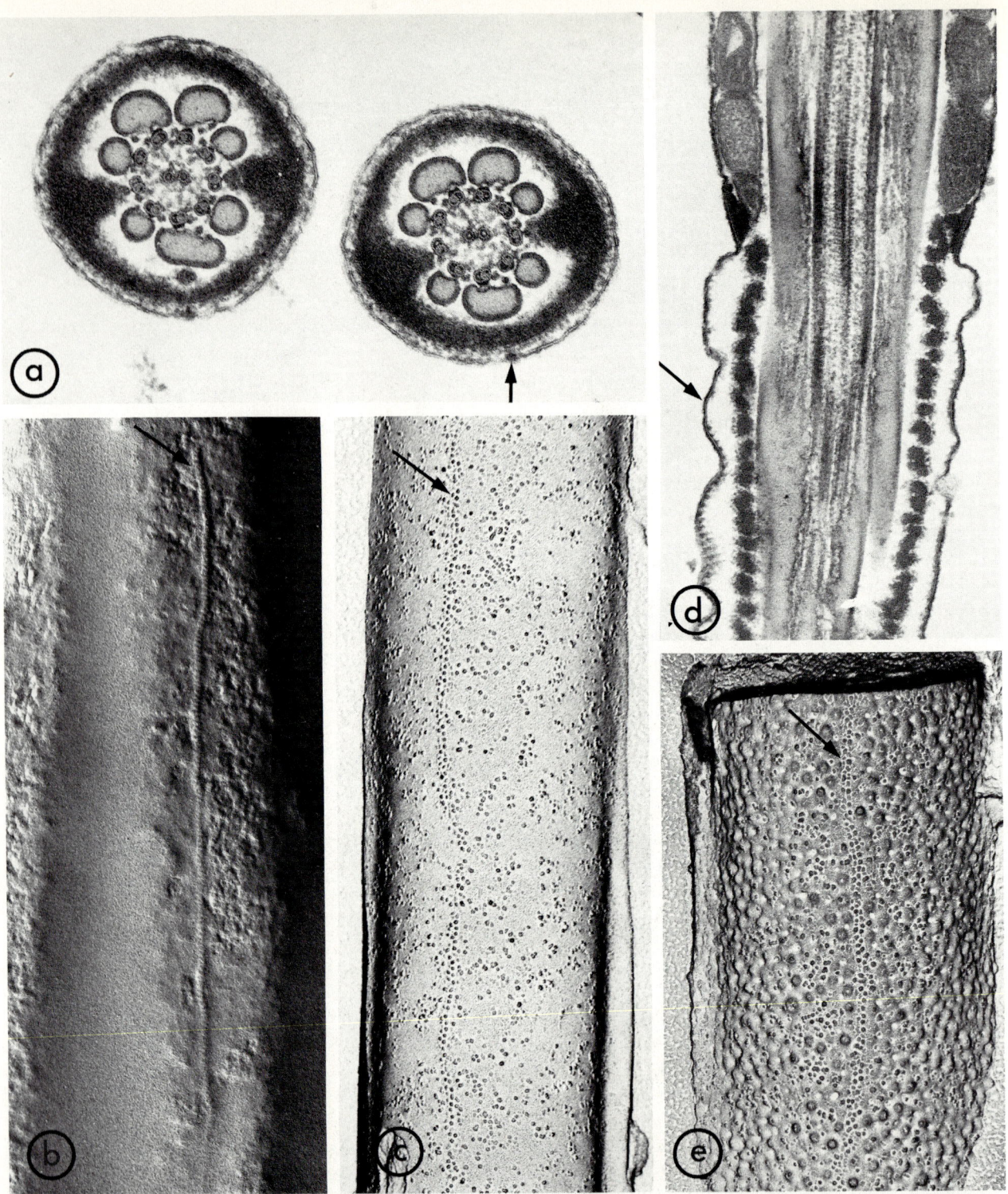

Figure 2. The principal piece of the guinea pig sperm tail. (a) Dense regions in the cross sections correspond to the zipper (arrow) opposite fiber No. 1. (b) The zipper (arrows) is also observed in surface and (c) freeze-fracture replicas. This freeze-fracture replica was rotary-shadowed (replica, courtesy of Dr. John Heuser, University of California). (d) Longitudinal section. (e) Filipin treatment, which induces 25-30-nm protuberances with 3-β-hydroxysterols, reveals the sterol-rich membrane surrounding the zipper. Cholesterol-containing portions of the membrane are vulnerable to disruption with digitonin and other saponin detergents (Rotary-shadowed replica, courtesy of Dr. John Heuser, University of California) (Elias et al., 1978a, b). (a) X58,000; (b) X50,000; (c) X64,000; (d) X50,000; (e) X84,000

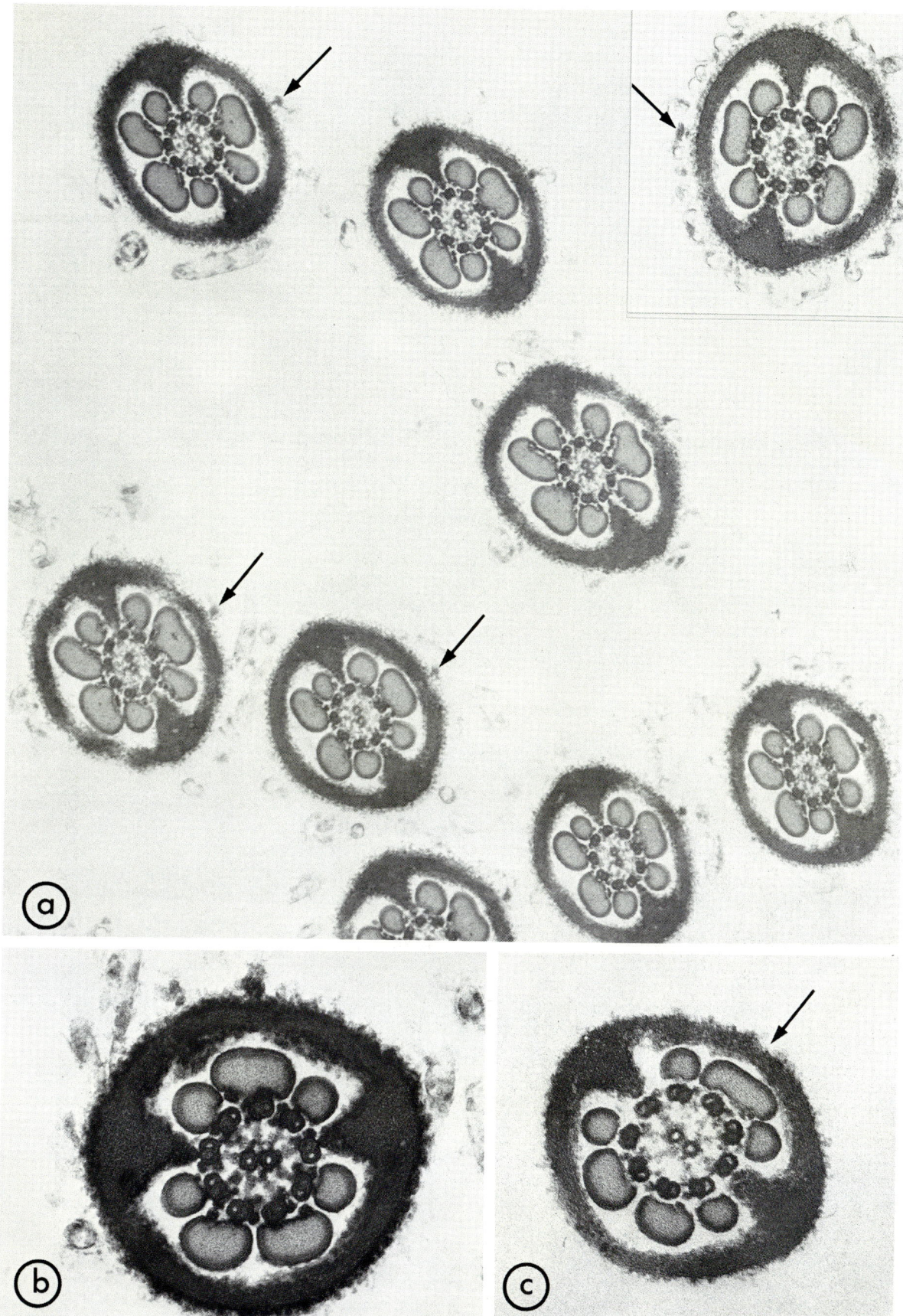

Figure 3. Digitonin-treated sperm. (a) Following treatment with 0.2% digitonin in buffered fixative for $<\frac{1}{2}$ h, the bulk of the membrane is stripped away, perhaps during later tissue processing, but the zipper persists (arrows). The inset depicts an intermediate stage of the membrane-scalloping effect. (b) Higher-magnification view of the attached zipper. (c) Triton X-100 treatment, 0.1% in Tyrode's solution (pH 7.9, 1 min), removes the zipper. The arrow indicates the site where the zipper was formerly located. (a) X50,000; (b) X114,000; (c) X88,000; inset, X56,000

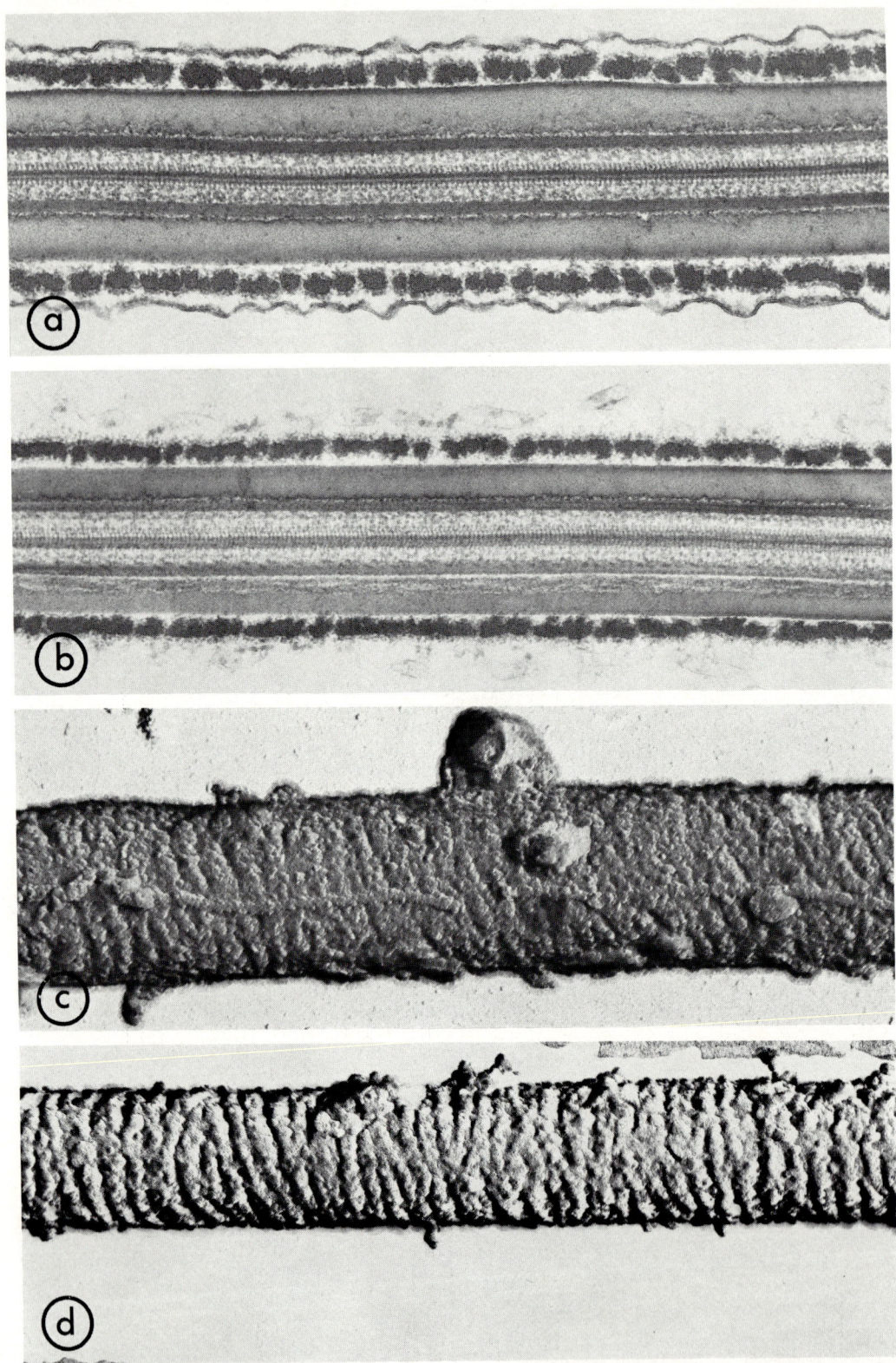

Figure 4. Digitonin-treated sperm. (a) Longitudinal section of the intact principal piece. (b) After digitonin treatment, the plasma membrane is gone, but the rest of the tail structure, including the axoneme and the fibrous sheath, remains intact. (c) Surface replicas confirm the persistence of the zipper, now overlying the fibrous ribs. (d) Triton X-100 removes the zipper. (a) X50,000; (b) X46,000; (c) X70,000; (d) X50,000

cles (Goodenough and Stoeckenius, 1972) are among the few such proteins isolated so far, and their analysis is important not only in regard to their specific compositions but to the general understanding of membrane organization. The characterization of any additional plasma-membrane protein is simply important *per se* in the context of membrane biology. Second, this structure cannot represent a merely trivial particulate array. With minor variations in contour, primarily involving the number of strands, it has been identified in the spermatozoa of man, *Drosophila*, earthworm, mouse, rat, guinea pig, opossum (Fawcett, 1975; Friend, 1977), and probably in more species. Indeed, this protein particle may prove to be common to all organisms that have internal fertilization. Its conservation in evolution as a structure as basic as the 9+2 axonemal microtubule configuration implies that it is functionally advantageous. Moreover, the isolation of this substance might provide relatively pure starting material for the induction of antibodies. Immunocytochemical localization would confirm its specificity. Antibody binding to the structure might prove to be a means of ablation, thereby providing evidence as to its function. In addition to its role as a structural reinforcement in the membrane and a site of attachment of the membrane to the fibrous sheath, more clues as to its chemical nature might enable us to further explore its functions.

Fortuitously, it was observed that n-butylamine dissociates the colchicine-resistant structures forming the axonemal complex. The reagent was employed as suggested by Cooper and Young (1977) for inducing sperm head and tail separation, which it does in the mouse. These investigators also noted that it disrupted microtubules (personal communication). The extent to which the agent dispersed microtubules after digitonin treatment of the sperm, after combined digitonin + Triton treatment, and also in freshly removed sperm (Fig. 5) was impressive. In the latter condition, the morphological preservation of the plasma membrane was good in a large percentage of the sperm examined. As in the case of zipper proteins, it is feasible to recover proteins from the n-butylamine extract by gel electrophoresis.

The Annulus

The behavior of the annulus (Fig. 6) is like that of the zipper in respect to its nonreactivity with filipin (Fig. 6c), resistance to dissolution with digitonin (Fig. 6e), and subsequent removal with Triton X-100 (Fig. 6f). This treatment also discloses an underlying dense filamentous mat. Unlike the zipper and the other plasmalemmal modifications discussed, the annular particles have a high affinity for the outer part (E-face) of the membrane (Fig. 6a, b)—its counterpart, the cytoplas-mic half, exhibits complementary linear depressions and scattered particles. Separation of the proteins derived from the annulus and from the zipper has not been undertaken.

The Midpiece

The strands of particles in the plasma membrane shrouding the mitochondrial sheath are lost in membrane extraction with digitonin. The sterol-rich character of the cytoplasmic droplet (Fig. 7a) is evidenced by its rapid destruction (Fig. 7b). Subsequent to the removal of these particles, Triton has a considerable effect on mitochondrial morphology—light, flocculent densities become commonplace in the matrix (Fig. 7c). As in the principal piece, n-butylamine swiftly dissolves the axonemal complex (Fig. 7d). It is of particular interest to us that n-butylamine also destroys the filaments adjacent to dense fibers in the midpiece (*cf.* Fig. 7c, 7d). Coupled with the observation that satellite filaments have a structure similar to microtubular protofilaments, this raises the question: Are satellite filaments composed of tubulin? Until proved otherwise, the assumption is that they are. Note that n-butylamine also perturbs the cortex of the dense fibers (Fig. 7d). Following treatment with this agent, mitochondria, too, often seem to be extracted. The plasma membrane and bulk of the dense fibers, however, are similar in control preparations.

SDS solubilizes all that remains of the tail except the major cores of the dense fibers (Fig. 8). When whole sperm are used, decondensed chromatin heavily contaminates the preparation.

CONCLUDING REMARKS

Considered in the aggregate, the step-wise procedures reported here may be utilized to dissolve particular portions of the spermatozoan tail. Recovery of both the solubilized and reagent-resistant components of the cell is therefore possible. These approaches certainly cannot supplant the careful, detailed biochemical procedures pioneered by other investigators (Clegg *et al.*, 1975; Gall *et al.*, 1974; Millette *et al.*, 1973; Olson and Linck, 1977) for dissection of the spermatozoon. Nevertheless the methods used on this study provide information necessary for isolating and identifying selected constituents of the plasma-membrane mosaic, such as the zipper and annulus, which have only been recognizable as intramembrane differentiations since the application of the freeze-fracture method. Earlier dissolution procedures therefore could not have been directed toward isolating these elements. Moreover, the techniques presented here permit the selective recovery of a class of colchicine-resistant microtubules and associated satellite filaments

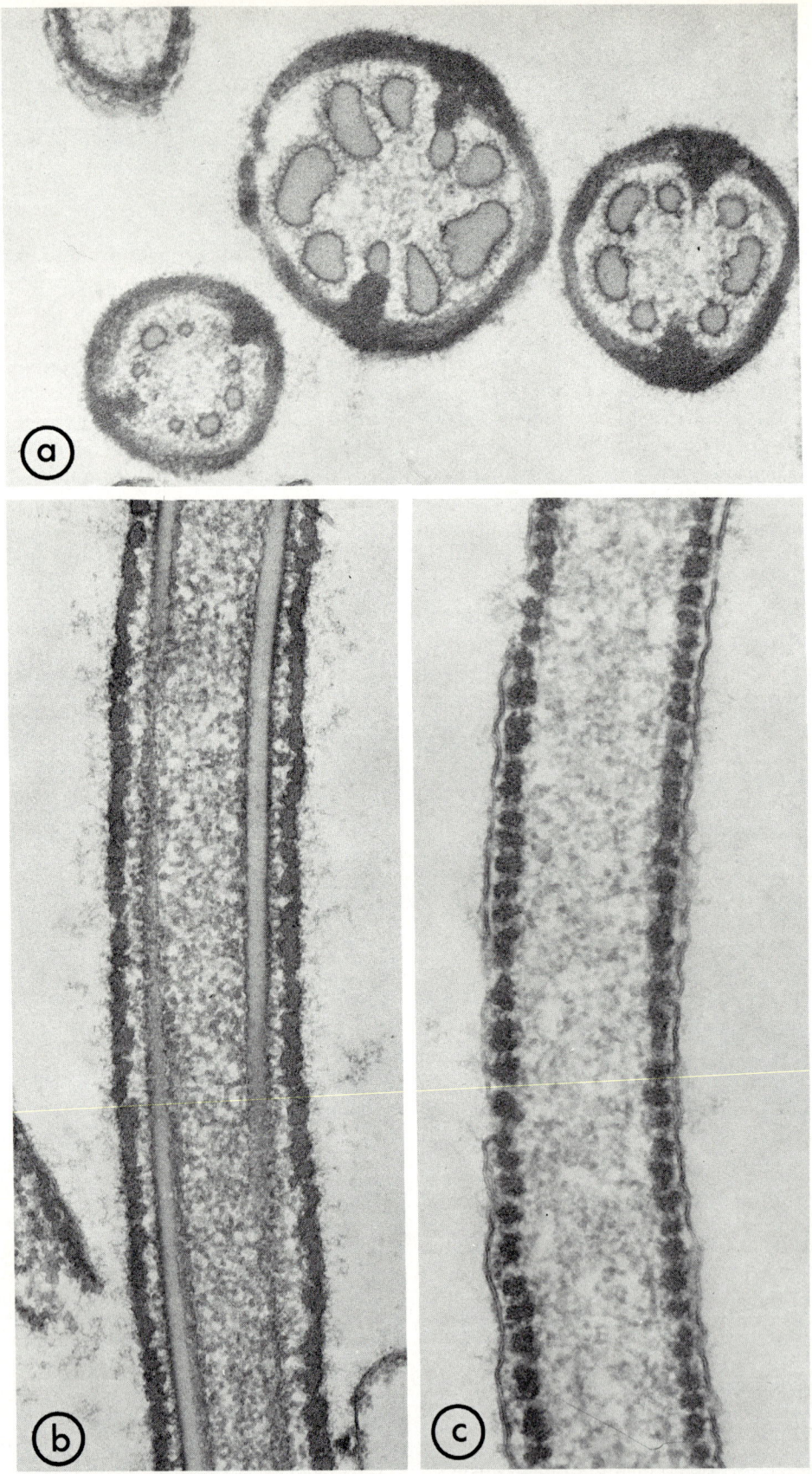

Figure 5. N-butylamine-treated sperm. Vortexing the sperm for 30 s in n-butylamine (0.01 ml/ml Tyrode's solution, pH 8-11) dissociates the microtubules of the axoneme. Retention of the plasma membrane is variable, lost in (a) and (b), but retained in (c), which is a portion of the principal piece distal to the termination of the outer dense fibers. (a) X75,000; (b) X50,000; (c) X80,000

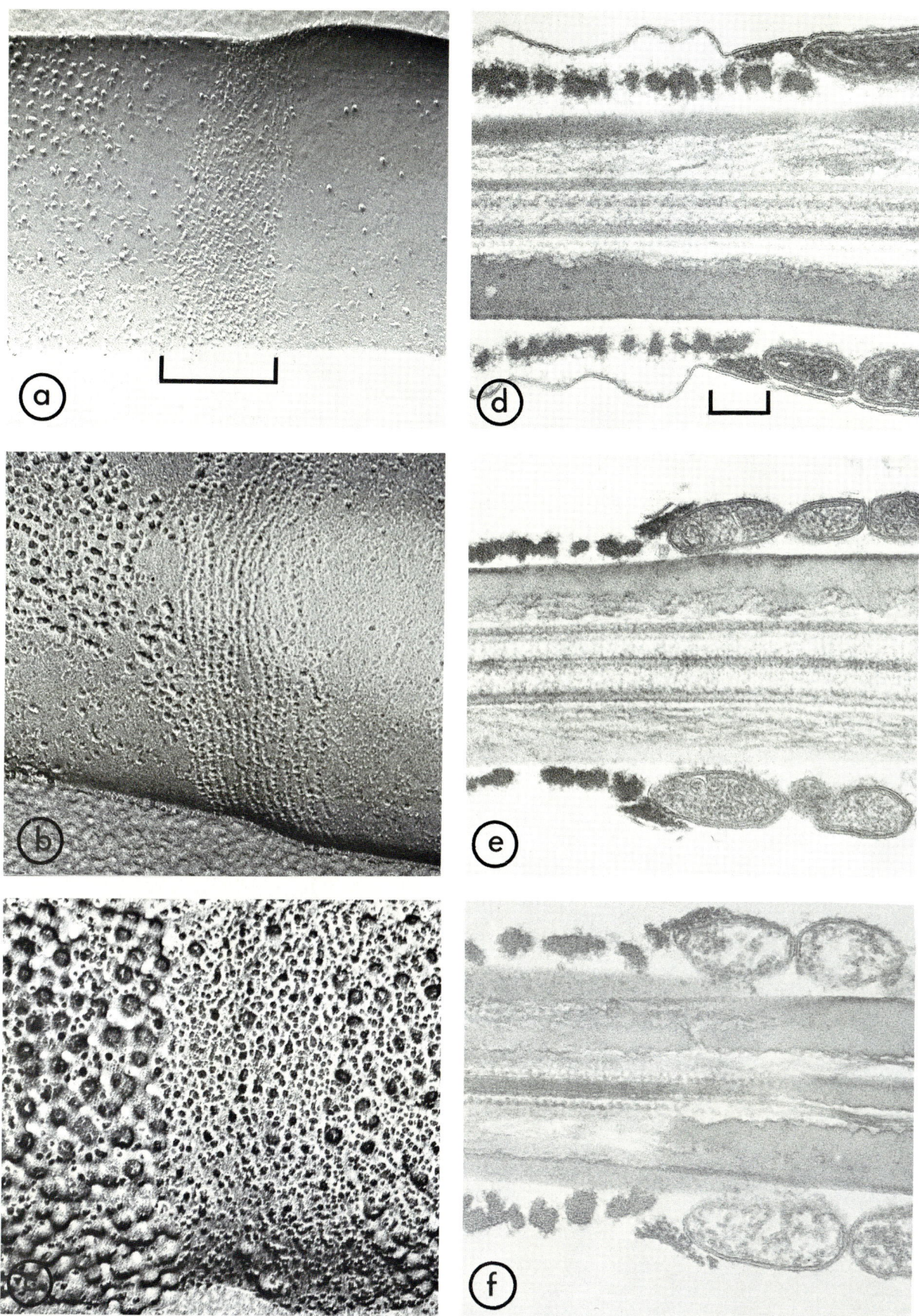

Figure 6. The annulus. (a) Unidirectional and (b) rotary-shadowed freeze-fracture replicas. The annulus contains lines of particles in the E-face of the plasma membrane (replica, courtesy of Dr. John Heuser, University of California). (c) Filipin treatment reveals that the annulus, like the zipper, is sterol-poor (rotary-shadowed replica, courtesy of Dr. John Heuser, University of California). (d) Longitudinal section. (e) The membrane of the annulus persists after digitonin treatment. (f) It is removed by Triton X-100. Both the zipper and the annulus are rich in proteins (particles) but probably deficient in sterols. (a) X70,000; (b) X110,000; (c) X120,000; (d) X70,000; (e) X62,000; (f) X76,000

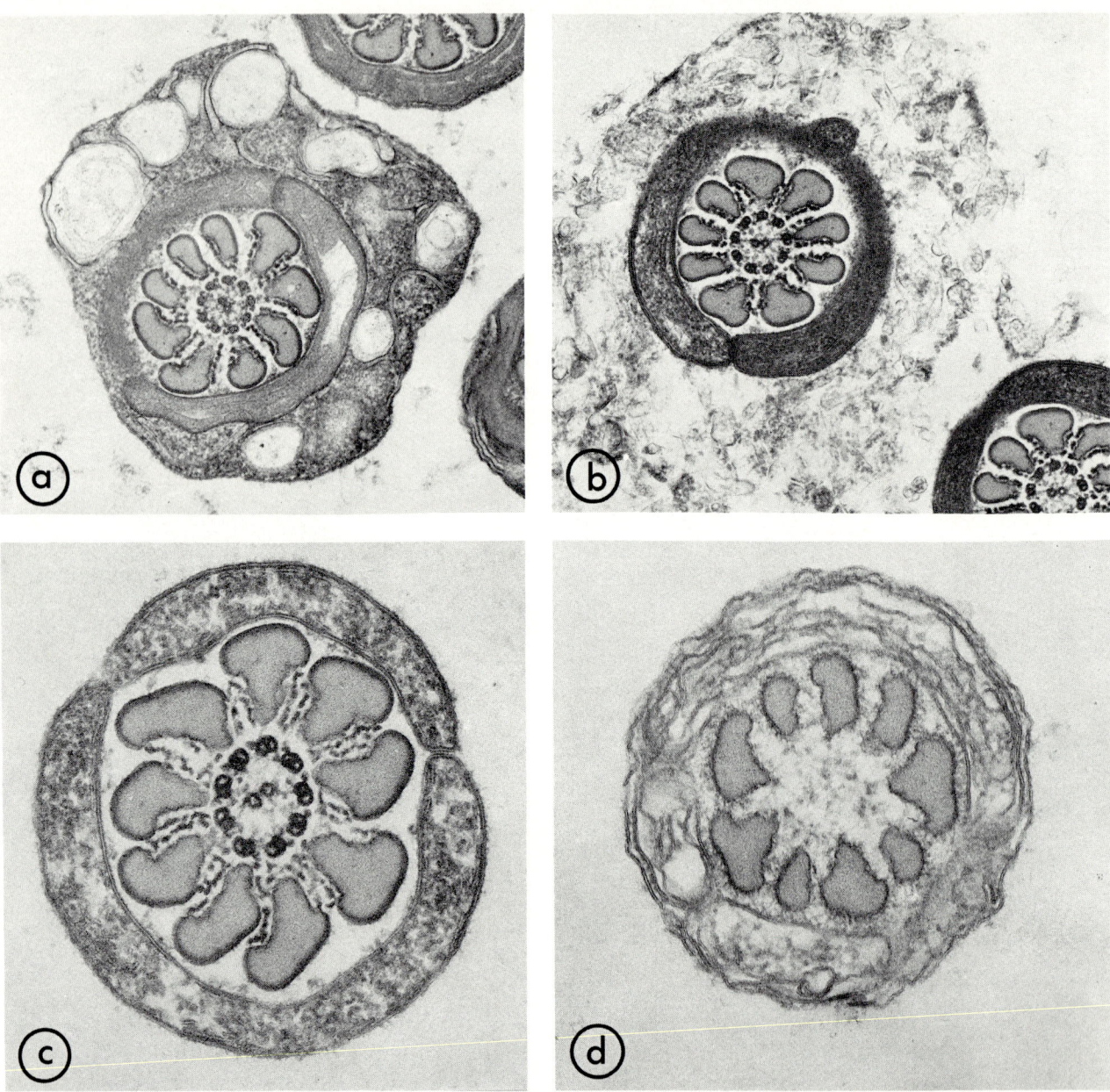

Figure 7. The midpiece. (a) Cytoplasmic droplet. (b) The droplet disintegrates in the digitonin solution, while the mitochondria and other tail organelles are left intact. (c) Subsequent treatment with Triton X-100 does not morphologically alter the axoneme, satellite filaments, or other midpiece organelles. (d) N-butylamine treatment removes the axonemal microtubules and satellite filaments. (a) X30,000; (b) X34,000; (c) X70,000; (d) X80,000

that have heretofore been accessible for exploration only by disruption of the entire cell. The ultimate value of these methods will be established by those who apply them to resolve significant questions in the fields of cell and reproductive biology.

REFERENCES

Branton, D.: Fracture Faces of Frozen Membranes. Proc Natl Acad Sci USA 55(1966)1048

Bullivant, S.: Freeze-Etching Techniques Applied to Biological Membranes. Phil Trans R Soc Lond [Biol] (1974)5-14

Clegg, E.D.; Morré, D.J.; Lunstra, D.D.: Porcine Sperm Membranes: *In Vivo* Phospholipid Changes, Isolation, and Electron Microscopy. In: The Biology of the Male Gamete, Vol. 7, pp. 321-335, ed. by J.G. Duckett and P.A. Racey. Supplement No. 1, Biological Journal of the Linnean Society, 1975

Cooper, G.W.; Young, R.J.: Mammalian Sperm are Dissociated into Heads and Tails by Primary Amines: Demonstration of Intermolecular Covalent Bonds between the Nuclear Membranes and Basal Plate of the Tail Connecting Piece. Anat Rec 187(1977)556A

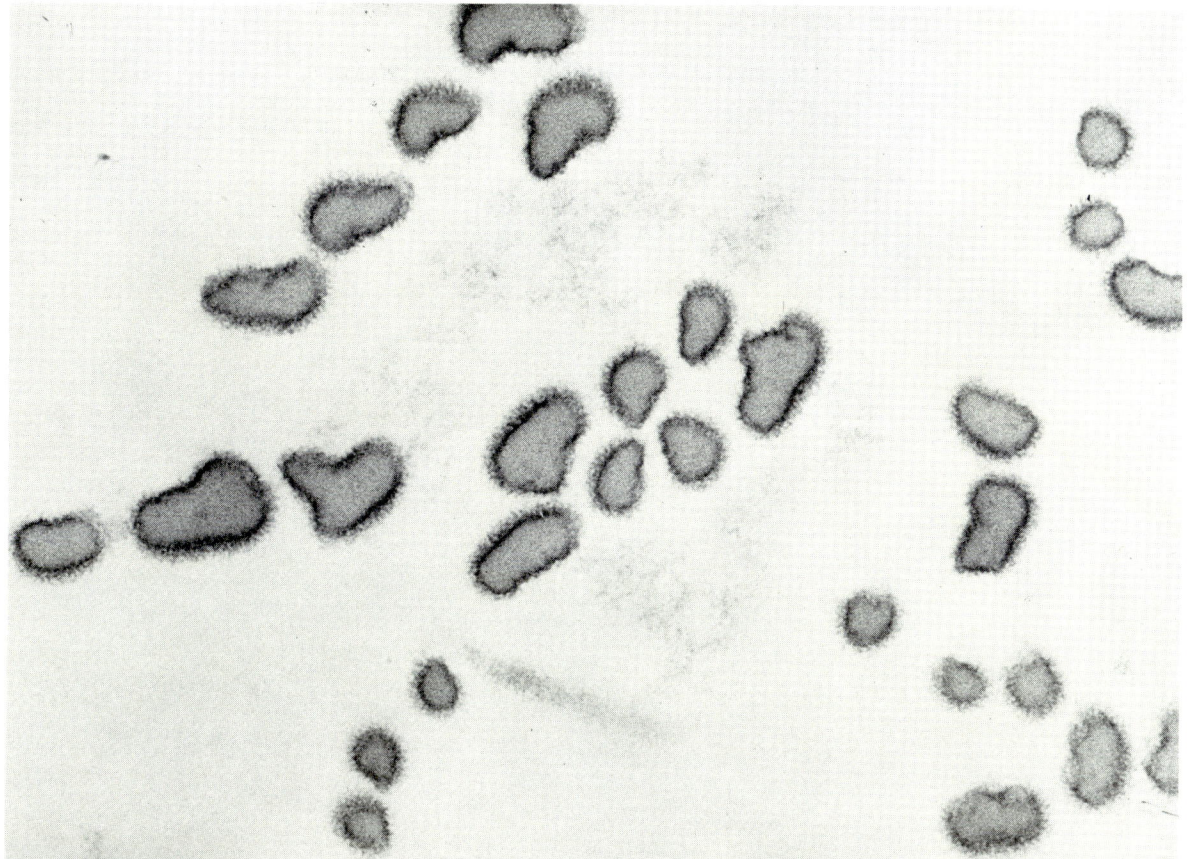

Figure 8. Sodium dodecyl sulfate dissolves all that is left of the tail save the outer dense fibers. Thus far, these are the only tail structures that have been recoverable in the form of a homogeneous pellet. X76,000

Elias, P.M.; Goerke, J.; Friend, D.S.: Freeze-fracture Identification of Sterol-Digitonin Complexes in Cell and Liposome Membranes. J Cell Biol 78(1978)577-596

Elias, P.M.; Friend, D.S.; Goerke, J.: Freeze-fracture Localization of Cholesterol in Cell and Liposome Membranes with Saponins and Filipin. J Cell Biol 79(1978)232a

Fawcett, D.W.: The Mammalian Spermatozoan. Dev Biol 44(1975)394-436

Fisher, K.A.; Stoeckenius, W.: Freeze-fractured Purple Membrane Particles: Protein Content. Science 197(1977)72-74

Flechon, J.E.: Freeze-fracturing of Rabbit Spermatozoa. J Microsc 19(1974)59-64

Friend, D.S.; Fawcett, D.W.: Membrane Differentiations in Freeze-fractured Mammalian Sperm. J Cell Biol 63(1974)641-664

Friend, D.S. Spermatozoan Membrane Organization. In: Immunobiology of the Gametes, pp. 5-30, ed. by M. Edidin and M.H. Johnson. Alden Press, Oxford, 1977

Friend, D.S.; Elias, P.M.: Heterogeneity of Filipin-Sterol Complexes in the Guinea Pig Sperm Plasma Membrane. J Cell Biol 79(1978)216a

Gall, W.E.; Millette, C.F.; Edelman, G.M.: Chemical and Structural Analysis of Mammalian Spermatozoa. In: Physiology and Genetics of Reproduction, pp. 241-257, ed. by E.M. Coutinho and F.Fuchs. Plenum Publishing Co., New York, 1974

Goodenough, D.A.; Stoeckenius, W.: The Isolation of Mouse Hepatocyte Gap Junctions: Preliminary Chemical Characterization and X-ray Diffraction. J Cell Biol 54(1972)646-656

Koehler, J.K.: An Unusual Filamentous Component Associated with the Guinea Pig Sperm Middle Piece. J de Microscopie 18(1973)263-266

Marchesi, V.T.; Furthmayr, H.; Tomita, M.: The Red Cell Membrane. Annu Rev Biochem 45(1976)667-698

McNutt, N.S.: Freeze-fracture Techniques and Applications to the Structural Analysis of the Mammalian Plasma Membrane. In: Dynamic Aspects of Cell Surface Organization, pp. 75-126, ed. by G. Poste and G.L. Nicolson. North-Holland Publishing Co., New York, 1977

Millette, C.F.; Spear, P.G.; Gall, W.E.; Edelman, G.M.: Chemical Dissection of Mammalian Spermatozoa. J Cell Biol 58(1973)662-675

Nicolson, G.L.: Transmembrane Control of the Receptors on Normal and Tumor Cells. I. Cytoplasmic Influence over Cell Surface Components. Biochim Biophys Acta 457(1976)57-108

Norman, A.Q.; Spielvogel, A.M.; Wong, R.G.: Polyene Antibiotic-Sterol Interaction. Adv Lipid Res 14(1976)127-170

O'Farrell, P.H.: High Resolution Two-Dimensional Electrophoresis of Proteins. J Cell Biol 250(1975)4007-4021

Olson, G.E.; Linck, R.W.: Observations of the Structural Components of Flagellar Axonemes and Central Pair of Microtubules from Rat Sperm. J Ultrastruct Res

61(1977)21-43

Olson, G.; Lifsics, M.; Hamilton, D.W.; Fawcett, D.W.: Structural Specializations in the Flagellar Plasma Membrane of Opossum Spermatozoa. J Ultrastruct Res 59(1977)207-221

Simionescu, N.; Simionescu, M.: Galloyl Glucoses of Low Molecular Weight as Mordants in Electron Microscopy. J Cell Biol 70(1976)608-621

Steck, T.L.: The Organization of Proteins in the Human Red Blood Cell Membrane. J Cell Biol 62(1974)1-19

Vail, W.J.; Papahadjopoulos, D.; Moscarello, M.A.: Interaction of a Hydrophobic Protein with Liposomes. Evidence for Particles Seen in Freeze-fracture as Being Proteins. Biochim Biophys Acta 345(1974)463-467

Verkleij, A.J.; DeKruijff, B.; Gerritsen, W.F.; Demel, R.A.; Van Deenen, L.L.M.; Verveergaert, P.H.J.: Freeze-etch Electron Microscopy of Erythrocytes, *Acholeplasma laidlawii* Cells and Liposomal Membranes after the Action of Filipin and Amphotericin B. Biochim Biophys Acta 291(1973)577-581

Yanagimachi, R.: Sperm-Egg Association in Mammals. In: Current Topics in Developmental Biology, pp. 83-105, ed. by A.A. Moscona and A. Monroy. Academic Press, New York, 1978

ELIMINATION OF THE ADVERSE EFFECT OF DILUTION ON HAMSTER SPERM MOTILITY *IN VITRO*

B.D. Bavister[1]

Department of Pathology, University of California at Los Angeles School of Medicine, Harbor General Hospital, Torrance, California 90509 USA

Motility is a fundamental characteristic of mature spermatozoa that appears to be intimately associated with their fertilizing ability (Nelson, 1969). Mature mammalian spermatozoa contained within the distal regions of the male reproductive tract exhibit little or no movement *in situ*, but can become highly motile following their release into suitable salt solutions (Mann, 1964; Turner and Howards, 1978).

A vast amount of information has been gathered since the early part of the 19th century on the motility characteristics and fertilizing ability of spermatozoa in culture solutions (Mann, 1964), and it has become evident that sperm motility can be beneficially or detrimentally influenced by a wide variety of physical and chemical factors. These factors include, among others, the ionic composition of the culture medium, pH, osmotic pressure, temperature, and the presence of colloids and chelating agents (Mann, 1964). One of the most pronounced adverse effects on sperm motility arises simply from excessive dilution of spermatozoa, whereupon, after an initial very brief burst of vigorous movement, spermatozoa can become completely immotile within a few minutes. This phenomenon, which has been recognized at least since the middle part of the 19th century, seems to be a common feature of spermatozoa, having been described in species of sea urchins, fish, frogs, birds, and mammals (Mann, 1964). Numerous attempts have been made to reduce or prevent the progressive loss of motility associated with dilution of spermatozoa, usually by adding various known chemical substances to the diluting medium, but these efforts appear to have had limited success (Mann, 1964). The precise reason for the adverse effect of dilution on sperm motility is unknown, but from observations with mammalian spermatozoa, it seems likely that excessive dilution (or washing) of sperm causes loss of cellular components needed for expression of motility (Emmens and Swyer, 1948; Cheng *et al.*, 1949; Blackshaw, 1953).

An understanding of the mechanisms underlying the effects of dilution on sperm motility could provide valuable insight into the physiology of spermatozoa. Moreover, elimination of the adverse effect of dilution (commonly termed the "sperm dilution effect") would obviate a practical problem that can severely hinder studies of mammalian fertilization *in vitro*. Very high sperm concentrations are usually needed under culture conditions in order to sustain sperm motility and viability, and thus to permit fertilization to occur; a range of approximately 10^4-10^7 sperm/ml has been used, depending on the species and the investigator (Fraser and Drury, 1975). The use of such high sperm concentrations often represents for practical reasons a sperm to egg ratio of 1000:1 or higher. This situation is in sharp contrast to that occurring at the natural site of fertilization in mammals, the oviductal ampulla, where sperm to egg ratios as low as 1:1 have been reported (Stefanini *et al.*, 1969). The high concentration of spermatozoa needed for the accomplishment of fertilization *in vitro* also creates a number of practical problems, including rapid dispersion of the granulosa cell mass that surrounds the freshly ovulated egg in most mammalian species, and which constitutes the initial barrier to sperm penetration. Polyspermic fertilization may well occur. In addition, high concentrations of spermatozoa profoundly influence the characteristics of their environment; the task of investigating the physical and chemical parameters that are important for gamete interaction is thus rendered very difficult. Finally, it is clearly impossible under these conditions to identify the fertilizing spermatozoon prior to its penetration of the

---

[1] Present Address: Department of Animal Physiology, University of California, Davis, California 95616 USA

The author thanks Drs. L. Zamboni and J. Marshall, and the Departments of Pathology and Obstetrics/Gynecology at Harbor General Hospital, for support during the course of this work. This study was also supported by NIH General Research Support Grant SO7-RR 0551-14.

© 1979 Urban & Schwarzenberg, Inc. Baltimore-Munich *The Spermatozoon*, edited by D.W. Fawcett and J.M. Bedford

egg; attempts to investigate motility and acrosomal changes (Yanagimachi, 1970a; Austin and Bishop, 1958) and their functional significance for fertilization in this class of spermatozoa are therefore precluded.

The problems associated with the "sperm dilution effect," as well as its intrinsic value, have provided the incentive for studies of the chemical factors that may regulate mammalian sperm motility. By incubating hamster epididymal spermatozoa in a culture medium containing naturally occurring sperm-motility-stimulating substances, the sperm dilution effect has now been virtually or completely eliminated in this species. This is thought to be the first time that elimination of the sperm dilution effect has been reported in any species of animal.

The sperm motility-stimulating substances used in these experiments were a partially purified preparation, derived from hamster adrenal glands, containing the "sperm motility factor" (SMF) (Bavister et al., 1976), and a catecholamine (epinephrine, norepinephrine, or isoproterenol). SMF is a low molecular weight, heat-stable substance found in a variety of body tissues (Bavister et al., 1976; Bavister and Yanagimachi, 1977; Bavister, 1975; Bavister et al., 1978); there can be little doubt that SMF corresponds to the sperm motility-sustaining substance(s) originally described in follicular fluid by Yanagimachi (1969). Recent work has shown that SMF is indispensable for the motility of epididymal hamster spermatozoa in vitro (Bavister and Yanagimachi, 1977). Very recently, it was found that catecholamines are also needed for hamster sperm motility (Cornett and Meizel, 1977; Bavister et al., 1979)[2] and it has now been found that in the presence of both SMF and a catecholamine, hamster sperm motility can be sustained for several hours at extremely high sperm dilutions; by contrast, all sperm flagellar movement ceased within a few minutes in the absence of these factors.

Partially purified SMF was obtained by homogenizing hamster adrenal glands and chromatographing the preparation on a Sephadex G-10 column, as previously reported (Bavister et al., 1976); the active SMF-containing fractions were pooled (active fractions pool = AFP). Drops (45 μl) of culture medium (TALP: Bavister and Yanagimachi, 1977) were prepared under mineral oil as previously described (Bavister and Yanagimachi, 1977), and after equilibration at 37°C with 5% CO_2 in air, 4 μl of AFP were added, together with either 1 μl of freshly prepared 1mM (−)-epinephrine or 1mM (−)-norepinephrine in phosphate-buffered saline or 1 μl of 0.81mM isoproterenol solution (ISUPREL, Winthrop Laboratories). Spermatozoa recovered from the hamster cauda epididymis were washed twice in a low ionic-strength medium (Bavister and Yanagimachi, 1977), and a primary sperm suspension containing roughly 10^6 cells/ml was made in a drop of equilibrated TALP. From this drop, a few spermatozoa were aspirated into a very finely drawn Pasteur pipette, the tip of which was then passed through several washing drops of medium to remove spermatozoa adhering to the outside. Finally, a small number (usually 5-10) of the spermatozoa in the pipette were ejected into one of the drops containing AFP and catecholamine while being observed under the dissecting microscope. After incubation of the inseminated drops at 37°C under 5% CO_2 in air for 3-4 h, the spermatozoa were examined and counted by direct observation of the drops with the dissecting microscope, or with an inverted phase-contrast microscope (total of 20 tests). Usually, careful scrutiny for several minutes was required to locate the spermatozoa. Typically, at least one-half of the inseminated spermatozoa were found to be actively motile, often displaying the vigorous "whiplash" form of motion ("activation") characteristic of capacitated hamster spermatozoa (Yanagimachi, 1970a). Moreover, by 5-6 h, some spermatozoa had undergone an "acrosome reaction."[3] Preliminary experiments have also demonstrated that minute numbers of spermatozoa pre-incubated under these conditions are able to penetrate and fertilize eggs in vitro.[4] By contrast, similar numbers of spermatozoa (5-10) incubated in medium TALP lacking both AFP and catecholamines lost their vigorous motility within a few minutes and did not regain it. In the absence of the AFP (SMF-containing) preparations, catecholamines were able to sustain feeble sperm motility (usually twitching) for 1-2 h only; the AFP prepara-

---

[2]In previous work (Bavister et al., 1976), column chromatography fractions (AFP) containing SMF were able to sustain hamster sperm motility without added catecholamines. However, more recent data (Bavister et al., unpublished data) suggest that small amounts of catecholamines or similar labile substance may be associated with SMF in these fractions, sufficient to sustain sperm motility when very freshly prepared fractions were used, as in the earlier experiments (Bavister et al., 1976). Moreover, in the present experiments, spermatozoa were washed free from male reproductive tract secretions (cauda epididymal plasma) in contrast to all earlier work in which unwashed sperm were used; this difference may also lead to the need for added catecholamines to supplement the SMF preparation.

[3]The occurrence of an acrosome reaction in mammalian spermatozoa is a prerequisite for fertilization (Austin and Bishop, 1958); the term here is defined as loss of the membranes overlying the anterior portion of the acrosome together with the acrosomal contents, insofar as these changes can be detected in motile spermatozoa with the phase-contrast microscope at 150 x magnification.

[4]Bavister, B.D.: Fertilization of Hamster Eggs in Vitro at Sperm:Egg Ratios Close to Unity. Submitted for publication.

tions alone supported very weak sperm motility for 2-4 h, but these spermatozoa could not penetrate eggs. These observations are consistent with those of Cornett and Meizel (1977) who have demonstrated that activation and the acrosome reaction of hamster spermatozoa are stimulated by catecholamines.

This study has demonstrated that spermatozoa from the hamster cauda epididymis can maintain their motility for several hours at extremely high sperm dilutions. The sperm concentrations used in this study were approximately 100-200/ml, which represents a dilution of $1/10^7$ relative to the sperm concentration in the cauda epididymis (Bavister, 1974). Viability of spermatozoa at lower concentrations was quite possible to achieve; the lower limits of sperm concentration appear to be dependent upon the expertise of the investigator in minimizing damage during sperm washing and insemination of individual spermatozoa. Maintenance of hamster sperm motility and fertilizing ability has previously been achieved only with sperm concentrations at least 3-5 orders of magnitude higher (Yanagimachi, 1970b; Talbot et al., 1974; Hanada and Chang, 1976; Bavister et al., 1976). Thus, in the present experiments, sperm concentration has been eliminated as a factor in sustaining sperm motility. By using such low concentrations of spermatozoa, it should be possible to avoid most if not all of the pitfalls outlined above that are associated with currently available *in vitro* fertilization methods.

Furthermore, the observations reported here that SMF and catecholamines can eliminate the sperm dilution effect provide a plausible explanation for the mechanism of this phenomenon in hamster spermatozoa. Both SMF and catecholamines are essential for sustained motility of hamster spermatozoa *in vitro* (Bavister and Yanagimachi, 1977; Bavister et al., 1979). SMF is found in hamster spermatozoa and in cauda epididymal plasma (Bavister and Yanagimachi, 1977; Bavister et al., 1978), while in several species catecholamines have been found in the female reproductive tract (Bodkhe and Harper, 1972; Dujovne et al., 1976) and (in substantial amounts) in distal regions of the male reproductive tract (Eliasson and Risley, 1968). Catecholamines might therefore be available to spermatozoa *in vivo*. In view of all these considerations, it may well be that the loss of SMF and catecholamines from spermatozoa during dilution or washing in solutions lacking these substances accounts for the associated progressive reduction in sperm motility.

REFERENCES

Austin, C.R.; Bishop, M.W.H.: Role of the Rodent Acrosome and Perforatorium in Fertilization. Proc R Soc Lond [Biol] 149(1958)241-248

Bavister, B.D.: The Effect of Variations in Culture Conditions on the Motility of Hamster Spermatozoa. J Reprod Fertil 38(1974)431-440

Bavister, B.D.: Properties of the Sperm Motility-stimulating Component Derived from Human Serum. J Reprod Fertil 43(1975)363-366

Bavister, B.D.; Chen, A.; Fu, P.C.: Catecholamine Requirement for Hamster Sperm Motility *in Vitro*. J Reprod Fertil, 1979 in press

Bavister, B.D.; Rogers, B.J.; Yanagimachi, R.: The Effects of Cauda Epididymal Plasma on the Motility and Acrosome Reaction of Hamster and Guinea Pig Spermatozoa *in Vitro*. Biol Reprod 19(1978) 358-363

Bavister, B.D.; Yanagimachi, R.: The Effects of Sperm Extracts and Energy Sources on the Motility and Acrosome Reaction of Hamster Spermatozoa *in Vitro*. Biol Reprod 16(1977)228-237

Bavister, B.D.; Yanagimachi, R.; Teichman, R.J.: Capacitation of Hamster Spermatozoa with Adrenal Gland Extracts. Biol Reprod 14(1976)219-221

Blackshaw, A.W.: The Motility of Ram and Bull Spermatozoa in Dilute Suspension. J Gen Physiol 36(1953)449-462

Bodkhe, R.R.; Harper, M.J.K.: Changes in the Amount of Adrenergic Neurotransmitter in the Genital Tract of Untreated Rabbits, and Rabbits Given Reserpine or Iproniazid during the Time of Egg Transport. Biol Reprod 6(1972)288-299

Cheng, P.; Casida, L.E.; Barrett, G.R.: Effects of Dilution on Motility of Bull Spermatozoa and the Relation Between Motility in High Dilution and Fertility. J Anim Sci 8(1949)81-88

Cornett, L.; Meizel, S.: Catecholamines Stimulate Acrosome Reactions of Hamster Sperm. J Cell Biol 75(1977)164a

Dujovne, A.R.; deLaborde, N.P.; Carril, L.M.; Cheviakoff, S.; Pedroza, E.; Rosner, J.M.: Correlation between Catecholamine Content of the Human Fallopian Tube and the Uterus and Plasma Levels of Estradiol and Progesterone. Am J Obstet Gynecol 124(1976)229-233

Eliasson, R.; Risley, P.L.: Adrenergic Innervation of the Male Reproductive Ducts of Some Mammals. III. Distributions of Noradrenaline and Adrenaline. Acta Physiol Scand 73(1968)311-319

Emmens, C.W.; Swyer, G.I.M.: Observations on the Motility of Rabbit Spermatozoa in Dilute Suspension. J Gen Physiol 32(1948)121-138

Fraser, L.R.; Drury, L.M.: The Relationship between Sperm Concentration and Fertilization *in Vitro* of Mouse Eggs. Biol Reprod 13(1975)513-518

Hanada, A.; Chang, M.C.: Penetration of Hamster and Rabbit Zona-free Eggs by Rat and Mouse Spermatozoa with Special Reference to Sperm Capacitation. J Reprod Fertil 46(1976)239-241

Mann, T.: Influence of Ion Concentration, Dilution, Temperature, and Other Extraneous Factors on Semen *in Vitro*. In: Biochemistry of Semen and of the Male Reproductive Tract, pp. 339-364. Wiley, New York, 1964

Nelson, L.: Sperm Motility. In: Fertilization. Vol. 1, pp. 27-97, ed. by C.B. Metz and A.B. Monroy. Academic Press, New York, 1969

Stefanini, M.; Oura, C.; Zamboni, L.: Ultrastructure of Fertilization in the Mouse. 2. Penetration of Sperm into the Ovum. J Submicros Cytol 1(1969)1-23

Talbot, P.; Franklin, L.E.; Fussell, E.N.: The Effect of the Concentration of Golden Hamster Spermatozoa on the Acrosome Reaction and Egg Penetration *in Vitro*. J Reprod Fertil 36(1974)429-432

Turner, T.T.; Howards, S.S.: Factors Involved in the Initiation of Sperm Motility. Biol Reprod 18(1978)571-578

Yanagimachi, R.: *In Vitro* Acrosome Reaction and Capacitation of Golden Hamster Spermatozoa by Bovine Follicular Fluid and Its Fractions. J Exp Zool 170(1969)269-280

Yanagimachi, R.: The Movement of Golden Hamster Spermatozoa before and after Capacitation. J Reprod Fertil 23(1970a)193-196

Yanagimachi, R.: *In Vitro* Capacitation of Golden Hamster Spermatozoa by Homologous and Heterologous Blood Sera. Biol Reprod 3(1970b)147-153

PART III
SURFACE PROPERTIES

Spermatozoa like other cells possess a continuous limiting plasma membrane, but the nature and properties of this membrane in spermatozoa are of special interest. The molecular character of its surface is an important determinant of the spermatozoon's ability to recognize and fuse with the ovum and is the primary determinant of its specificity in fertilization.

In mammals at least, the plasmalemma of the spermatozoon must be considered unusual in that it possesses consistent defined regional characteristics. These domains may be expressed by regionally specific antigens and by affinities for surface markers that reflect terminal oligosaccharides of intrinsic glycoproteins. They are revealed also in different regional charge densities or simply by differential adhesiveness that may cause spermatozoa to agglutinate either head-to-head or tail-to-tail. Such regional specialization of the surface is generally defined in relation to structures underlying it. The purpose of such surface differentiation resides at least in part in the sequential participation of different regions of the plasmalemma of the sperm head during penetration of the egg; and in the tail, it may perhaps reflect special qualities required for ion fluxes in that region overlying the mitochondria. Also of considerable interest is the fact that the character of the surface of the male germ cell undergoes a programmed sequence of changes during spermatogenesis, during epididymal transit and later within the female tract. Notwithstanding recent increased awareness of the character of the sperm plasmalemma and its fate during fertilization, there is still little understanding of its changing state in the male and the female tracts, and of the nature of the components that contribute to it. This section is concerned with some of these gaps in our knowledge.

SYMPOSIUM PAPERS

APPEARANCE AND PARTITIONING OF PLASMA MEMBRANE ANTIGENS DURING MOUSE SPERMATOGENESIS

C.F. Millette

Department of Anatomy, Harvard Medical School, Boston, Massachusetts 02215 USA

The role of the cell surface in the regulation of mammalian spermatogenesis has remained largely unexplored even though this complex process provides a unique system for the molecular analysis of cellular proliferation and differentiation. During spermatogenesis there exist a variety of dynamic cellular interactions that may be governed, at least in part, by initial recognition events at the plasma membranes of cells comprising the seminiferous epithelium. These interactions may involve cells at all stages of spermatogenesis, from spermatogonia to spermatozoa. In addition, the interaction of germ cells and Sertoli cells may also be regulated by signals modulated at the cell surface.

Sertoli cells are interconnected by extensive occluding junctions that form the blood-testis barrier (Gilula et al., 1976; Nagano and Suzuki, 1976), creating an adluminal compartment in the seminiferous tubule which presumably provides the milieu necessary for the continued growth and development of spermatocytes, spermatids, and testicular spermatozoa. Sertoli cells are also interconnected by both gap junctions (Gilula et al., 1976) and septate junctions (Connell, 1978) which could allow their coordinated activity in the translocation of germ cells from the basal to the luminal aspects of the seminiferous tubule. Finally, junctional complexes may be involved in the direct interactions of Sertoli cell membranes with the surfaces of germ cells themselves (Ross, 1976) although the physiological significance of these findings is not yet clear. To date, virtually all studies of junctional complexes during spermatogenesis have been conducted using morphological procedures. No biochemical investigations of particular cell surface components constituting these membrane specializations have been attempted and as a result the functional roles of cell-cell junctions in sperm development are poorly understood.

The regulation of spermatogonial proliferation and of meiotic cell division is a second feature of mammalian spermatogenesis that presently remains obscure. The mitotic proliferation of spermatogonia is highly orchestrated with respect to the number, timing, and positioning of successive cell divisons (Clermont and Leblond, 1953; Clermont, 1972; Huckins, 1971). Even the selective degradation of some differentiating spermatogonia seems to be rigidly controlled (Huckins, 1978). Similarly, the known morphological and biochemical events occurring during the long meiotic prophase follow a well defined sequence of cell growth, cell division, and in some instances cell destruction. The regulatory mechanisms coordinating mitosis and meiosis in the seminiferous tubule have not been determined, but they may relate directly to changes in cell surface components. Many alterations in somatic cell surfaces have been shown to be correlated with the cell cycle (Nicolson, 1976) and it is postulated that these alterations are important timing devices somehow ensuring successful cell division. Moreover, the induction of mitosis by antibodies or by lectins must be initiated by specific receptor molecules in the plasma membrane (Edelman, 1976). These analogies strongly suggest that unique membrane receptors may be present on developing spermatogonia and spermatocytes. Such receptors require identification and biochemical characterization in order to facilitate studies of their physiological role in the mammalian testis.

The molecular constituents of spermatozoan membranes must also be identified and analyzed in detail. Mature mammalian spermatozoa exhibit a polar distribution of some glycoproteins and cell surface antigens (Millette, 1976). Furthermore, unlike most somatic cells this localized distribution of membrane components on spermatozoa is maintained at least until capacitation (Friend et al., 1977). Spermatozoa in transit down the male reproductive tract do not show extensive lateral mobility of cell surface molecules (Millette, 1976). The molecular constraints limiting the fluidity of sperm membrane proteins have not been described and it is not yet evident at what stage of spermatogenesis these constraints develop, although a recent report documents events occurring during spermatogenesis in the rabbit (Romrell and O'Rand, 1978).

Mammalian spermatozoa are distinguished from many somatic cells not only with regard to the fluid

© 1979 Urban & Schwarzenberg, Inc. Baltimore-Munich *The Spermatozoon*, edited by D.W. Fawcett and J.M. Bedford

mobility of membrane constituents, but also with regard to particular molecules comprising the sperm membrane itself. A number of sperm surface molecules seem to be either unique to spermatozoa or found also only on certain types of somatic cells, especially those of the central nervous system. The F9 teratocarcinoma antigen (Vitetta et al., 1975), H-Y antigen (Wachtel, 1977), and the NS antigens (Schachner, 1975) are examples of surface components already described for spermatozoa. Recently, workers have detailed the appearance of the F9 antigen on spermatogonial membranes (Felous et al., 1976) and the intracellular appearance of the testis-specific enzymes LDH-X (Meistrich et al., 1977; Hintz and Goldberg, 1977) and cytochrome c_t (Goldberg et al., 1977) in primary pachytene spermatocytes. It is necessary, however, to identify and characterize other molecular components unique to spermatogenic cells. Such components should most likely include specific regulatory agents which when analyzed could be exploited for both a better understanding of the general principles of cell differentiation as well as potential points of intervention for the development of male contraceptives.

The major reason for the relative paucity of experimental data concerning the structure and function of mammalian spermatogenic cell membranes has been the inability to obtain purified populations of the different spermatogenic cell types, including spermatogonia, primary spermatocytes, and maturing spermatids. However, over the past few years this technical difficulty has been largely overcome using a variety of procedures. Centrifugal elutriation, for example, seems to be suited for the isolation of particular stages of condensing spermatids (Meistrich, 1977). The satisfactory purification of earlier spermatogenic cell types, however, requires cell sedimentation at unit gravity. For details of the sedimentation procedures as applied in this laboratory, the reader is referred to the contribution of Romrell to this symposium and also Romrell et al., (1976) and Bellvé et al. (1977a, b). For all studies described in this chapter the enzyme concentrations used to achieve single cell suspensions of seminiferous cells have been reduced to 0.5 mg/ml. Adult and prepuberal mice have been used as donor animals as detailed in Bellvé et al. (1977a). Using sedimentation at unit gravity the following cell populations and purities are readily obtained: primitive type-A spermatogonia (day 6 animals, 90% purity), type-A spermatogonia (day 8, 91%), type-B spermatogonia (day 8, 76%), preleptotene spermatocytes (day 18, 93%), leptotene/zygotene spermatocytes (day 18, 52%), prepuberal pachytene spermatocytes (day 18, 89%), adult pachytene spermatocytes (day 60-90, 92%), round spermatids (day 60-90, spermatid stages 1-8, 95%), and residual bodies (day 60-90, 91%). In addition, prepuberal Sertoli cells have been obtained from day-6 animals at 99% purity. All cell populations are isolated in quantities (10^6-10^8 per experiment) sufficient for biochemical and immunological analysis.

The major aim of these studies is the identification of plasma membrane components of spermatogenic cells, particularly components that are not found on any somatic cell types. For the initial analysis of spermatogenic cell surfaces, antibodies have been raised in rabbits by the intravenous injection of purified classes of mouse germ cells. The immunologically privileged character of the mammalian testis allows the generation of heterologous antibody recognizing antigens specific to seminiferous tissue (Millette and Bellvé, 1977). In this chapter two aspects of cell membrane involvement in spermatogenesis are discussed: first discussed is the temporal appearance of surface membrane antigens at the pachytene stage of the first meiotic prophase using four different immunoglobulin preparations as molecular probes. Second is the selective partitioning of membrane components during spermiogenesis. The results indicate that germ cells undergo dramatic alterations in the composition and organization of their plasma membranes during spermatogenesis. These changes seem amenable to study using serological and biochemical procedures.

TEMPORAL APPEARANCE OF CELL SURFACE ANTIGENS

Four antibody preparations were used to examine the expression of cell surface antigens on isolated germ cells. The immunoglobulin preparations were made against: 1) purified adult pachytene spermatocytes (AP), 2) purified round spermatids (ARS), 3) a mixture of cells from the adult mouse seminiferous epithelium (ASC), and 4) spermatozoa obtained from the vas deferens (AVDS). Analysis of unabsorbed IgG preparations by fluorescence microscopy and by complement-mediated cytotoxicity revealed that very little antibody activity was directed against mouse somatic cells and that all activity against nongerminal cells could be removed by standard techniques (Millette and Bellvé, 1977). Following absorption, the binding of the antibodies to purified populations of spermatogenic cells was examined by indirect fluorescence microscopy, by cytotoxicity and by quantitative assays using radioiodinated immunoglobulin.

All four antibody preparations bound to mouse germ cells in a similar fashion when examined by immunofluorescence. The results obtained using AP are representative (Fig. 1). Only adult pachytene spermatocytes, round spermatids and residual bodies were labelled; all cells in these populations showed strong, uniform binding on the cell surface. No spermatogenic cell type prior to the late pachytene stage showed any reactivity by immunofluorescence. Primitive type-A spermatogonia, type-A spermatogonia, type-B spermatogonia, preleptotene spermatocytes, leptotene/zygotene spermatocytes, and prepuberal pachytene spermatocytes were all unlabelled as were Sertoli cells and Leydig cells.

To confirm the initial expression of membrane components during the late phases of pachynema, purified germ cells were examined by complement mediated cytotoxicity. Results of these experiments corroborated the data obtained by immunofluorescent microscopy. Table 1 lists the cytotoxicity assays and demonstrates that early germ cells, from primitive type-A spermatogonia to leptotene/zygotene spermatocytes, were not lysed in significant numbers under any conditions tested. Pachytene spermatocytes, round spermatids, and residual bodies, however, were all lysed in significant numbers indicating that the membrane constituents recognized by the antibodies first appeared during pachynema.

As a third measure of antibody reactivity to germ cell surfaces, purified populations of intact spermatogenic cells were incubated with radioiodinated preparations of IgG antibody under saturating conditions to quantitate the number of antibody receptors per cell. As shown in Table 2, fewer than 1000 receptors per cell were detected on primitive type-A spermatogonia, type-A spermatogonia, type-B spermatogonia, preleptotene spermatocytes, or leptotene/zygotene spermatocytes. Pachytene spermatocytes, however, had approximately 2×10^5 receptors per cell while round spermatids, residual bodies, and vas deferens spermatozoa exhibited from 6×10^4 to 1.5×10^5 receptors per cell depending upon the particular antibody and cell type examined.

Using all assays—immunofluorescence, cytotoxicity, and quantitation—control experiments with normal rabbit immunoglobulin indicated that the binding detected was immunologically specific (Millette and Bellvé, 1977). These results, then, demonstrate that new components are inserted into the plasma membrane of pachytene spermatocytes and that these components are retained on mature spermatozoa in the vas deferens. Similar findings have been reported by O'Rand and Romrell (1977) in rabbit and by Tung and Fritz (1978) in the rat. The present investigations do not indicate the number or the molecular nature of those components that first appear on the pachytene spermatocyte surface. Other experiments suggest, however, that the four antibodies (AP, ARS, ASC, and AVDS) recognize different antigens and, therefore, that the germ cell components detected by these reagents represent multiple molecular species. Vas deferens spermatozoa were labelled with each of the IgG preparations and examined by indirect fluorescent microscopy. AVDS labelled the entire sperm surface except for the lateral

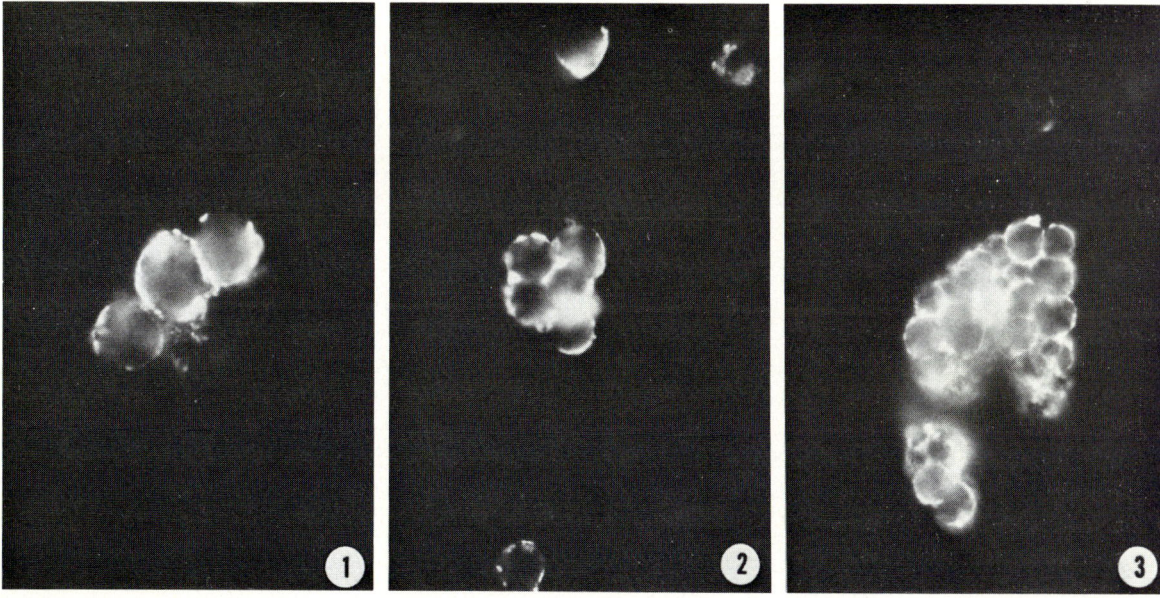

Figure 1. Labelling of purified mouse spermatogenic cells by rabbit antibody against adult mouse pachytene spermatocytes (AP). (1) Isolated pachytene spermatocytes. X885 (2) Isolated round spermatids. X885 (3) Isolated residual bodies. X885 No spermatogenic cell types prior to late primary pachytene spermatocytes are labelled by AP.

Table 1. Cytotoxic Effect of Antibody Preparations on Spermatogenic Cell Populations

Cell Type	Percent Dead Cells			
	AP	ARS	ASC	AVDS
Primitive type-A spermatogonia	<5	6	<5	<5
Type-A spermatogonia	<5	14	<5	7
Type-B spermatogonia	14	19	5	7
Preleptotene spermatocytes	<5	<5	<5	<5
Leptotene/zygotene spermatocytes*	<5	<5	<5	<5
Pachytene spermatocytes	85	65	66	80
Round spermatids	55	90	76	80
Residual bodies	25	22	22	36

Data represent the maximum percentage of killed cells at an immunoglobulin concentration of 100 µg/ml. All results are the average of three independent determinations, which differ by less than 5%.
*This cell population contained 10% Sertoli cells.
AP: Antibody against adult pachytene spermatocytes.
ARS: Antibody against round spermatids (steps 1-8).
ASC: Antibody against adult seminiferous cells.
AVDS: Antibody against vas deferens spermatozoa.

postacrosomal region of the sperm head. ASC bound only to the sperm principal piece, while AP bound to the sperm membrane overlying the acrosome and the midpiece. ARS labelled sperm in a manner similar to that detected for AVDS, although binding to the principal piece was weaker than binding to the midpiece. Each antibody, then, exhibited a different labelling pattern when tested on spermatozoa, suggesting that a variety of surface antigens are responsible for the prior observations.

Further studies are required to quantitate the exact number of cell surface components recognized by each antibody and to establish the molecular nature of each plasma membrane antigen. Although it seems apparent that the surface moieties discussed in this report are not components previously described by other investigators (cf. Millette and Bellvé, 1977), postulates regarding possible regulatory functions for those spermatogenic cell membrane antigens that first appear during pachynema must await functional assays.

SELECTIVE PARTITIONING OF SURFACE ANTIGENS DURING SPERMIOGENESIS

The molecular mechanisms responsible for the release of spermatozoa into the tubule lumen are not known. Spermiation is initiated with the dissolution of mem-

Table 2. Quantitation of Antibody Receptors on Spermatogenic Cell Populations

Cell Type	Sites per Cell ($\times 10^3$)			
	AP	ARS	ASC	AVDS
Primitive type-A spermatogonia	<1	<1	<1	<1
Type-A spermatogonia	<1	<1	<1	<1
Type-B spermatogonia	<1	<1	<1	<1
Preleptotene spermatocytes	<1	<1	<1	<1
Leptotene/zygotene spermatocytes*	<1	<1	<1	<1
Pachytene spermatocytes	274	180	241	183
Round spermatids	98	75	63	89
Residual bodies	103	86	99	106
Spermatozoa	62	61	90	147

Data represent the average of triplicate determinations that differed by less than 10%. Background labelling, as defined by the binding of ^{125}I-labelled normal rabbit IgG, has been subtracted from these data. Nonspecific labelling was always less than 5% of the total binding.
*This cell population contained 15% Sertoli cells.
AP: Antibody against adult pachytene spermatocytes.
ARS: Antibody against round spermatids (steps 1-8).
ASC: Antibody against adult seminiferous cells.
AVDS: Antibody against vas deferens spermatozoa.

brane junctional specializations interposed between Sertoli cells and condensing spermatids (Ross, 1976). As the sperm gradually loosens from the surrounding Sertoli cell the spermatid cytoplasm becomes lobulated, but remains attached to the spermatid neck by a thin stalk (Fawcett and Phillips, 1969). Eventually this cytoplasmic connection is broken to release the spermatozoon, while the cytoplasmic remnant or residual body is phagocytized by the Sertoli cell. The process of spermiation, therefore, results in the physical separation of two segments of the spermatid plasma membrane.

It is possible that the segregation of cell surface components into the residual body membrane is a nonrandom process. For example, specific membrane receptors responsible for continued adhesion of germ cell to Sertoli cell could be sequestered on the residual body to allow sperm release. Preliminary data demonstrating a greater density of concanavalin-A sites on the surfaces of residual bodies in comparison with spermatids support the idea that individual membrane components are, in fact, partitioned selectively during late spermiogenesis (Millette, 1976). In order to examine this question directly a number of rabbit anti-mouse germ cell IgG preparations were assayed for binding to purified spermatogenic cells. Particular emphasis was placed on determining the relative binding of the antibodies to round spermatids, residual bodies, and maturing spermatozoa.

Surprisingly, an IgG fraction directed against purified type-B spermatogonia provided clear evidence for the selective partitioning of spermatogenic cell surface antigens. The specificity of the rabbit anti-mouse type-B spermatogonia IgG (ATBS), unabsorbed and absorbed preparations, was first assayed by fluorescence microscopy on a number of mouse germ cells and somatic cells. Unabsorbed ATBS labelled all mouse somatic and germ cells examined (Fig. 2). Mouse thymocytes and splenocytes were strongly labelled by ATBS in a patchy fashion. With the noted exception of spermatozoa, mouse germ cells were labelled diffusely. Spermatozoa from the testis, the caput epididymidis, cauda epididymidis and vas deferens were all labelled in a distinctive pattern. The entire cell surface, except for lateral areas of the sperm head anterior and posterior to the postacrosomal segment, was labelled uniformly (Fig. 2).

Immunofluorescence indicated that unabsorbed ATBS was not specific for spermatogenic cell surface antigens, since mouse thymocytes and splenocytes were labelled strongly. This was in contrast to results obtained for AP, ARS, ASC, and AVDS where unabsorbed IgG preparations labelled few somatic cells. The difference in immunological specificities may be explained by the respective cell populations used as immunogens. Spermatogonia lie on the basal side of the Sertoli cell junctional complexes which form the blood-testis barrier (Dym and Fawcett, 1970) and are not protected from the immune system as are pachytene spermatocytes, round spermatids, and spermatozoa. Spermatogonia, therefore, would not be expected to express cell surface components that could engender an autoimmune response.

Absorption of ATBS with mouse thymocytes or splenocytes abolished all labelling of thymocytes, splenocytes, peripheral blood lymphocytes, erythrocytes, and Leydig cells as assayed by immunofluorescence. Mouse Sertoli cells, however, from both prepuberal and adult animals were still labelled strongly in a diffuse fashion. The significance of this binding activity is not yet clear. Experiments conducted using purified populations of mouse spermatogenic cells revealed that primitive type-A spermatogonia, type-A spermatogonia, type-B spermatogonia, preleptotene primary spermatocytes, leptotene/zygotene primary spermatocytes, prepuberal pachytene spermatocytes, adult pachytene spermatocytes, round spermatids, and residual bodies were all labelled. In contrast, spermatozoa obtained from the testis, caput epididymidis, cauda epididymidis, or vas deferens showed no labelling by absorbed ATBS.

These results suggest that ATBS recognizes at least two classes of cell-surface antigenic determinants. One class of antigens is shared by germ cells and somatic cells. These components are present on testicular, epididymal, and vas deferens spermatozoa and show a nonrandom topographical distribution on these cells. Other surface antigens are found only on Sertoli cells, on spermatogonic cells at early stages of differentiation, and on residual bodies. This class of antigens is not found on spermatozoa at any stage of maturation.

Complement-mediated cytotoxicity assays were used to obtain further information on the binding specificity of unabsorbed and absorbed antibody. All germ cell populations tested, in addition to prepuberal mouse Sertoli cells, were lysed by ATBS before and after absorption (Table 3). No significant differences were obtained in the maximum percentage of dead cells between the two antibody preparations. With the exception of residual bodies, all testicular cell populations were killed in significant numbers (77-90%). Residual bodies, however, were not killed at levels greater than 50% by any concentration of either antibody preparation. The membrane of residual bodies has been found previously to be relatively resistant to complement-mediated lysis (Table 1).

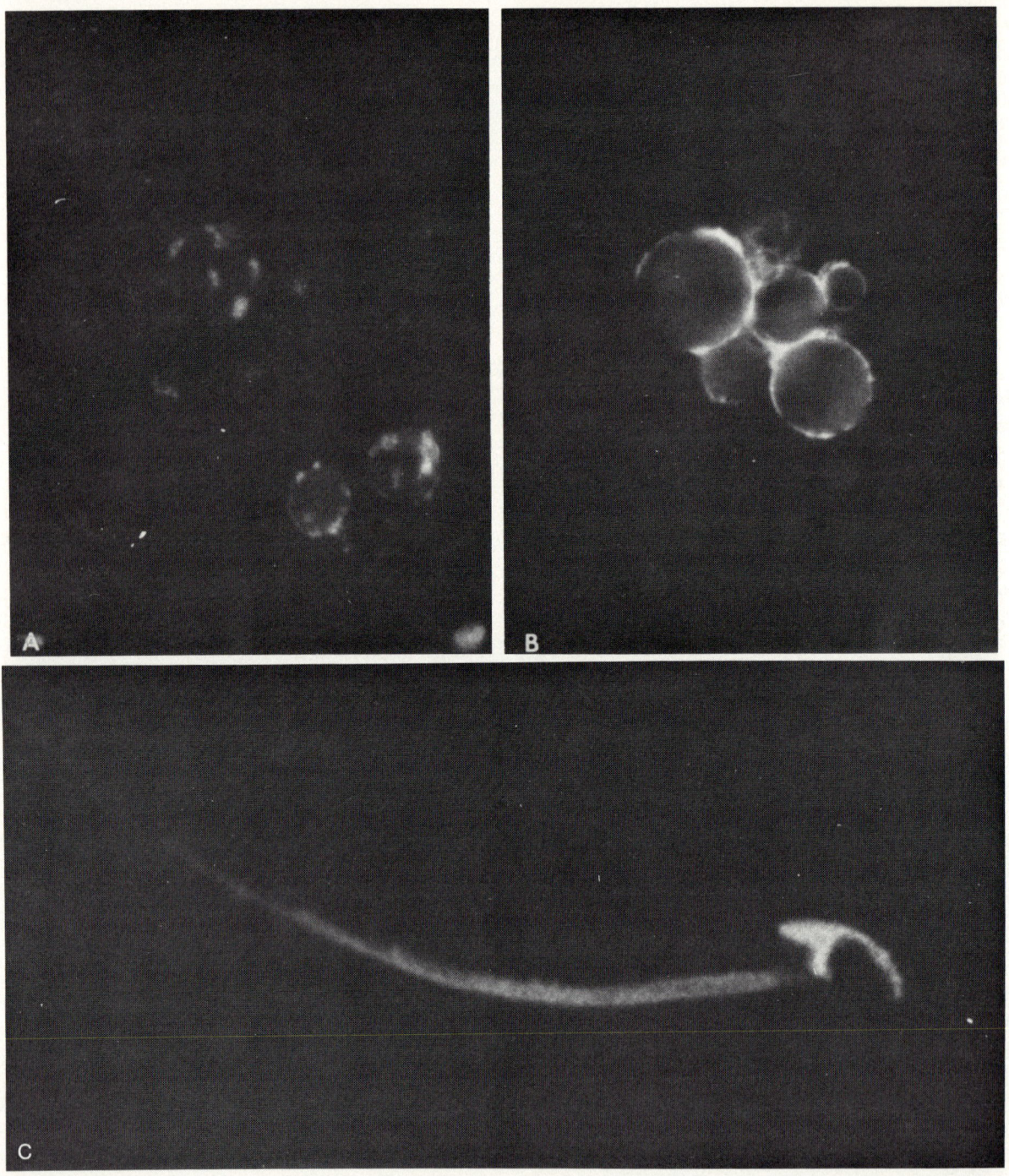

Figure 2. Labelling of mouse cells by unabsorbed rabbit antibody against purified mouse type-B spermatogonia (ATBS) (A) Splenocytes are labelled in distinct patches. X990 (B) Mixed spermatogenic cells from adult mouse seminiferous epithelium, including pachytene spermatocytes, round spermatids, and residual bodies, are labelled uniformly. X990 (C) Spermatozoon from the vas deferens shows uniform labelling of the cell surface, except for lateral areas of the sperm head anterior and posterior to the post-acrosomal region. X2190

Table 3. Effect of Absorption on Binding of ATBS to Isolated Seminiferous Epithelial Cells

Cell Type	Dead Cells	
	Unabsorbed IgG (%)	Absorbed IgG (%)
Primitive type-A spermatogonia	86	85
Type-A spermatogonia	87	77
Type-B spermatogonia	86	88
Preleptotene spermatocytes	83	79
Leptotene/zygotene spermatocytes*	77	81
Prepuberal pachytene spermatocytes	83	85
Adult pachytene spermatocytes	89	90
Round spermatids (steps 1-8)	90	84
Residual bodies	50	50
Sertoli cells	83	82

Data represent the maximum percentage of killed cells at an immunoglobulin concentration of 100 µg/ml. All results are the average of three independent determinations.
*This cell population contained 11% Sertoli cells.
ATBS: Antibody against type B spermatogonia.

Finally, radioiodinated ATBS IgG, after absorption, was used to quantitate cell surface receptor sites on isolated mouse germ cells. After absorption of ATBS with mouse thymocytes or splenocytes to remove reactivity shared with somatic cells, primitive type-A spermatogonia bound the greatest number of absorbed ATBS molecules, 2.7 million per cell, while round spermatids and residual bodies each had about 1 million surface receptor sites (Table 4). Estimations were made of the cell membrane density of antigenic receptors for absorbed antibody based upon the data shown in Table 4, and the cell surface area calculated from the respective volumes of isolated spermatogenic cells (Bellvé et al., 1977b). These calculations indicate that the density of antibody receptors per cell increases approximately two and one-half-fold during the mitotic proliferation of spermatogonia. In contrast, the density of surface receptors decreases approximately fourfold during the first meiotic prophase as the developing primary spermatocytes increase in size without concomitant cell division.

Vas deferens spermatozoa bound very low levels of absorbed ATBS. Only 0.003 million sites per cell were detectable (Table 4). Contrasted with the 1 million sites per cell seen on both round spermatids and residual bodies, these data are in good agreement with the immunofluorescent results already presented. Some cell-surface antigens detected on mouse spermatogenic cells appear to be partitioned during spermiogenesis so that they are excluded from the spermatozoon.

Spermatozoa from the caput epididymidis, cauda epididymidis, and vas deferens were examined to quantitate the temporal disappearance of binding sites for absorbed ATBS. Only minor quantitative differences were detected between epidymal spermatozoa and vas deferens spermatozoa (Table 5). Thus, the most dramatic alteration in the number of membrane receptors for ATBS, as depicted by the disparity in antigenic sites between round spermatids and vas deferens spermatozoa (Table 4), occurs before the cells enter the caput epididymis. Furthermore, the immunofluorescent data obtained for testicular spermatozoa demonstrate that these membrane components assume a discrete topographical regionalization prior to spermiation.

Table 4. Quantitation of Cell Surface Receptor Sites for Absorbed ATBS

Cell Type	Sites per Cell ($\times 10^3$)
Primitive type-A spermatogonia	2670
Type-A spermatogonia	2150
Type-B spermatogonia	1510
Preleptotene spermatocytes	2050
Leptotene/zygotene spermatocytes*	2480
Prepuberal pachytene spermatocytes	1430
Adult pachytene spermatocytes	2230
Round spermatids (steps 1-8)	1030
Residual bodies	920
Vas deferens spermatozoa	3

Data represent the average of triplicate determinations which invariably differed by less than 10%. Background labelling, as defined by the binding of ^{125}I-labelled normal rabbit IgG, has been subtracted from these data. Nonspecific labelling was always less than 5% of the total binding.
*This cell population contained 11% Sertoli cells.
ATBS: Antibody against type-B spermatogonia.

In contrast to other spermatogenic cells, vas deferens spermatozoa bound less of the absorbed antibody (Table 4). It was important to test the possibility that sperm surface receptors for ATBS were peripheral as opposed to integral plasma membrane components. Fluid secretions of the epididymis or the vas deferens could be adsorbed onto the sperm surface, thereby

Table 5. Quantitation of ATBS Receptors during Sperm Maturation

Cell Type	Sites per Cell ($\times 10^3$)	
	Unabsorbed IgG	Absorbed IgG
Caput spermatozoa	8542	4
Cauda spermatozoa	8710	4
Vas deferens spermatozoa	9720	3

Cells were washed three times in EKRB before labelling. Data represent the average of triplicate determinations which differed by less than 7%. Background labelling represented less than 5% and was subtracted from these data.

ATBS: Antibody against type-B spermatogonia.

either creating peripheral binding sites for unabsorbed ATBS or nonspecifically masking integral binding sites for the absorbed antibody. Therefore, vas deferens spermatozoa were first washed extensively in a variety of suspension media known to remove peripheral cell membrane constitutents. Quantitation of antibody receptor sites was then conducted as described previously.

The normal washing procedure in enriched Krebs Ringer biocarbonate buffer (EKRB) resulted in values of 10 million receptor sites per cell for unabsorbed ATBS and only 0.003 million sites per cell for absorbed antibody. Treatment of vas deferens spermatozoa in five other media had only a minimal effect on the number of binding sites for unabsorbed ATBS (Table 6). The greatest decrease in surface binding sites obtained was 25% using 200mM NaCl in Toyoda's medium (Toyoda et al., 1971). Although the small differences seen between EKRB and the other incubation media were reproducible, these data strongly imply that the binding of unabsorbed ATBS to mouse vas deferens spermatozoa secretions was not due to components adsorbed from epididymal secretions.

Conversely, the alteration of incubation media had little or no effect on the binding of absorbed ATBS to mouse vas deferens spermatozoa (Table 6). In all instances, only 0.003-0.005 million receptor sites per cell were detected. These values are just above the sensitivity limit of the quantitative assay used for these experiments. The incubation media tested included physiological fluids (EKRB, phosphate buffered saline (PBS), and 0.15M NaCl), slightly hypertonic conditions known to remove decapacitation factors from mouse spermatozoa (200mM NaCl/Toyoda), strongly hypertonic conditions (3M KCl), and chelating agents (10mM ethylenediaminetetraacetate (EDTA)/NaCl). It does not appear, therefore, that receptor sites for absorbed ATBS are masked on spermatozoa by epididymal secretions. Instead, these receptors seem to be entirely absent from the sperm surface, having been partitioned selectively to the residual body membrane.

Several mechanisms could account for the apparent redistribution of plasma membrane components prior to spermiation. Receptors for ATBS may be masked nonspecifically by newly adsorbed peripheral surface molecules. Alternatively, the antigenic sites may be selectively removed from specific areas of the developing sperm plasma membrane by proteolysis or by internalization. A third and more plausible explanation is that these antigenic determinants are partitioned by lateral translocation in the plane of the membrane. The nonselective masking of ATBS receptors by adsorbed peripheral proteins appears unlikely for two reasons: first, the results of membrane partitioning are evident even on testicular spermatozoa that show no binding of absorbed ATBS. Testicular cells are not exposed to the membrane-coating components present in epididymal secretions (Gordon et al., 1975). Second, extensive washing of spermatozoa in media known to remove adsorbed peripheral membrane constituents and decapacitation factors failed to expose additional binding sites for the absorbed antibody (Table 6). The selective removal of surface receptors for absorbed ATBS by hydrolytic processes or internalization cannot be ruled out completely. It should be noted, however, that the number of surface receptors detected on round spermatids is quantitatively similar to the number found on purified re-

Table 6. Quantitation of ATBS Receptors on Washed Vas Deferens Spermatozoa

Wash Solution	Sites per Cell ($\times 10^3$)	
	Unabsorbed IgG	Absorbed IgG
EKRB	9720	3
PBS	8535	3
0.15 M KCl	8100	5
3 M KCl	7475	3
10 mM EDTA/NaCl	7370	4
200 mM NaCl/Toyoda	7355	4

Cells were washed three times in the indicated medium before resuspension in EKRB and the addition of ^{125}I-ATBS. Data represent the average of triplicate determinations which differed by less than 11%. Background labelling as assayed by the binding of ^{125}I-normal rabbit IgG was always less than 5% of the total binding and was subtracted from these data.

EKRB: Enriched Krebs Ringer bicarbonate buffer, pH 7.25.
PBS: Phosphate buffered saline, pH 7.4.

sidual bodies (Table 4). It seems unlikely that residual bodies are able to synthesize plasma membrane receptors in order to replace quantitatively any molecules lost from round spermatids by proteolysis. There is no evidence for protein synthesis by residual bodies.

A selective and differential partitioning of membrane molecules is a more plausible explanation for the present observations. Selective lateral translocation of surface components has been demonstrated to occur during erythroid cell differentiation. Chan and Oliver (1976) have described the asymmetric distribution of concanavalin-A receptors during the transition from proerythroblast to erythroblast in the chicken. Also, following enucleation during rabbit erythropoiesis, the residual membrane overlying the extruded nucleus is selectively enriched in both concanavalin-A receptors and antigenic sites (Skutelsky and Danon, 1970). Finally, a discrete segregation of two intrinsic membrane glycoproteins and of acetylcholinesterase has been demonstrated during the vesiculation of erythrocytes (Lutz *et al.*, 1977). The selective partitioning of plasma membrane components, therefore, is not limited to spermatogenic cell differentiation and may be of general importance for the membranes of diverse cell types.

The physiological function of those spermatogenic cell surface antigens that are partitioned to the residual body must remain speculative at present. Current experiments are designed to isolate plasma membranes of purified spermatogenic cells for the fractionation and identification of cell membrane constituents using isotopic labelling techniques and immunocoprecipitation procedures. Preliminary results indicate that cell membranes may be readily prepared in high purity and in quantities sufficient to allow the biochemical analysis of individual surface molecules, including those that are selectively segregated during mammalian spermiogenesis.

REFERENCES

Bellvé, A.R.; Cavicchia, J.C.; Millette, C.F.; O'Brien, D.A.; Bhatnagar, Y.M.; Dym, M.: Spermatogenic Cells of the Prepuberal Mouse: Isolation and Morphological Characterization J Cell Biol 74(1977a)68-85

Bellvé, A.R.; Millette, C.F.; Bhatnagar, Y.M.; O'Brien, D.A.: Dissociation of the Mouse Testis and Characterization of Isolated Spermatogenic Cells. J Histochem Cytochem 25(1977b)480-494

Chan, L.-N.L.; Oliver, J.M.: Changes in Number, Mobility and Topographical Distribution of Lectin Receptors during Maturation of Chick Erythroid Cells. J Cell Biol 69 (1976)647-658

Connell, C.J.: A Freeze-fracture and Lanthanum Tracer Study of the Complex Junction between Sertoli Cells of the Canine Testis. J Cell Biol 76(1978)57-75

Clermont, Y.; Leblond, C.P.: Renewal of Spermatogonia in the Rat. Am J Anat 93(1953)475-501

Clermont, Y.: Kinetics of Spermatogenesis in Mammals: Seminiferous Epithelial Cycle and Spermatogonial Renewal. Physiol Rev 52(1972)198-236

Dym, M.; Fawcett, D.W.: The Blood Testis Barrier in the Rat and the Physiological Compartmentation of the Seminiferous Epithelium. Biol Reprod 3(1970)308-326

Edelman, G.M.: Surface Modulation in Cell Recognition and Cell Growth. Science 192(1976)218-226

Fawcett, D.W.; Phillips, D.M.: Observations on the Release of Spermatozoa and on Changes in the Head during Passage through the Epididymis. J Reprod Fertil [Suppl] 6(1969)405-418

Fellous, M.; Erickson, R.P.; Gachelin, G.; Dubois, P.; Jacob, F.: The Time of Appearance of Ia Antigens during Spermatogenesis in the Mouse, Relationship between Ia Antigens and H-2, B2 Microglobulin and F9 Antigens. Folia Biol 22(1976)381-383

Friend, D.S.; Orci, L.; Perrelet, A.; Yanagimachi, R.: Membrane Particle Changes Attending the Acrosome Reaction in Guinea Pig Spermatozoa. J Cell Biol 74(1977)561-577

Gilula, N.B.; Fawcett, D.W.; Aoki, A.: The Sertoli Cell Occluding Junctions and Gap Junctions in Mature and Developing Mammalian Testis. Dev Biol 50(1976)142-168

Goldberg, E.; Sberna, D.; Wheat, T.E.; Urbanski, G.L.; Margoliash, E.: Cytochrome *c*: Immunofluorescent Localization of the Testis-specific Form. Science 196(1977)1010-1011

Gordon, M.; Dandekar, P.V.; Bartoszewicz, W.: The Surface Coat of Epididymal, Ejaculated and Capacitated Sperm. J Ultrastruct Res 50(1975)199-207

Hintz, M.; Goldberg, E.: Immunohistochemical Localization of LDH-X during Spermatogenesis in Mouse Testis. Dev Biol 57(1977)375-384

Huckins, C.: The Spermatogonial Stem Cell Population in Adult Rat. I. Their Morphology, Proliferation, and Maturation. Anat Rec 169(1971)533-558

Huckins, C.: The Morphology and Kinetics of Spermatogonial Degeneration in Normal Rats: An Analysis Using a Simplified Classification of the Germinal Epithelium. Anat Rec 190(1978)905-926

Lutz, H.U.; Lomant, A.J.; McMillan, P.; Wehrli, E.: Rearrangements of Integral Membrane Components during *in Vitro* Aging of Sheep Erythrocyte Membranes. J Cell Biol 74(1977)389-398

Meistrich, M.L.: Separation of Spermatogenic Cells and Nuclei from Rodent Testes. In: Methods in Cell Biology, Volume XV, pp. 15-54, ed. by D.M. Prescott. Academic Press, New York, 1977

Meistrich, M.L.; Trostle, P.K.; Frapart, M.; Erickson, R.P.: Biosynthesis and Localization of Lactate Dehydrogenase X in Pachytene Spermatocytes and Spermatids of Mouse Testes. Dev Biol 60(1977)428-441

Millette, C.F.: Distribution and Mobility of Lectin Binding Sites on Mammalian Spermatozoa. In: Immunobiology of Gametes, pp. 51-71, ed. by M. Edidin and M.H. Johnson. Cambridge University Press, Cambridge, 1976

Millette, C.F.; Bellvé, A.R.: Temporal Expression of Membrane Antigens during Mouse Spermatogenesis. J Cell Biol 74(1977)86-97

Nagano, T.; Suzuki, F.: The Postnatal Development of the Junctional Complexes of the Mouse Sertoli Cells as Revealed by Freeze Fracture. Anat Rec 185(1976)403-418

Nicolson, G.L.: Trans-membrane Control of the Receptors on Normal and Tumor Cells. II. Surface Changes Associated with Transformation and Malignancy. Biochim Biophys Acta 458(1976)1-72

O'Rand, M.G.; Romrell, L.J.: Appearance of Cell Surface Auto- and Iso-Antigens during Spermatogenesis in the Rabbit. Dev Biol 55(1977)347-358

Romrell, L.J.; Bellvé, A.R.; Fawcett, D.W.: Separation of Mouse Spermatogenic Cells by Sedimentation Velocity. A Morphological Characterization. Dev Biol 49(1976)119-131

Romrell, L.J.; O'Rand, M.G.: Capping and Ultrastructural Localization of Sperm Surface Isoantigens during Spermatogenesis. Dev Biol 63(1978)76-93

Ross, M.H.: The Sertoli Cell Junctional Specialization during Spermiogenesis and at Spermiation. Anat Rec 186(1976)79-104

Schachner, M.; Wortham, K.A.; Carter, L.D.; Chaffee, J.K.: NS-4 (Nervous System Antigen-4), a Cell Surface Antigen of Developing and Adult Mouse Brain and Sperm. Dev Biol 44(1975)313-325

Skutelsky, E.; Danon, D.: Electron Microscopical Analysis of Surface Charge Labelling Density at Various Stages of the Erythroid Line. J Membr Biol 2(1970)173-179

Toyoda, Y.; Yokoyama, M.; Hosi, T.: Fertilization of Mouse Eggs *in Vitro* 1. By Fresh Epididymal Sperm 2. Effects of *in Vitro* Preincubation of Spermatozoa on Time of Spermatozoa Penetration. Jpn J Anim Reprod 16(1971)147-157

Tung, P.S.; Fritz, I.B.: Specific Surface Antigens on Rat Pachytene Spermatocytes and Successive Classes of Germinal Cells. Dev Biol, 64(1978)297-315

Vitetta, E.S.; Artzt, K.; Bennett, D.; Boyse, E.A.; Jacob, F.: Structural Similarities between a Product of the T/t Locus Isolated from Sperm and Teratoma, and H-2 Antigens Isolated from Splenocytes. Proc Natl Acad Sci USA 72(1975)3215-3219

Wachtel, S.S.: H-Y Antigen and the Genetics of Sex Determination. Science 198(1977)797-799

CELL SURFACE CHANGES ASSOCIATED WITH THE EPIDIDYMIDAL MATURATION OF MAMMALIAN SPERMATOZOA

G.L. Nicolson and R. Yanagimachi

Department of Developmental and Cell Biology, University of California, Irvine, California 92717 USA; Department of Anatomy and Reproductive Biology, University of Hawaii School of Medicine, Honolulu, Hawaii 96822 USA

Epididymidal maturation is a term that has been used to describe biological and biochemical changes that occur when spermatozoa progressively gain the ability to fertilize ova during their passage through the epididymidis (review: Bedford, 1978). In the rabbit, spermatozoa isolated from the caput epididymidis are essentially unable to fertilize ova, but when isolated from the cauda epididymidis, spermatozoa are fully capable of fertilization similar to ejaculated sperm. During their passage to the middle corpus epididymidis, rabbit spermatozoa begin to acquire their fertilization capacity (Bedford, 1966; Orgebin-Crist, 1967).

Epididymidal maturation is associated with a variety of morphological, physiological, and biochemical changes. Differences in the size, shape, and internal structure of the acrosome (Bedford, 1963, 1965; Bedford and Nicander, 1971; Fawcett and Phillips, 1969; Flechon, 1973) and midpiece (Olson and Hamilton, 1976) of spermatozoa have been revealed by electron microscopy. In addition, modifications in the cohesiveness between the outer acrosomal membrane and the underlying plasma membrane (Bedford, 1975; Fawcett and Phillips, 1969) and migration of the cytoplasmic droplet (Branton and Salisbury, 1947; Nicander, 1957) have been seen in some species of spermatozoa during epididymidal passage. Lavon et al. (1970) have found differences in lipoprotein content between caput and cauda epididymidal spermatozoa. Variations have also been noted in the susceptibility of spermatozoa to modification of iodoacetamide (Bedford et al., 1973), carboxyphenol-maleimide (Reyes et al., 1976), and nigrosine-eosin stain (Glover, 1962; Ortavant, 1953; Brochert and Debatene, 1953) during epididymal passage.

The specific properties of the cell surface of spermatozoa are probably important in epididymidal maturation. Bedford (1963) noted increases in electrophoretic mobility of rabbit sperm during passage through the epididymidis, and Chulavatnotol and Yindepit (1976) found decreases in the activity of a membrane ATPase between caput and cauda epididymidal spermatozoa.

Ultrastructural examination of cell surface anionic sites by the binding of positively charged colloidal particles has revealed biochemical changes during epididymidal passage (Bedford et al., 1972; Flechon, 1973; Yanagimachi et al., 1972). In these studies modifications in the binding of colloidal iron hydroxide (CIH) particles were found between caput epididymidal, cauda epididymidal, and ejaculated spermatozoa. Bedford et al. (1972) found that the binding of CIH at pH 3.0-4.6 to rabbit sperm heads was far greater on spermatozoa isolated from cauda epididymidis than on those isolated from caput epididymidis; Yanagimachi et al. (1972) noted that CIH binding at pH 1.8 to rabbit sperm tails increased during epididymidal passage of spermatozoa; and Flechon (1973) has shown that CIH particles are bound in a more dense, discontinuous distribution on ejaculated spermatozoa compared with spermatozoa isolated from caput or corpus epididymidis.

During their passage through the epididymidis and vas deferens, spermatozoa are known to be modified by absorption of epididymidal material (Baker and Aman, 1970; Hunter and Hafs, 1964; Killian and Aman, 1973). Binding these epididymidal materials is associated with changes in the antigenic properties of the sperm surface (Edwards et al., 1964; Hunter, 1969; Johnson and Hunter, 1972; Baker and Aman, 1970; Killian and Aman, 1973; Weil, 1965). Some of these absorbed materials are tightly bound and are not readily removed by washing in physiological saline or by treatment with organic solvents (Weil, 1965), and these antigenic components have been collectively called sperm-coating antigens (Boettcher, 1969; Edwards et al., 1964; Weil, 1965, 1967). Certain spermatozoa-bound substances are known plasma membrane proteins such as lactoferrin, an iron-bound protein found in human seminal plasma (Hekman and Rümke, 1969). In addition to the acquisition of spermatozoa-bound substances, certain spermatozoa-coating antigens may be lost during epididymidal maturation. The functional significance of the spermatozoa-bound substances, or their binding and release during epididymidal maturation, and the role these substances play in fertilization remain to be determined.

© 1979 Urban & Schwarzenberg, Inc. Baltimore-Munich *The Spermatozoon*, edited by D.W. Fawcett and J.M. Bedford

LECTIN-MEDIATED AGGLUTINATION AND EPIDIDYMAL MATURATION

Plant lectins have been used to identify saccharide components on the surfaces of a variety of mammalian cells (review: Nicolson, 1974). Uhlenbruck and Herrmann (1972) and Nicolson and Yanagimachi (1972) were the first to examine mammalian spermatozoa for the presence of lectin-binding sites. The former authors found a variety of different lectin-binding sites on ejaculated human spermatozoa before and after treatment with trypsin and neuraminidase. Trypsin treatment was found to enhance *Evonymus europaeus*-mediated agglutination of some human sperm samples, while neuraminidase treatment unmasked *Helix pomatia*-binding sites on other specimens. Nicolson and Yanagimachi (1972) utilized concanavalin A, wheat germ agglutinin, and *Ricinus communis* agglutinin to study the surfaces of hamster and rabbit caput and cauda epididymal spermatozoa as well as rabbit ejaculated spermatozoa. When ejaculated spermatozoa or spermatozoa obtained from caput or cauda epididymidis were washed and mixed with various concentrations of the lectins, agglutination occurred (Nicolson and Yanagimachi, 1972). When lectin-mediated agglutination of rabbit caput epididymal spermatozoa was compared with agglutination of ejaculated spermatozoa or cauda epididymal spermatozoa, the caput spermatozoa were consistently more agglutinable with wheat germ agglutinin and *Ricinus communis* agglutinin (Nicolson et al., 1977). Rabbit caput epididymal spermatozoa were agglutinated strongly by wheat germ agglutinin down to low lectin concentrations, while cauda epididymal and ejaculated spermatozoa were agglutinable only at the highest lectin concentrations used (Fig.1). Similar but less pronounced differences were found with *Ricinus communis*-mediated agglutination of rabbit spermatozoa at various stages of epididymal maturation. Only a small difference was found concanavalin A-mediated agglutination among cauda epididymal, caput epididymal, and ejaculated spermatozoa, the last being slightly less agglutinable compared with cauda epididymal spermatozoa (Nicolson et al., 1977). Thus, we have determined that the cell surface N-acetylglucosamine-like or N-acetylneuraminic acid-like and galactose-like residues in oligosaccharides recognized by wheat germ agglutinin and *Ricinus communis* agglutinin were modified after contact of spermatozoa with seminal plasma, and the spermatozoa became less agglutinable.

LOCALIZATION OF LECTIN-BINDING SITES AND EPIDIDYMAL MATURATION

Lectin-binding sites have been ultrastructurally localized using lectin peroxidase (Gordon et al., 1975), lectin-ferritin (Nicolson and Yanagimachi, 1974; Nicolson et al., 1977), and lectin-hemocyanin (Kinsey and Koehler, 1976) techniques (review: Nicolson, 1978). Gordon et al. (1975) found that the surfaces of washed rabbit caput spermatozoa were not labelled by the indirect concanavalin A-peroxidase technique, However, using ferritin-conjugated concanavalin A, Nicolson et al. (1977) were able to demonstrate that the surfaces of rabbit caput sperm contain large numbers of accessible concanavalin A-binding oligosaccharides. Labelling unfixed, washed spermatozoa from caput epididymidis with ferritin-*Ricinus communis* agglutinin at 25°C resulted in a dense uniform ferritin-lectin localization in the acrosome region and patchy labelling in the postacrosomal region of rabbit spermatozoa (Fig. 2). The presence of a patchy distribution of lectin receptors in the postacrosomal region of unfixed rabbit spermatozoa labelled at 25°C is probably due to lectin-induced redistribution and perhaps to some ligand-induced receptor shedding (Nicolson and Yanagimachi, 1974). In contrast with these results, unfixed caput epididymal rabbit spermatozoa labelled at 0°C or labelled after formaldehyde fixation at 25°C were uniformly labelled with ferritin-lectin conjugates (Nicolson et al., 1977). Unfixed spermatozoa isolated from rabbit caput epididymidis, cauda epididymidis, and ejaculate were compared after labelling with ferritin-conjugated *Ricinus communis* agglutinin, and distinct differences in ferritin-lectin binding and distribution were found. Specifically, head regions of caput epididymal spermatozoa bound relatively more ferritin-lectin than those of cauda epididymal or ejaculated spermatozoa (cf. Fig. 2 and 3).

Differences were also found on the tail regions of unfixed rabbit spermatozoa during epididymal passage. On caput and cauda epididymal spermatozoa both middle piece and principal piece regions were almost equally labelled with ferritin-conjugated *Ricinus communis* agglutinin, whereas in ejaculated spermatozoa the middle piece region was much more densely labelled than the principal piece region (Nicolson et al., 1977). Comparisons of spermatozoa from caput epididymidis, cauda epididymidis, and ejaculate have shown that the binding of ferritin-*Ricinus communis* agglutinin was most prominent in caput epididymal spermatozoa and least prominent in ejaculated spermatozoa, although the differences were not as dra-

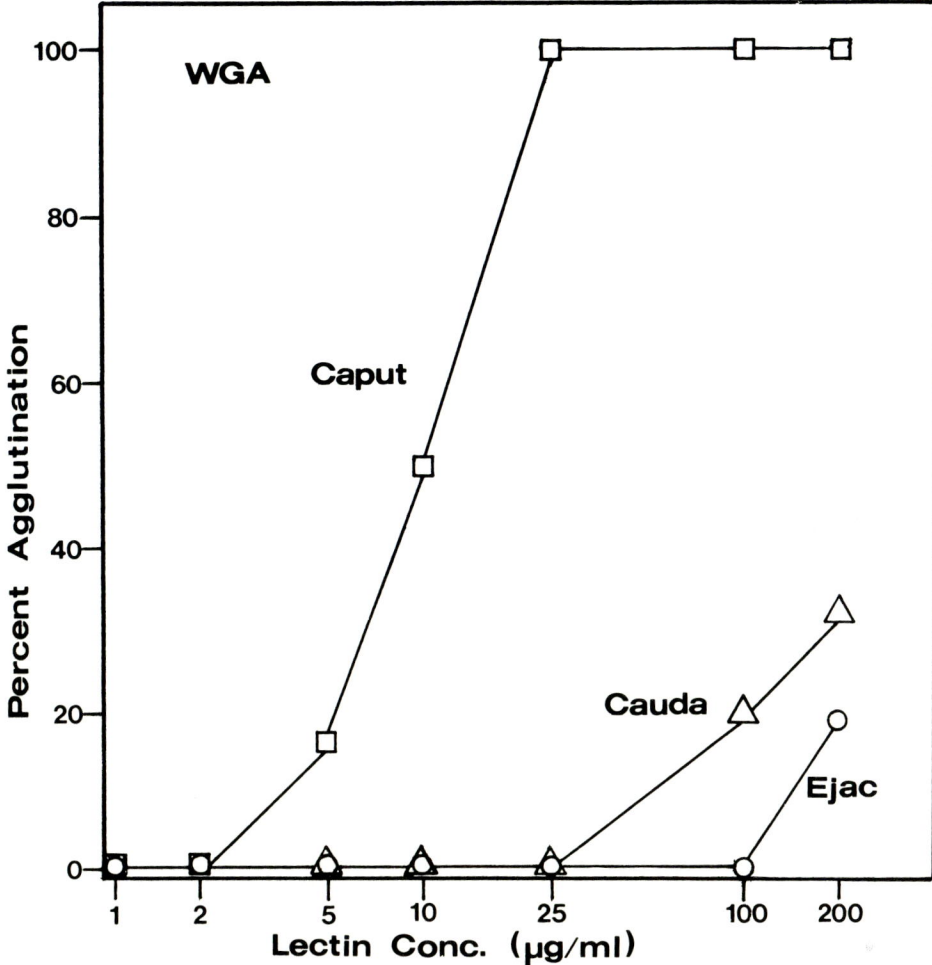

Figure 1. Agglutination by wheat germ agglutinin (WGA) of caput epididymal (□), cauda epididymal (△), and ejaculated (○) rabbit spermatozoa. For details see Nicolson et al., (1977).

matic as those seen in the head regions (Nicolson et al., 1977).

Similar results were found with ferritin-wheat germ agglutinin labelling of rabbit spermatozoa. Ferritin-wheat germ agglutinin bound densely to the acrosomal and postacrosomal regions of caput epididymal spermatozoa. However, labelling of cauda epididymal spermatozoa was quite sparse except for the apical area of the acrosomal region. Ejaculated spermatozoa bound only a few molecules of ferritin-wheat germ agglutinin (Nicolson et al., 1977).

In contrast to *Ricinus communis* and wheat germ agglutinins, ferritin-concanavalin-A conjugates bound well to all head and tail regions of the caput, cauda, and ejaculated spermatozoa, in disagreement with Gordon et al. (1975). The authors' results indicate that concanavalin-A receptors are not drastically altered during epididymal maturation or after ejaculation of rabbit spermatozoa.

The apparent decrease in lectin receptors for *Ricinus communis* and wheat germ agglutinins during epididymal passage and after ejaculation of rabbit spermatozoa could be due to a variety of cell surface changes. For example: (a) degradation of sperm surface glycoproteins by proteases or alterations in oligosaccharides by glycosidases; (b) absorption of coating substances that mask available lectin receptors at the surface; and (c) completion of oligosaccharide chains by glycosyltransferases resulting in an alteration of the lectin-binding sites (for instance, addition of sialic acid to terminal galactose residues via a sialotransferase would be expected to block binding of *Ricinus communis* agglutinin [Nicolson, 1973]). It is interesting that the increased binding of CIH to low pK_a anionic sites on sperm surfaces (Bedford et al., 1972; Yanagimachi et al., 1972) suggests that residues such as sialic acid or its derivatives might be added to terminal D-galactose residues by glycosyltransferases present in epididymal

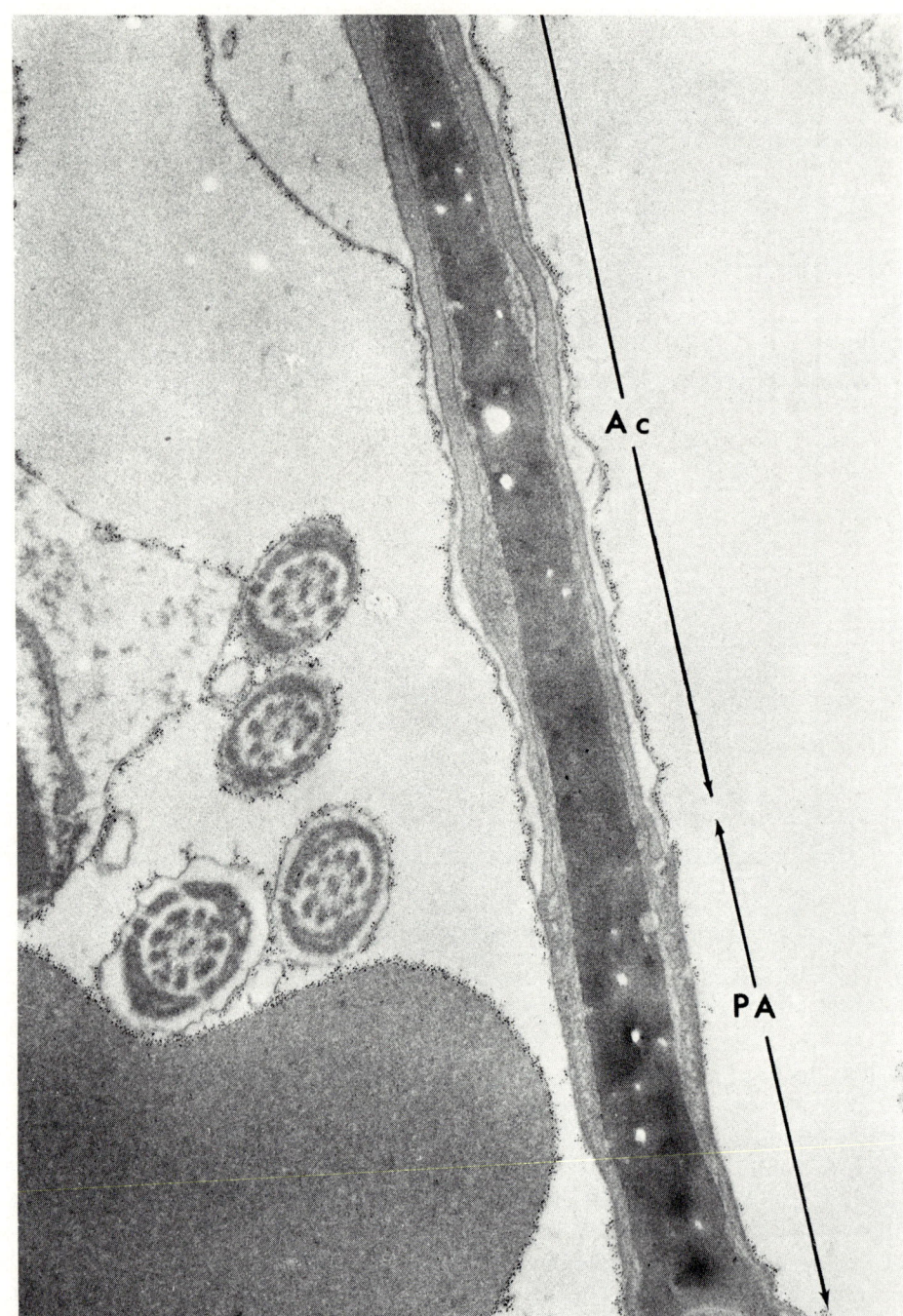

Figure 2. Unfixed, washed rabbit spermatozoon isolated from caput epididymidis and labelled with ferritin-conjugated *Ricinus communis* agglutinin. Ac, acrosomal region; PA, postacrosomal region. X35,500

secretions. Fouquet (1972) found that epididymal secretions in the hamster contain high concentrations of sialic acid plus two unidentified sialic acid derivatives. If these derivatives are nucleotide sugars, they might serve as donors in glycosyltransferase reactions (Shur and Roth, 1975).

SURFACE PROTEINS AND EPIDIDYMAL MATURATION

The surface proteins of mammalian spermatozoa have been identified by surface labelling techniques. Differences in the exposure or display of rat spermatozoa surface proteins during epididymal maturation have

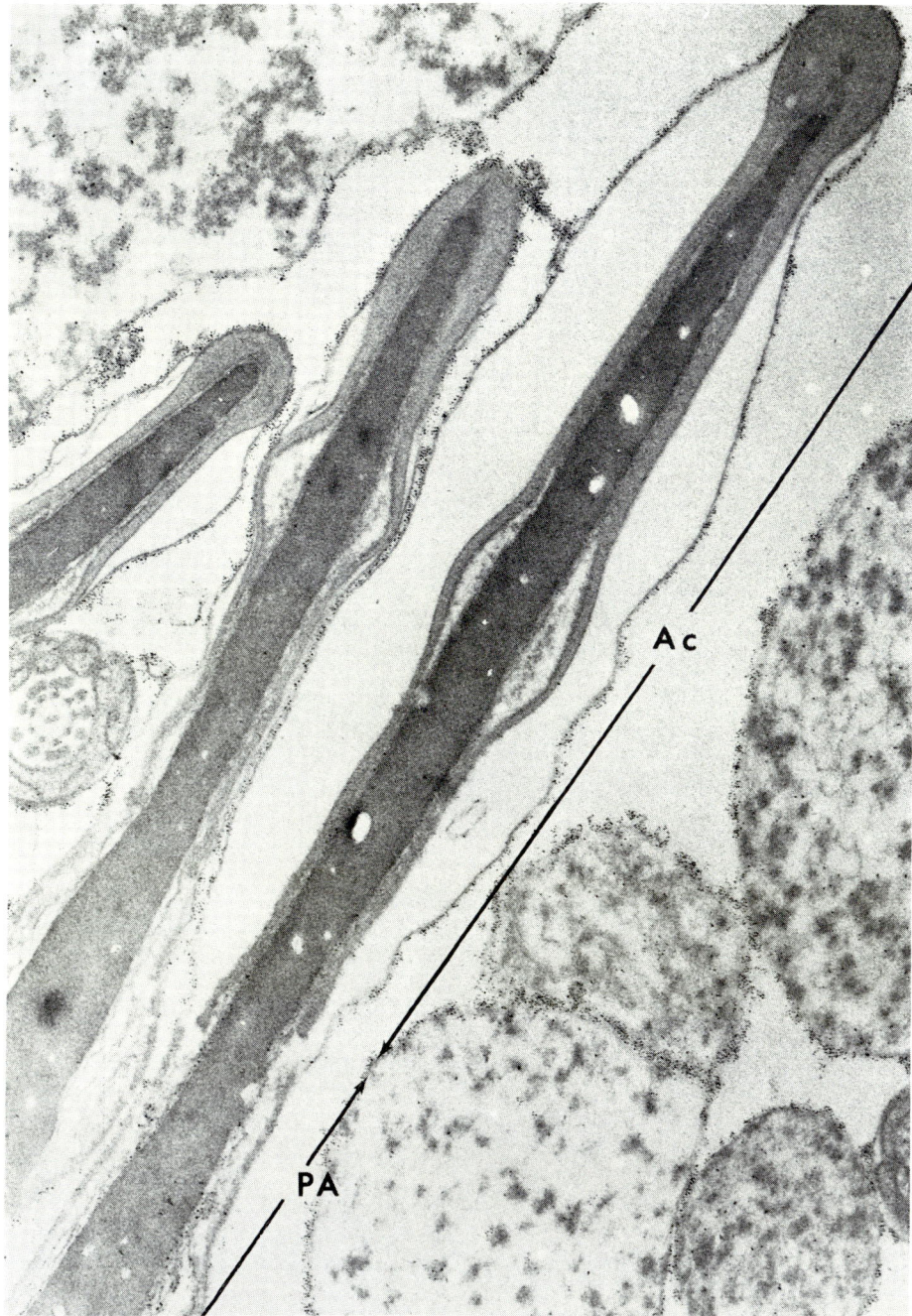

Figure 3. Unfixed, washed rabbit spermatozoon isolated from ejaculate and labelled with ferritin-conjugated *Ricinus communis* agglutinin. Ac, acrosomal region; PA, postacrosomal region. X35,500

been obtained using surface labelling with galactose oxidase or metaperiodate followed by ^{3}H borohydride reduction (Olson and Hamilton, 1978). Galactose oxidase modifies terminal galactosyl or N-acetyl-galactosaminyl residues on glycoproteins and sodium metaperiodate alters sialic acid residues on sialoglycoproteins. Aldehydes that form by these procedures can be reduced with ^{3}H-borohydride resulting in the incorporation of tritium into surface glycoproteins. When Olson and Hamilton (1978) isolated rat spermatozoa membranes and examined total protein compositions by sodium dodecylsulfate polyacrylamide gel electrophoresis, they found little differences in the Coomassie blue-stained protein bands. However, when radioactivity was determined on the gels, they found that galactose oxidase-^{3}H-borohydride or metaperiodate-^{3}H-

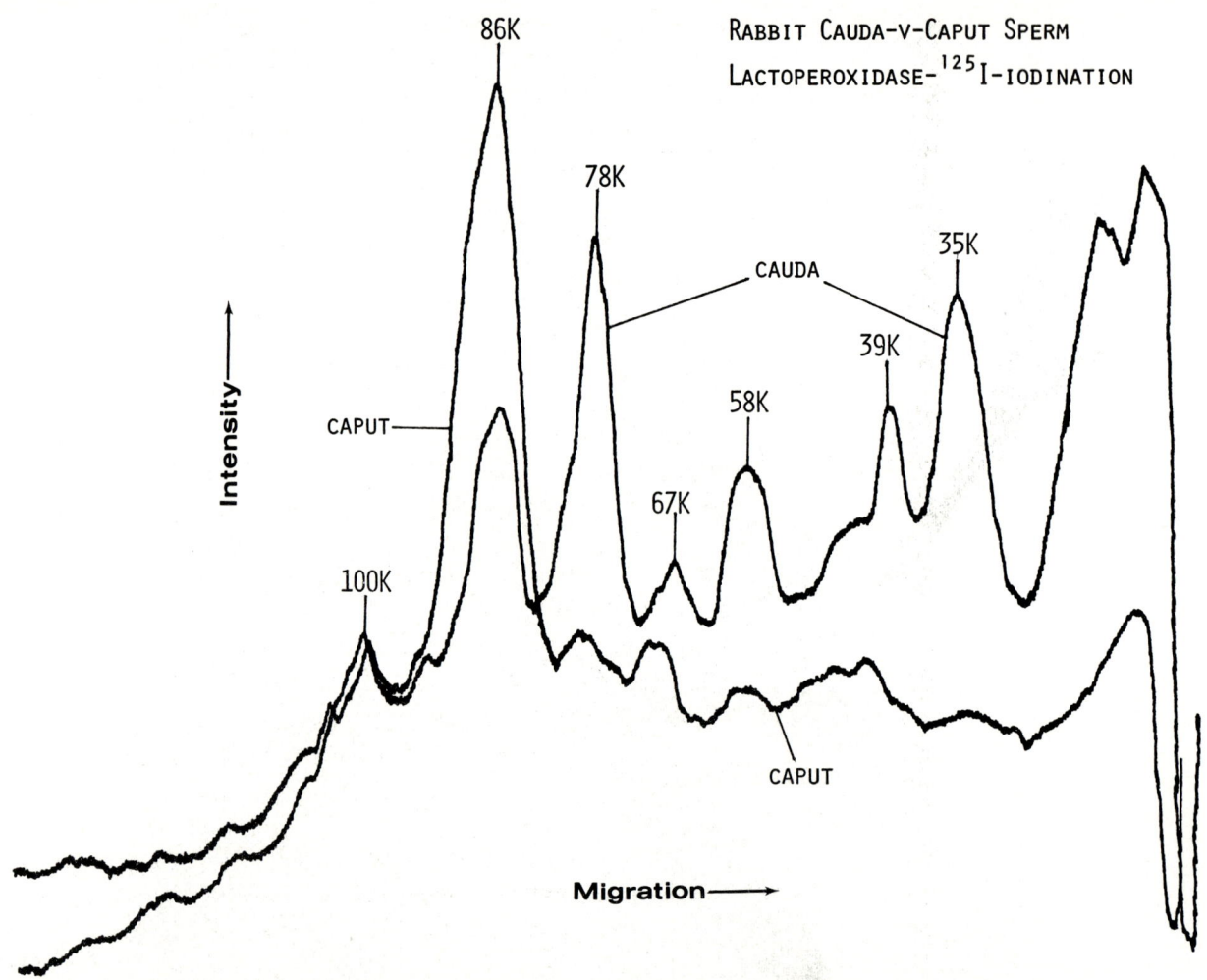

Figure 4. Lactoperoxidase-catalyzed ^{125}I-iodination of rabbit caput epididymidal spermatozoa. Radio-labelled spermatozoa were washed and dissolved in sodium dodecylsulfate (SDS) and then electrophoresed on a 7.5% polyacrylamide gel slab in buffered SDS containing 2-mercaptoethanol. Electrophoresis was from left to right, and the results are presented as densitometer tracings made from autoradiograms of the dried gels. For details on the techniques see Robbins et al. (1977).

borohydride reactions resulted in specific labelling of an approximate 37,000 M_r sialoglycoprotein on cauda but not caput epididymidal spermatozoa. Labelling caput epididymidal spermatozoa with galactose oxidase-^{3}H-borohydride followed by membrane solubilization in Triton X-100, affinity chromatography on immobilized *Ricinus communis* agglutinin and specific elution by D-galactose yielded only a 37,000 M_r galactoprotein, indicating that this was the major galactoprotein bound on the rat caput epididymidal spermatozoa surface.

Somewhat similar results have been found using lactoperoxidase-catalyzed ^{125}I-iodination techniques and rabbit spermatozoa (Nicolson et al., 1979). Lactoperoxidase-catalyzed iodination results in the introduction of ^{125}I into the exposed tyrosine residues in proteins and glycoproteins of rabbit caput and cauda epididymidal spermatozoa (Fig. 4). Using these techniques it was possible to identify an approximate 35,000 M_r protein component on the surface of rabbit cauda but not caput epididymidal spermatozoa. However, it was also possible to identify components of approximately 58,000 and 39,000 and some lower molecular weight proteins labelled more heavily on the cauda epididymidal spermatozoa. Since these components are probably glycoproteins that can migrate anomalously in sodium dodecyl sulfate polyacrylamide gel electrophoresis (Segrest et al., 1971), these molecular weights may not be accurate. The exact locations of the iodinated surface proteins on caput and cauda epididymidal spermatozoa are unknown, but the modifications described above may occur on spermatozoa head glycoproteins involved in sperm capacitation and egg recognition.

Future approaches on spermatozoa membrane changes associated with epididymidal maturation will undoubtedly focus on the role of specific surface proteins and glycoproteins in this process. It is now feasible to consider the bulk isolation and purification of most, if not all, of the sperm surface glycoproteins using newly developed techniques for lectin immobilization and affinity chromatography in buffered detergent solutions (Lotan et al., 1977). Specific antibodies made against these components should be useful in identifying their location, exposure, and mobility on spermatozoa during epididymidal passage. In addition, the functional roles of these components in the subsequent steps of capacitation and fertilization could be probed by the use of antibodies or their Fab fragments directed against specific spermatozoa head proteins and glycoproteins.

REFERENCES

Baker, L.D.S.; Amann, R.P.: Epididymal Physiology. I. Specificity of Antisera against Bull Spermatozoa and Reproductive Fluid. J Reprod Fertil 22(1970)441-452

Bedford, J.M.: Morphological Changes in Rabbit Spermatozoa during Passage through the Epididymis. J Reprod Fertil 5(1963)169-177

Bedford, J.M.: Changes in the Fine Structure of Rabbit Sperm Head during Passage through the Epididymis. J Anat 99(1965)891-906

Bedford, J.M.: Development of the Fertilizing Ability of Spermatozoa in the Epididymis of the Rabbit. J Exp Zool 163(1966)319-329

Bedford, J.M.: Maturation, Transport, and Fate of Spermatozoa in the Epididymis. In: Handbook of Physiology, Vol. 5, sect. 7, pp. 303-317, ed. by D.W. Hamilton and R.O. Greep. Williams and Wilkins Co., 1975

Bedford, J.M.; Calvin, H.; Cooper, G.W.: The Maturation of Spermatozoa in the Human Epididymis. J Reprod Fertil 18(1973)199-213

Bedford, J.M.; Cooper, G.W.: Membrane Fusion Events in the Fertilization of Vertebrate Eggs. In: Membrane Fusion, Vol. 5 of Cell Surface Reviews, pp. 65-125, ed. by G. Poste and G.L. Nicolson. North-Holland Publishing Co., New York, 1978

Bedford, J.M.; Cooper, G.W.; Calvin, H.I.: Postmeiotic Changes in the Nucleus and Membranes of Mammalian Spermatozoa. In: The Genetics of the Spermatozoa, pp. 69-89, ed. by R.A. Beatty and S. Glueckson-Waelsch. Bogtrykeriet Forum, Copenhagen, Denmark, 1972

Bedford, J.M.; Nicander, L.: Ultrastructural Changes in the Acrosome and Sperm Membranes during Maturation of Spermatozoa in the Testis and Epididymis of the Rabbit and Monkey. J Anat 108(1971)527-543

Boettcher, G.: Blood Group Antigens in Seminal Plasma, and the Nature of Human Sperm-coating Antigen. In: Immunology and Reproduction, pp. 148-167, ed. by R.G. Edwards. International Planned Parenthood Federation, 1969.

Branton, C.; Salisbury, G.W.: Morphology of Spermatozoa from Different Levels of the Reproductive Tract of the Bull. J Anim Sci 6(1947)154-160

Brochert, M.; Debatene, D.: Diminution de la Perméabilité a l'Eosine de la Capsule Lipoidique de la Tête des Spermatozoides de Ruminants Domestiques après de l'Ejaculation. C R Soc Biol (Paris) 147(1953)20-25

Chulavatnatol, M.; Yindepit, S.: Changes in Surface ATPase of Rat Spermatozoa in Transit from the Caput to the Cauda Epididymis. J Reprod Fertil 48(1976)91-97

Edwards, R.G.; Ferguson, L.C.; Combs, R.R.A.: Blood Group Antigens on Human Spermatozoa. J Reprod Fertil 7(1964)153-161

Fawcett, D.W.; Phillips, D.H.: Observations on the Release of Spermatozoa and on Changes in the Head during Passage through the Epididymis. J Reprod Fertil Suppl 6(1969)405-418

Flechon, J.E.: Modifications Ultrastructurals et Cytochimiques des Spermatozoides de Lapin au Cours du Transit Epididymaire. INSERM (Inst Natl Santé Rech Med) Colloq 26(1973)115-140

Fouquet, J.P.: Free Sialic Acids in the Seminal Vesicle Secretion of the Golden Hamster. J Reprod Fertil 28(1972)273-275

Glover, T.D.: The Reaction of Rabbit Spermatozoa to Nigrosin Eosin following Ligation of the Epididymis. Int J Fertil 7(1962)1-9

Gordon, M.; Dandekar, P.V.; Bartoszewicz, W.: The Surface Coat of Epididymal, Ejaculated and Capacitated Sperm. J Ultrastruct Res 50(1975)199-207

Hekman, S.; Rümke, P.: The Antigens of Human Seminal Plasma: With Special Reference to Lactoferrin as a Spermatozoa-coating Antigen. Fertil Steril 20(1969)312-323

Hunter, A.G.; Hafs, H.D.: Antigenicity and Cross-reactions of Bovine Spermatozoa. J Reprod Fertil 7(1964)357-365

Hunter, R.H.F.: Capacitation in the Gold Hamster with Special Reference to the Influence of the Uterine Environment. J Reprod Fertil 20(1969)223-237

Johnson, W.L.; Hunter, A.G.: Seminal Antigens: Their Alteration in the Genital Tract of Female Rabbits and during Partial in Vitro Capacitation with β-Amylase and β-Glucuronidase. Biol Reprod 7(1972)332-340

Killian, G.J.; Amann, R.P.: Immunophoretic Characterization of Fluid and Sperm Entering and Leaving the Bovine Epididymis. Biol Reprod 9(1973)489-499

Kinsey, W.H.; Koehler, J.K.: Fine Structural Localization of Concanavalin A Binding Sites on Hamster Spermatozoa. J Supramol Struct 5(1976)185-198

Lavon, U.; Volcani, R.; Davon, D.: The Lipid Content of Bovine Spermatozoa during Maturation and Aging. J Reprod Fertil 23(1970)215-222

Lotan, R.; Beattie, G.; Hubbell, W.; Nicolson, G.L.: Activities of Lectins and Their Immobilized Derivatives in Detergent Solutions. Implications on the Use of Lectin Affinity Chromatography for the Purification of Membrane Glycoproteins. Biochemistry 16(1977)1787-1794

Nicander, L.: On the Regional Histology and Cytochemistry of the Ductus Epididymis in the Rabbit. Acta Morphol Neerl Scand 1(1957)99-118

Nicolson, G.L.: Neuraminidase "Unmasking" and the Failure of Trypsin to "Unmask" β-D-Galactose-like Sites on Erythrocyte, Lymphoma and Normal and SV40-transformed 3T3 Fibroblast Cell Membranes. J Natl Cancer Inst 50(1973)1443-1451

Nicolson, G.L.: The Interactions of Lectins with Animal Cell Surfaces. Int Rev Cytol 39(1974)89-190

Nicolson, G.L.: Ultrastructural Localization of Lectin Receptors. In: Advanced Techniques in Biological Electron Microscopy, pp. 1-38, ed. by J.K. Koehler. Springer-Verlag, New York, 1978

Nicolson, G.L.; Brodginski, A.B.; Beattie, G.; Yanagimachi, R.: Cell Surface Changes in the Proteins of Rabbit Spermatozoa during Epididymal Passage. Gamete Res. (in press) (1979)

Nicolson, G.L.; Usui, N.; Yanagimachi, R.; Yanagimachi, H.; Smith, J.R.: Lectin-binding Sites on the Plasma Membranes of Rabbit Spermatozoa. Changes in Surface Receptors during Epididymal Maturation and after Ejaculation. J Cell Biol 74(1977)950-962

Nicolson, G.L.; Yanagimachi, R.: Terminal Saccharides on Sperm Plasma Membranes: Identification by Specific Agglutinins. Science 177(1972)276-279

Nicolson, G.L.; Yanagimachi, R.: Mobility and the Restriction of Mobility of Plasma Membrane Lectin-binding Components. Science 184(1974)1294-1296

Olson, G.E.; Hamilton, D.W.: Morphological Changes in the Midpiece of Wooly Opossom Spermatozoa during Epididymal Transit. Anat Rec 186(1976)387-404

Olson, G.E.; Hamilton, D.W.: Characterization of the Surface Glycoproteins of Rat Spermatozoa. Biol Reprod 19(1978)26-35

Orgebin-Crist, M-C.: Maturation of Spermatozoa in the Rabbit Epididymis: Fertilizing Ability and Embryonic Mortality in Does Inseminated with Epididymal Spermatozoa. Ann Biol Anim Biochim Biophys 7(1967)373-389

Ortavant, R.: Existence d'une Phase Critique dans la Maturation Epididymaive des Spermatozoides de Bélier et de Taureau. C R Soc Biol (Paris) 147(1953)1552-1556

Reyes, A.; Mercado, E.; Goicoechea, G.; Rosado, A.: Participation of Membrane Sulfhydryl Groups in the Epididymal Maturation of Human and Rabbit Spermatozoa. Fertil Steril 27(1976)1452-1458

Robbins, J.C.; Hyman, R.; Stallings, V.; Nicolson, G.L.: Cell Surface Changes in a *Ricinus communis* Toxin (Ricin)-Resistant Variant of a Murine Lymphoma. J Natl Cancer Inst 58(1977)1027-1033

Segrest, J.P.; Jackson, R.L.; Andrews, E.P.; Marchesi, V.T.: Human Erythrocyte Membrane Glycoprotein: A Re-evaluation of the Molecular Weight as Determined by SDS-Polyacrylamide Gel Electrophoresis. Biochem Biophys Res Commun 44(1971)390-395

Shur, B.D.; Roth, S.: Cell Surface Glycosyltransferases. Biochim Biophys Acta 415(1975)473-512

Uhlenbruck, G.; Herrmann, W.P.: Agglutination of Normal, Coated and Enzyme-treated Human Spermatozoa with Heterophile Agglutinins. Vox Sang 23(1972)444-451

Weil, A.J.: The Spermatozoa-coating Antigen (SCA) of the Seminal Vesicle. Ann NY Acad Sci 124(1965)267-269

Weil, A.J.: Antigens of the Seminal Plasma. J Reprod Fertil Suppl 2(1967)25-34

Yanagimachi, R.; Noda, Y.D.; Fujimoto, M.; Nicolson, G.L.: The Distribution of Negative Surface Charges on Mammalian Spermatozoa. Am J Anat 135(1972)497-520

CHANGES IN SPERM SURFACE PROPERTIES CORRELATED WITH CAPACITATION

M.G. O'Rand

Department of Anatomy, College of Medicine, University of Florida, Gainesville, Florida 32610 USA

Capacitation, an endogenous, physiological change of the spermatozoon necessary for mammalian fertilization (Bedford, 1972; Austin, 1975), has remained a poorly understood phenomenon since its discovery in 1951 (Austin, 1951; Chang, 1951). The question of mechanism remains unanswered and this is perhaps explained by the underlying assumption that capacitation is a single, discrete event like the activation of an enzyme or the removal of a surface protein. More probably it is not one step but a series of steps, only the sum of which is equal to capacitation. With recent advances in membrane biology, capacitation can now be approached as a membrane phenomenon at the molecular level. This chapter deals with capacitation as a sperm surface phenomenon and proposes a model that can be tested and used, it is hoped, to inspire further experimentation.

NONMAMMALIAN CAPACITATION

Almost all animal phyla have some representatives that possess internal fertilization. However, as Lillie pointed out (1919), there are too few gametes available from these organisms and they do not lend themselves to experimental manipulation and easy observation. As a result, animals with internal fertilization, other than mammals, have been neglected from the viewpoint of gamete interaction and capacitation.

Three organisms (Table 1) have been found to show capacitation-like interaction; the coelenterate *Campanularia* (O'Rand, 1972), the housefly *Musca* (Leopold and Degrugillier, 1973), and the frog *Rana* (Shivers and James, 1970). In each of these cases the female environment (cells or their extracellular product) is in some way necessary for fertilization. This is perhaps exemplified by *Campanularia,* the best studied example and the one most similar to mammalian capacitation.

In *Campanularia* a specific interaction must occur between the surface of the female epithelial cells lining the female gonangium funnel (gonoduct) and the surface of the spermatozoon (O'Rand, 1972, 1974). This interaction is specific for the homologous spermatozoon and allows release of acrosome-like vesicles from the sperm's head (O'Rand and Miller, 1974).

The *Campanularia* sperm-female interaction as well as the interactions observed in *Musca* and *Rana* can best be characterized as primitive mechanisms (in an evolutionary sense) to allow the basic parameters of fertilization to operate at the proper time and place. Thus, this interaction allows the three basic features of the fertilization reaction to occur, namely sperm-egg recognition specificity, irreversibility, and activation (Lillie, 1919). The point is that in a number of different species and particularly in those with internal fertilization there is a mechanism for conferring upon the sperm the ability to penetrate and fuse with the egg at the proper time and place.

Seen in this light, mammalian capacitation fits into a better evolutionary perspective. The time requirements and specific environmental conditions (*e.g.,* ionic strength, hormonal status of the female, etc.) that exist in mammals are, in a hierarchial sense, imposed upon the basic parameters of fertilization. There does not seem to be any exacting species-specificity to mammalian capacitation (Bedford, 1972) and this might be expected since specificity is a property of the fertilization reaction itself. However, a final species-specific step during capacitation, affecting the sperm's postacrosomal region and operating at the level of sperm-egg fusion cannot be ruled out. Consequently, in both mammalian and nonmammalian systems the proper end point of capacitation would seem to be not only the acrosome reaction but necessarily the sperm's ability to fertilize the egg.

SURFACE CHANGES DURING MAMMALIAN CAPACITATION

Important observations of sperm surface changes during capacitation in mammals have been made. This section describes a number of these but is not exhaustive. The reader is referred to several recent reviews for more details (Austin, 1975; Barros, 1974; Bedford, 1972; Chang and Hunter, 1975).

This work was supported by the United States Public Health Service, National Institutes of Health Grant HD-10618. The author gratefully acknowledges P. Sandow for her excellent assistance during all phases of this study, Dr. L. Romrell for reading the manuscript, and Drs. L. Eng and G. Oliphant for providing a copy of their unpublished manuscript.

© 1979 Urban & Schwarzenberg, Inc. Baltimore-Munich *The Spermatozoon,* edited by D.W. Fawcett and J.M. Bedford

Table 1. Capacitation and Capacitation-like Interaction in the Animal Kingdom

Phyla	Capacitation-like Interaction	
	Genus Species	Responsible Structure
Colenterata	*Campanularia flexuosa*	female epithelial-cell surface (gonoduct)
Insecta	*Musca domestica*	female accessory gland secretions
Amphibia	*Rana pipiens*	egg jelly
	Capacitation	
Mammalia	Various species	uterine and/or oviduct environment

As demonstrated by Chang (1957), capacitated sperm can be decapacitated by the supernatant from centrifuged semen and then recapacitated. This discovery led to the search for decapacitation factors (Bedford and Chang, 1962) and their chemical characterization (Williams, 1972). Decapacitation factors are present in epididymal fluid (Weinman and Williams, 1964) and seminal plasma, at least one factor having a low molecular weight (Pinsker and Williams, 1967) and another a high molecular weight (115,000) (Reyes et al., 1975; Eng and Oliphant, personal communication). Both epididymal and seminal fluid components are present on ejaculated spermatozoon surfaces (Weinman and Williams, 1964; Weil, 1967) and are removed, along with possibly other peripheral membrane components, from the sperm's surface during its sojourn in the female tract (Johnson and Hunter, 1972; Oliphant and Brackett, 1973a; Davis, 1974; Koehler, 1976). The modification or removal of surface components can be brought about by various ionic changes in the medium (Oliphant and Brackett, 1973b; Brackett and Oliphant, 1975). Additionally, follicular fluid or serum factors (Barros and Austin, 1967; Yanagimachi, 1969; Barros and Garavagno, 1970; Lui et al., 1977) evidently modify surface components since they are known to capacitate spermatozoa. Enzymes (Gwatkin et al., 1974) also may contribute to the sperm's surface alterations. However, when the critical test for capacitation is fertilization, the argument that these treatments simply accelerate capacitation cannot be completely excluded. Nevertheless, the removal and modification of surface components undoubtedly has profound consequences for the sperm's plasma membrane.

In addition to the removal of peripheral membrane components other changes have been noted. ATPase is activated (Gordon and Dandekar, 1977) and the newly capacitated sperm surface shows a decreased net negative charge (Vaidya et al., 1971; Rosado et al., 1973); however, after capacitation in the hamster, no change in the density or relative distribution of CIH particles has been observed (Yanagimachi et al., 1973). Decreases in free surface-active —SH and —NH_2 groups (Rosado et al., 1973) and modified lectin binding (Gordon et al., 1975; Talbot and Franklin, 1978) also occur. An increase in the permeability of the plasma membrane has been suggested to occur in the guinea pig as a result of capacitation (Summers et al., 1976). Finally, changes in the sperm's postacrosomal surface region may occur following capacitation or alternatively these changes may be a result of the acrosome reaction (Yanagimachi, 1977; Barros, 1974).

Whether these observed changes in mammalian capacitated spermatozoa are specific steps in the capacitation process or only secondary changes in membrane components remains to be determined. Furthermore, the variety of changes may only reflect species differences. Nevertheless, as pointed out previously (O'Rand, 1977), the relationship between an individual peripheral component and an intrinsic one is important and would seem to be an area for future research. In this connection, peripheral components of other cell types have been implicated in internal cellular changes (Yamada and Weston, 1974; Johnson and Epel, 1975).

INTRINSIC MEMBRANE CHANGES DURING CAPACITATION

Recently two lines of evidence have suggested intrinsic sperm membrane changes during capacitation, namely changes in the lateral mobility of proteins (O'Rand,

1977) and changes in intramembranous particles (Friend et al., 1977). In the plasma membrane over the acrosomal region of rabbit spermatozoa, the lateral mobility of a single sperm surface glycoprotein became restricted following incubation of the spermatozoa in utero (O'Rand, 1977). It was concluded from this study that the restricted mobility reflected a membrane fluidity change that was an intrinsic physiological change occurring during capacitation. In the plasma membrane over the acrosomal region of guinea pig spermatozoa as well as in the underlying outer acrosomal membrane, areas free of the intramembranous particles seen in freeze-fracture became apparent during capacitation (Friend et al., 1977).

Additional data on the mobility of sperm surface proteins has been obtained by utilizing rabbit anti-rabbit-sperm autoantisera. Using indirect labelling, rabbit sperm autoantibodies show a patchy distribution on ejaculated spermatozoa (Fig. 1a) and a uniform distribution on capacitated spermatozoa (Table 2; Fig. 1c, d). Ejaculated spermatozoa fixed prior to labelling also show a uniform distribution of label (Fig. 1b). There is distinct similarity in the label distribution between pre-fixed and capacitated spermatozoa (Fig. 1b, d). Control treated sperm do not label (Fig. 1e, f). Thus, the ability of intrinsic membrane autoantigens to move laterally within the plasma membrane after capacitation appears restricted.

The binding of sperm autoantibody Fab fragments to the plasma membrane over the acrosomal region has been further examined in the electron microscope by utilizing ferritin labelled goat anti-rabbit IgG antibodies. As shown in Figure 2 the label is patchy on ejaculated spermatozoa but uniform (Fig. 4) on spermatozoa fixed prior to labelling. Control treated spermatozoa do not label (Fig. 3). On capacitated spermatozoa labelled at 37°C (Fig. 5), the label which appears uniformly distributed under the fluorescence microscope appears as small patches under the electron microscope.

These small patches are approximately 8×10^4 $(Å)^2$ in contrast to the larger patches (190×10^4 $(Å)^2$) seen on ejaculated spermatozoa labelled under the same conditions. Ejaculated spermatozoa fixed prior to labelling show a patch size of approximately 10×10^4 $(Å)^2$, comparable to that seen following capacitation. Although the entire periacrosomal plasma membrane is labelled on both ejaculated (prefixed) and capacitated spermatozoa, it is not known whether the number of autoantibody plasma membrane binding sites over the acrosome changes after capacitation. Significantly, the distribution of labelled intrinsic membrane components after capacitation is seen to be different on the ultrastructural level from that seen on the light microscopic level. These observations are consistent, however, with a restricted mobility of intrinsic membrane proteins (O'Rand, 1977) and the formation of areas depleted of membrane proteins (Friend et al., 1977).

SURFACE CHANGES CORRELATED WITH CAPACITATION: A MODEL

To incorporate the changes already observed and to help in determining further experiments, a molecular model of surface changes in the periacrosomal plasma membrane is proposed (Fig. 6). In this model the plasma membrane prior to capacitation (Fig. 6A) is identified as having at least four classes of molecules involved in the surface change: 1) glycoproteins that are mobile within the plane of the membrane, 2) nonmobile glycoproteins, 3) glycolipids, and 4) peripheral membrane components.

Several observations are consistent with this precapacitation model. Antibodies to seminal plasma (class 4) will bind to the sperm surface (Oliphant and Brackett, 1973a). Antibodies to whole sperm or whole semen (all classes) will not show patching or capping because both mobile and nonmobile classes are involved (Romrell and O'Rand, 1978). Lectin binding of class 1, 3, or 4 to class 2 will not show patching (Koehler, 1976). Antibodies or lectins binding to class 1 will show some degree of patching (MGP, O'Rand, 1977; autoantigens, O'Rand, 1978). Complement-dependent antibody im-

Table 2. Indirect[1] Immunofluorescent Staining Pattern of Fab-autoantibody Labelled Rabbit Spermatozoa

	Patchy (%)	Uniform (%)	Labelled (%)
Ejaculated			
Fab-I[2]; 37°	90	10	80
Fab-I; Prefix	0	100	100
Fab-C[3]; 37°	0	0	0
Fab-C; Prefix	0	All dull yellow fluorescence	
Capacitated[4]			
Uterine			
Fab-I; 37°	0	100	64
Fab-C; 37°	0	0	0
Oviduct			
Fab-I; 37°	0	100[5]	80
Fab-C; 37°	0	0	0

[1] Fluorescein-conjugated goat (IgG) anti-rabbit IgG
[2] Fab fragment of IgG fraction of rabbit anti-rabbit-sperm serum. Incubation at 37°C or prefixed with glutaraldehyde before labelling.
[3] Fab fragment of IgG fraction of rabbit adjuvant control serum. Incubation at 37°C or prefixed with glutaraldehyde before labelling.
[4] Sperm were recovered from the uterus or oviduct 6 and 12 hours after artificial intravaginal insemination and 100 IU HCG i.v. injection.
[5] Strong postacrosomal fluorescence was observed.

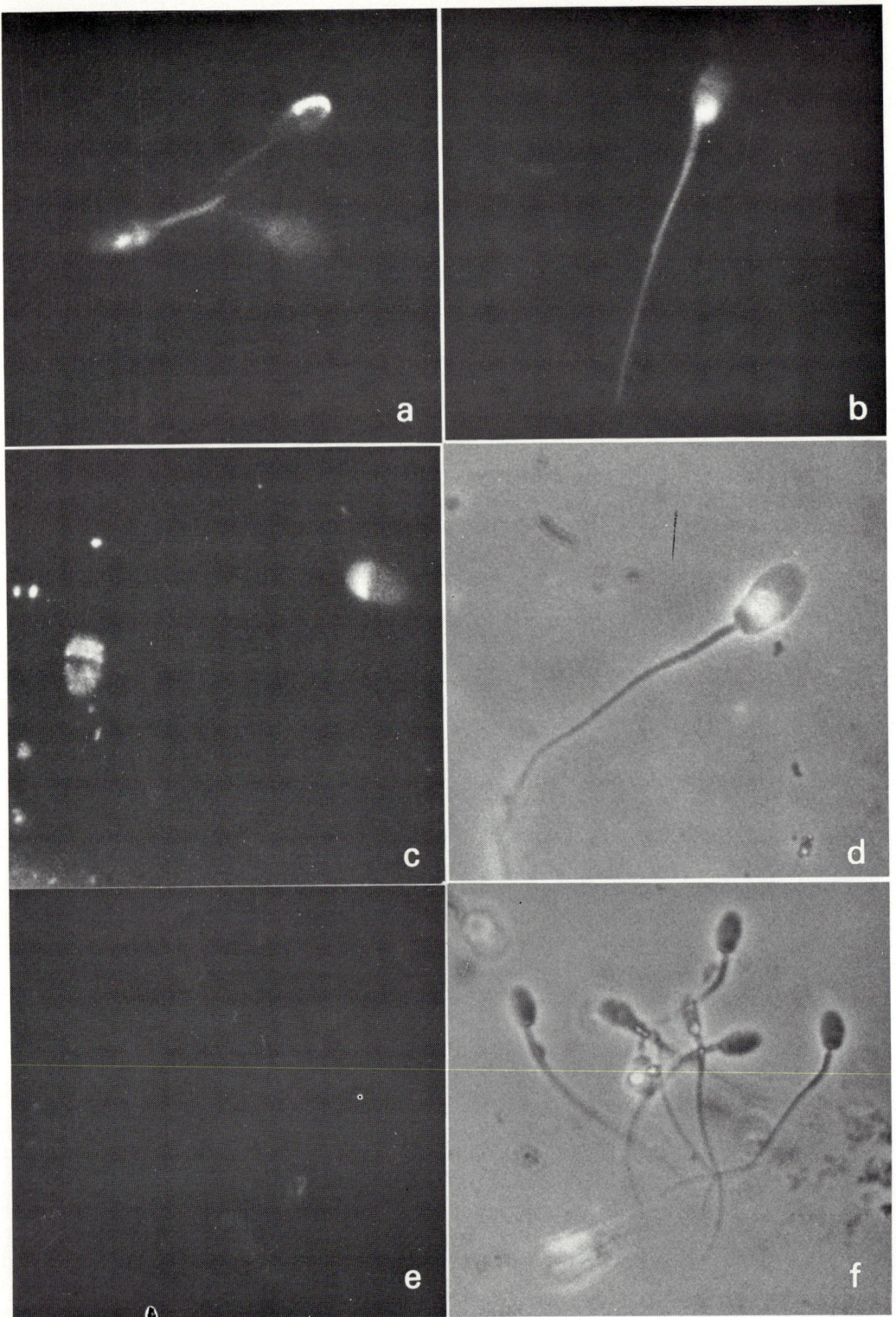

Figure 1. Rabbit spermatozoa labelled with rabbit anti-rabbit-sperm autoantibodies (Fab fragment of IgG fraction) and secondarily labelled with fluorescein-conjugated goat (IgG) anti-rabbit IgG (O'Rand, 1977). a) Live, ejaculated spermatozoa. Note fluorescent patch over the acrosome. X3100 b) Ejaculated spermatozoa fixed with glutaraldehyde prior to labelling. X2100 c) Live, capacitated spermatozoa recovered from the uterus. X2700 d) Live, capacitated spermatozoa recovered from the oviduct. X4000 The tungsten light was turned on to emphasize the bright postacrosomal fluorescence. e, f) Fluorescence and phase-contrast micrographs of live, ejaculated spermatozoa labelled with Fab fragments from adjuvant control IgG. X2100

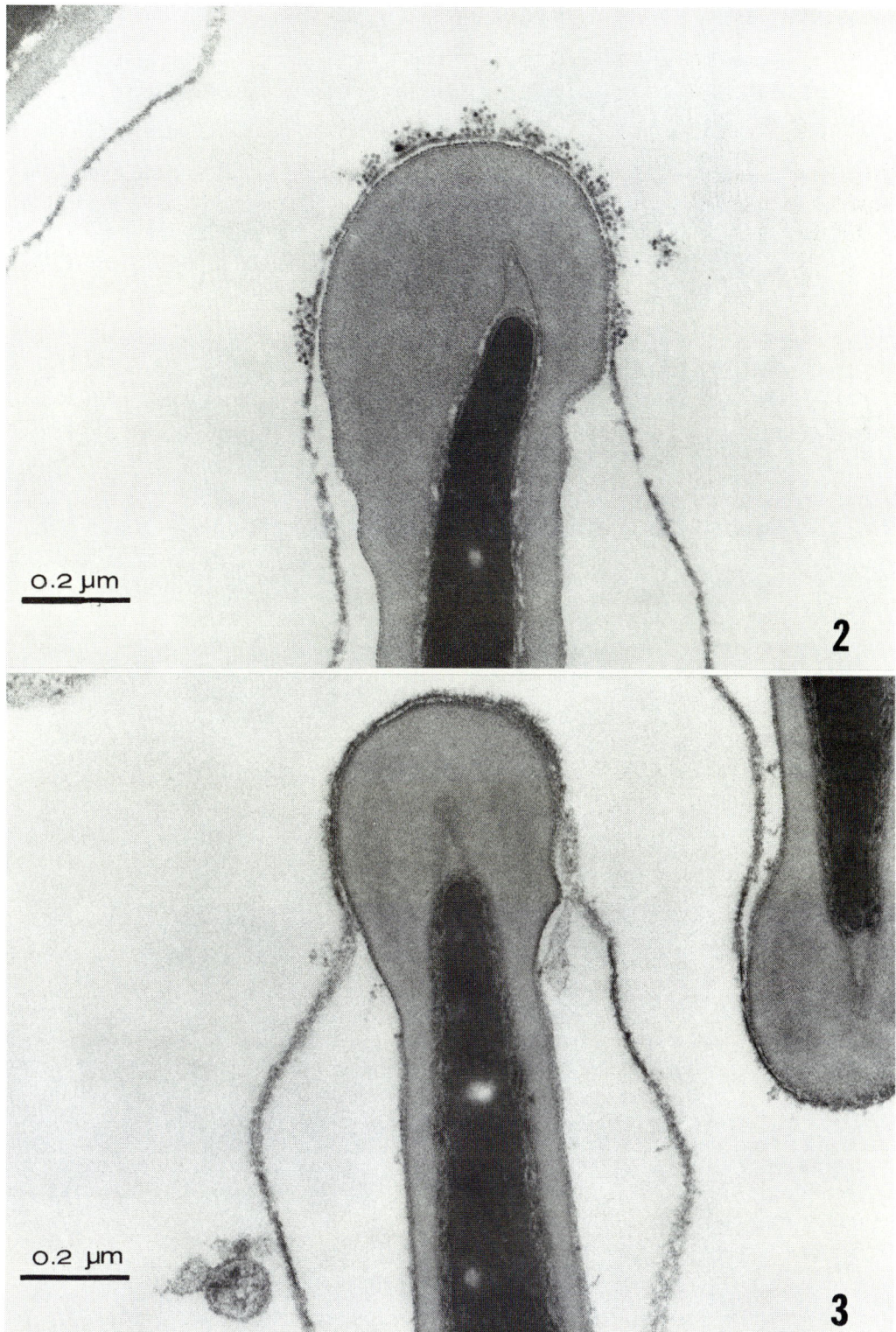

Figure 2. Ejaculated rabbit spermatozoon labelled with rabbit anti-rabbit-sperm autoantibodies (Fab fragment of IgG fraction) and secondarily labelled with ferritin-conjugated goat (IgG) anti-rabbit IgG. All labelling performed on live spermatozoa. X84,600

Figure 3. Ejaculated rabbit spermatozoon labelled with Fab fragments from rabbit adjuvant control IgG and secondarily labelled with ferritin-conjugated goat (IgG) anti-rabbit IgG. All labelling performed on live spermatozoa. X84,600

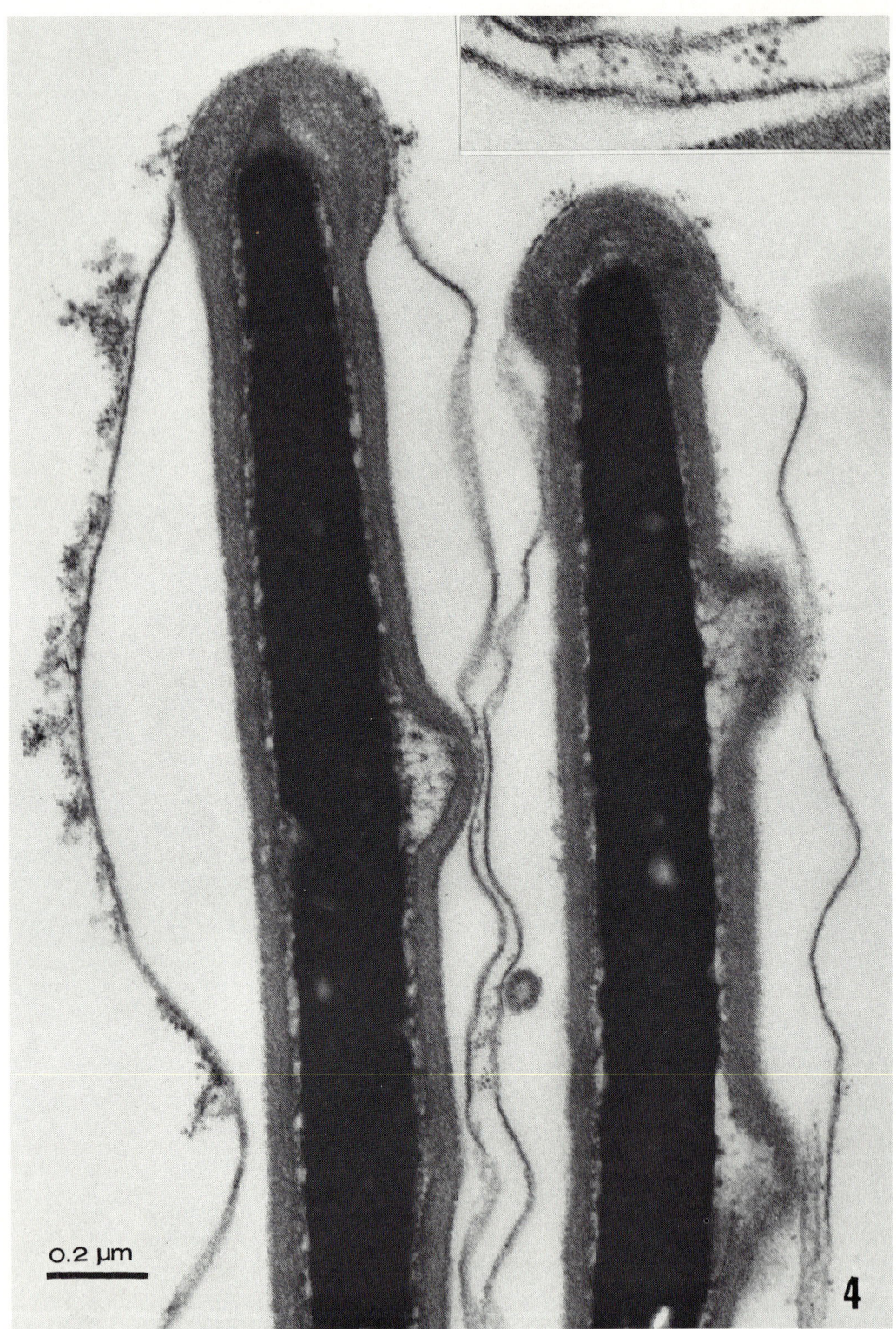

Figure 4. Ejaculated rabbit spermatozoa fixed with glutaraldehyde prior to labelling. Labelling conditions were identical to those in Figure 2. X77,800
Insert: Higher magnification of ferritin-labelled antibodies on the external side of the plasma membrane. X181,300

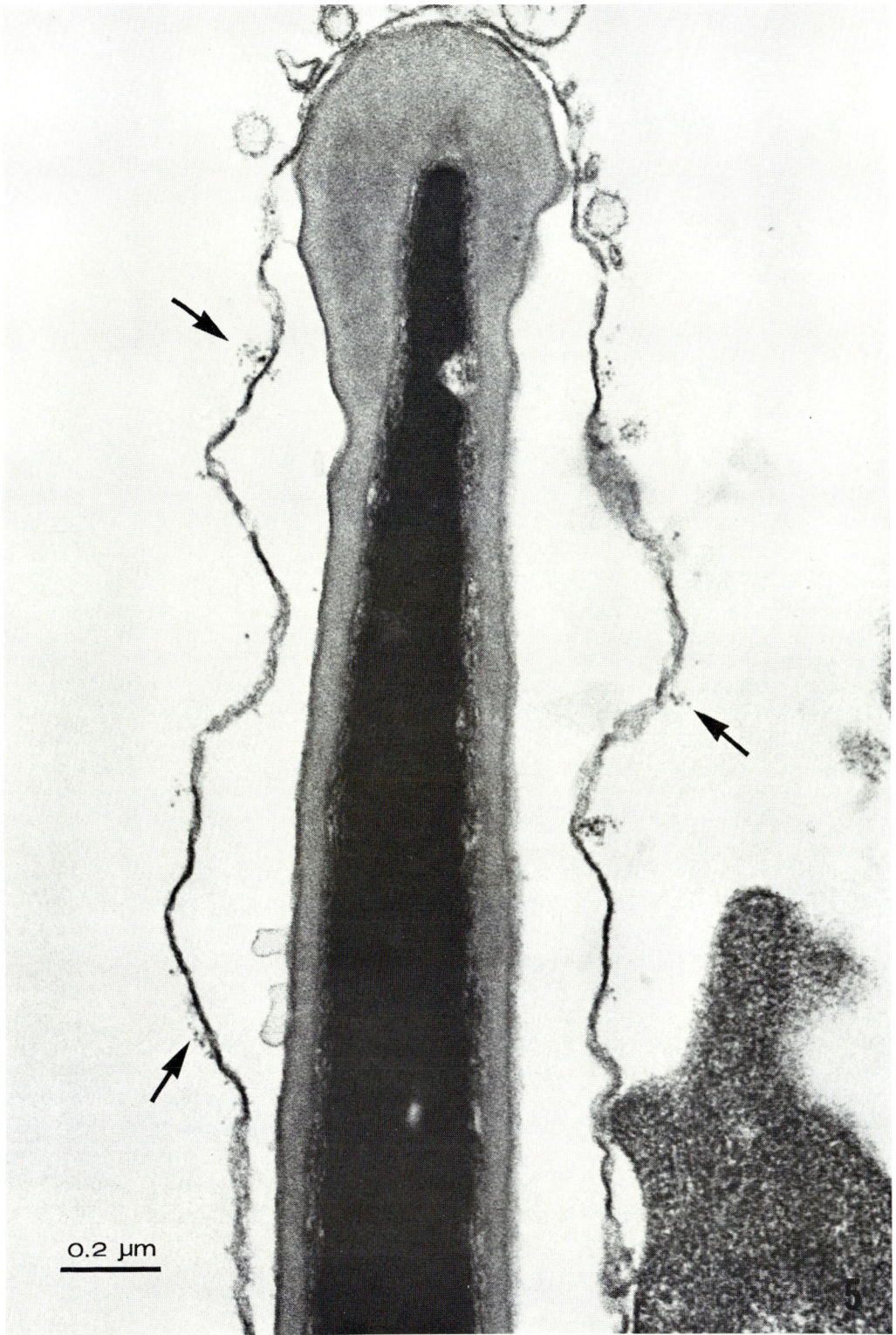

Figure 5. Capacitated rabbit spermatozoon recovered from the uterus 7 h after artificial intravaginal insemination and injection of HCG (75 IU, i.v.). Arrows indicate ferritin label. X77,000 human chorionic gonadotropin

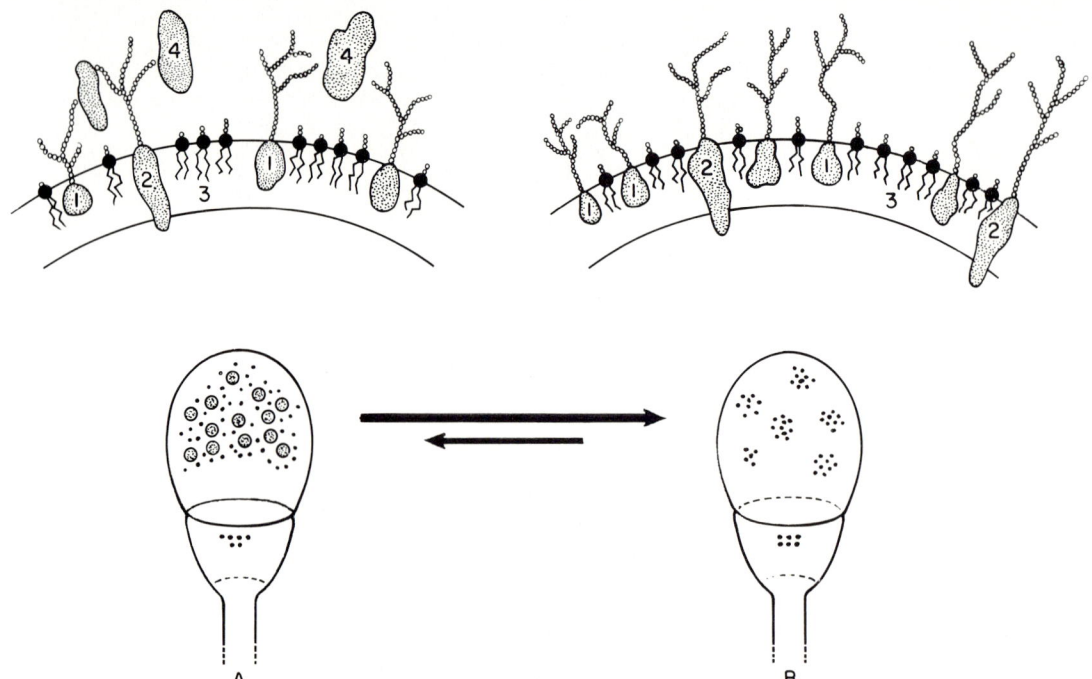

Figure 6. A model for the surface changes in the periacrosomal plasma membrane associated with capacitation. A) Prior to capacitation. B) After capacitation. Four classes of molecules are shown: 1) mobile glycoproteins, 2) nonmobile glycoproteins, 3) glycolipids, and 4) peripheral components. The lower sketches show the surface pattern expected for intrinsic mobile glycoproteins (class 1) in association with peripheral components (class 4) before capacitation (A) and without peripheral components after capacitation (B). Sperm outlines are not drawn to scale.

mobilization of ejaculated spermatozoa depends upon the relationship between the intrinsic surface antigen and class 4 (O'Rand and Metz, 1976).

After capacitation the relationship between the four classes of molecules changes (Fig. 6B). Peripheral components have been modified or removed (e.g., decapacitation factor, Eng and Oliphant, personal communication) and the mobile and nonmobile classes (1 and 2) have re-associated. This is consistent with several observations. Antiserum to seminal plasma (class 4) and whole semen (all classes) show decreased binding as does concanavalin A (Brackett and Oliphant, 1975; Koehler, 1976; Gordon et al., 1974). Immobilization becomes more rapid and is not blocked by class 4 (O'Rand and Metz, 1976). Smaller patches of antigen are visualized using electron microscopy (Fig. 5) with antibodies to class 1 because the receptors have a restricted mobility (O'Rand, 1977).

The reasons for the restricted mobility of membrane components after capacitation are not clear, although a segregation of membrane lipids has been suggested (O'Rand, 1977). Additionally, some intrinsic components could be removed from the plasma membrane. Whatever the reason, the model shows that there should be regions of membrane glycoproteins and separate domains relatively free of glycoproteins. Thus protein-poor, high fluidity areas ready for membrane fusion (Friend et al., 1977) may coexist with protein-rich areas of decreased fluidity (O'Rand, 1977) in a patchwork quilt-like topography. This would be consistent with the pattern of membrane fusion seen during the acrosome reaction (Franklin et al., 1970).

Changes in the postacrosomal region have been observed (Friend et al., 1977; Fig. 1a, d). However, they have not been studied in as much detail. Presumably, the postacrosomal surface changes during capacitation in preparation for sperm-egg fusion. But these postacrosomal changes may occur as a result of the acrosome reaction (Barros and Berrios, 1977; Friend et al., 1977) and be a final step in the capacitation process. The mixing of intrinsic inner acrosomal membrane components with those of the postacrosomal plasma membrane could lead to the formation of a new membrane ready for sperm-egg fusion. Such a newly constituted membrane might be much more analogous to the invertebrate sperm inner acrosomal membrane than is now thought (Austin, 1975). More experimental data will be necessary to resolve this question.

CONCLUSIONS

The phenomenon of capacitation is now amenable to experimentation at the molecular level. The endogenous, physiological change seems to be a membrane change related to the rearrangement of intrinsic components. Probes for regions of high and low fluidity as well as elucidation of the specific lipid composition and topography will lend support to or modify the model presented. Whatever the outcome, the goal of understanding the fertilization process is certainly closer at hand.

REFERENCES

Austin, C.R.: Observations on the Penetration of Sperm into the Mammalian Egg. Aust J Sci Res B 4(1951)581-596

Austin, C.R.: Membrane Fusion Events in Fertilization. J Reprod Fertil 44(1975)155-166

Barros, C.: Capacitation of Mammalian Spermatozoa. In: Physiology and Genetics of Reproduction, Part B, pp. 3-24, ed. by E.M. Coutinho and F. Fuchs. Plenum Press, New York, 1974

Barros, C.; Austin, C.R.: *In Vitro* Fertilization and the Sperm Acrosome Reaction in the Hamster. J Exp Zool 166(1967)317-324

Barros, C.; Berrios, M.: Is the Activated Spermatozoon Really Capacitated? J Exp Zool 201(1977)65-72

Barros, C.; Garavagno, A.: Capacitation of Rabbit Spermatozoa with the Blood Sera. J Reprod Fertil 22(1970)381-384

Bedford, J.M.: Sperm Transport, Capacitation and Fertilization. In: Reproductive Biology, pp. 338-392, ed. by H Balin and S. Glasser. Exerpta Medica Monograph, Amsterdam, 1972

Bedford, J.M.; Chang, M.C.: Removal of Decapacitation Factor from Seminal Plasma by High Speed Centrifugation. Am J Physiol 202(1962)179-181

Brackett, B.G.; Oliphant, G.: Capacitation of Rabbit Spermatozoa *in Vitro*. Biol Reprod 12(1975)260-274

Chang, M.C.: Fertilizing Capacity of Spermatozoa Deposited into the Fallopian Tubes. Nature 168(1951)697-698

Chang, M.C.: A Detrimental Effect of Seminal Plasma on the Fertilizing Capacity of Sperm. Nature 179(1957)258-259

Chang, M.C.; Hunter, R.H.F.: Capacitation of Mammalian Sperm: Biological and Experimental Aspects. In: Handbook of Physiology. Vol. V, Sect. 7, chap. 16, pp. 339-351. ed. by D.W. Hamilton and R.O. Greep. Williams and Wilkins Co., Baltimore, 1975

Davis, B.K.: Decapacitation and Recapacitation of Rabbit Spermatozoa Treated with Membrane Vesicles from Seminal Plasma. J Reprod Fertil 41(1974)241-244

Franklin, L.E.; Barros, C.; Fussell, E.N.: The Acrosomal Region and the Acrosome Reaction in Sperm of the Golden Hamster. Biol Reprod 3(1970)180-200

Friend, D.S.; Orci, L.; Perrelet, A.; Yanagimachi, R.: Membrane Particle Changes Attending the Acrosome Reaction in Guinea Pig Spermatozoa. J Cell Biol 74(1977)561-577

Gordon, M.; Dandekar, P.V.: Fine-structural Localization of Phosphatase Activity on the Plasma Membrane of the Rabbit Sperm Head. J Reprod Fertil 49(1977)155-156

Gordon, M.; Dandekar, P.V.; Bartoszewicz, W.: The Surface Coat of Epididymal, Ejaculated and Capacitated Sperm. J Ultrastruct Res 50(1975)199-207

Gwatkin, R.B.L.; Andersen, O.F.; Williams, D.T.: Capacitation of Mouse Spermatozoa *in Vitro*: Involvement of Epididymal Secretions and Cumulus Oophorus. J Reprod Fertil 41(1974)253-256

Johnson, J.D.; Epel, D.: Relationship between Release of Surface Proteins and Metabolic Activation of Sea Urchin Eggs at Fertilization. Proc Natl Acad Sci USA 72(1975)4474-4478

Johnson, W.L.; Hunter, A.G.: Seminal Antigens: Their Alteration in the Genital Tract of Female Rabbits and during Partial *in Vitro* Capacitation with β-Amylase and β-Glucuronidase. Biol Reprod 7(1972)332-340

Koehler, J.K.: Changes in Antigenic Site Distribution on Rabbit Spermatozoa after Incubation in "Capacitating" Media. Biol Reprod 15(1976)444-456

Leopold, R.A.; Degrugillier, M.E.: Sperm Penetration of Housefly Eggs: Evidence for Involvement of a Female Accessory Secretion. Science 181(1973)555-557

Lillie, F.R.: Problems of Fertilization. University of Chicago Press, Chicago, 1919.

Lui, C.W.; Cornett, L.E.; Meizel, S.: Identification of the Bovine Follicular Protein Involved in the *in Vitro* Induction of the Hamster Sperm Acrosome Reaction. Biol Reprod 17(1977)34-41

Oliphant, G.; Brackett, B.G.: Immunological Assessment of Surface Changes of Rabbit Sperm Undergoing Capacitation. Biol Reprod 9(1973a)404-414

Oliphant, G.; Brackett, B.G.: Capacitation of Mouse Spermatozoa in Media with Elevated Ionic Strength and Reversible Decapacitation with Epididymal Extracts. Fertil Steril 24(1973b)948-955

O'Rand, M.G.: *In Vitro* Fertilization and Capacitation-like Interaction in the Hydroid *Campanularia flexuosa*. J Exp Zool 182(1972)299-306

O'Rand, M.G.: Gamete Interaction during Fertilization in *Campanularia*-the Female Epithelial Cell Surface. Am Zool 14(1974)487-493

O'Rand, M.G.: Restriction of a Sperm Surface Antigen's Mobility during Capacitation. Dev Biol 55(1977)260-270

O'Rand, M.G.: Capping of Sperm-specific Autoantigens on Spermatids, Residual Bodies and Ejaculate Spermatozoa. Anat Rec 190(1978)497

O'Rand, M.G.; Metz, C.: Isolation of an "Immobilizing Antigen" from Rabbit Sperm Membranes. Biol Reprod 14(1976)586-598

O'Rand, M.G.; Miller, R.L.: Spermatozoon Vesicle Loss during Penetration of the Female Gonangium in the Hydroid, *Campanularia flexuosa*. J Exp Zool 188(1974)179-194

Pinsker, M.C.; Williams, W.L.: Properties of Spermatozoon Antifertility Factor. Arch Biochem Biophys 122(1967)111-117

Reyes, A.; Oliphant, G.; Brackett, B.: Partial Purification and Identification of a Reversible Decapacitation Factor from Rabbit Seminal Plasma. Fertil Steril 26(1975)148-157

Romrell, L.J.; O'Rand, M.G.: Capping and Ultrastructural Localization of Sperm Surface Isoantigens during Spermatogenesis. Dev Biol 63(1978)76-93

Rosado, A.; Velazquez, A.; Lara-Ricalde, R.: Cell Polarography. II. Effect of Neuraminidase and Follicular Fluid upon

Surface Characteristics of Human Spermatozoa. Fertil Steril 24(1973)349-354

Shivers, C.A.; James, J.M.: Capacitation of Frog Sperm. Nature 227(1970)183-184

Summers, R.G.; Talbot, P.; Keough, E.M.; Hylander, B.L.; Franklin, L.E.: Ionophore A23187 Induces Acrosome Reactions in Sea Urchin and Guinea Pig Spermatozoa. J Exp Zool 196(1976)381-385

Talbot, P.; Franklin, L.E.: Surface Modification of Guinea Pig Sperm during *in Vitro* Capacitation: An Assessment using Lectin-induced Agglutination of Living Sperm. J Exp Zool 203(1978)1-14

Vaidya, R.A.; Glass, R.H.; Dandekar, P.; Johnson, K.: Decrease in the Electrophoretic Mobility of Rabbit Spermatozoa following Intrauterine Incubation. J Reprod Fertil 24(1971)299-301

Weil, A.J.: Antigens of the Seminal Plasma. J Reprod Fertil Suppl 2(1967)25-34

Weinman, D.E.; Williams, W.L.: Mechanism of Capacitation of Rabbit Spermatozoa. Nature 203(1964)423-424

Williams, W.L.: Biochemistry of Capacitation of Spermatozoa. In: Biology of Mammalian Fertilization and Implantation, pp. 19-53, ed. by K.S. Moghissi and E.S.E. Hafez. C.C Thomas, Springfield, Ill., 1972.

Yamada, K.; Weston, J.A.: Isolation of a Major Cell Surface Glycoprotein from Fibroblasts. Proc Natl Acad Sci USA 71(1974)3492-3496

Yanagimachi, R.: *In Vitro* Acrosome Reaction and Capacitation of Golden Hamster Spermatozoa by Bovine Follicular Fluid and its Fractions. J Exp Zool 170(1969)269-280

Yanagimachi, R.: Specificity of Sperm-Egg Interaction. In: Immunobiology of Gametes, pp. 255-295, ed. by M. Edidin and M.H. Johnson. Cambridge University Press, Cambridge, 1977.

Yanagimachi, R.; Nicolson, G.L.; Noda, Y.D.; Fujimoto, M.: Electron Microscopic Observations of the Distribution of Acidic Anionic Residues on Hamster Spermatozoa and Eggs before and during Fertilization. J Ultrastruct Res 43(1973)344-353

CHARACTERIZATION OF SPERM SURFACES USING PHYSICAL TECHNIQUES

R.H. Hammerstedt

Department of Biochemistry & Biophysics, The Pennsylvania State University, University Park, Pennsylvania 16802 USA

Characterization of spermatozoan surface structure is essential to a full understanding of sperm maturation within the epididymis and the subsequent modifications that occur in sperm during passage through the female reproductive tract. Sperm structure has been examined in detail using thin-section, freeze-fracture, and scanning electron microscopy (Bedford, 1975; Fawcett, 1975; Fléchon and Morstin, 1975; Yanagimachi et al., 1972). Careful analysis of these observations has provided information about regional differences on the sperm surface (e.g., head versus tail) and established relationships among membranes and other cell components. However, such studies cannot characterize the molecules imparting the unique physical characteristics to the surface. Cell fractionation experiments have provided samples for careful chemical analyses (Ebenshade and Clegg, 1976; Lunstra et al., 1974; Zahler and Doak, 1975; Herman et al., 1976), but assignment of cellular location was often difficult. Physical characterization of intact cells, using techniques believed to uniquely sample specific zones of the cell surface, represents another experimental approach.

The schematic representation of a plasma membrane surface (Fig. 1) is based on results obtained from chemical analysis of isolated membrane components and depicts the generally accepted concept. Three zones (the phospholipid bilayer, the phospholipid-water interface, and the glycocalyx) representing chemically unique layers of the surface are emphasized. The overall functions of the membrane are distributed among the molecules of these three zones.

The lipid bilayer is composed of polar phospholipids oriented with hydrocarbon chains directed to the interior of this zone and the charged polar groups directed toward the polar solvent, water. Proteins within these lipids are considered either intrinsic (integral and essential for structure) or extrinsic (associated with the membrane but easily removed by mild physical treatments). This zone provides a general permeability barrier to charged molecules. Specific transport systems are required to exchange intracellular and extracellular molecules. The chemical composition of this zone defines the ability of the cell to maintain permeability barriers when subjected to physical stress; changes in composition result in changes in bilayer strength. The phospholipid-water interface, between the bilayer and the medium, has a fixed electrical charge located in the bilayer which represents the mixture of functional groups found on lipid and protein. Counter-ions located in the solution are attracted by these charges. Change in either the polar lipids or proteins of the phospholipid bilayer results in a redistribution of the fixed charge at this interface. Finally, some glycoproteins and glycolipids extend out from the bilayer interface and constitute the glycocalyx zone. These macromolecules have a net negative charge (due to sialic acid or sulfate residues) and form a fixed electrical charge extending possibly 150 Å from the phospholipid-water interface. Counter-ions to these molecules may be either small ions (hydrogen or metal ions) or macromolecules.

A molecular description of the surface requires precise analyses to locate specific molecules in these zones to within 5-50 Å. The physical techniques presented below enable study of the general characteristics of the zones represented in Figure 1. Permeability barriers to small molecules are provided by the lipid bilayer (verticle lines); the phospholipid-water interface (dotted area) represents a unique charge domain; and the glycocalyx (grid area) comprises another charged zone. Techniques specific for analysis of each zone were used in these studies.

METHODS USED TO CHARACTERIZE SPERM SURFACES

Preparation of Sperm

Three types of ram sperm were used. Testicular sperm leaving the testis were diverted from entering the caput epididymidis by placing a catheter within the rete testis and collecting the cells ($>10^8$/h) at

---

The results reported herein represent a collaborative effort with other Pennsylvania State University faculty (Drs. A.D. Keith, P. Todd, and R.P. Amann) and staff (S. Hay and N. DeLuca). Partial financial support was provided by NIH grant HD-05859 (RHH), ERDA grant AT (11-1)-3419 (ADK), NIH contract NO1-CB-43984 (PT) and WHO contract 76,173 (RPA).

© 1979 Urban & Schwarzenberg, Inc. Baltimore-Munich *The Spermatozoon*, edited by D.W. Fawcett and J.M. Bedford

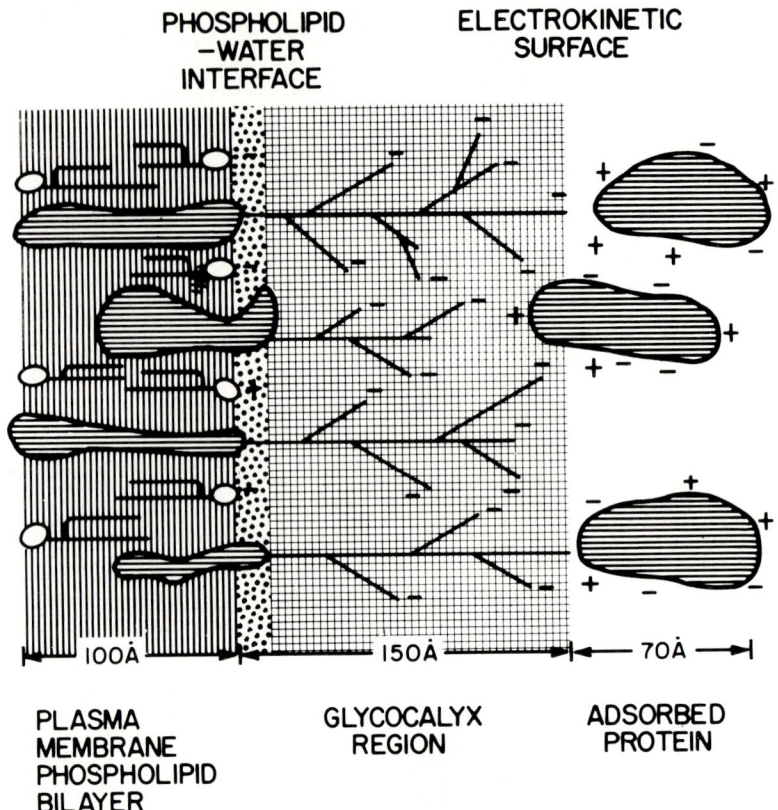

Figure 1. Schematic representation of the sperm plasma membrane showing zones sampled in these experiments. The phospholipid bilayer is composed of polar lipids with their charged groups directed to the surface and proteins (horizontal lines) extending partially or completely across the membrane. These proteins can extend out of the membrane into the aqueous solvent around the cell. The phospholipid-water interface has a characteristic electrical charge. The glycocalyx region consists of glycoproteins anchored in the plasma membrane and extending 100-150 Å from the phospholipid-water interface. The glycoproteins have a net negative charge, due to sialic acid or sulfate residues attached to the carbohydrate side chains, which produces an electrokinetic surface to which extracellular proteins may be absorbed. Only fixed electrical charges are represented.

ambient temperature (20°C) or 5°C. The technique used was similar to that described by Suominen and Setchell (1972), except that an L-shaped rather than a T-shaped catheter was used. Cauda epididymidal sperm ($>2 \times 10^{10}$) were obtained at hemi-castration by retrograde flushing of the proximal ductus deferens and distal cauda epididymidis with buffer. Ejaculated sperm ($\sim 3 \times 10^9$) were collected by artificial vagina. The preparations were free of extraneous cells and the sperm were washed once in buffer (Hammerstedt, 1975) prior to dilution and use. All experiments with ram sperm were conducted between August and January. Bull and rabbit ejaculated sperm were collected by artificial vagina and washed as described (Hammerstedt, 1975).

Electron Spin Resonance Techniques

Resonance spectroscopy has been used extensively in recent years to study biological systems. The principal techniques are nuclear magnetic and electron spin resonance (ESR) spectroscopy. Recent reviews describe the principles of ESR (Keith et al., 1973; Griffith and Wagner, 1969; Azzi and Montecucco, 1977) and the essential details are outlined below.

ESR requires that the molecule or species being detected have paramagnetic properties. Molecules, ions, and other species with unpaired electrons satisfy this requirement; nitroxide compounds have been extensively used in recent years (Fig. 2). These molecules have a stable, unpaired electron associated with the nitroxide group ($N \rightarrow O$). Steric hindrance within the molecule is provided by organic substituents. A variety of organic compounds can be attached to the nitroxide group to yield useful "spin labelled" molecules or spin labels.

An ESR spectrometer consists of a sample cavity, an external magnetic field of known but variable intensity, a microwave energy source, and a microwave

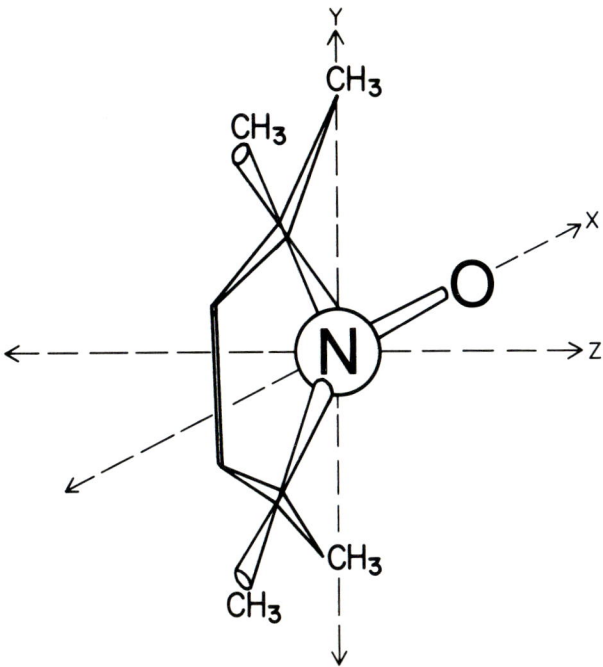

Figure 2. Schematic representation of a spin label molecule emphasizing the nitroxide group (N → O) and the steric hindrance provided by the substituents located adjacent to the nitroxide group.

detector. When a population of spin label is placed in an ESR spectrometer under appropriate conditions, energy absorption results. The ESR equation describing this condition is

$$h\vec{v} = g\beta\vec{H}$$

where h is Boltzman's constant, $\vec{v}$ is the applied microwave frequency, g is a constant characteristic of the paramagnetic species, β is the Bohr mageton and $\vec{H}$ is the intensity of the applied magnetic field. In principle, either $\vec{v}$ or $\vec{H}$ can be varied. In practice, $\vec{H}$ is varied ± 50 G for the study of nitroxides.

The characteristics of the ESR spectrum result from the ^{14}N-nucleus operating on the energy absorbed by the unpaired electron. Since the nuclear spin factor of ^{14}N is 1, the energy absorption of the unpaired electron is split into -1, 0, and $+1$ energy states. These absorption lines are recorded as first derivatives to maximize signal-to-noise ratio (Fig. 3).

Analyses of these three first derivative lines yield four types of information relating to local viscosity, solvent polarity, translational diffusion, and relative solubility between two solvent phases of a heterogeneous preparation. Local viscosity is determined via a derived parameter known as rotational correlation time (Γ_c). This parameter is calculated from spectral measurements and its physical basis is the time-depend-

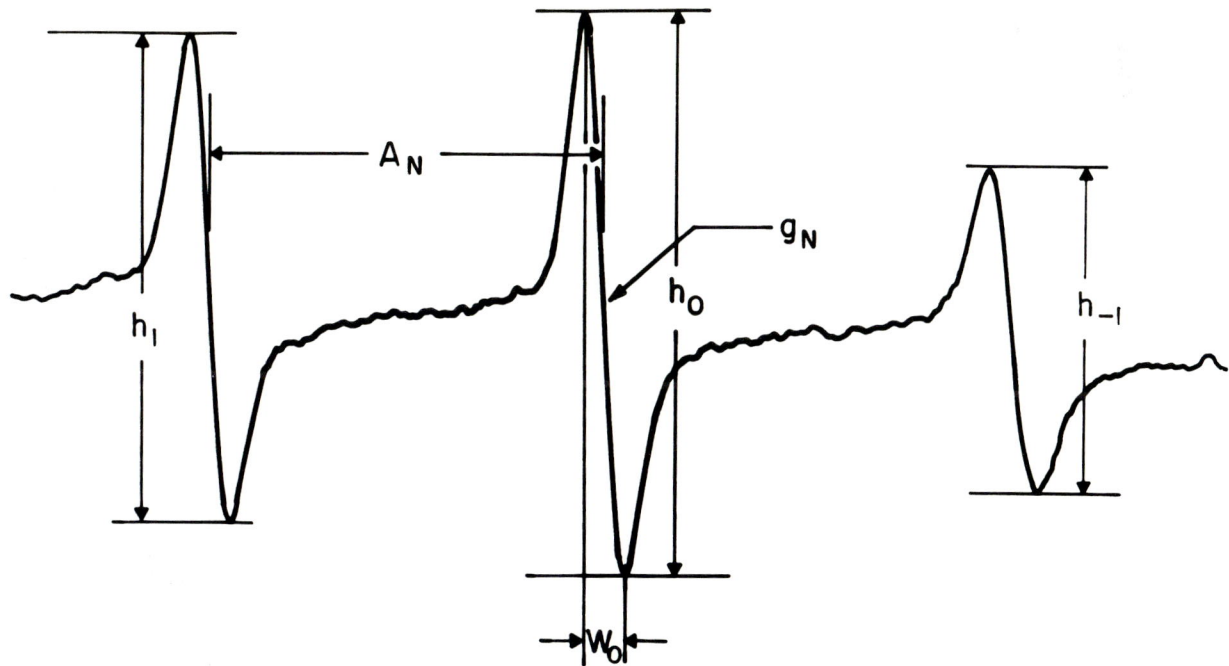

Figure 3. First derivative of an ESR spectrum of a spin label, showing height (h), nitrogen hyperfine coupling (A_n) and widths (W) of the absorption lines. Low-, mid- and high-field lines are designated by subscripts 1, 0, and -1. Taken from Hammerstedt et al. (1976) with permission of the publisher.

ent averaging of hyperfine and g-matrix tensor terms. Solvent polarity is determined by measuring perturbations on the isotropic component of the hyperfine coupling and g-value terms. Its physical basis is the delocalization of the unpaired electron with respect to the N-nucleus caused by nearby solvent molecules. This delocalization causes a measurable increase or decrease in the effect of the N-nucleus on the unpaired electron. Translational diffusion is determined by measuring the collision frequency between spin-labelled molecules. The collision frequency is controlled by the concentration of spin label and properties of the solvent matrix. Near encounters between two spin-labelled molecules result in transfer of spin angular momentum from one spin-labelled molecule to another; uniform broadening of each of the three hyperfine lines is observed. Partitioning of spin-labelled molecules between two environments in a heterogeneous preparation can be studied; the basis for these determinations is presented in the previous discussion of polarity. Two signals are observed. For example, one could originate from a spin-labelled population located in the nonpolar lipid and the second signal from the spin-labelled population in the aqueous medium. The relative intensity of these two signals, best seen in the high field line, describes the partitioning.

Electronic interactions with other spin-labelled molecules or paramagnetic ions such as Ni^{2+} or $Fe(CN)_6^{3-}$ result in a uniform line broadening due to spin exchange during collisional events or near encounters. Since paramagnetic ions such as Ni^{2+} or $Fe(CN)_6^{3-}$ do not have a detectable signal under assay conditions, increasing their concentration in the presence of spin label effectively removes all signal from the spin label. A schematic representation of the distribution of selected spin labels in sperm and the effect of Ni^{2+} on their spectral characteristics have been published (Hammerstedt et al., 1976).

By controlling properties of the spin-label probe and using paramagnetic broadening agents, distinction between the interior and exterior surfaces of a membrane is possible. Furthermore, the polarity and viscosity of the local microenvironment, the state of molecular ordering, and the ease of molecular diffusion can be obtained from carefully designed ESR experiments (Hammerstedt et al., 1978).

Initial studies revealed that for sperm with intact membranes, small water soluble spin labels localized within the cells are inaccessible to paramagnetic ions (Hammerstedt et al., 1976). Quantitative measurements of spin-label signal intensity from the total aqueous compartment of sperm from several species were made (Hammerstedt et al., 1978). Comparisons of these data with dimensions obtained by microscopic measurements of sperm were consistent with the conclusion that the intracellular compartment sampled by a water-soluble spin label is a large, relatively homogenous, compartment that is inaccessible to Ni^{2+}. Probably this total aqueous compartment is dominated by the sperm head, but the tail represents a small portion of the total volume. The viscosity of this compartment can be determined from the spectra (Hammerstedt et al., 1978). Loss of spin-label signal intensity from the total aqueous compartment probably reflects damage to both the plasma membrane and membranous structures within the head and tail. Water soluble spin labels have been used in the experiments presented below to determine the integrity of the plasma membrane bilayer after various physical treatments. Butylated hydroxytoluene (BHT) was shown to protect many sperm cells from cold-induced membrane damage (Hammerstedt et al., 1976, 1978).

Surface-directed spin labels have been developed (Lepock et al., 1975)[1] to detect changes in charge at the phospholipid-water interface. The spin labels must be amphiphilic (partition between water and lipid) to localize specifically at this zone. These spin labels are anchored to the membrane by their long hydrocarbon side chains but cannot pass through the membrane because of charged bridge groups (e.g., a phosphodiester). The nitroxide group is located at the phospholipid-water interface. Thus, the ESR signal from this class of spin labels reflects the physical environment in the phospholipid-water interface zone of the membrane. Factors that could alter the ESR signal from these spin labels include their partitioning between bulk water of solution and water associated with membrane, charge density at the phospholipid-water interface, and freedom of motion within this zone. The surface location of these spin labels was verified since their ESR spectra were broadened by Ni^{2+} and the spin label was removed from the cells by repeated washing without destroying the integrity of the plasma membrane. Two different spin labels were prepared, but the most useful was octa-decylphosphoryl-3-methylene-2,2,5,2-tetramethylpyrroline-N-oxyl (18PP). This spin label exists free in solution (yielding a sharp-lined spectral component) and associated with the membrane (broad spectral component reflecting relatively immobilized spin-labelled molecules).

---

[1]Hammerstedt, R.H.; Keith, A.D.; Boltz, R.C., Jr.; Todd, P.W.: Use of Amphiphilic Spin Labels and Whole Cell Isoelectric Focusing to Assay Charge Characteristics of Sperm Surfaces. Arch Biochem Biophys: in press.

Whole-cell Isoelectric Focusing

Electrokinetic methods respond to the charge characteristics of the glycocalyx. Electrophoretic measurements are hydrodynamic assays of individual cells in a medium of relatively high ionic strength. Estimates of charge per mass unit are obtained. The charge and mass are determined by the plane of cleavage between the fixed electrical charges of the glycocalyx plus absorbed ions and the movable charges of the suspending medium. In most cases, this plane of cleavage is 150-200 Å from the phospholipid-water interface. Electrophoretic studies of bull, ram, and rabbit sperm have been published (Bangham, 1961; Bey, 1965; Hafs and Boyd, 1971). Caput epididymal sperm have a lower mobility than do cauda epididymal sperm and the regional distribution of charge over the cell surface may change. Since the mass of the sperm changes only slightly, the change in electrophoretic mobility probably reflects a change in charge density.

The reported study used a different electrokinetic technique—whole-cell isoelectric focusing, to evaluate the charge characteristics of the glycocalyx zone of the sperm surface (Fig. 1). Isoelectric focusing evaluates the equilibrium state of cells in a very low ionic strength medium. The balance of fixed positive and negative charges at the boundary limit of the cell is measured. This boundary limit is about 50 Å from the phospholipid-water interface in the low ionic strength medium used.

Isoelectric focusing of whole cells is accomplished by establishing a pH gradient within a density-stabilized liquid column. Constant osmotic strength is maintained throughout the solution. A central sampling-tube allows determination of the point within the gradient where the pH is appropriate for sample introduction and also serves as the channel to introduce sperm into the column. Upon application of an electrical current, the cells migrate from the position of introduction to the position within the pH gradient where the charge on their boundary limit is neutralized. A schematic representation is presented (Fig. 4). Extensive preliminary experiments defined the limits of this technique.[1] No difference in the isoelectric focusing pH value was noted when washed and unwashed sperm were compared. However, the pH of insertion had an effect on the isoelectric focusing pH values of rabbit ejaculated sperm but not bull ejaculated sperm. Samples to be compared should be inserted at the same pH

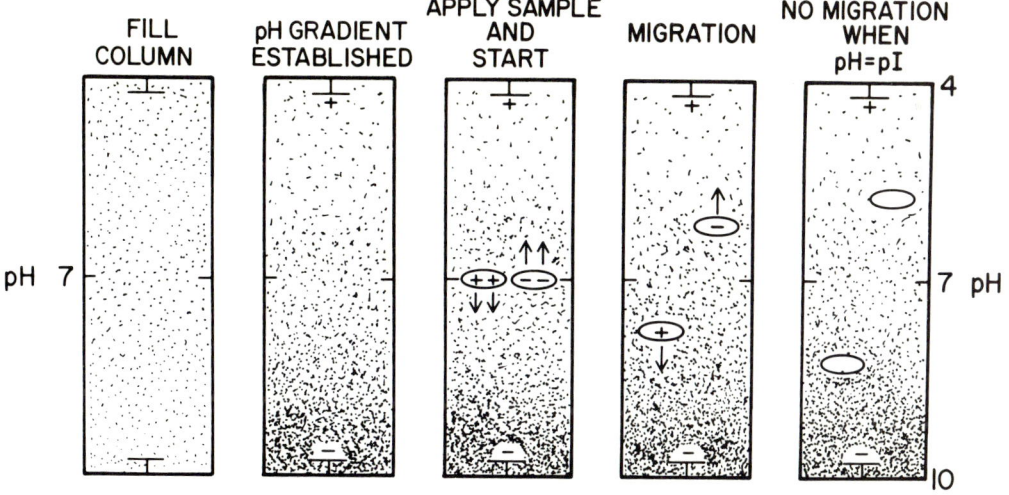

Figure 4. Schematic representation of whole-cell isoelectric focusing technique used with sperm. The isoelectric focusing column is filled with a solution of synthetic ampholites (LKB, AS) and a complex gradient of both Ficoll (Pharmacia) and sucrose; the resulting solution column has a density gradient (to prevent sedimentation of cells) yet is isoosmotic. Passing a current through the column for 18-24 h establishes a pH gradient. The sperm are applied at neutral pH and the glycocalyx is charged; the magnitude of this surface charge reflects the difference between the pH of insertion and the isoelectric point (pI) of the sperm. When power is reapplied the sperm move toward their isoelectric point and then stop moving when the charge at the boundary limit reaches zero. Details of the technique have been described.[1]

(between pH 6-8). Plasma and acrosomal sperm membranes appeared to be intact when examined by phase-contrast and differential interference-contrast microscopy.

Analysis of Subcompartments within Sperm

Electron microscopic analyses of sperm structure emphasize several membrane-limited structures or compartments within the cell. For this discussion, a more simplistic view of the sperm is used. The plasma membrane surrounds the entire cell. The head compartment includes the nucleus, acrosome, their respective membranes, and the postacrosomal lamina. Integrity of this compartment can be determined by measuring the total aqueous compartment (see above). The tail compartment includes the axoneme and dense fibers surrounded by mitochondria of the middle piece and the fibrous sheath of the principal piece. Adenine nucleotides are associated with metabolically active compartments and may be exclusively associated with the tail. Loss of intracellular nucleotides is considered an indication of membrane damage in this compartment. The integrity of these two compartments and their surrounding plasma membrane was examined in a series of experiments described below.

CHARACTERISTICS OF THE SPERM SURFACES

Species Differences in Membranes

Initial experiments optimized conditions for the use of water soluble spin labels to study the aqueous compartment of ejaculated bull sperm (Hammerstedt et al., 1976). These studies were later expanded to examine ejaculated sperm from other species (Hammerstedt et al., 1978). Surprisingly, the optimum conditions for analysis of ejaculated sperm from boar, bull, rabbit, rooster, and stallion all differ. Preliminary experiments using techniques optimized for bull sperm were unsatisfactory for sperm from guinea pig, man, mouse, and rat.

Experiments were designed to test for differential lability of membranes surrounding the head and tail compartments of ejaculated rabbit and bull sperm.[1] Sperm were treated with increasing concentrations of either a negative detergent (octadecylphosphate, $18PO_4$) or a positive detergent (cetyltrimethylammonium bromide, CTAB). The total aqueous compartment and the intracellular adenine nucleotide content were measured for control and detergent-treated sperm (Fig. 5). Rabbit sperm lost permeability barriers to Ni^{2+} when treated with increasing concentrations of CTAB; adenine nucleotide content was drastically reduced. Treatment with the negative detergent $18PO_4$ had no effect. Thus, membranes limiting the head and tail compartments of rabbit sperm apparently responded similarly to detergent treatment. Bull sperm responded differently. Both detergents broke the membranes surrounding the head, resulting in loss of ESR signal. Adenine nucleotides were lost from the tail compartment of bull sperm after CTAB treatment but not $18PO_4$ treatment. It can be concluded that membranes surrounding compartments of bull sperm have a differential lability. This example illustrates how combinations of physical and biochemical measurements can be used to quantitatively describe characteristics of both inner and plasma membranes of multi-compartmented cells.

The charge at the phospholipid-water interface of sperm apparently differed among species. The charge density at the phospholipid-water interface of ejaculated sperm was much more negative for bull and rabbit sperm than for ram sperm. This was evident in comparisons of spectra for each sperm type (Fig. 6 and 7). When total 18PP concentration was $0.2mM$ for bull and rabbit sperm, "free" 18PP was the dominant feature of the spectrum. $NiCl_2$ had to be added to eliminate this spectral feature and emphasize the relatively immobilized, membrane-associated population of 18PP (Fig. 6). When ram sperm were tested under these same conditions, virtually no "free" 18PP was found. The concentration of 18PP had to be raised to $1mM$ before the sharp-lined spectral component was observed (control in Fig. 7).

The isoelectric focusing pH values were different for ejaculated sperm from various species. The values obtained for boar sperm (Moore and Hibbitt, 1975) and rabbit sperm[1] were approximately pH 7 while those for bull[1] and ram[2] were below pH 5.

Evaluation of Sperm Maturation

Similar ESR techniques were used to detect changes in ram spermatozoan membranes during epididymal transit. The ability of the sperm plasma membrane to withstand abrupt temperature changes and retain the ability to exclude Ni^{2+} was studied.[2] From representative spectra for ram sperm (Fig. 8), it was evident that the increased porosity of the plasma membrane induced by temperature shock resulted in progressive loss of low-viscosity (sharp-line) components until only a broad signal remained. However, this susceptibility of cauda epididymidal sperm to rapid cooling to 0°C was

---

[2]Hammerstedt, R.H.; Keith, A.D.; Hay, S.; DeLuca, N.; Amann, R.P.: Changes in Ram Sperm Membranes during Epididymidal Transit, Arch Biochem Biophys: in press.

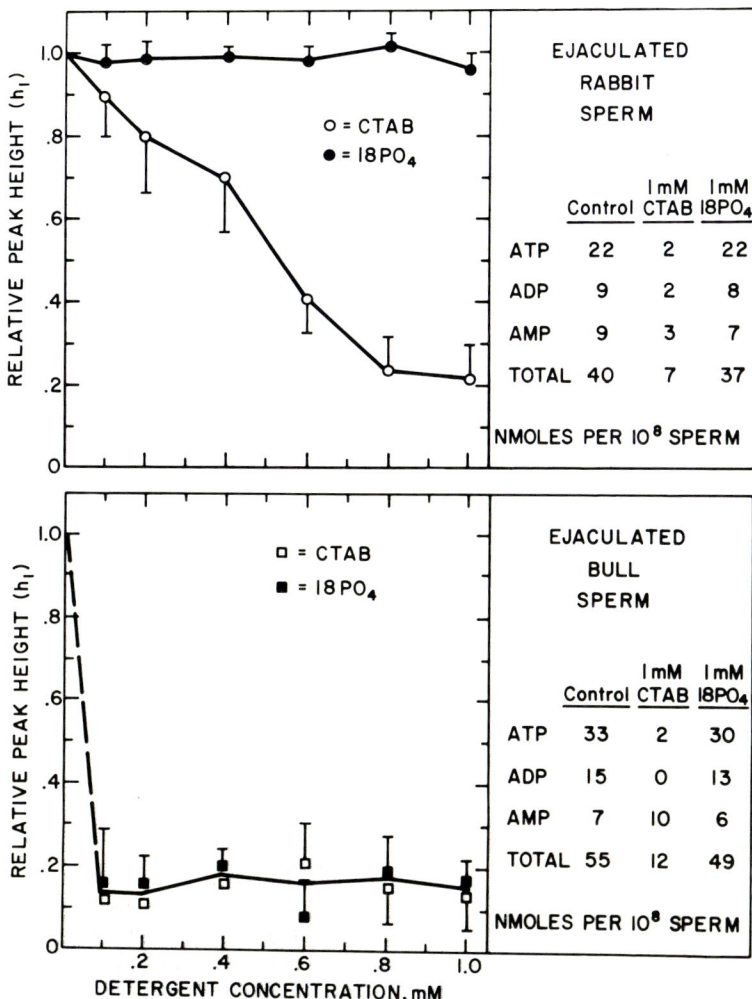

Figure 5. Effects of detergents on the membrane permeability of sperm. Washed ejaculated sperm were incubated with increasing concentrations of negative (octadecylphosphate [18PO$_4$]) or positive (cetyltrimethylammonium bromide [CTAB]) detergent. The loss of the total intracellular aqueous compartment of the sperm was estimated from the peak height of the high-field line of spectra from a water-soluble spin label in treated sperm relative to nondetergent treated (control) sperm preparations. The effect of 1mM detergent on adenine nucleotide levels also was determined. Experimental details are provided elsewhere.[1]

in marked contrast to the resistance of testicular sperm (Fig. 9). Thus, maturation-associated changes in sperm membranes can be detected by ESR.

Volume of the total aqueous compartment of untreated (control) testicular, cauda epididymidal and ejaculated sperm were similar (P>0.05; Fig. 9). Values ranged from 20-24 μm^3 per cell. Volume of the total aqueous compartment of testicular sperm was maintained (>90%) after rapid cooling to 0°C (cold shock) but reduced ~50% by freezing (on solid CO$_2$) and thawing. Addition of BHT at <4mM did not protect testicular sperm against membrane damage from freezing. Cauda epididymidal and ejaculated sperm retained only 20-30% of their isolated intracellular aqueous volume after cold shock and 10% after freezing. However, BHT at 1mM prevented membrane damage to both cells during cold shock. A BHT concentration of 2-4mM prevented freeze damage to ejaculated sperm but not cauda epididymidal sperm. It was concluded that the composition of the lipid bilayer portion of the sperm membrane must change during epididymal transit and that further changes must occur upon contact of sperm with accessory sex gland fluids. A molecular explanation for these changes of physical properties is not available.

Inspection of the spectra obtained when 18PP was used to study the sperm surface suggested that the charge density at the phospholipid-water interface changed during epididymal transit. To more precisely quantify differences in charge density at the phos-

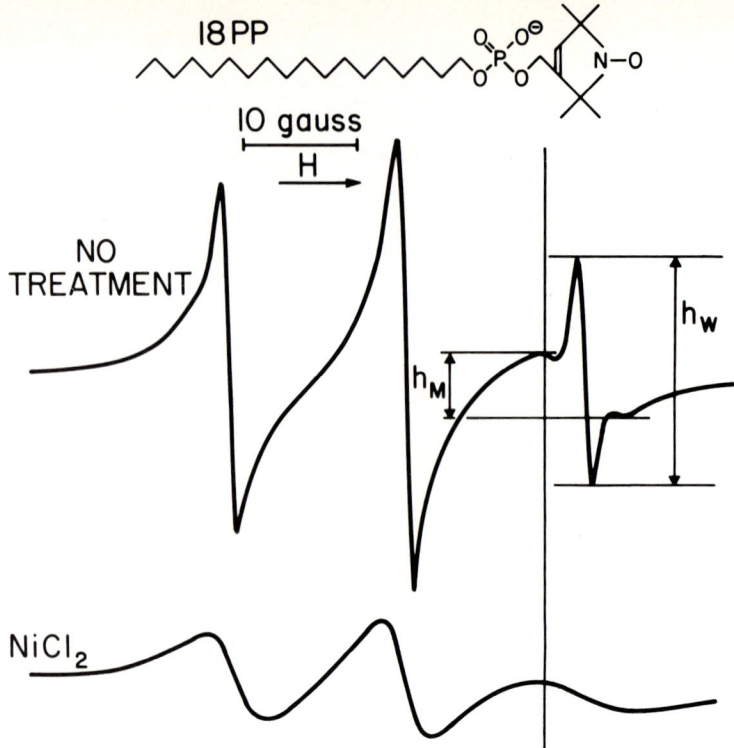

Figure 6. Distribution of the surface spin label 18PP on rabbit ejaculated sperm. Suspensions of sperm were made 0.2mM in 18PP and ESR spectra were recorded. A complex spectrum resulted (control) and the high-field components were assigned to 18PP within an immobilized zone (h_M) and a free, unrestricted zone (h_W). Addition of 100mM NiCl$_2$ was required to remove the contribution of the free 18PP revealing the immobilized signal. Data for bull ejaculated sperm were similar. Experimental details are provided elsewhere.[1]

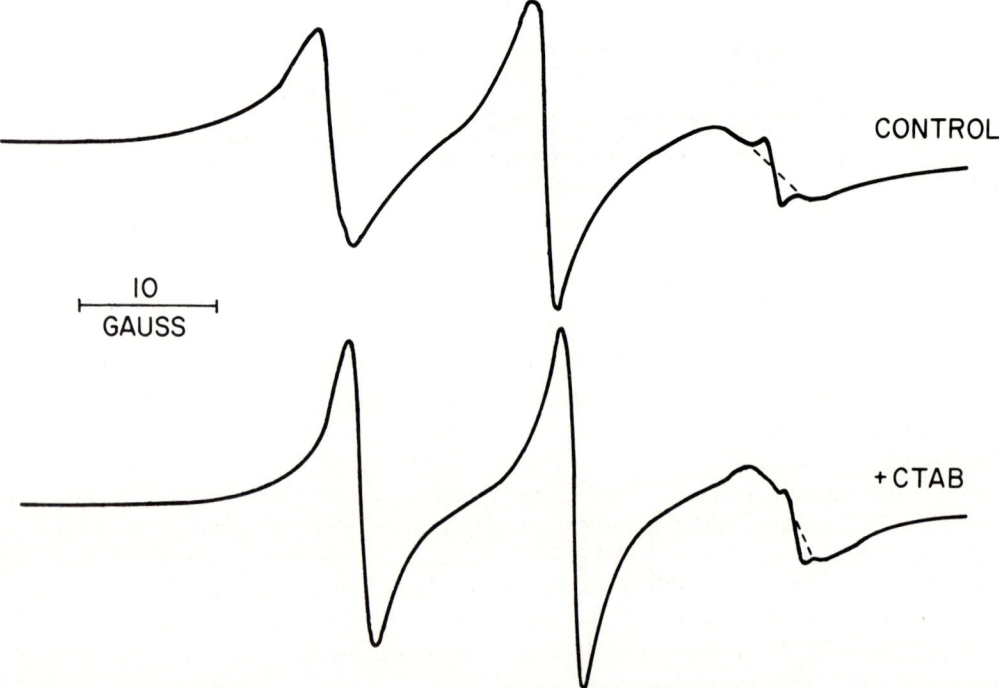

Figure 7. Distribution of the surface spin label 18PP in ram ejaculated sperm. Sperm suspensions were prepared and evaluated using 1mM 18PP without (control) or with 1mM CTAB (cetyltrimethylammonium bromide). The high-field components of the spectra were analyzed and the relative contributions of the "free" (or sharp spectral component) and "immobilized" (or broad spectral component) components to the total peak area were determined. Addition of NiCl$_2$ was not required because the dominant feature of the spectra was the immobilized component. Spectra for testicular and cauda epididymidal sperm were qualitatively similar. Experimental details are provided elsewhere.[2]

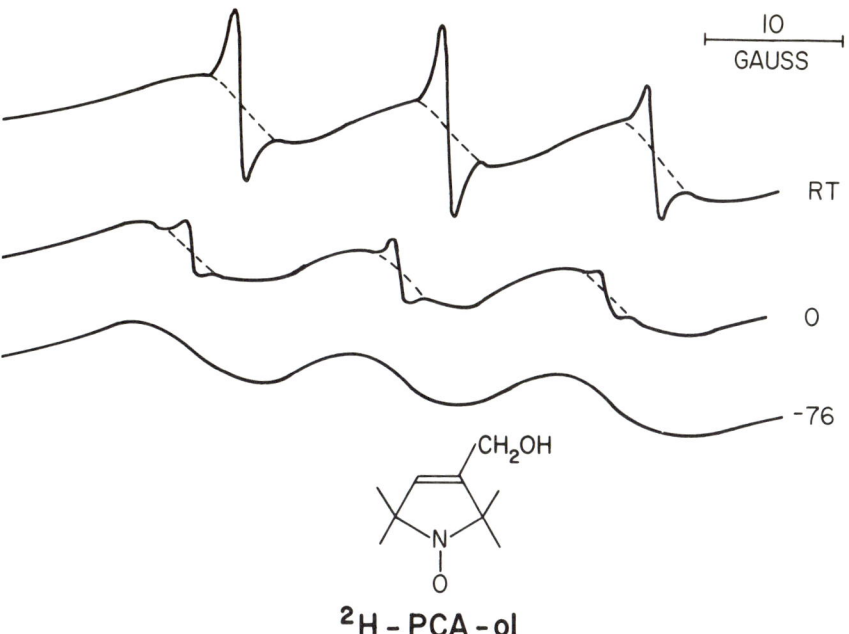

Figure 8. ESR spectra of ram cauda epididymal sperm containing ^{2}H-PCA-ol. Suspensions of ram cauda epididymidal sperm were made 100mM in NiCl$_2$ and 1mM in ^{2}H-PCA-ol (3-hydroxymethyl-2,2,5,5-tetra[^{2}H]methylpyrroline-N-oxyl). Sperm were held at either room temperature (RT), cooled rapidly to 0°C or frozen on solid CO$_2$ (−76°C) and then warmed to room temperature. The size of the low field spectral component, reflecting a low viscosity, Ni^{+2}-inaccessible compartment, was measured to determine the total aqueous compartment. Experimental details are provided elsewhere.[2]

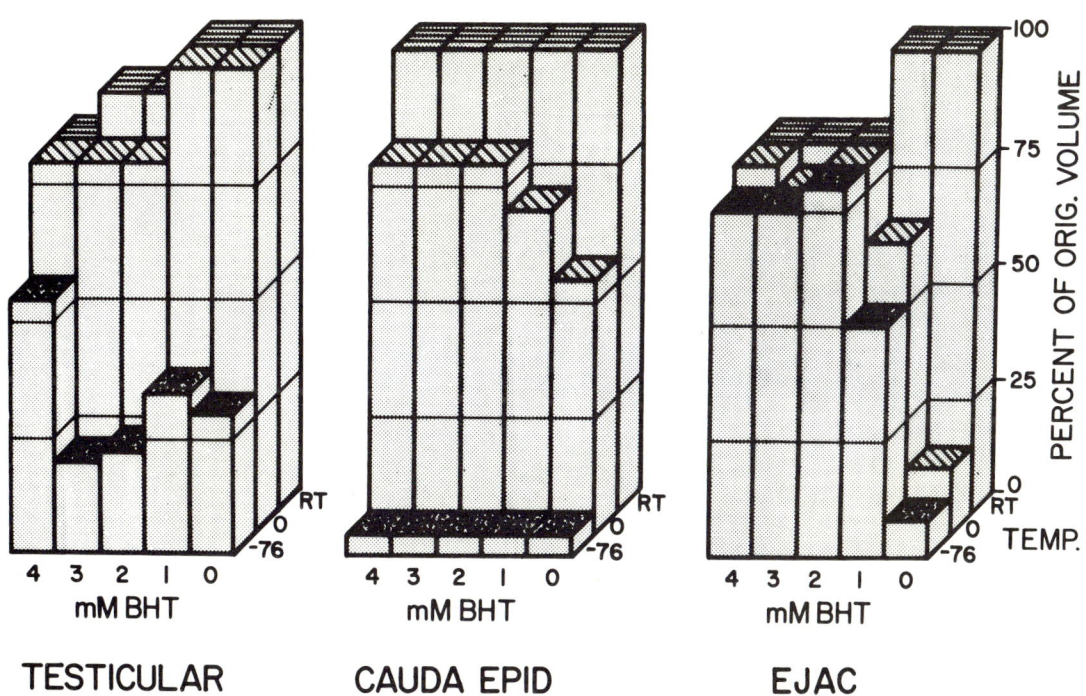

Figure 9. Effects of BHT and rapid temperature change on the total aqueous compartment of ram sperm. Testicular, cauda epididymidal, and ejaculated sperm were treated with 0-4mM BHT and held at room temperature (RT), subjected to rapid cooling (0°C) or rapid freezing (−76°C) and thawing. Volume of the total aqueous compartment was determined as described in Figure 5. The volume for each treated sample was expressed as a percentage of its control (no BHT at RT). Experimental details are provided elsewhere.[2]

pholipid-water interface, an alternate method of comparing spectra was developed. The spectra were recorded in the presence and absence of CTAB. This positive detergent disrupts the plasma membrane of testicular, cauda epididymal, and ejaculated ram sperm as assessed from Ni^{2+} broadening of the ESR signal from 3H—PCA—0l (unpublished data). It appears that the CTAB-treated sperm provide a common reference point for comparisons since cells with a disrupted plasma membrane have a maximum membrane surface and binding of CTAB to these membranes would provide a maximum positive charge domain to interact with the negative spin label. The changes occurring at this zone in ram sperm during epididymal transit were determined.[3]

The ratios ($h_W:h_M$) of the spectral components (Fig. 7) for control sperm (18PP) and for treated sperm (18PP + CTAB) were calculated for each sample pair as $[(h_W/h_M) \text{control}/(h_W/h_M)\text{CTAB}] \times 100$. These values were: testicular sperm, 58; cauda epididymal sperm, 44; and ejaculated sperm, 34 (ejaculated sperm different from testicular sperm, $P<0.05$). The interpretation of the different spectral characteristics of the surface-directed spin-label patterns was that the phospholipid-water interface increases in negative charge density as sperm pass through the epididymis and become mixed with seminal plasma. This could be accomplished by removal of positive charges (phosphatidylcholine) and/or addition of negative charges (phosphatidylinositol, sterol sulfate, or ganglioside).

In detailed experiments[2] it was found that the isoelectric focusing pH values for ram testicular, cauda epididymal, and ejaculated sperm were 5.2, and 4.7, and 4.8. The similarity of the values for cauda epididymal and ejaculated ram sperm were surprising since it had previously been found[1] that the isoelectric focusing pH of rabbit sperm differed for cells from the cauda epididymidis and ejaculated semen. Moore and Hibbitt (1975) described differences in the isoelectric focusing pH values of cauda epididymal and ejaculated boar sperm.

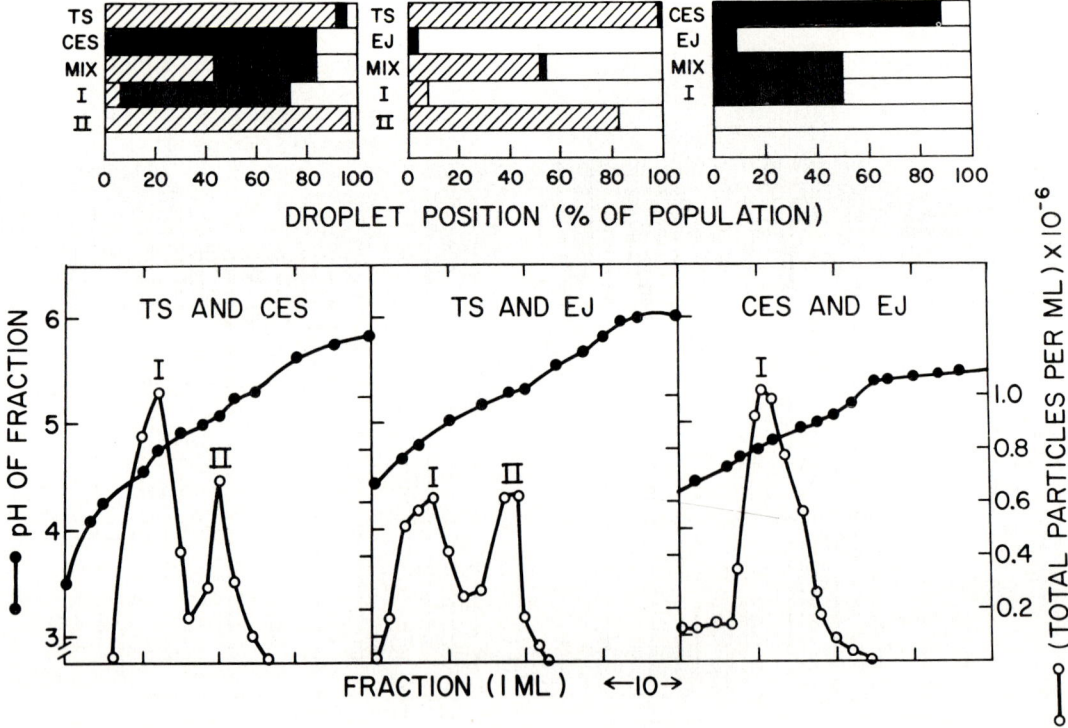

Figure 10. Separation of ram sperm by isoelectric focusing. Testicular (TS), cauda epididymal (CES), and ejaculated (EJ) sperm, obtained by rete testis cannulation, retrograde flush of the vas deferens-distal cauda epididymidis and artificial vagina, were prepared and focussed. The position of the cytoplasmic droplet was determined by phase-contrast microscopy and served as a marker to distinguish TS, CES, and EJ. The percentages of the population having a proximal (diagonal), distal (solid bar), or no (open bar) droplet were determined. Characterized mixtures (MIX) of each paired combination of sperm types were prepared and applied at pH 6 to the preformed pH gradient. After 3 h, 1-ml fractions were collected and analyzed for pH and particle content. Droplet position was noted for the peak (I or II) fraction(s). This separation is representative of four separations of each mixture using sperm from two to four animals. Experimental details are provided elsewhere.[2]

Testicular sperm are characterized by the presence of a proximal cytoplasmic droplet in the neck region. By use of a phase-contrast microscope, testicular sperm can be distinguished readily from cauda epididymidal sperm, most of which have a cytoplasmic droplet at the distal end of the middle piece. Since the distal cytoplasmic droplet normally is lost upon admixture of cauda epididymidal semen with seminal fluid at ejaculation (Bedford, 1975), the two preceding cell types can be distinguished from ejaculated sperm. Mixtures of all paired combinations of these sperm types were characterized. As anticipated from studies of the individual cell types, it was possible to separate testicular from cauda epididymidal sperm, and testicular from ejaculated sperm while cauda epididymidal and ejaculated sperm were isolated as a single peak (Fig. 10). The ability to separate testicular and cauda epididymidal sperm is evidence of an alteration of the glycocalyx of ram sperm during epididymal transit.

GENERAL COMMENTS AND CONCLUSIONS

Physical techniques have been developed that ultimately will be useful for the molecular characterization of three selected zones of the sperm surface. These techniques measure the integrity of the membrane phospholipid bilayer, charge density at the phospholipid-water interface, and charge at the boundary limit of the glycocalyx region. Results of detailed experiments were interpreted as evidence that changes induced in one zone of the plasma membrane do not alter measurements of the other two zones. Thus, physiological or *in vitro* modifications of sperm surfaces can be localized to specific zones of the sperm surface.

Striking differences in ejaculated sperm from different species were detected by ESR spectroscopy. These differences include strength of the phospholipid bilayer, degree of internal compartmentation, protoplasmic viscosity within the cell and charge at the phospholipid-water interface. Whole-cell isoelectric focusing revealed differences in the charge of the glycocalyx zone. Further interspecies comparisons should aid our understanding of the function of sperm membranes. However, since differences among species were found for each parameter examined, great caution should be used when applying these techniques to new systems or when making general physiological interpretations.

All three zones of the plasma membrane are altered during epididymal transit of sperm and further changes probably occur during passage through the female reproductive tract. A molecular explanation of the species differences and maturation-associated changes which were observed is not available. If one accepts the premise that a change in physical properties of a membrane zone results from changes in its chemical composition, then methods have been established that will enable monitoring modification of the sperm surface. These techniques should be useful for studying all phases of the complex events between spermiation and semination by enabling a precise quantification of the changes occurring in the sperm plasma membrane.

REFERENCES

Azzi, A.; Montecucco, C.: Spin Labels and Biological Membranes. Horizons Biochem Biophys 4(1977)266-294

Bangham, A.D.: Electrophoretic Characteristics of Ram and Rabbit Spermatozoa. Proc R Soc, Lond [Biol] 155(1961)292-305

Bedford, J.M.: Maturation, Transport and Fate of Spermatozoa in the Epididymis. In: Handbook of Physiology. Vol. V, Sect. 7, Male Reproductive System, pp. 303-318, ed. by D.W. Hamilton and R.O. Greep. Am Physiol Soc, Washington, D.C., 1975

Bey, E.: The Electrophoretic Mobility of Sperm Cells. In: Cell Electrophoresis, pp. 142-151, ed. by E.J. Ambrose. Brown, Little and Co., Boston, 1965

Ebenshade, K.L.; Clegg, E.D.: Electrophoretic Characterization of Proteins in the Plasma Membrane of Porcine Spermatozoa. J Reprod Fertil 47(1976)333-337

Fawcett, D.W.: The Mammalian Spermatozoon. Dev Biol 44(1975)394-436

Fléchon, J.-E.; Morstin, J.: Localisation des Glycoproteines et des Charges Négatives et Positives dans le Revêtement de Surface des Spermatozoides Ejaculés de Lapin et de Taureau. Ann Histochim 20(1975)291-300

Griffith, O.H.; Wagner, A.S.: Nitroxide Free Radicals: Spin Labels for Probing Biomolecular Structure. Accts Chem Res 2(1969)17-24

Hafs, H.D.; Boyd, L.L.: Galvanic Separation of X- and Y-Chromosome-bearing Sperm. In: Sex Ratio at Birth Prospects for Control, pp. 85-97, ed. by C.A. Kiddy and H.D. Hafs. American Society of Animal Sciences, Champaign, Ill., 1971

Hammerstedt, R.H.: Tritium Release from D[2-^{3}H]Glucose as a Method of Measuring Glucose Consumption by Bovine Sperm. Biol Reprod 12(1975)545-551

Hammerstedt, R.H.; Amann, R.P.; Rucinsky, T.; Morse, P.D., II; Lepock, J.; Snipes, W.; Keith, A.D.: Use of Spin Labels and Electron Spin Resonance Spectroscopy to Characterize Membranes of Bovine Sperm: Effect of Butylated Hydroxytoluene and Cold Shock. Biol Reprod 14(1976)381-397

Hammerstedt, R.H.; Keith, A.D.; Snipes, W.; Amann, R.P.; Arruda, D.; Griel, L.C., Jr.: Use of Spin Labels to Evaluate Effects of Cold Shock and Osmolality on Sperm. Biol Reprod 18(1978)686-696

Herman, C.A.; Zahler, W.L.; Doak, G.A.; Campbell, B.J.: Bull Sperm Adenylate Cyclase: Localization and Partial Characterization. Arch Biochem Biophys 177(1976)622-629

Keith, A.D.; Sharnoff, M.; Cohn, G.: A Summary and Evaluation of Spin Labels used as Probes for Biological Membrane Structure. Biochim Biophys Acta (Biomembrane Reviews) 300(1973)379-419

Lepock, J.R.; Morse, P.D., II; Mehlhorn, R.J.; Hammerstedt, R.H.; Snipes, W.; Keith, A.D.: Spin Labels For Cell Surfaces. FEBS Lett 60(1975)185-189

Lunstra, D.D.; Clegg, E.D.; Morré, D.J.: Isolation of Plasma Membrane from Porcine Spermatozoa. Prep Biochem 4(1974)341-352

Moore, H.D.M.; Hibbitt, K.G.: Isoelectric Focusing of Boar Spermatozoa. J Reprod Fertil 44(1975)329-332

Suominen, J.; Setchell, B.P.: Enzymes and Trypsin Inhibitor in the Rete Testis Fluid of Rams and Boars. J Reprod Fertil 30(1972)235-245

Yanagimachi, R.; Noda, Y.O.; Fujimoto, M.; Nicholson, G.L.: The Distribution of Negative Surface Charges on Mammalian Spermatozoa. Am J Anat 135(1972)497-520

Zahler, W.L.; Doak, G.A.: Isolation of the Outer Acrosomal Membrane from Bull Sperm. Biochim Biophys Acta 406(1975)479-488

CONTRIBUTED PAPERS

PERSISTENCE OF SPERM SURFACE COMPONENTS IN THE EARLY EMBRYO

C.A. Gabel*, E.M. Eddy,** and B.M. Shapiro*

Departments of Biochemistry* and Biological Structure.** University of Washington, Seattle Washington 98195 USA

Spermatozoa are structurally and functionally asymmetric, and their surface heterogeneity presumably reflects the different activities of the plasma membrane in various regions of the cell. The sperm plasma membrane is topographically heterogeneous in terms of lectin binding (Edelman and Millette, 1971; Nicolson et al., 1977; Aketa, 1975), antigen distribution (Koo et al., 1973; Fellous et al., 1975; Koehler, 1975), charge characteristics (Yanagimachi et al., 1972), and intramembranous particle distribution (Koehler and Gaddum-Rosse, 1975; Friend and Fawcett, 1974; Friend, 1977). However, with the paucity of information about the molecular composition of the sperm membrane, nothing is known of the components responsible for its topographic heterogeneity. In addition, despite the many studies showing that the sperm plasma membrane fuses with the egg plasma membrane at fertilization (Franklin, 1965; Colwin and Colwin, 1963; Barros and Franklin, 1968), the fate of the sperm membrane after fusion is unknown. The authors are interested in determining the fate of sperm membrane components, since some of these may play a role in the initiation and continuation of development of the embryo. For example, the site of sperm entry in amphibian eggs partially determines the location of the grey crescent (Clavert, 1962), and this area undergoes subsequent invagination at gastrulation. Since the grey crescent is a fertilization-induced feature of the egg cortex (Curtis, 1960, 1962), sperm surface components may participate, either directly or indirectly, in its formation.

In order to study some components of the sperm surface that might be important in its function, a unique probe has been developed for covalently labelling the exterior of living sperm. With such a reagent, it has been possible to directly and quantitatively determine which sperm components are labelled and to trace their fate after fertilization, by a combination of morphological and biochemical techniques. The authors' approach followed a previous observation that fluorescein isothiocyanate (FITC) could be used to label mammalian spermatozoa without causing loss of motility (Mellish and Baker, 1970; Overstreet and Bedford, 1974). FITC was found to label the sperm of sea urchin and fish, as well as that of mammals, without affecting viability. In order to make the label useful for biochemical analyses of the labelled components as well as for fluorescence microscopy, a radioactive derivative of the fluorochrome has been synthesized (Gabel and Shapiro, 1978). The reagent, ^{125}I-diiodofluorescein isothiocyanate (^{125}I-diI-FITC), has been used in this study to identify the labelled sperm components and to study their transfer to the egg at fertilization.

CHARACTERISTICS OF THE LABELLING REAGENT

When sperm from either the golden hamster or the sea urchin *Strongylocentrotus purpuratus* are treated with FITC or its iodinated derivative, the cells become fluorescent, as shown in Figure 1. However, when the fluorescence micrographs of labelled sperm are compared to the cellular morphology, as seen by scanning electron microscopy (Fig. 1), the binding is seen to be non-uniform, with the majority of the fluorescence occurring in the midpiece region of both kinds of sperm. Therefore, it appears that this region of the sperm is differentiated in terms of its ability to bind the fluorescent probes. Figure 2 shows the structures of two fluorescein derivatives used in this study. FITC is useful for fluorescence microscopy because of its high quantum yield of fluorescence. Diiodo-FITC has a lower quantum yield than FITC as a result of the iodine substitution reaction. However, the derivative can be obtained at a high specific radioactivity, which is useful for biochemical characterization of the labelled cellular components. Figure 3 depicts the reaction by which ^{125}I-diI-FITC combines with amino groups on cells or proteins to produce covalent thiourea derivatives. Although isothiocyanates may also react with sulfhydryl groups (Cecil and McPhee, 1959), the authors believe that the binding of the fluorescein derivatives to sperm is via amino groups. Pretreatment of sea urchin sperm with iodoacetic acid, a reagent that blocks sulfhydryl groups,

---

This research was supported by Grants GM 23910 from the NIH and PCM 7621727 from the NSF; C.A.G. was supported by a National Research Service Award from the National Institutes of Health (GM 07270).

© 1979 Urban & Schwarzenberg, Inc. Baltimore-Munich *The Spermatozoon*, edited by D.W. Fawcett and J.M. Bedford

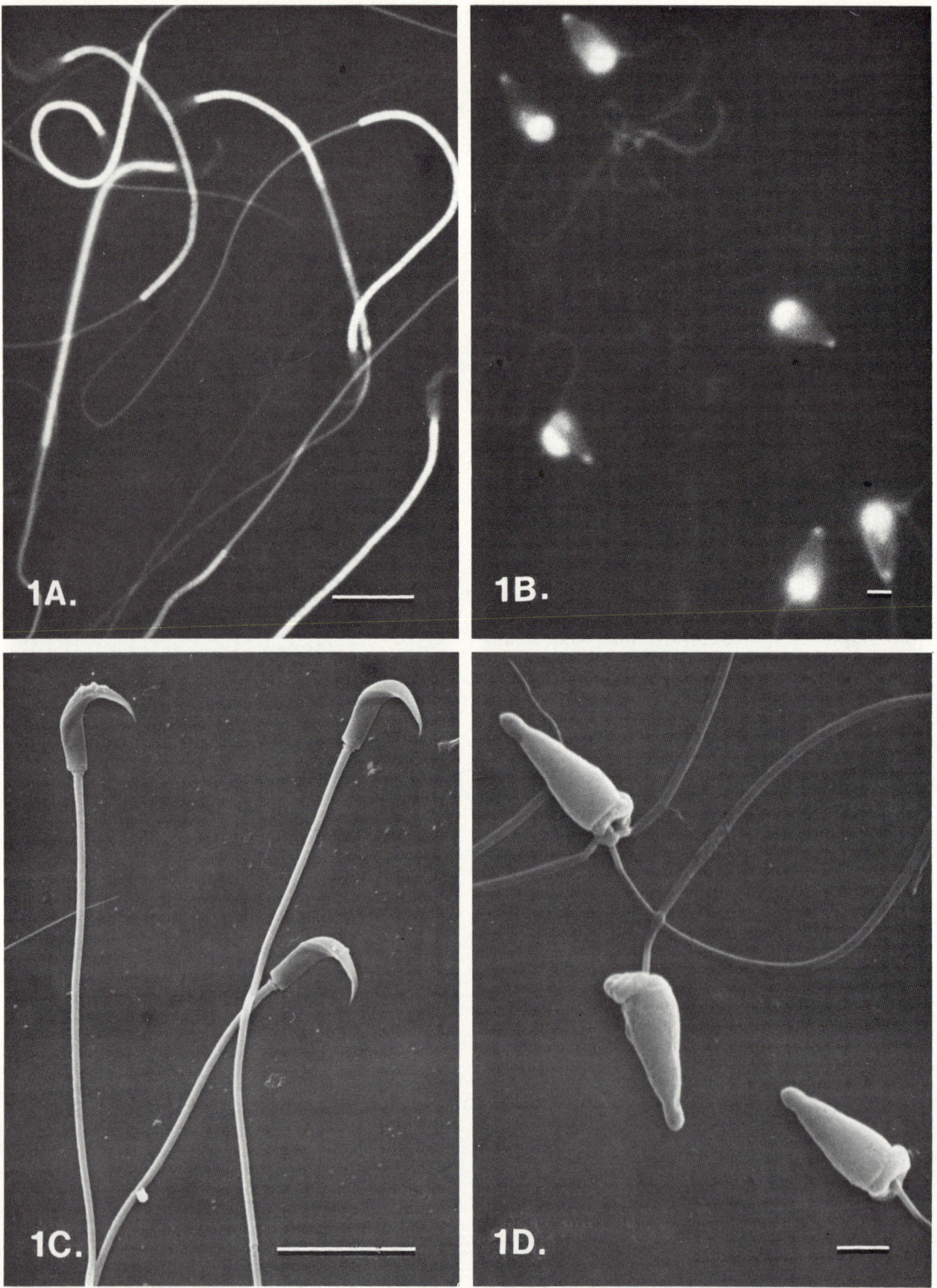

Figure 1. Fluorescent labelling of sperm. Fluorescence micrographs of hamster (A) and sea urchin (B) sperm treated with FITC. Sea urchin sperm (5×10^8/ml) were incubated with 30 μM FITC in 10 mM Tris (hydroxymethyl) aminomethane (TRIS) buffered sea H_2O, pH 8, for 30 min at 12°C. Hamster cauda epididymides sperm (4×10^7/ml) were treated with 13 μM FITC in Tyrodes for 5 min at 37°C. In both cases, excess FITC was removed by centrifuging the sperm and washing the pellets repeatedly. The scanning electron micrographs show the cellular morphology for hamster (C) and sea urchin (D) sperm. The bar equals 10 μM in (A and C) and 1 μM in (B and D).

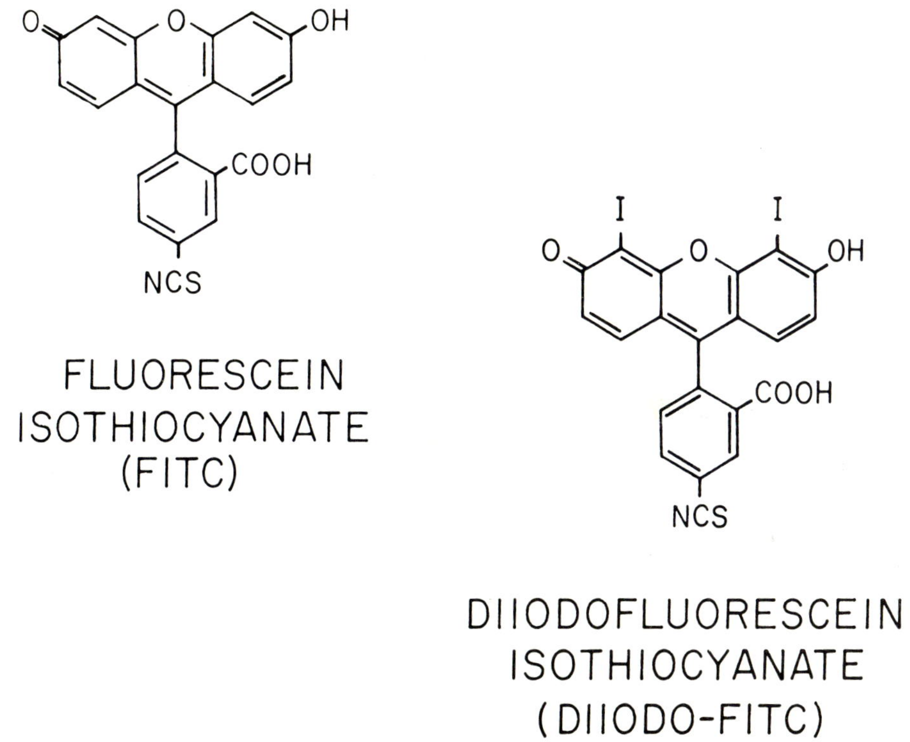

Figure 2. Structure of the fluorescein derivatives.

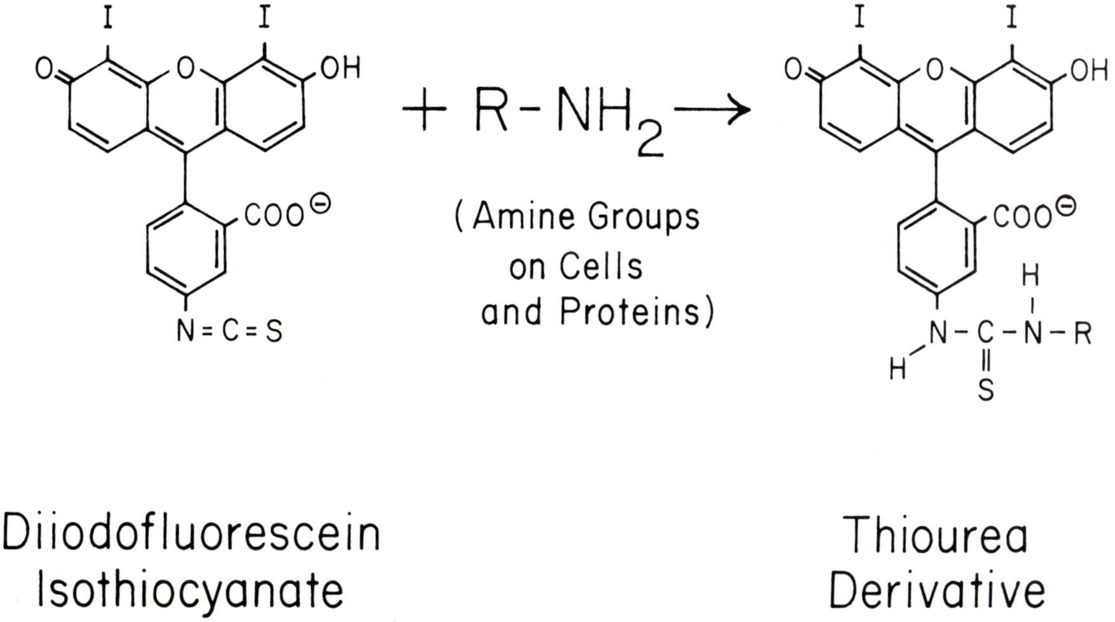

Figure 3. Primary reaction involved in the covalent attachment of diI-FITC to cells and proteins.

did not affect the binding of FITC, whereas pretreatment with acetic anhydride, a reagent that blocks amino groups, prevented FITC from binding.

To trace the fate of the labelled sperm components after fertilization, it was necessary to establish that neither the label, nor the conditions used during labelling, affected the viability of the cells. As shown in Figure 4, sea urchin sperm may be labelled with ^{125}I-diI-FITC under physiological conditions of temperature, pH, and ionic strength, with no loss of viability. This is in contrast to the iodination of sperm by lactoperoxidase, a common surface-labelling technique (Phillips and Morrison, 1970), which is spermicidal to both mammalian (Smith and Klebanoff, 1970) and sea urchin (Shapiro, unpublished results) sperm.

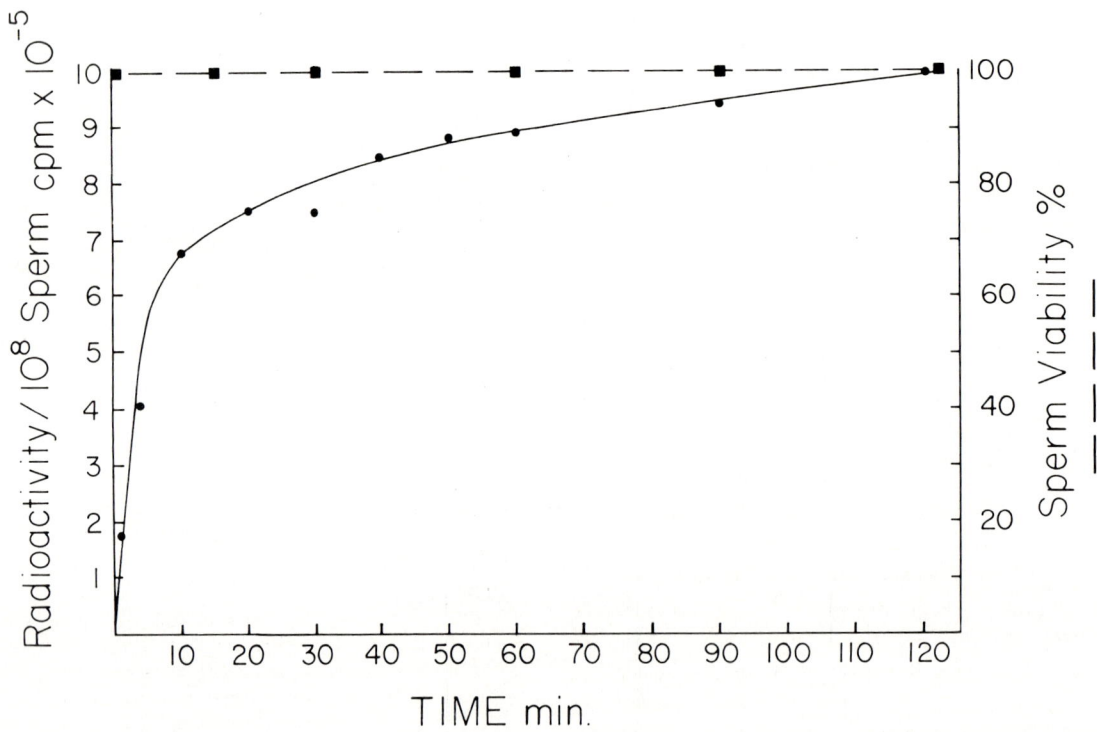

Figure 4. Kinetics of sperm labelling by ^{125}I-diI-FITC. Sea urchin sperm (5×10^8/ml) were incubated with 16 μM ^{125}I-diI-FITC in 10mM Tris-buffered sea H$_2$O, pH 8.0. For estimation of radioactivity, aliquots of the reaction mixture were removed, spotted onto glass-fiber filters, and dropped into an ice bath of 10% trichloroacetic acid (TCA). After all the time points were taken, the filters were washed with two changes of cold 5% TCA, one change of 5% TCA at room temperature, and with one change each of 95% ethanol, acetone, and ether. The filters were dried and counted in a liquid scintillation counter. For estimation of viability, aliquots (containing just enough sperm to give 100% fertilization at time 0) were removed, added to 5 ml of a 1% egg solution, and the % fertilization scored on the basis of the number of eggs elevating fertilization membranes.

NATURE AND LOCATION OF LABELLED SPERM COMPONENTS

The proteins responsible for binding the fluorescent probes were detected by disaggregating ^{125}I-diI-FITC–labelled sperm with sodium dodecyl sulfate (SDS) and analyzing them by polyacrylamide gel electrophoresis. Figures 5A and 6A show the total protein patterns of labelled sea urchin and hamster sperm, respectively, as detected by Coomassie brilliant blue staining of the gels. The corresponding radioautograms (Fig. 5B and 6B) show that only a limited number of polypeptides are labelled by ^{125}I-diI-FITC, as expected, since labelling as seen by fluorescence microscopy is restricted to a specific region of each cell and only surface proteins should be labelled (Gabel and Shapiro, 1978). Also, note in Figure 5B that a large amount of radioactivity bound to sea urchin sperm is associated with a low molecular weight material that does not stain for protein. This probably represents ^{125}I-diI-FITC attached to phospholipids, since 25% of the bound radioactivity of sea urchin sperm is extractable with chloroform/methanol.

It was important to determine whether proteins labelled by ^{125}I-diI-FITC were surface constituents, or components of the sperm cytoplasm. FITC is generally thought not to penetrate cell membranes (Edidin et al., 1976; Peters et al., 1974) and, as shown previously, ^{125}I-diI-FITC does not enter human red blood cells (Gabel and Shapiro, 1978) where labelling is restricted to a surface component.

Because it is difficult to isolate pure preparations of sperm plasma membranes, an immunological approach was used to determine whether diI-FITC was binding to the sperm plasma membrane. Antibodies against diI-FITC were prepared by coupling the label to porcine-γ-globulin and immunizing rabbits with the haptenized protein. The isolated antisera (RADIF) was then used as an indirect immunocytochemical reagent, as described in Figure 7, to determine whether diI-FITC was binding to the surface of sperm. Hamster sperm were treated with diI-FITC, then exposed sequentially to RADIF and goat anti-rabbit IgG conjugated to horseradish peroxidase. The sperm samples were subsequently treated with diaminobenzidine (DAB) and then osmium tetroxide to localize the peroxidase (Graham and Karnovsky, 1966) and the samples were processed for electron microscopy. As shown in Figures 8A and 8B, diI-FITC–labelled sperm treated as described above display a dense, uniform layer of DAB reaction product over the midpiece region of the cells but the staining is faint and patchy elsewhere. Conversely,

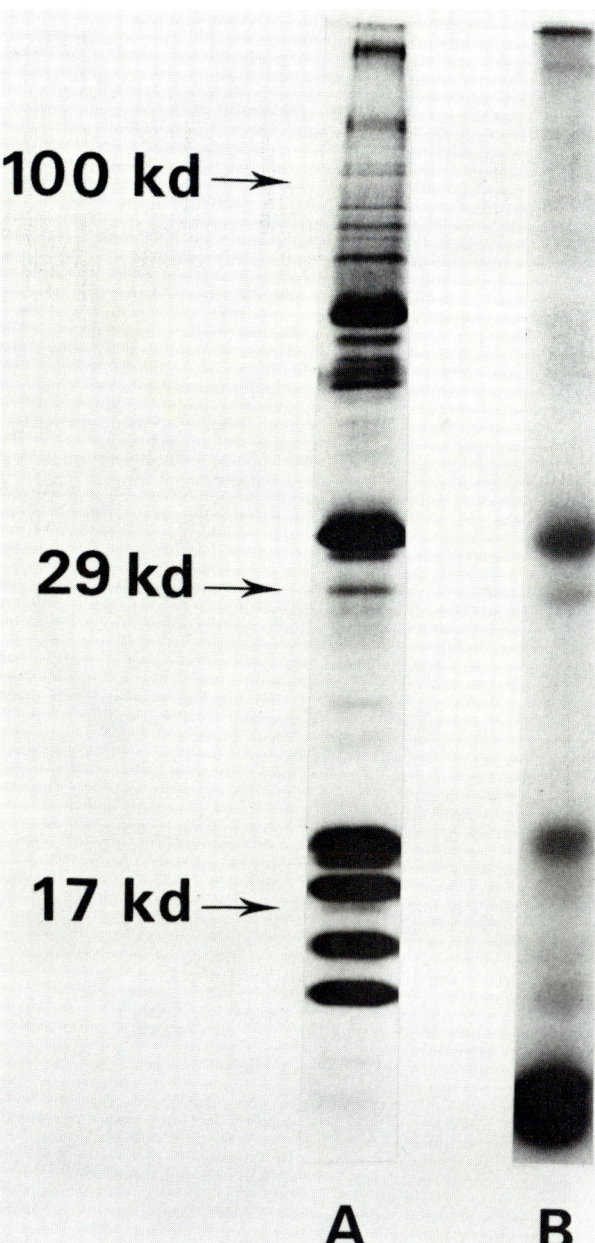

Figure 5. Fractionation of ^{125}I-diI-FITC–labelled sea urchin sperm by SDS-polyacrylamide gel electrophoresis. Sperm (3×10^8/ml) were incubated with 11 μM ^{125}I-diI-FITC in 10mM Tris-buffered sea H$_2$O for 30 min at 12°C. To remove excess label, the reaction mixture was applied to a small Sephadex G-25 column equilibrated in sea H$_2$O. The labelled sperm pass directly through the column, whereas free label is absorbed to the Sephadex resin and remains at the top of the column. The eluted sperm were subsequently disaggregated and electrophoresed (as described earlier, Gabel and Shapiro, 1978) on a 12.5% polyacrylamide slab gel. (A) Protein pattern detected by Coomassie brilliant blue staining. (B) Radioautogram of the gel showing the proteins labelled by ^{125}I-diI-FITC.

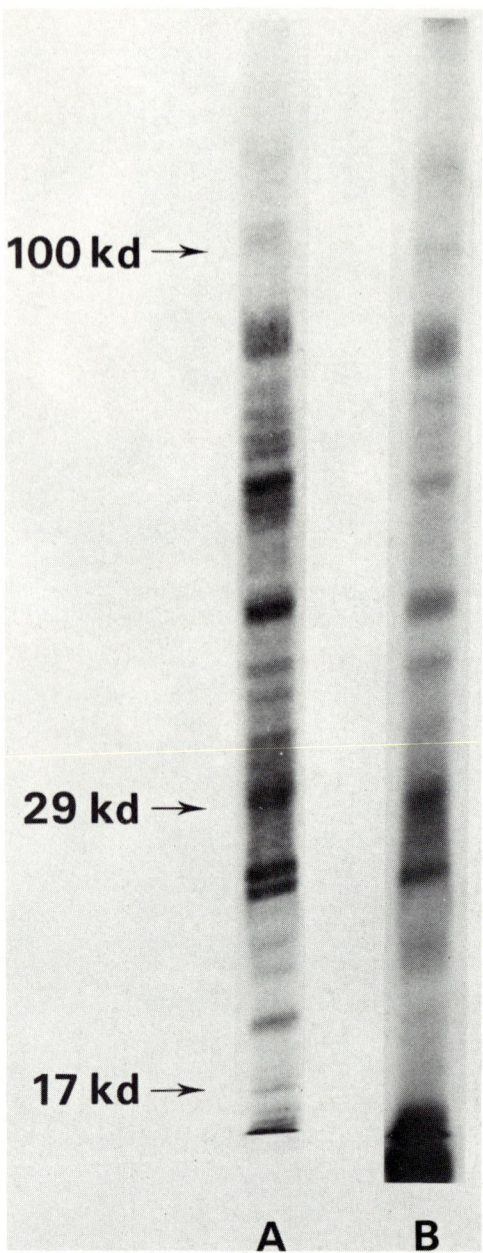

Figure 6. Fractionation of ^{125}I-diI-FITC labelled hamster sperm by SDS-polyacrylamide gel electrophoresis. Sperm were labelled as described in the legend to Figure 1, except ^{125}I-diI-FITC was used in place of FITC. The labelled cells were electrophoresed, as described in the legend to Figure 5, on a 10-15% polyacrylamide gradient slab gel. (A) Protein pattern detected by Coomassie brilliant blue staining. (B) Radioautogram of the same gel.

when unlabelled sperm are treated with the antibodies and DAB, little, if any, staining is detected (Figure 8C). Therefore, the localization of diI-FITC to the midpiece by the indirect immunocytochemical method agrees with the fluorescence localization and suggests that the plasma membrane is differentiated in this region of the cell in terms of its ability to bind diI-FITC.

In a final test as to whether diI-FITC is labelling surface components of spermatozoa, sea urchin sperm were used in an agglutination assay. Table 1 shows that diI-FITC–labelled, RADIF-treated sperm could be agglutinated, in a concentration-dependent manner, by goat anti-rabbit IgG, whereas, unlabelled cells could not be agglutinated. Hence, as with hamster sperm, at least some of the diI-FITC–labelled sperm components are on the surface where they are accessible to antibody molecules.

PERSISTENCE OF THE LABEL THROUGH EARLY DEVELOPMENT

Since ^{125}I-diI-FITC–labelled sea urchin sperm remain viable, it allows us to ask whether the labelled sperm surface components are transferred to the egg at fertilization. As shown in Figure 9, not only are the labelled sperm components transferred to the fertilized egg, but the specific radioactivity of the embryos remains constant throughout early development, suggesting that the labelled sperm components remain associated with the developing embryos. It should be noted that the specific radioactivity of the embryos corresponds to one sperm per fertilized egg, a ratio that agrees well with the known biology of the system.

To obtain additional evidence as to whether the radioactivity associated with these eggs is due to ^{125}I-diI-FITC–labelled components contributed by the fertilizing spermatozoa, sea urchin eggs were fertilized with labelled sperm and then fixed and sectioned for radioautography. Figure 10 shows a cross section of an egg in which the fertilizing sperm has fused with, but not completely penetrated, the egg surface. Silver grains are present in the vicinity of the penetrating spermatozoa. This can be interpreted as direct evidence that the fertilizing sperm is transferring ^{125}I-diI-FITC–labelled components to the egg at fertilization.

The transfer of radioactive sperm components was further analyzed by fertilizing sea urchin eggs with ^{125}I-diI-FITC–labelled sperm at different sperm per egg ratios. One would intuitively predict that prior to the sperm concentration at which polyspermy begins to occur, the amount of radioactivity transferred should be constant and independent of the sperm per egg ratio at fertilization, since only one sperm fertilizes each egg. However, as shown in Figure 11, the amount of radioactivity transferred is dependent upon the sperm per egg ratio, even at values that should not (and did not, since normal development occurred) result in polyspermic eggs. To exclude the possibility that the egg-

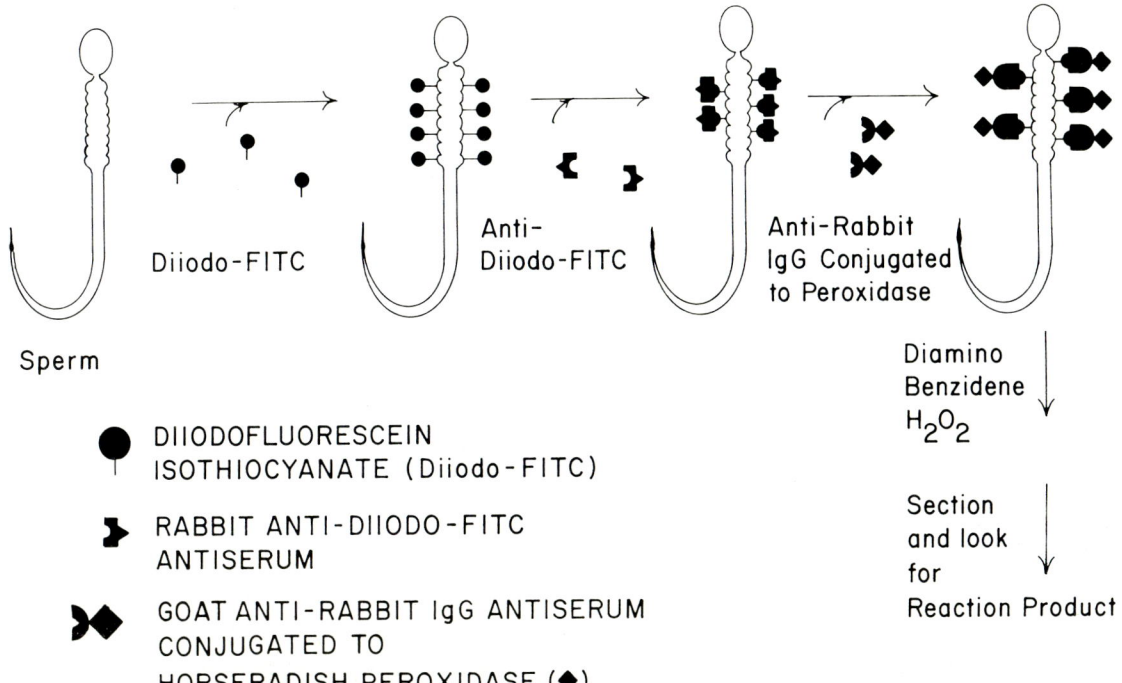

Figure 7. Scheme of the indirect immunoelectron microscopic sandwich labelling method used to detect diI-FITC on hamster sperm.

associated radioactivity was due to the binding of free ^{125}I-diI-FITC, which might be present in association with the sperm, labelled sperm were heat treated to destroy their fertilizing capacity and then added to unfertilized eggs. After incubation of the dead sperm and eggs for 7 min, viable, nonlabelled sperm were added to initiate development. As shown in Figure 11, although there was some radioactivity associated with these embryos after hatching (possibly due to contaminating sperm), it was much less than the amount present in eggs fertilized with viable, labelled cells. Therefore, at ratios of sperm per egg greater than 100/1, spermatozoa other than the fertilizing one may contribute labelled components to the egg. This may indicate that the many sperm that transiently bind to an egg during fertilization can contribute components to the egg surface prior to being dislodged as the result of activation of the systems possessed by sea urchin eggs to prevent polyspermy (Foerder and Shapiro, 1977).

Finally, to demonstrate that the radioactivity associated with developing sea urchin embryos is not due to free ^{125}I-diI-FITC or to labelled protein degradation products, embryos developing from eggs fertilized with ^{125}I-diI-FITC–labelled sperm were homogenized and the insoluble components were separated by centrifugation. As shown in Table 2, the majority of the radioactivity associated with both blastula and pluteus larvae is not soluble, as would be expected for free label or labelled amino acids, but rather, is associated with insoluble cellular material. In addition, a large percentage of the soluble radioactivity in pluteus larvae is acid precipitable, suggesting that it is protein bound. Furthermore, if the ^{125}I-diI-FITC–labelled sperm proteins were degraded by enzymes within the egg, the labelled

Table 1. Agglutination of diI-FITC Labelled Sea Urchin Sperm

Dilution of Goat Anti-rabbit Antiserum	$1/3$	$1/9$	$1/27$	$1/81$	$1/243$	$1/729$	$1/2187$
Labelled Sperm	−	+	+	+	+	+	−
Unlabelled Sperm	−	−	−	−	−	−	−

DiI-FITC–labelled (or unlabelled) sperm were treated with RADIF (60 min at 12°C) and then washed three times with sea H_2O to remove excess antibody. The final sperm pellets were re-suspended in sea H_2O; then, 25 μl of each sperm solution was added to 50 μl of sea H_2O containing goat anti-rabbit IgG, at the indicated dilution. After 30 min at 12°C, the sperm solutions were scored under a dissecting microscope for agglutination (+ indicates agglutination did occur).

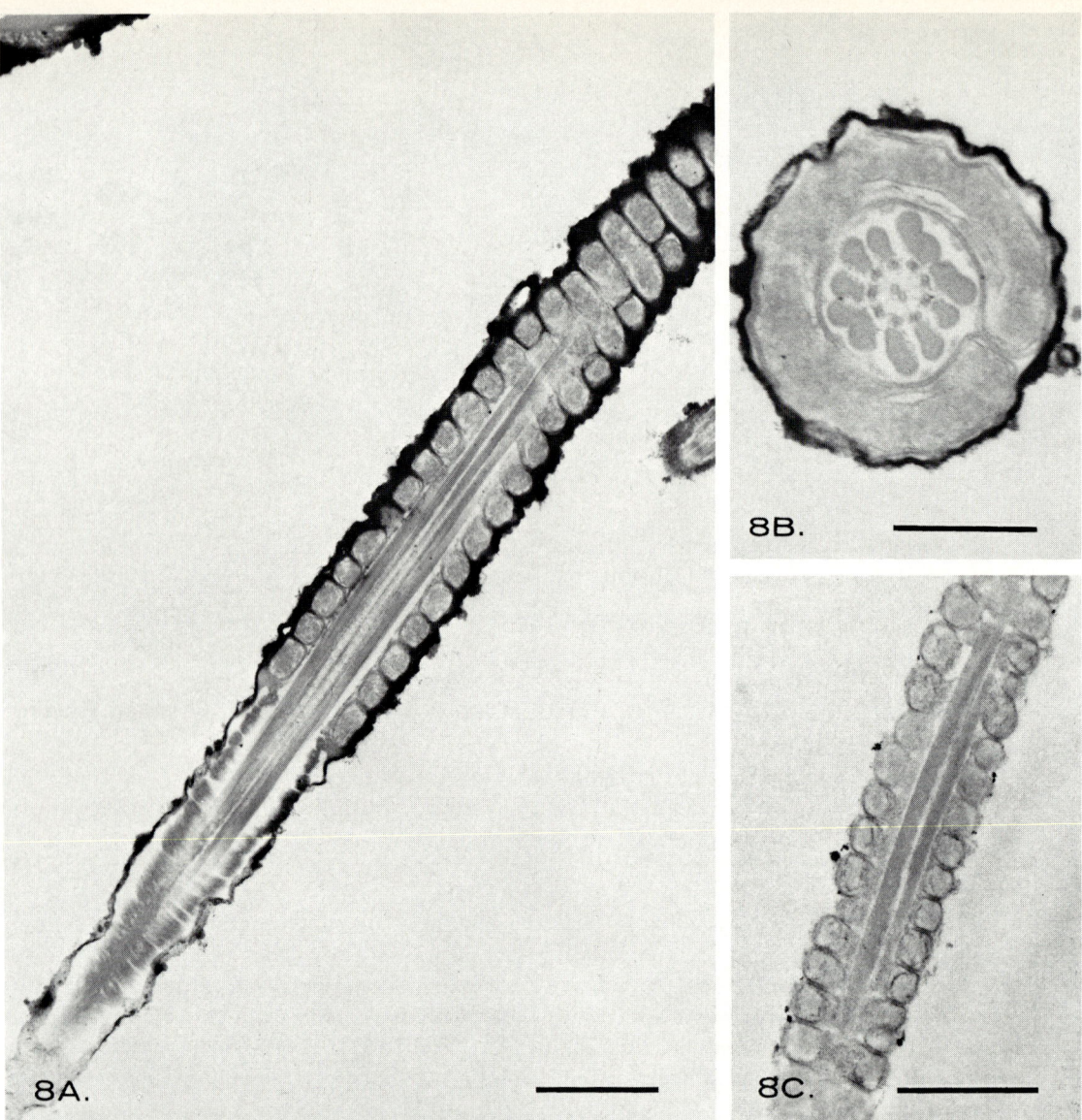

Figure 8. Electron microscopic cytochemical localization of diI-FITC to the hamster sperm surface. Hamster sperm, treated as described in Figure 7, were sectioned (but not stained) and scored for the presence of the DAB-reaction product. (A) Longitudinal section through the posterior end of the midpiece and anterior portion of the principal piece showing the dense layer of DAB-reaction product associated with the midpiece. (B) Cross section through the sperm midpiece. (C) Longitudinal section through the midpiece of a sperm that was treated as above except that the sperm preparation was not labelled with diI-FITC. Note the absence of the DAB-reaction product. The bar equals 1 μM in (A and C) and 0.5 μM in (B).

Figure 10. Radioautography of sea urchin eggs fertilized with ^{125}I-diI-FITC labelled sperm. Eggs were treated with 1 M glycerol, adjusted to pH 9.0 with NH_4OH, to induce polyspermy then fertilized with ^{125}I-diI-FITC-labelled sperm. After 3 min, the eggs were fixed and sections were prepared for radioautography. (A) Section of a ^{125}I-diI-FITC-labelled sea urchin sperm. (B) Section of an egg with a fertilizing sperm still visible. Note the silver grains in the area of the penetrating sperm. The bar equals 10 μM in both (A) and (B).

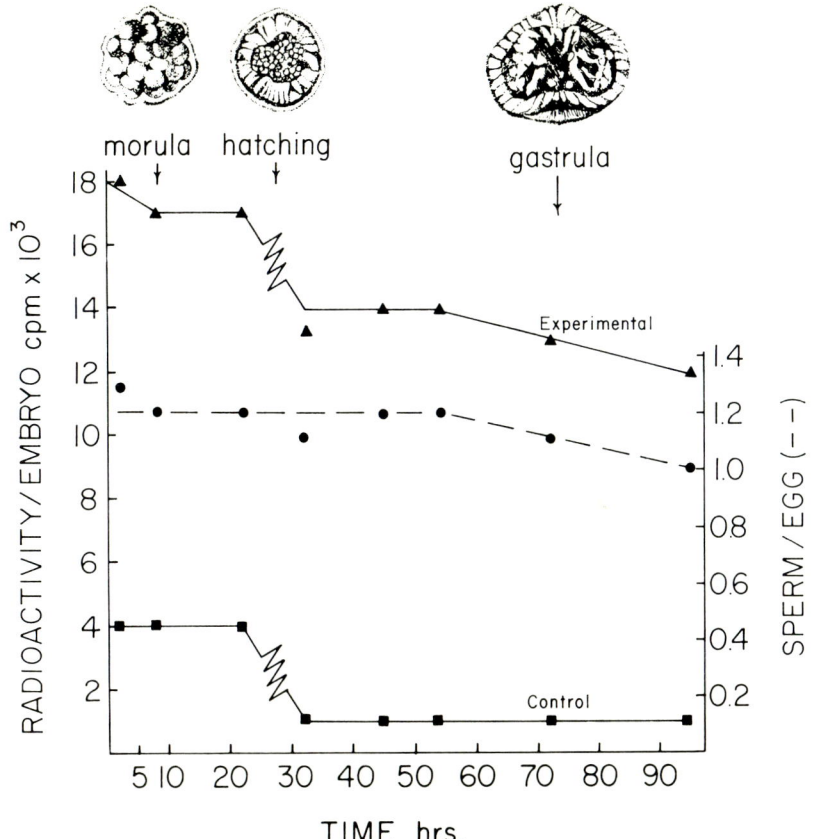

Figure 9. Persistence of ^{125}I-diI-FITC labelled sperm components with the developing sea urchin embryo. Sperm labelled with ^{125}I-diI-FITC were added to unfertilized eggs and, after 7 min, the eggs were diluted in a large volume of sea H$_2$O. When the eggs settled, the supernatant was removed and the eggs were resuspended in fresh sea H$_2$O. The washing was repeated four times, after which the eggs were resuspended in sea H$_2$O containing 50 µg/ml of penicillin and streptomycin and allowed to develop at 12°C. At the indicated times, aliquots of the culture were removed and the embryos were killed by the addition of CN$^-$. The dead embryos were collected by hand centrifugation, resuspended in a small volume of sea H$_2$O, layered onto 10 ml of 5% Ficoll in sea H$_2$O, and again collected by centrifugation. The final embryo pellet was washed once with sea H$_2$O, then aliquots were removed and counted to determine the radioactivity present/embryo (—▲—▲—). For the control curve (—■—■—), the eggs were fertilized with unlabelled sperm and, after 7 min, ^{125}I-diI-FITC labelled sperm, equivalent to the amount used in the experimental culture, were added and the eggs treated as described above. The sperm per egg curve (—●—●—) was calculated by subtracting the control curve from the experimental and dividing by the specific radioactivity of the sperm solution (1.1 x 10^{-2} cpm/sperm).

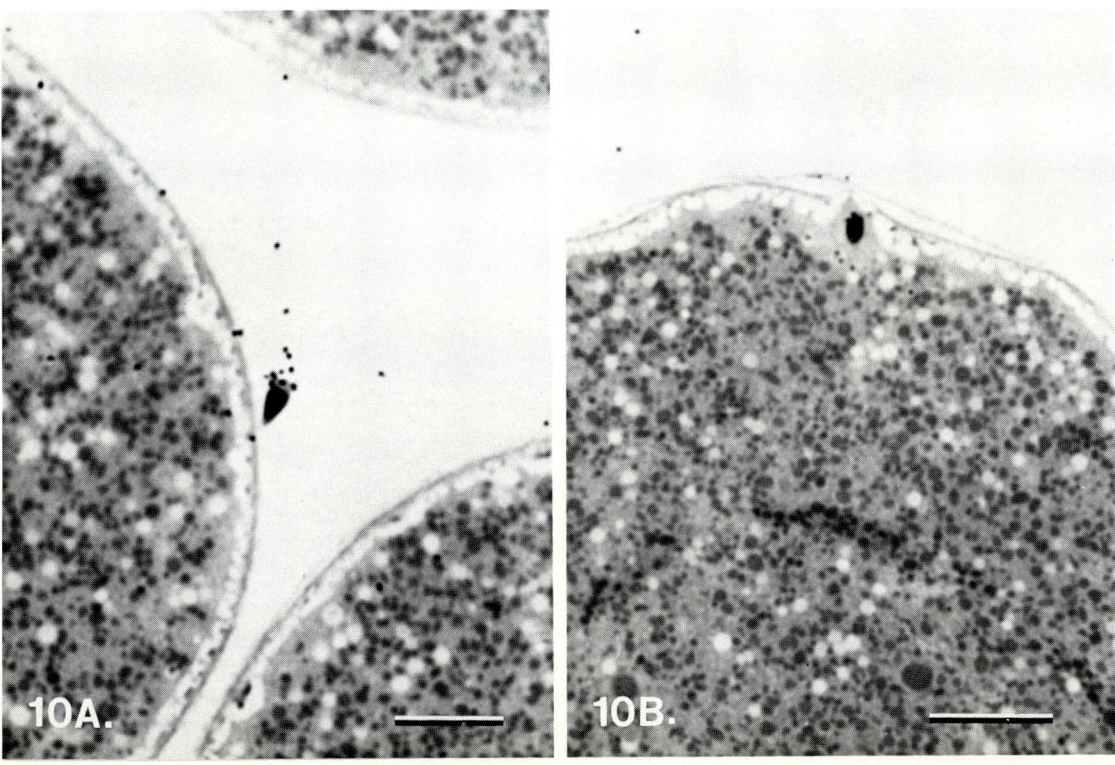

Table 2. Fractionation of Labelled Embryos

	CPM	%
Experiment 1		
Total Gastrula Larvae	447	100
Supernatant (27,000 g)	113	25
Pellet (27,000 g)	280	63
Experiment 2		
Total Pluteus Larvae	2545	100
Supernatant (100,000 g)	270	11
Pellet (100,000 g)	2063	81
TCA Precipitate of 100,000 g Supernatant	250	—

Sea urchin eggs were fertilized with ^{125}I-diI-FITC–labelled sperm and washed and cultured as described in Figure 9. The embryos were harvested by hand centrifugation at either the gastrula (Experiment 1) or pluteus (Experiment 2) larval stages and homogenized with 50 mM Tris, pH 6.8, containing 0.1 mM phenylmethyl sulfonyl fluoride, and 10 mM ethylenediaminetetraacetic acid. The homogenates were subsequently centrifuged at the indicated speeds, and counted to determine the amount of radioactivity present in each fraction. In Experiment 2, the supernatant was made 10% with TCA after counting and the precipitated protein was collected by centrifugation and re-counted.

amino acids would probably not be re-incorporated into other egg proteins due to the specificity of the protein synthesizing machinery (von Ehrenstein, 1970) which should not recognize the derivatized residues. However, the radioactivity associated with the developing embryos is not soluble, and the ^{125}I-diI-FITC–labelled sperm components remain as macromolecules. Additionally, the finding that a large amount of radioactivity is associated with the pellet fractions of homogenized embryos is consistent with the other evidence that ^{125}I-diI-FITC is labelling membrane components.

SUMMARY

The use of ^{125}I-diI-FITC as a covalent probe for components of the sperm surface offers several advantages over other currently available techniques for studying cell surfaces. First, because the probe forms stable covalent linkages with the modified cellular components, the nature of these components may be determined by standard biochemical fractionations and, by analysis of

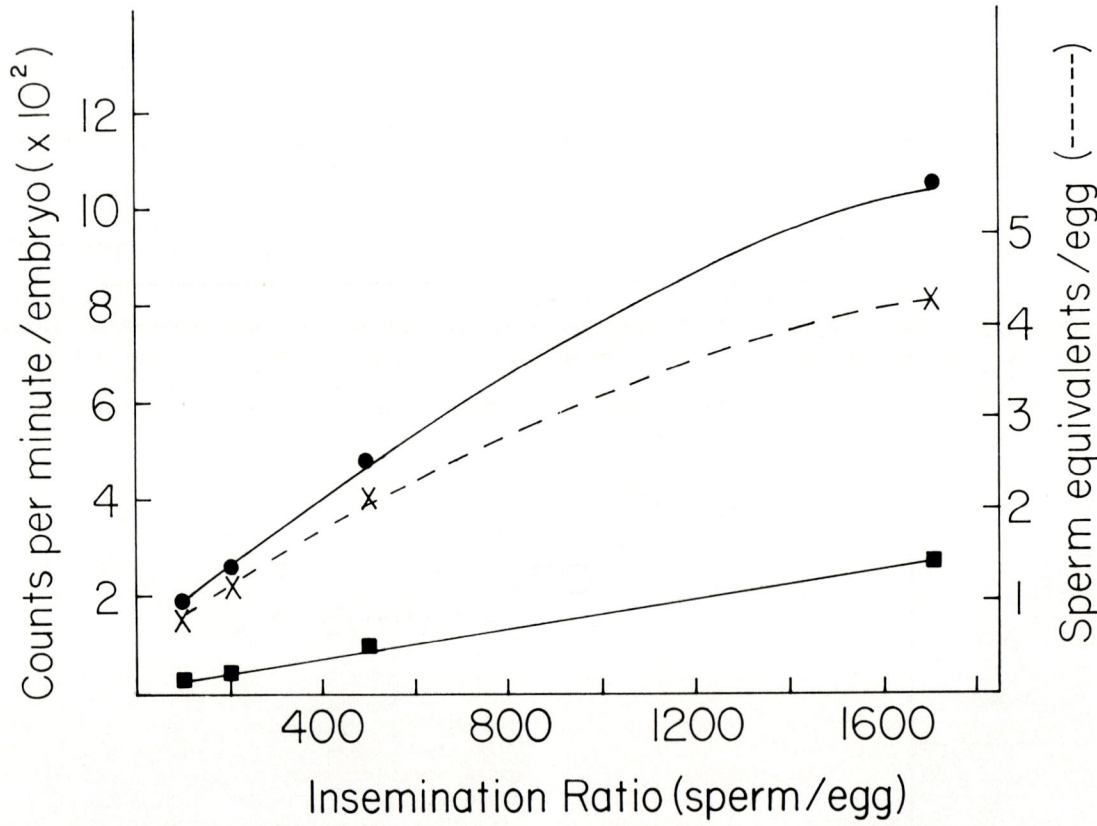

Figure 11. Effect of the ratio of ^{125}I-diI-FITC labelled sperm/egg at fertilization on the specific activity of hatched blastulae. Experimental embryos (—●—●—) were fertilized with ^{125}I-diI-FITC–labelled sperm at the indicated ratios, washed to remove supernumerary sperm, then allowed to develop. After hatching, the embryos were harvested, as described in the legend to Figure 9, and counted to determine the specific radioactivity of the embryos (counts per minute per embryo). Control embryos (—■—■—) were incubated for 7 min with ^{125}I-diI-FITC–labelled sperm which had previously been heat treated (56°C for 5 min) to kill them. The eggs were subsequently fertilized with unlabelled sperm and processed as above. The number of sperm equivalents per egg present at each point (—x—x—) was arrived at by taking the difference of the two curves and dividing that by the specific radioactivity of the sperm solution (1.9 x 10^{-2} cpm/sperm).

radioactivity, the amount of binding to a specific component can be easily quantitated. Second, because diI-FITC is both fluorescent and antigenic, the location of the modified components within the cell can be determined by a combination of fluorescence and immuno-electron microscopy. Finally, because the probe reacts with surface components under physiological conditions, labelled sperm can be obtained which are viable and capable of effecting fertilization.

Preliminary data presented in this Chapter indicate that plasma membrane components in the region of the midpiece of sperm from two animals in widely separated phyla preferentially bind the fluorescein derivative. The significance of this binding is unknown, but it may indicate that there are common characteristics in the midpiece region of spermatozoa from these animals. Additionally, ^{125}I-diI-FITC-labelled components of sea urchin sperm are transferred to the egg at fertilization and remain associated with the developing embryo. It thus is of interest to localize these components within the embryo and to determine what role, if any, they play in development.

REFERENCES

Aketa, K.: Physiological Studies and the Sperm Surface Components Responsible for Sperm-Egg Bonding in Sea Urchin Fertilization. Exp Cell Res 90(1975)56-62

Barros, C.; Franklin, L.E.: Behavior of the Gamete Membranes during Sperm Entry into the Mammalian Egg. J Cell Biol 37(1968)c13-c18

Cecil, R.; McPhee, J.R.: The Sulfur Chemistry of Proteins. Adv Protein Chem 14(1959)255-390

Clavert, J.: Symmetrization of the Egg of Vertebrates. Adv Morphol 2(1962)27-60

Colwin, L.H.; Colwin, A.L.: Role of the Gamete Membrane in Fertilization in *Saccoglossus kowalevskii* (Enteropneusta). J Cell Biol 19(1963)501-518

Curtis, A.S.G.: Cortical Grafting in *Xenopus laevis*. J Embryol Exp Morph 8(1960)163-173

Curtis, A.S.G.: Morphogenetic Interactions before Gastrulation in the Amphibian *Xenopus laevis*—the Cortical Field. J Embryol Exp Morphol 10(1962)410-423

Edelman, G.M.; Millette, C.F.: Molecular Probes of Spermatozoan Structures. Proc Natl Acad Sci USA 68(1971)2436-2440

Edidin, M.; Zagyansky, Y.; Lardner, T.J.: Measurement of Membrane Protein Lateral Diffusion in Single Cells. Science 191(1976)466-468

Fellous, M.; Gachelin, G.; Buc, M.H.; Dubois, P.; Jacob, F.: Similar Location of an Early Embryonic Antigen on Mouse and Human Spermatozoa. Dev Biol 41(1975)331-337

Foerder, C.M.; Shapiro, B.M.: Release of Ovoperoxidase from Sea Urchin Eggs Hardens the Fertilization Membrane with Tyrosine Crosslinks. Proc Natl Acad Sci USA 74(1977)4214-4218

Franklin, L.E.: Morphology of Gamete Membrane Fusion and of Sperm Entry into Oocytes of the Sea Urchin. J Cell Biol 25(1965)81-100

Friend, D.S.: The Organization of the Spermatozoal Membrane. In: Immunobiology of Gametes, pp. 5-30, ed. by M. Edidin and M.H. Johnson. Cambridge University Press, Cambridge-London-New York-Melbourne, 1977.

Friend, D.S.; Fawcett, D.W.: Membrane Differentiations in Freeze-fractured Mammalian Sperm. J Cell Biol 63(1974)641-664

Gabel, C.A.; Shapiro, B.M.: [^{125}I]Diiodofluorescein Isothiocyanate: Its Synthesis and Use as a Reagent for Labelling Proteins and Cells to High Specific Radioactivity. Anal Biochem 86(1978)396-406

Graham, R.C.; Karnovsky, M.J.: The Early Stages of Absorption of Injected Horseradish Peroxidase in the Proximal Tubules of Mouse Kidney: Ultrastructural Cytochemistry by a New Technique. J Histochem Cytochem 14(1966)291-302

Koehler, J.K.: Studies on the Distribution of Antigenic Sites on the Surface of Rabbit Spermatozoa. J Cell Biol 67(1975)647-659

Koehler, J.K.; Gaddum-Rosse, P.: Media-induced Alterations of the Membrane-associated Particles of the Guinea Pig Sperm Tail. J Ultrastruct Res 51(1975)106-118

Koo, G.C.; Stackpole, C.W.; Boyse, E.A.; Hammerling, U.; Lardis, M.P.: Topographical Location of H-Y Antigen on Mouse Spermatozoa by Immunoelectronmicroscopy. Proc Natl Acad Sci USA 70(1973)1502-1505

Mellish, K.S.; Baker, R.D.: Marking Boar Spermatozoa with Fluorochromes for Evaluating Spermatozoan Transport Within Gilts. J Anim Sci 31(1970)917-922

Nicolson, G.L.; Usui, N.; Yanagimachi, R.; Yanagimachi, H.; Smith, J.R.: Lectin Binding Sites on the Plasma Membranes of Rabbit Spermatozoa. J Cell Biol 74(1977)950-962

Overstreet, J.W.; Bedford, J.M.: Transport, Capacitation and Fertilizing Ability of Epididymal Spermatozoa. J Exp Zool 189(1974)203-213

Peters, R.; Peters, J.; Tews, K.H.; Bähr, W.: A Microfluorimetric Study of Translational Diffusion in Erythrocyte Membranes. Biochim Biophys Acta 367(1974)282-294

Phillips, D.R.; Morrison, M.: The Arrangement of Proteins in the Human Erythrocyte Membrane. Biochem Biophys Res Commun 40(1970)284-289

Smith, D.C.; Klebanoff, S.Y.: A Uterine Fluid-mediated Sperm-inhibitory System. Biol Reprod 3(1970)229-235

von Ehrenstein G.: Transfer RNA and Amino Acid Activation. In: Aspects of Protein Biosynthesis, pp. 139-214, ed. by C.B. Anfinsen, Jr. Academic Press, New York and London, 1970

Yanagimachi, R.; Noda, Y.D.; Fujimoto, M.; Nicolson, G.L.: The Distribution of Negative Surface Charges on Mammalian Spermatozoa. Am J Anat 135(1972)497-520

SEROLOGICAL ANALYSIS OF THE EXPRESSION OF T/t LOCUS ANTIGENS ON SPERMATOGENIC CELLS OF THE MOUSE

G.B. Dooher

Sloan-Kettering Institute for Cancer Research, New York, New York 10021 USA

Mouse spermatozoa display unique, serologically detectable surface antigens specified by both mutant and wild-type genetic factors at the T/t locus on chromosome 17 (Bennett et al., 1972; Yanagisawa et al., 1974). Mutations within this complex genetic region have two seemingly paradoxical effects on male germ cells. Most recessive embryonic lethal t-factors in heterozygous males must impart some sort of functional advantage to spermatozoa that carry them since these gametes fertilize a much higher proportion of oocytes than their +−bearing counterparts, a phenomenon known as transmission ratio distortion (Bennett and Dunn, 1971). On the other hand, males that carry two different lethal or semi-lethal t-factors are invariably sterile. Spermatozoa develop abnormally (Dooher and Bennett, 1977) and appear unable to interact successfully with oocytes even under conditions of artificial insemination (Olds, 1971). The reproductive biology of female mice is unaffected by T/t mutations.

Despite the deleterious effects of many t-haplotypes, these factors occur in high frequency in most wild populations of mice; thus they are important constituents of the mouse genome, not mere laboratory curiosities. Recessive lethal mutations can be placed into one of six complementation groups; members of each complementation group produce similar syndromes of embryonic lethality in homozygotes and distort their own transmission through heterozygous males in a characteristic way. Members of different complementation groups permit viability in a proportion of double heterozygotes (t^x/t^y).

Genetical analysis of the T/t locus has been hampered because many recessive mutations suppress recombination within a large stretch of chromosome extending from the T-region to the H-2 complex (the major histocompatibility complex of the mouse). Clues to the organization of the T/t locus have been obtained recently, however, by taking advantage of the fact that t-factors specify antigens on spermatozoa that can be analyzed using serological probes. It has been shown previously by complement-mediated cytotoxicity tests and by absorption analysis with spermatozoa and t-specific antisera, that antigens coded by two different lethal t-factors (t^0, t^{w18}) share certain "public" serological specificities while also retaining unique specificities that appear to be related to embryonic lethality (Artzt and Bennett, 1977). Thus serological techniques provide another approach for defining member-haplotypes within complementation groups as well as providing new criteria by which different complementation groups may be distinguished.

The observation that t-specific antigens occur only on spermatozoa and not on any somatic cells, as well as the phenomena of transmission ratio distortion and of male sterility suggest a role for the T/t locus in the differentiation of male germ cells. Therefore, the author and colleagues have begun to examine the expression of t-antigens during spermatogenesis. Using this approach they have begun to determine whether t-antigens are continuously displayed on the surfaces of male germ cells during spermatogenesis or appear in association with specific differentiative events. They have continued to explore the serological interrelationships among antigenic determinants specified by t-haplotypes of different complementation groups with an aim to illuminating the genetics of this complex region. Finally they have asked whether antiserum, specific for cell surface components determined by one member of a complementation group can distinguish antigenic differences among other member mutations which, by genetic and embryological criteria, are identical.

MATERIALS AND METHODS

Antisera were prepared by immunizing normal female mice (+/+ with respect to the T/t locus) with testicular cells from males heterozygous for the lethal t-factor t^{w12} (genotype $T\,tf/t^{w12}+$). *Tufted* (tf) is a linked recessive marker which in homozygotes produces a characteristic pattern of hair loss and replacement in adults. This t-mutation is a member of the t^{w1} complementation group which also contains the independently derived

---

This work was supported by NSF Grant BMS 16354 and NIH Grants HD 10669-01 and CA 08748-12. The author thanks Althea Dimeo, Marilyn Lockwood, and Florence Morgenstern for technical assistance.

© 1979 Urban & Schwarzenberg, Inc. Baltimore-Munich *The Spermatozoon*, edited by D.W. Fawcett and J.M. Bedford

haplotypes designated t^{w1} and t^{w71}. To remove nonspecific activity against testicular cells serum was absorbed with testicular cells ($T\,tf/++$ or $+/+$) prior to use in cytotoxicity tests and absorption analysis. To circumvent the possibility that sera might also recognize antigens shared by somatic cells, preabsorption with $T\,tf/t^{w12}+$ and $T\,tf/++$ splenocytes was also performed. Testicular cells were prepared as targets for cytotoxocity tests and absorption analysis by sequential incubation of seminiferous tubules in collagenase and trypsin, followed by mechanical dissociation according to the methods of Romrell et al. (1976) with modifications developed by the author. Cytotoxicity tests were performed using absorbed rabbit serum (Boyse et al., 1970) as the source of complement, and trypan blue exclusion as the criterion for viability.

OBSERVATIONS

Antiserum obtained from a hyperimmunized female mouse (#64, BTBRTF/Nev $+/+$) showed significant reactivity specific for $T\,tf/t^{w12}+$ testicular cells after appropriate absorptions were carried out to remove nonspecific cytotoxic activity. Figure 1 shows a typical titration of this serum tested against $T\,tf/t^{w12}+$ and $T\,tf/++$ testicular cells. Results are given as cytotoxic indices which show the proportion of cells lysed specifically after the percentage of dead cells in the complement controls has been subtracted. A cytotoxic index of 0.10 or less is considered to be negative. Although this serum is still active against $T\,tf/t^{w12}+$ testicular cells at a dilution of 1/128, the serum kills less than half of the cells available for killing at all serum dilutions tested, a characteristic feature of anti-t-antisera since this system is, serologically speaking, a weak one.

To test the possibility that t-haplotypes function in very early germ cells (spermatogonia) as well as at later stages of differentiation, spermatogonia were obtained from testes of 10-day old $T\,tf/t^{w12}+$ mice. Testes at this age contain no later stages of spermatogenesis. Anti-t^{w12} serum shows cytotoxic activity against spermatogonia comparable to that seen when testicular cells from adult

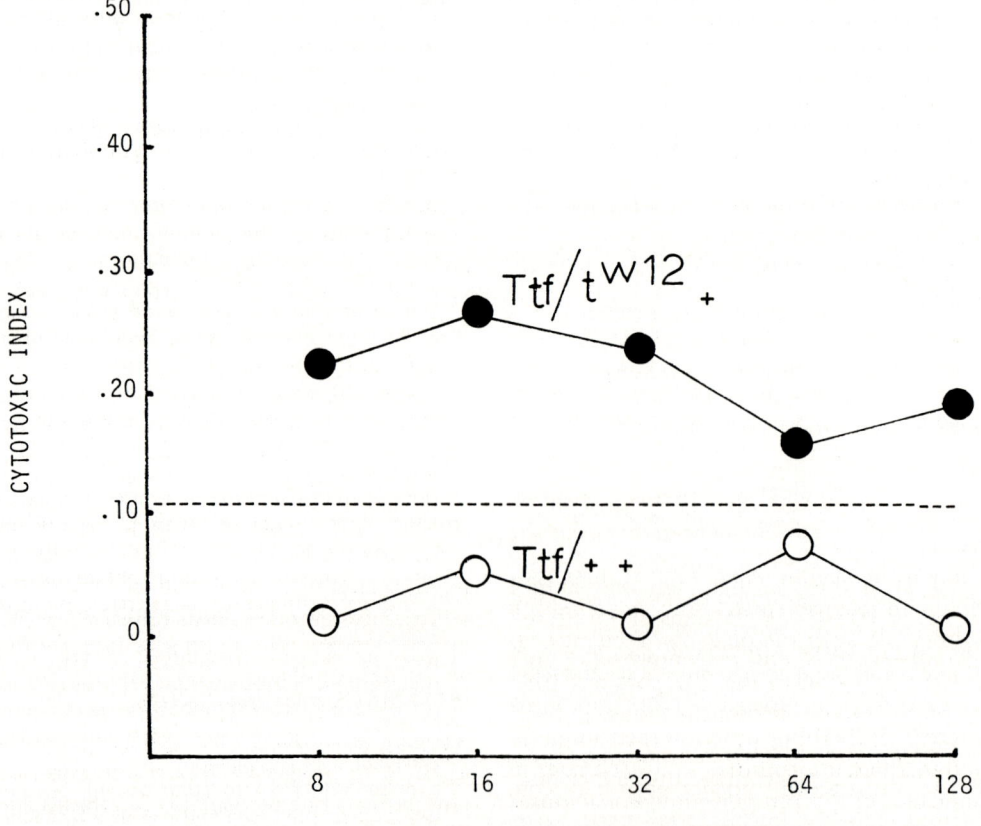

Figure 1. Cytotoxic indices obtained after complement controls have been subtracted with anti-t^{w12} serum No. 64 tested against testicular cells from $T\,tf/t^{w12}+$ and $T\,tf/++$ mice showing weak specific activity characteristic of anti-t sera.

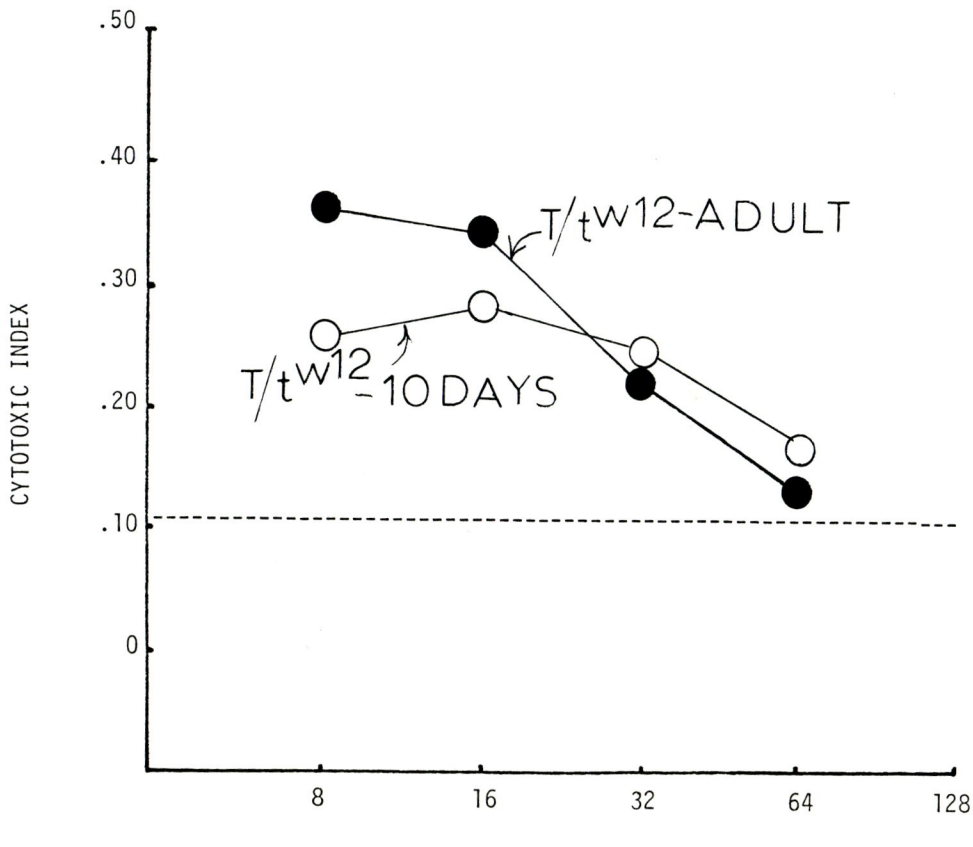

Figure 2. Cytotoxic indices of anti-t^{w12} serum No. 64 tested on testicular cells from an adult mouse heterozygous for t^{w12} and from a 10-day-old heterozygote.

animals are used (Fig. 2). Thus, at least for the t^{w12} haplotype, antigenic determinants appear to arise early in the differentiation of the germ line.

Testicular cells from a panel of T/t genotypes, including at least one member of each known lethal and semilethal complementation group, were screened by direct cytotoxicity tests to determine whether t-factors of other complementation groups shared serologically detectable characteristics in common with t^{w12}. Unlike previous findings which showed serological similarities between the lethal factors t^0 and t^{w18}, however, (Artzt and Bennett, 1977) this serum did not appear to contain specificities common to t-factors other than those within the t^{w1} complementation group (Table 1).

Finally, this serum was tested by direct cytotoxicity and by absorption analysis on testicular cells from mice heterozygous for each of the other members of the t^{w1} complementation group maintained in the colony. Four separate closed colonies of mice heterozygous for member-haplotypes of the t^{w1} complementation group are maintained and bred in the genetic configuration

Table 1. Cytotoxic Indices Obtained With anti-t^{w12} Serum No. 64 in Representative Cytotoxicity Tests Against Testicular Cells From Mice Carrying T/t-haplotypes[a]

Genotype	Cytotoxic Index		
T tf/+ +	0.05,	0.08,	0.03
T tf/t^{w12} +	0.26,	0.26,	0.49
T tf/t^{w1} +	0.41,	0.31,	0.26
T tf/t^{w71} +	0.09,	0.16,	0.21
T tf/t^{w12} tf	0.01,	0.00,	0.16
T tf/t^{w32} +	0.11,	0.03,	0.04
T tf/t^{12} +	0.07		
T tf/t^0 +	0.10,	0.00	
T tf/t^{w5} +	0.06,	0.04,	0.05
T tf/t^{w18} +	0.02,	0.03,	0.07
T tf/t^{w73} +	0.09,	0.09	
T tf/t^{w2} +	0.07,	0.06,	0.03
T tf/t^{w8} +	0.07		

[a] Each index is from a separate test and reflects specific kill at a serum dilution of 1:32.

T tf/t +. Three of these stocks carry mutations of the t^{w1} type independently derived from different wild populations of mice and thus have different designations, i.e., t^{w1}, t^{w12}, and t^{w71}. A fourth stock is also maintained (presumed genotype T tf/t^{w12} tf) which originated in the laboratory from the parent T tf/t^{w12} + stock about 20 years ago. A male mouse that expressed the tf phenotype formed the basis for this new t-bearing stock. Ordinarily the acquisition of tf by the t-bearing chromosome is via crossing over, an event that also includes the transformation of t to one of another complementation group, usually a viable mutation (Bennett, 1975). In this instance, however, by both embryological and genetic criteria, t^{w12} remained unchanged. The two most obvious etiologies for the origin of the t^{w12} tf chromosome are either a mutation to tf, or a deletion including the tf locus that leads to the expression of the tf phenotype as a consequence of pseudodominance. The correct explanation remains to be determined.

Not surprisingly, anti-t^{w12} serum showed significant cytotoxic activity against T tf/t^{w1} + testicular cells (Fig. 3). Furthermore, absorption of this serum with a relatively small number of T tf/t^{w1} + testicular cells removed all cytotoxic activity against both T tf/t^{w12} + and T tf/t^{w1} + testicular cells from the serum (Fig. 4). These findings suggest that t^{w12} and t^{w1} are identical mutations. Unusual results were obtained, however, when the same analysis was performed for the other member haplotypes.

Although anti-t^{w12} antiserum was cytotoxic for T tf/t^{w71} + testicular cells, comparative tests consistently showed lower activity against T tf/t^{w71} + testicular cells than T tf/t^{w12} + cells (Table 1, Fig. 5). Quantitative absorptions of the anti-t^{w12} serum with testicular cells from T tf/t^{w71} + mice also failed to reduce cytotoxic activity against T tf/t^{w12} + testicular cells although all cytotoxic activity against T tf/t^{w71} + testicular cells was easily removed (Fig. 6). These findings show that this anti-t^{w12} serum contains antibodies directed against cell surface components, specified by the t^{w12} haplotype, that are not expressed by the similar mutation t^{w71}.

Testicular cells from mice of the T tf/t^{w12} tf stock were

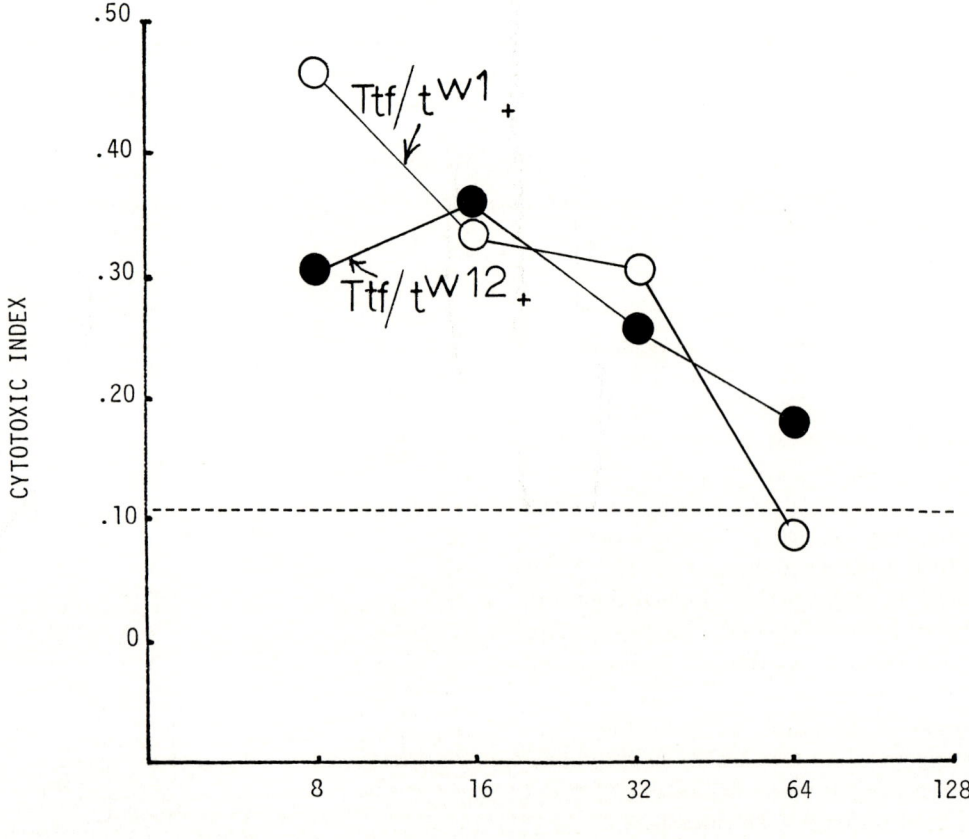

Figure 3. Cytotoxic indices of anti-t^{w12} serum No. 64 on testicular cells from mice heterozygous for two different members of the t^{w1} complementation group, t^{w1} and t^{w12}.

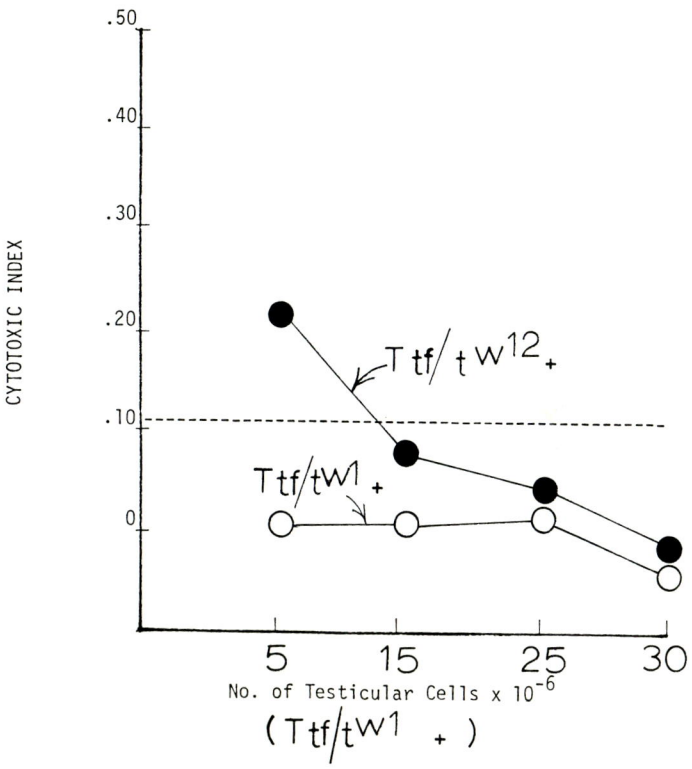

Figure 4. Results of a quantitative absorption of anti-t^{w12} serum No. 64 with testicular cells from $T\ tf/t^{w1}+$ mice and retest of the serum against $T\ tf/t^{w12}+$ and $T\ tf/t^{w1}+$ testicular cells. Specific activity against both $T\ tf/t^{w12}+$ and $T\ tf/t^{w1}+$ testicular cells is removed when $15 \times 10^6\ T\ tf/t^{w1}+$ testicular cells are used to absorb 0.05 ml of serum diluted 1:8.

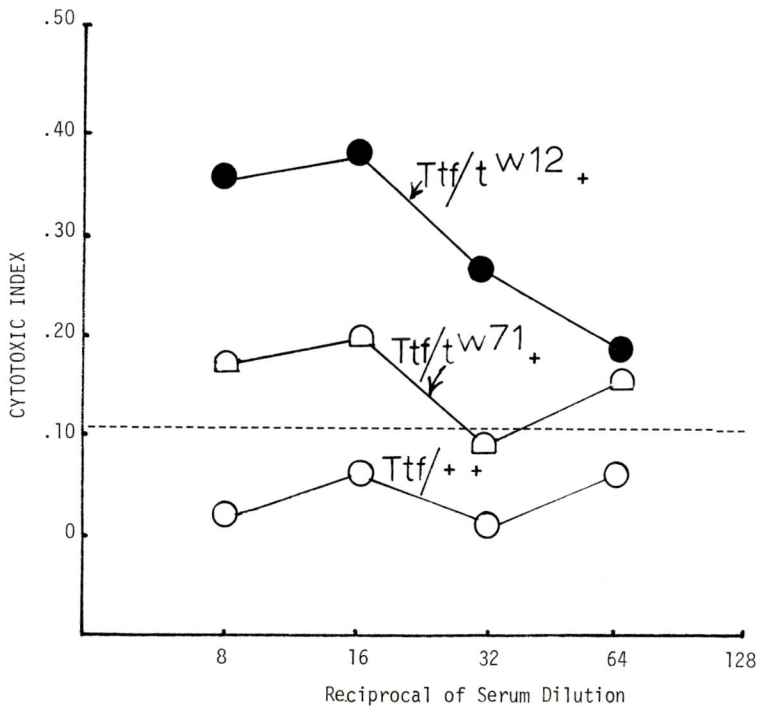

Figure 5. Results of a cytotoxic test of anti-t^{w12} serum No. 64 tested on $T\ tf/t^{w12}+$, $T\ tf/t^{w71}+$, and $T\ tf/++$ testicular cells.

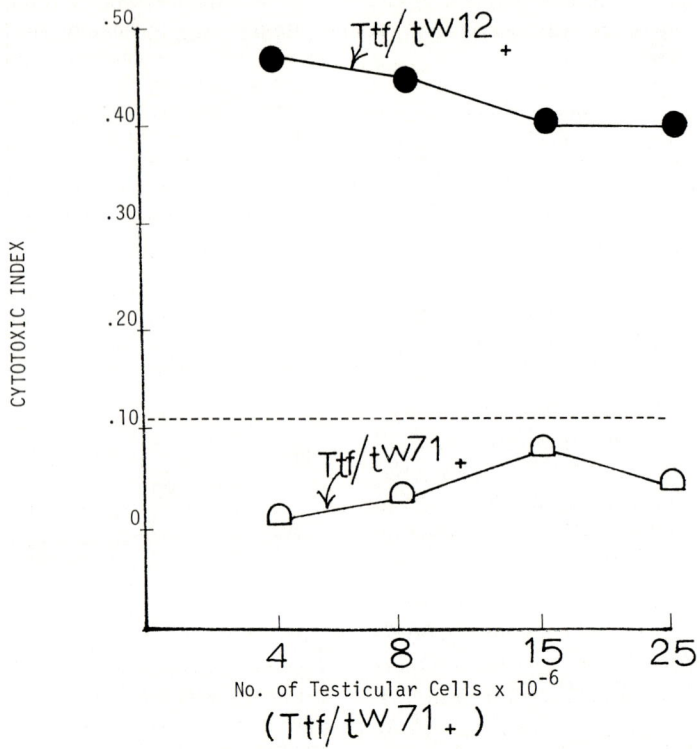

Figure 6. Results of a quantitative absorption of anti-t^{w12} serum No. 64 with testicular cells from $T\ tf/t^{w71}+$ mice, and retest on testicular cells from $T\ tf/t^{w12}+$ and $T\ tf/t^{w71}+$ mice.

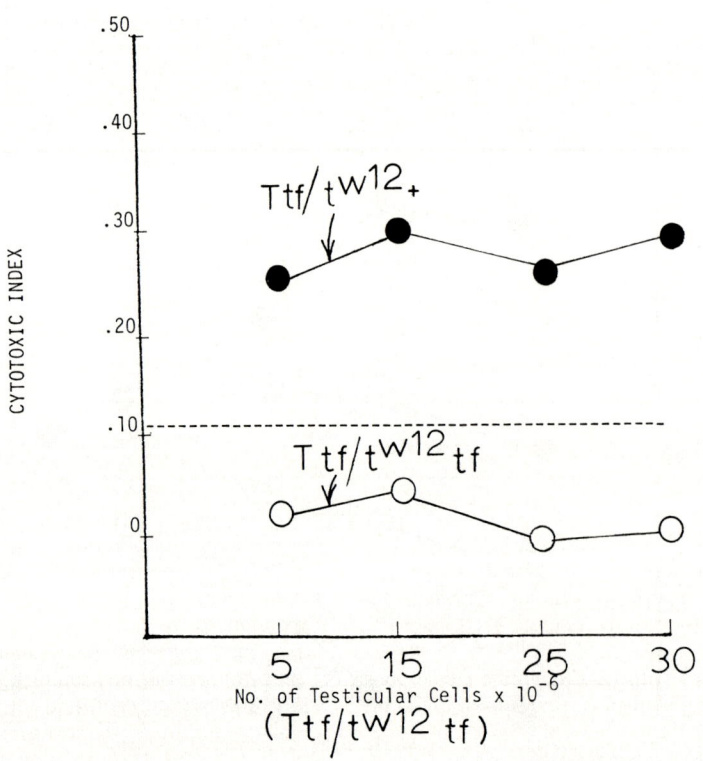

Figure 7. Results of a representative cytotoxicity test of anti-t^{w12} serum No. 64 against $T\ tf/t^{w12}+$ and $T\ tf/t^{w12}\ tf$ testicular cells.

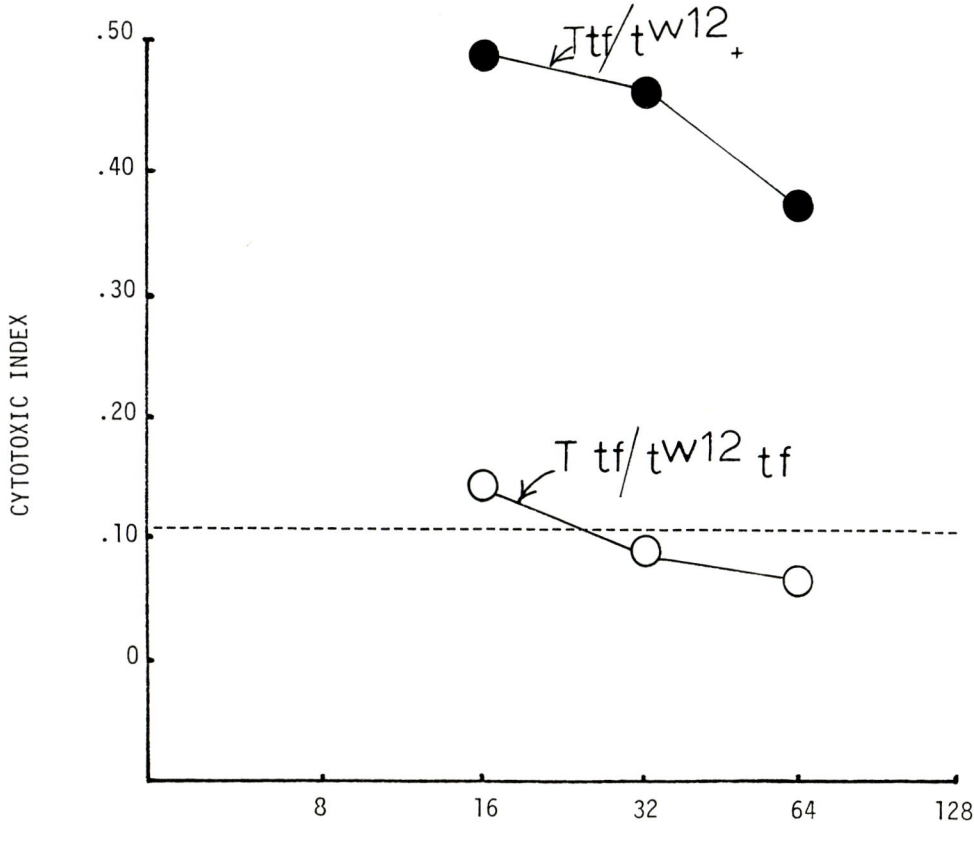

Figure 8. Results of a quantitative absorption of anti-t^{w12} serum No. 64 with $T\,tf/t^{w12}\,tf$ testicular cells and retest on $T\,tf/t^{w12}\,+$ and $T\,tf/t^{w12}\,tf$ cells. Activity of the serum remains high against $T\,tf/t^{w12}\,+$ testicular cells after absorption with 30×10^6 $T\,tf/t^{w12}\,tf$ cells whereas absorption with 4×10^6 cells is sufficient to remove activity against $T\,tf/t^{w12}\,tf$ cells.

consistently refractory to lysis by anti-t^{w12} serum No. 64 (Table 1, Fig. 7). Furthermore, quantitative absorption of the anti-t^{w12} serum #64 with testicular cells from $T\,tf/t^{w12}\,tf$ animals failed to reduce cytotoxic activity against $T\,tf/t^{w12}\,+$ testicular cells (Fig. 8). By these criteria, therefore, the derived t^{w12} mutation behaves as a member of a complementation group other than the t^{w1} group.

CONCLUSIONS

Most lethal t-mutations produce a unique syndrome leading to embryonic death, seemingly confined to a specific population(s) of cells and limited to a discrete phase of early embryogenesis. Death of the embryo, therefore, occurs predictably at a particular time during gestation depending upon the genotype (review: Bennett, 1975). Members of the t^{w1} complementation group are exceptional in this regard, however; although a specific defect, degeneration of the ventral roof of the hind brain, can be recognized at approximately nine days of gestation, embryos may die at intervals thereafter. A few embryos even come to term, although they are invariably microcephalic and edematous (Bennett et al., 1959). Abnormalities of the skull are frequently observed. These homozygotes, therefore, more closely resemble homozygotes for semilethal rather than lethal t-factors, for which a proportion of homozygous embryos also dies, at various times during embryogenesis and manifest a variety of morphological abnormalities (Bennett and Dunn, 1969).

Valid correlations between embryological observations and serological data are, of course, difficult to draw; nevertheless, it is interesting and perhaps significant that t^{w12} specifies serologically detectable determinants that are not shared by members of other lethal complementation groups. The unique serological specificities of t^{w12} may be related to the pleomorphic defects observed in homozygous embryos. The findings presented here also suggest that the t^{w1} complementation group is genetically heterogeneous, a possibility that has previously defied genetic and embryological analysis.

REFERENCES

Artzt, K.; Bennett, D.: Serological Analysis of Sperm of Antigenically Cross-Reacting T/t Haplotypes and Their Recombinants. Immunogenetics 5(1977)97-107

Bennett, D.: The T-Locus of the Mouse. Cell 6(1975)441-454

Bennett, D.; Dunn, L.C.: Transmission Ratio Distorting Genes on Chromosome IX and Their Interactions. In: Proceedings of the Symposium on the Immunogenetics of the H-2 System; Eds., A. Lengerova and M. Vojtiskova, pp. 90-103. Karger, Basel, 1971

Bennett, D.; Badenhausen, S.; Dunn, L.C.: The Embryological Effects of Four Late Lethal t Alleles in the Mouse Which Affect the Neural Tube and Skeleton. J Morphol 105(1959)105-143

Bennett, D.; Goldberg, E.; Dunn, L.C.; Boyse, E.A.: Serological Detection of a Cell-Surface Antigen Specified by the T (Brachyury) Mutant Gene in the House Mouse. Proc Natl Acad Sci 69(1972)2076-2080

Boyse, E.A.; Hubbard, L.; Stockert, E.; Lamm, M.E.: Improved Complementation in the Cytotoxic Test. Transplantation 10(1970)446-449

Dooher, G.B.; Bennett, D.: Spermiogenesis and Spermatozoa in Sterile Mice Carrying Different Lethal T/t Locus Haplotypes: A Transmission and Scanning Electron Microscopic Study. Biol Reprod 17(1977)269-288

Olds, P.J.: Effect of the T Locus on Fertilization in the House Mouse. J Exp Zool 177(1971)417-434

Romrell, L.J.; Bellvé, A.R.; Fawcett, D.W.: Separation of Mouse Spermatogenic Cells by Sedimentation Velocity. A Morphological Characterization. Dev Biol 49(1976)119-131

Yanagisawa, K.; Bennett, D.; Boyse, E.A.; Dunn, L.C.; Dimeo, A.: Serological Identification of Antigens Specified by Lethal t Alleles in the Mouse. Immunogenetics 1(1974)57-67

PART IV
COMPARATIVE ASPECTS

Contemporary biology is dominated by a reductionist approach that assigns exceptional merit to analysis of the molecular mechanisms underlying cell functions. Regrettably, purely descriptive accounts of familiar structures or developmental events in yet another species are often disparaged as redundant and unimaginative. But it cannot be denied that such studies occasionally identify species uniquely suitable for the resolution of specific problems in cell physiology. Moreover, comparative studies of the same process in several unrelated species often reveal constant features or distinctive differences that lead to valid generalizations. Detailed analysis of the unusual not infrequently forces us to reexamine and revise long accepted interpretations based upon the study of a few common laboratory species. The evolution of animals and of their organ systems is widely accepted and the paleontological and ontological evidence for phylogeny forms a large part of the classical literature of biology, but the evolution of cells and their components has received little attention. Examination of specific differences in sperm structure offers an unusual opportunity to trace through phylogeny the influence of the changing environment of fertilization on the morphological adaptations of this complex cell. This section addresses some of the intriguing problems of comparative anatomy and evolution at the cellular level.

SYMPOSIUM PAPERS

SPERM STRUCTURE IN RELATION TO PHYLOGENY IN LOWER METAZOA

B.A. Afzelius

Wenner-Gren Institute, University of Stockholm, Stockholm, Sweden

In the beginning of this century the Swedish biologist Gustaf Retzius (1904, 1905) studied spermatozoa from several hundred animal species. He was surprised to find a species specificity imprinted on the structure of the sperm cell. There were sometimes small, but always recognizable, differences in size and shape between the spermatozoa from each of the many mussel species or each of the many sea urchin species. The variations followed some rules: related species tend to have spermatozoa of rather similar type; many primitive metazoa have spermatozoa of a certain, characteristic architecture (this well-defined sperm type, Retzius called "the primitive spermatozoon.") The primitive spermatozoon needs no extensive presentation: a round or bullet-shaped sperm head with acrosome and nucleus, a short midpiece, and a long, thin sperm tail.

It is also well-known that Franzén (1956) discovered that only those animal species that discharge semen into the ambient water have the primitive type of spermatozoon. Usually, the semen discharge leads to an external fertilization, but in some species the spermatozoa are sucked into the body of the female and the eggs are "internally" fertilized. Animal species with other modes of fertilization have spermatozoa with some other morphology. This rule of Franzén thus shows that there is a relationship between sperm structure and fertilization biology, and that the shape of the sperm cell is influenced not only by phylogenetic relationships but also by existing functional demands on the spermatozoa at fertilization.

In retrospect, this conclusion is hardly surprising. The anatomy of an animal is determined both by the previous history of the phylum and genus, and by the actual pressure of the environment on the species. The same can be expected to be valid for any of its organs and cells. There are differences in degree however. Whereas the body colors or the arrangement of the sensory organs show an enormous variation between different, yet related species, other structures show a lesser variability.

The spermatozoa can be regarded as being evolutionarily rather stable cells, and the primitive spermatozoon seems unique in that it occurs in rather similar shape in most branches in the animal phylogenetic tree.

Because sperm structure is determined both by phylogeny and fertilization biology, it is necessary to keep one of these factors constant, when analyzing the causes of variation. Spermatozoa from closely related species may be compared in a study of the influence of the fertilization biology. An example is the study by Chia et al. (1975), who were able to relate certain features in the morphology of echinoderm spermatozoa to some factors in their reproduction biology. Another example concerns the shipworms, where the internally fertilizing species have been shown to have smaller acrosomes and shorter acrosomal rods than the externally fertilizing species (Popham, 1974). Further examples can be found in the monograph by Baccetti and Afzelius (1976).

The other alternative is to analyze spermatozoa from animal species with a similar fertilization biology. Differences can then be expected to have phylogenic causes. A good example is the study by Baccetti and Dallai (1976) concerning the cecidomyid flies. It may be possible to construct a phylogenetic tree for another insect group, the true bugs (Hemiptera, Heteroptera), based on sperm features. A common characteristic of the spermatozoa within this group is the existence of bridges between two of the ciliary tubules (No. 1 and 5) and the mitochondrial derivatives; another characteristic is the presence of not one but two or three crystals within these derivatives. Other examples can be found in the monograph by Baccetti and Afzelius (1976).

The above examples have been taken from animal groups with internal fertilization, and by necessity the examined species have been closely related in any single study; i.e., they belong to a single family or order. By contrast, a study of animals with external fertilization may be extended to include a major part of the animal kingdom. The fertilization biology of species from over half of the animal phyla is identical as far as can be evaluated: in all cases, a cloud of spermatozoa is emitted from the male and the spermatozoon fuses with a small, naked egg upon a collision with it. This mode of fertilization undoubtedly is the original one for metazoa.

The study has been supported by the Swedish Natural Science Research Council. The author thanks Dr. A.L. Colwin for permission to use his micrographs of the *Saccoglossus* spermatozoon.

© 1979 Urban & Schwarzenberg, Inc. Baltimore-Munich *The Spermatozoon*, edited by D.W. Fawcett and J.M. Bedford

The purpose of this chapter is to examine the ultrastructure of as many types of primitive spermatozoa as possible and to see whether any structural characteristics can be found that are related to the phylogenetic position of the species. Any characteristics that can be found and that are common to two or more phyla would be welcome, since the reconstructions of the evolutionary history of the major metazoan phyla are very uncertain. The phylogenetic tree given in Table 1 is essentially that by Marcus (1958) and is modified only by omitting branches of the tree where there are no primitive spermatozoa. This reconstruction of the evolutionary pattern is just one of several current ones. Valentine (1977) gives four other schemes and discusses their relative merits.

The lowest metazoans are the three cnidarian groups Hydrozoa, Scyphozoa, and Anthozoa. It is typical for spermatozoa from these groups, that a true acrosome does not exist, but that there are Golgi-derived vesicles in the sperm head that may function as acrosomes. The spermatozoon of the primitive scyphozoan *Nausithoe* spec. may be taken as a type example (Afzelius and Franzén, 1971). It has a midpiece containing two centrioles which are located perpendicularly to each other, four mitochondria, and a prominent anchoring fiber apparatus which apparently keeps the distal centriole anchored to the plasma membrane.

The anchoring fiber apparatus is a rather complicated fabric of striated fibers, and forms a nine-pointed star with a diameter of about 1 μ and a skewed nine-pointed star with about half this diameter. The nine primary fibers or lamellae in the anchoring fiber apparatus have three secondary processes (Fig. 1).

In the more evolved scyphozoans (*Aurelia, Cyanea*) the anchoring fiber apparatus is slightly reduced in size, but each primary lamellae has three secondary processes (Fig. 2). There is no proximal centriole. In other respects the midpiece has the same organization as that of *Nausithoe*.

Examined spermatozoa from the hydrozoans have two centrioles, which are on line rather than perpendicular to each other (Fig. 8), and four mitochondria (Fig. 11) (Afzelius, 1971; Hinsch and Clark, 1973). The anchoring fiber apparatus may appear as described above, *e.g.*, in *Hydractinia*, or may be simplified, *e.g.*, in *Tubularia*.

Anthozoan spermatozoa (*Protanthea, Metridium*, a.o.) are peculiar in having many mitochondria, which have been fused by narrow bridges to form a single sleeve of mitochondrial material (Fig. 13 and 14). The two centrioles are perpendicular to each other. There are nine primary processes radiating from the distal centriole, but no proper anchoring fiber apparatus.

The remaining coelenterate group Ctenophora has one species *Beroë ovata*, whose spermatozoa have been examined with electron microscopy (Franc, 1973). An acrosome is present in this species, there are also two perpendicularly oriented centrioles and an anchoring fiber apparatus with three short secondary processes extending from the primary ones. In many other respects the spermatozoon is unusual; thus there is no fixed location or number of mitochondria.

All the other metazoan phyla have three primary germ layers and are derived from the coelenterates. It is believed that two main courses have been followed during the evolution of these phyla. One line has given rise to the phyla which usually are called the protostome animals, the other to the deuterostome animals. The four lowest phyla of the protostomes are Sipuncula, Aschelmintha, Plathelmintha, and Nemertina. No primitive spermatozoa have been found in the plathelminth phylum, unless the genus *Xenoturbella* belongs to this phylum. (Spermatozoa from this animal genus have not been examined with the electron microscope.) The sperm tail from all advanced plathelminths has a characteristic 9+1 structure. Primitive spermatozoa from the other three phyla are remarkably similar. The midpiece of the aschelminth *Priapulus caudatus* thus has four mitochondria and two perpendicularly oriented centrioles (Afzelius and Ferraguti, 1978a). The nine primary processes of the anchoring fiber apparatus each have two secondary processes (Fig. 5). Spermatozoa from the nemertine worm *Micrura fasciolata* have the same number and arrangement of the mitochondria and centrioles (Fig. 9 and 12). The nine primary processes each have three short secondary processes. The same is true of the sipunculid worm *Golfingia gouldi*, which has been examined by Baccetti (1977), except that it is not quite clear whether there are any secondary branches of the anchoring fiber apparatus.

The four higher phyla in the protostome line are Mollusca, Echiura, Annelida, and Arthropoda. In all these phyla there are some animal species which have the primitive type of spermatozoon and others which have not. Thus within the mollusc phylum the lowest classes, the most primitive representatives of the gastropod class (*e.g., Calliostoma linnei*)[1] and most or all of the lamellibranch class (*e.g.,* Popham, 1974) have the primitive type of spermatozoon. Many lamellibranch spermatozoa and some gastropod spermatozoa have been examined with electron microscopy. Again, the number of mitochondria commonly is four, and the two centrioles are perpendicular to each other. There is no complex anchoring fiber apparatus; nine rather short primary processes extend from the distal centriole.

---

[1] Afzelius, B.A.: unpublished data

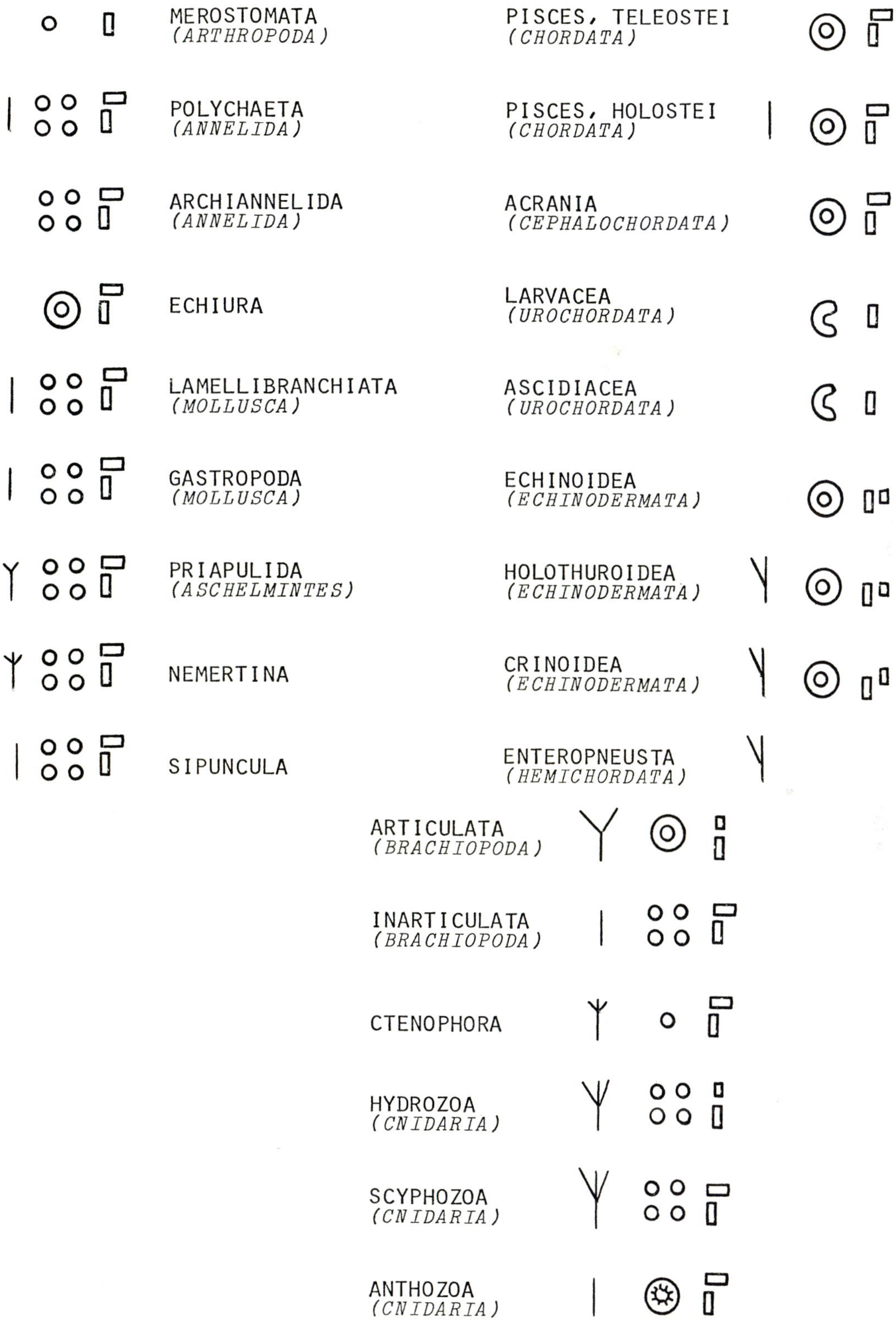

o ▯	MEROSTOMATA (ARTHROPODA)		PISCES, TELEOSTEI (CHORDATA)	⊙ ▯
│ ᵒᵒᵒᵒ ▯	POLYCHAETA (ANNELIDA)		PISCES, HOLOSTEI (CHORDATA)	│ ⊙ ▯
ᵒᵒᵒᵒ ▯	ARCHIANNELIDA (ANNELIDA)		ACRANIA (CEPHALOCHORDATA)	⊙ ▯
⊙ ▯	ECHIURA		LARVACEA (UROCHORDATA)	⊂ ▯
│ ᵒᵒᵒᵒ ▯	LAMELLIBRANCHIATA (MOLLUSCA)		ASCIDIACEA (UROCHORDATA)	⊂ ▯
│ ᵒᵒᵒᵒ ▯	GASTROPODA (MOLLUSCA)		ECHINOIDEA (ECHINODERMATA)	⊙ ▯▫
Y ᵒᵒᵒᵒ ▯	PRIAPULIDA (ASCHELMINTES)		HOLOTHUROIDEA (ECHINODERMATA)	Y ⊙ ▯▫
Y ᵒᵒᵒᵒ ▯	NEMERTINA		CRINOIDEA (ECHINODERMATA)	Y ⊙ ▯▫
│ ᵒᵒᵒᵒ ▯	SIPUNCULA		ENTEROPNEUSTA (HEMICHORDATA)	Y
		ARTICULATA (BRACHIOPODA)	Y ⊙ ▯	
		INARTICULATA (BRACHIOPODA)	│ ᵒᵒᵒᵒ ▯	
		CTENOPHORA	Y o ▯	
		HYDROZOA (CNIDARIA)	Y ᵒᵒᵒᵒ ▯	
		SCYPHOZOA (CNIDARIA)	Y ᵒᵒᵒᵒ ▯	
		ANTHOZOA (CNIDARIA)	│ ⊛ ▯	

Table 1. A phylogenetic tree according to the model by Marcus where only branches of the tree are shown that have spermatozoa of the primitive type. Symbols for three components of the sperm midpiece are given: to the left, one of the nine processes of the anchoring fiber apparatus. (No data available from the groups Archiannelida, Echiura, and Acrania.) In the middle, the mitochondria, which may be small and irregular in number (Merostomata, some Polychaeta, although not shown here, and Ctenophora). (No data available from Enteropneusta.) To the right, the centrioles. (No data available from Enteropneusta.)

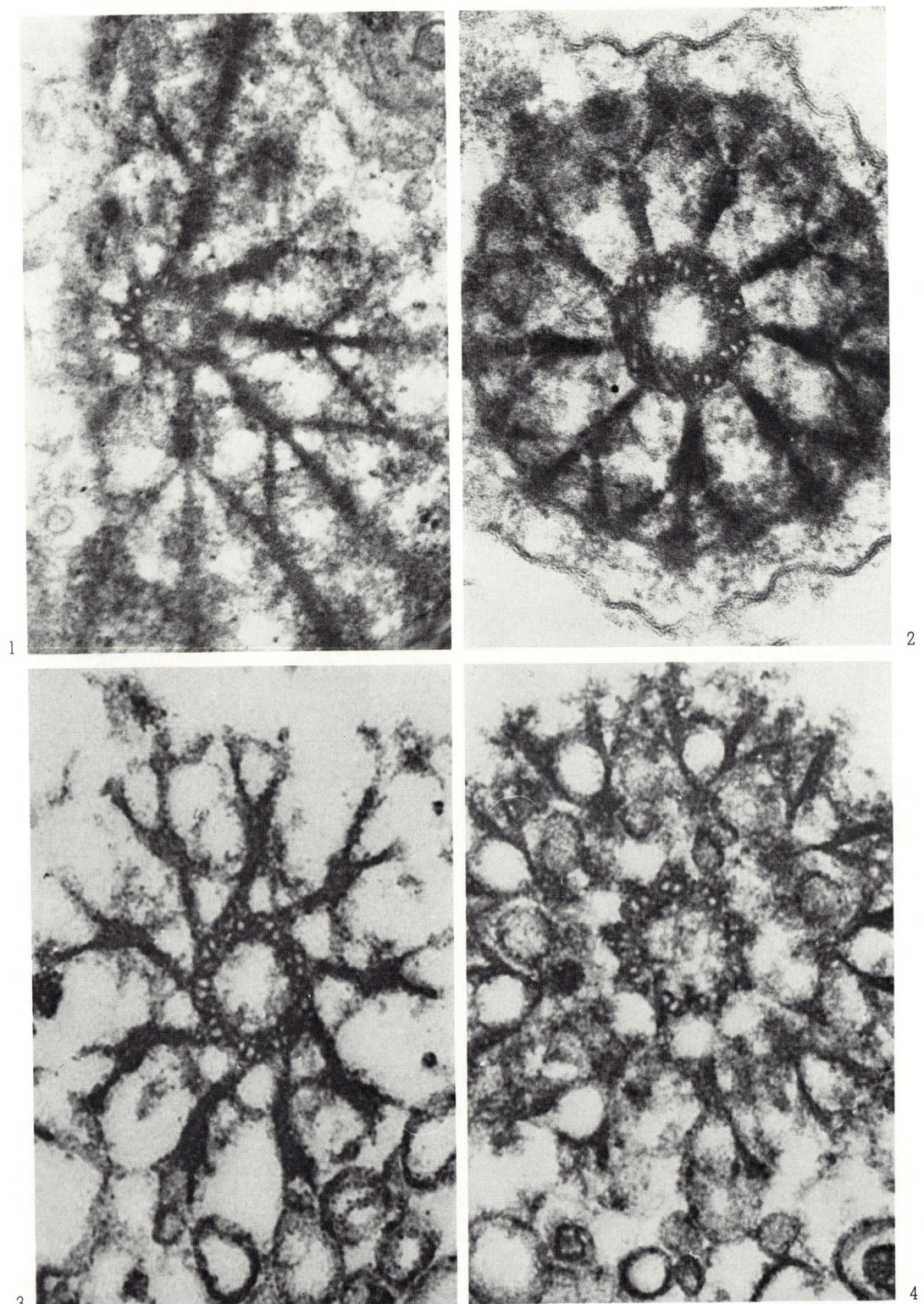

Figures 1-4. The anchoring fiber apparatus in the sperm midpiece. This fabric of striated fibers is particularly prominent in the lower metazoa, as represented here by two scyphozoans, *Nausithoe* (Fig. 1), and *Aurelia* (Fig. 2), and an enteropneust *Saccoglossus* (Fig. 3 and 4). Figures 3 and 4 are from serial sections, and show that the nine primary processes branch into two secondary processes and that one of them divides further into tertiary processes. Magnifications: Fig. 1: 80,000x; Fig. 2-4: 100,000x.

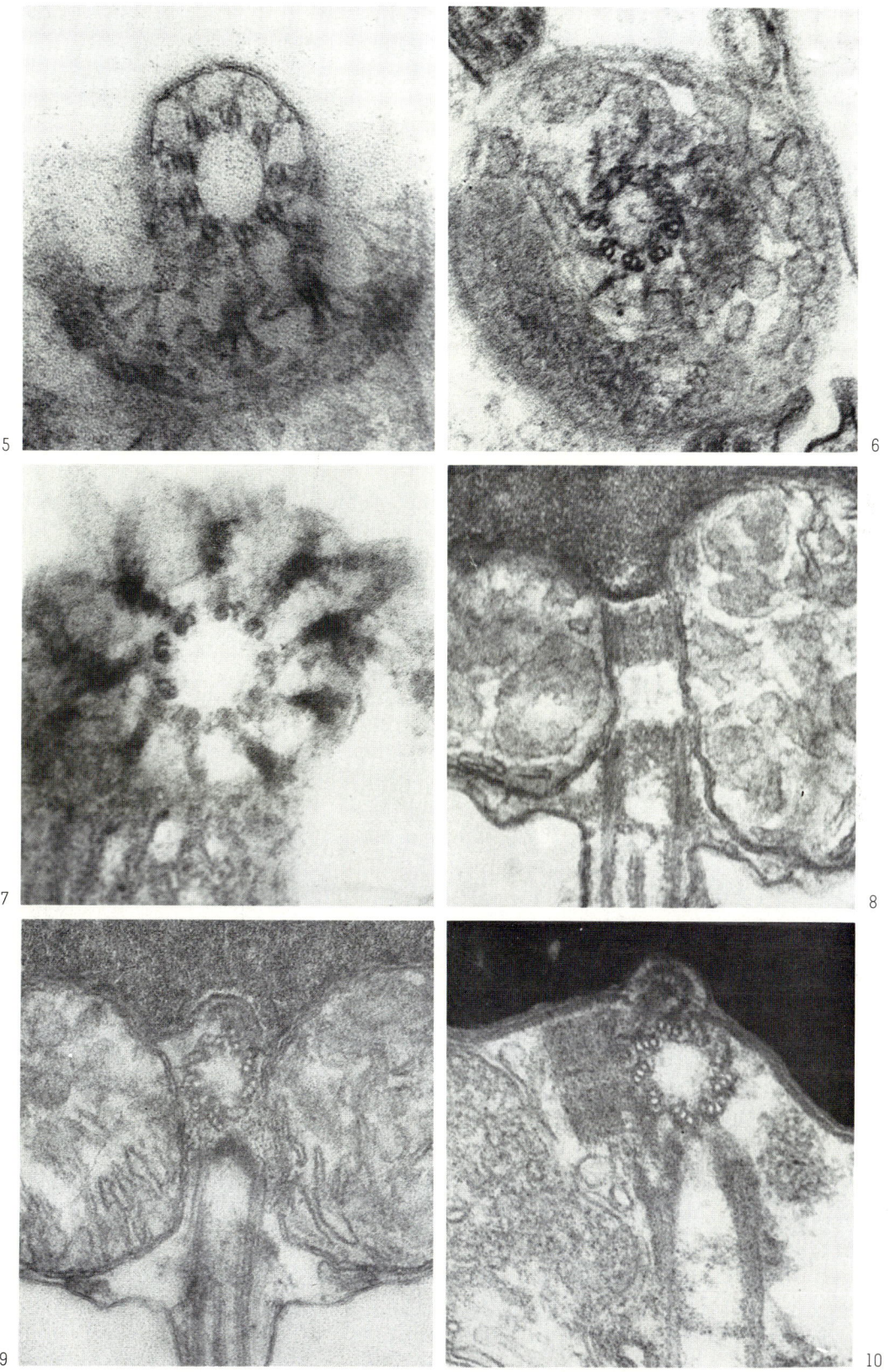

Figures 5-10. The anchoring fiber apparatus and the centrioles in some primitive types of spermatozoa. The secondary branches from the nine primary ones are small in the nemertine *Micrura* (Fig. 5), and lacking in the garpike *Lepisosteus* (Fig. 6). In the articulate brachiopod *Terebratulina* the two secondary processes from neighboring primary processes join to form a star-like figure. In the hydrozoan *Tubularia* (Fig. 8) the two centrioles are on line, whereas in the nemertine *Micrura* (Fig. 9) and in the garpike *Lepisosteus* (Fig. 10) they are oriented perpendicularly to each other. Magnifications: Fig. 5: 100,000x; Fig. 6: 80,000x; Fig. 7: 90,000x; Fig. 8: 55,000x; Fig. 9 and 10: 75,000x.

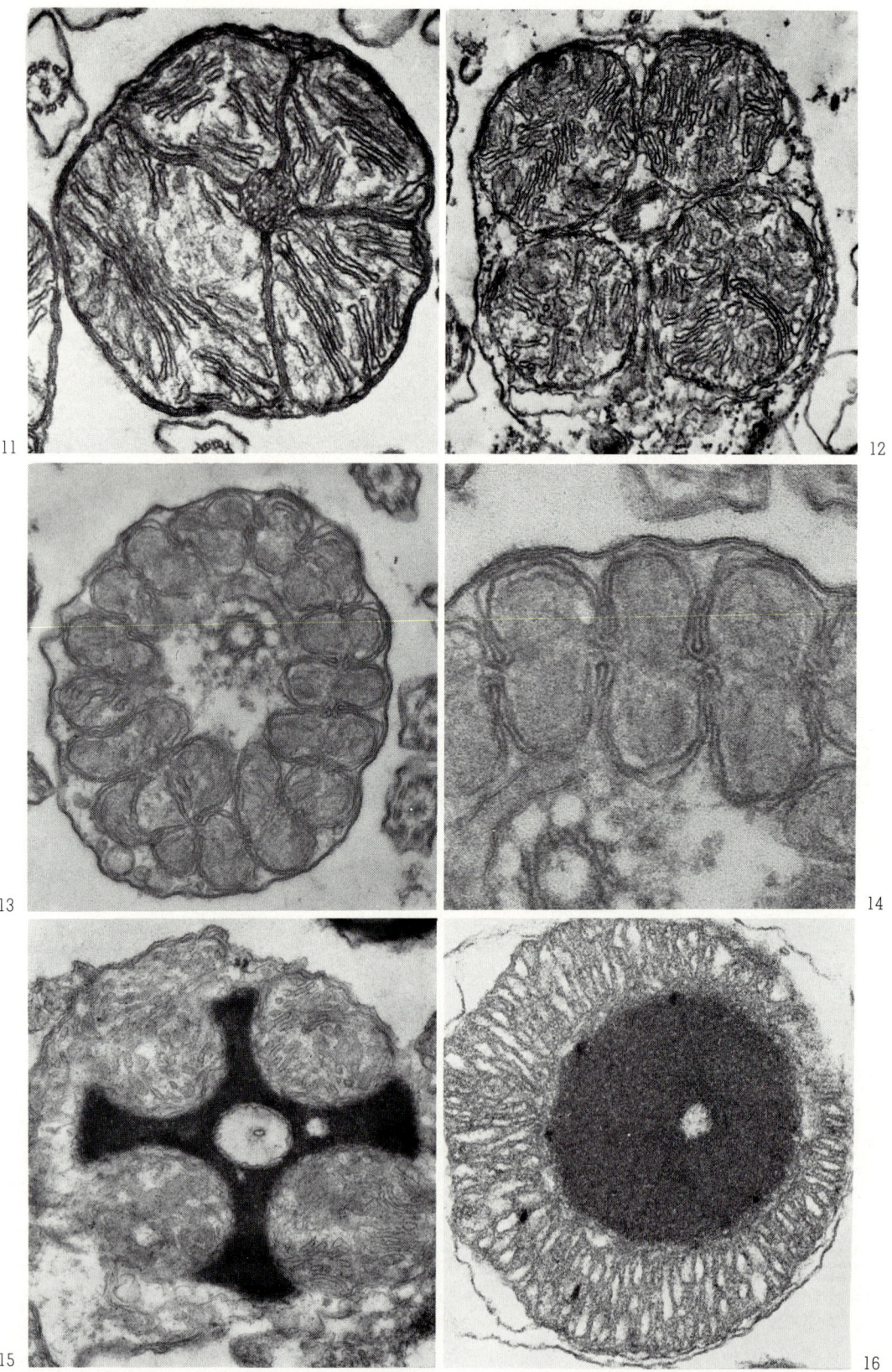

Figures 11-16. Midpiece mitochondria in some spermatozoa. There are four mitochondria in the hydrozoan *Tubularia* (Fig. 11), the nemertine *Micrura* (Fig. 12), and the archiannelid *Polygordius* (Fig. 15). In the anthozoan *Metridium* there is a single ring-shaped one, which apparently is derived from several partially fused mitochondria (Fig. 13 and 14). The crinoid *Antedon* (Fig. 16) also has a single ring-shaped mitochondrion, although there are no traces from the fusion of the many original, smaller mitochondria. Magnifications: Fig. 11: 55,000x; Fig. 12: 35,000x; Fig. 13: 40,000x; Fig. 14: 85,000x; Fig. 15: 28,000x; Fig. 16: 40,000x.

With the echiurid group a new feature appears. The midpiece consists of a single ring-shaped mitochondrion. This feature has been found both in the species *Ikedosoma gogoshimense* (Sawada *et al.*, 1975) and the species *Urechis caupo*.[2] The arrangement of centrioles and an eventual anchoring fiber apparatus has not been examined.

Within the annelid phylum, primitive spermatozoa are found in one archiannelid genus *Polygordius* and in many polychaete genera. The sperm cells of *Polygordius lacteus* have four mitochondria (Fig. 15) and two perpendicularly oriented centrioles. Polychaete spermatozoa usually have this arrangement too, and the existence of four mitochondria seems to be the rule. However, in one genus, *Nereis,* the midpiece mitochondria have other arrangements, usually irregular, as can be seen in four different *Nereis* species (Fallon and Austin, 1967; Bass and Brafield, 1972; Defretin and Wissocq, 1974; Bertout, 1976). The same is true of the species *Perinereis brevicirris* (Kubo and Sawada, 1977). There are radiating processes from the distal centriole (Fallon and Austin, 1967), but secondary processes appear to be lacking.

Within the largest animal phylum, that of the arthropods, a primitive type of spermatozoon has been described from one species only, the horseshoe crab *Limulus polyphemus* (Fahrenbach, 1973). Its spermatozoon is not constructed according to the same plan as the sperm types described above. The mitochondria do not have a fixed number and arrangement. There is only one centriole and no anchoring fiber apparatus. A unique feature is the very long preformed acrosome filament. The fertilization biology in *Limulus* is different from those which characterize animals with primitive spermatozoa (Cavanaugh, 1975). Thus there is some kind of mating, although fertilization is external. The eggs are fairly large and covered by an egg shell.

Animals within the deuterostome phyla form a rather homogeneous group. The Hemichordata probably is the most primitive group with external fertilization and spermatozoa of the primitive type. The ultrastructure of their sperm cells is only partially described. However, A.L. Colwin's hitherto unpublished micrographs of the spermatozoa from *Saccoglossus kowalewskii* show that the anchoring fiber apparatus is as large and complicated as that of the lower scyphozoa or hydrozoa (Fig. 3 and 4). The nine primary lamellae have two secondary processes each; these are the middle one and the one that is directed away from the centriolar microtubules A (terminology as in Gibbons, 1961). A skewed nine-pointed star is visible just as in the *Nausithoe* anchoring fiber apparatus.

The next deuterostomian phylum to be described is the Echinodermata. Spermatozoa from more than 100 species from this phylum have been examined, many with electron microscopy (Chia *et al.*, 1975). At least in all the sperm cells that conform to the primitive type of spermatozoa, the midpiece consists of one single mitochondrion which forms a ring around the two centrioles. These centrioles may have many different types of arrangement, but usually are not perpendicular (Summers *et al.*, 1975; Afzelius, 1977). The anchoring fiber apparatus is fairly large in the crinoid *Antedon petasus* thus a representative of the lowest echinoderm class. In the higher echinoderm classes the anchoring fiber apparatus may have the same appearance, as in some holothurians and ophiuroids Fontaine and Lambert, 1976), or it may be completely lost as in the sea urchins. It is of interest in this connection that a rather large anchoring fiber apparatus exists in the sea urchin spermatocytes and spermatids but disappears before maturation (Longo and Anderson, 1969). Also, the centrioles have a perpendicular orientation in spermatids but not in mature spermatozoa.

The next group to be treated in Urochordata or Tunicata. It has three classes, Ascidiacea, Thaliacea, and Larvacea. Spermatozoa from the first have been examined (Woollacott, 1977) and found to have just one mitochondrion which in a cross section through the spermatozoon is C-shaped. There is only one centriole and no anchoring fiber apparatus. The same is true of the larvacean *Oikopleura dioica* (Flood and Afzelius, 1978), although in respects other than mitochondria, centrioles, and anchoring fiber apparatus, this type of spermatozoon differs from that of the investigated ascidian spermatozoa. The *Oikopleura* spermatozoon is thus peculiar in having a nuclear chromatin that is smaller than that of other primitive or modified spermatozoa by a factor of 10. No ultrastructural data from thaliacian spermatozoa are available.

The group Acrania, with the species *Branchiostoma lanceolatum,* has spermatozoa with a single ring-shaped mitochondrion (Baccetti *et al.*, 1972). The two centrioles have a perpendicular orientation. No processes from the distal centrioles have been described.

Within the subphylum Vertebrata the primitive type of spermatozoon occurs only in two fish groups, Holostei and Teleostei. The spermatozoon of the holostean fish *Lepisosteus osseus* has been described by Afzelius (1978); it has a ring-shaped or C-shaped mitochondrion, two perpendicularly oriented centrioles (Fig. 10), and nine rather slender processes from the distal centriole (Fig. 6). The proximal centriole is adjoined to

---

[2]Holland, L.: personal communication

a fibrous body which has an equivalent in selachian, chondrost, and teleost spermatozoa, but is evidently not found elsewhere. The same description as given for *Lepisosteus* is valid for some primitive representatives of the teleosts, except that radiating processes from the distal centrioles have not yet been found.

This survey of primitive spermatozoa among metazoan animals has taken us through the protostomian and the deuterostomian lines, but has omitted one group with a position somewhat in between these two lines. This is the phylum Brachiopoda, which has two classes termed Inarticulata and Articulata. The inarticulate brachiopods are considered to be the most primitive ones. One of its species *Crania anomala* has a midpiece consisting of four mitochondria and two perpendicularly oriented centrioles. There are nine primary processes from the distal centriole but no secondary ones. A representative from the other brachiopod class, *Terebratulina caput-serpentis,* has spermatozoa of quite a different morphology. There is a rather prominent anchoring fiber apparatus; each one of the nine primary processes has two secondary processes which meet and form a star-like figure (Fig. 7). There is only one ring-shaped mitochondrion. The two centrioles are on line rather than perpendicular to each other (Afzelius and Ferraguti, 1978b).

The presented data are summarized in Table 1. No data on the nucleus or acrosome structure are given in the table or in most of the text above. The author believes that the nucleus, acrosome vesicle, and subacrosomal material show a greater morphological variation within each phylum than the mitochondria, centrioles, and anchoring fiber apparatus, and that they thus are less useful than these as indicators of the relationship between the phyla. An analysis of their morphology within the phyla will probably be rewarding however.

What conclusions can be drawn from all these data? With the understanding that the data are provisional and may be invalidated when new data accumulate, it seems fair to summarize the findings as follows:

1. The spermatozoan prototype in Metazoa must have had a midpiece very similar to that of *Nausithoe,* four mitochondria, two perpendicularly oriented centrioles, and a prominent anchoring fiber apparatus of a complex appearance.
2. Modifications of the spermatozoa have proceeded differently within the protostomian and deuterostomian lines. Sperm data are thus consistent with a dichotomy of the coelomate metazoa.
3. The available sperm data are compatible with the evolutionary scheme proposed by Marcus (1958). The scheme by Hyman is difficult to accept since the base of the coelomate animals is a group, the acoel turbellarians, which do not have primitive spermatozoa.
4. Within the protostomian line there is a gradual loss of the anchoring fiber apparatus, but the arrangement of mitochondria and centrioles is retained in all phyla but the echiurids (mitochondria) and the horseshoe crab (mitochondria, centrioles).
5. Within the deuterostomian line the anchoring fiber apparatus is retained within some phyla, but the arrangement of mitochondria and centrioles is lost in all phyla.
6. The brachiopods have a position which is intermediate between the protostomes and the deuterostomes. The inarticulate class is closer to the protostomian line, the articulate class to the deuterostomian line.

REFERENCES

Afzelius, B.A.: The Fine Structure of the Spermatozoon of *Tubularia larynx* (Hydrozoa, Coelenterata). J Ultrastruct Res 37(1971)679-689

Afzelius, B.A.: Spermatozoa and Spermatids of the Crinoid *Antedon petasus* with a Note on Primitive Spermatozoa from Deuterostome Animals. J Ultrastruct Res 59(1977)272-281

Afzelius, B.A.: Fine Structure of the Garfish Spermatozoon. J Ultrastruct Res, 64(1978)309-314

Afzelius, B.A.; Ferraguti, M.: The Spermatozoon of *Priapulus caudatus* Lamarck. J Submicrosc Cytol 10(1978a)71-79

Afzelius, B.A.; Ferraguti, M.: Fine Structure of Brachiopod Spermatozoa. J Ultrastruct Res, 63(1978)308-315

Afzelius, B.A.; Franzén, Å.: The Spermatozoon of the Jellyfish *Nausithoe.* J Ultrastruct Res 37(1971)186-199

Baccetti, B.: Lo Spermatozoo dei Sipunculidi. Atti Accad Lincei 62(1977)89-92

Baccetti, B.; Afzelius, B.A.: The Biology of the Sperm Cell, Karger, Basel, 1976

Baccetti, B.; Burrini, A.; Dallai, R.: The Spermatozoon of *Branchiostoma lanceolatum.* J Morphol 136(1972)211-226

Baccetti, B.; Dallai, R.: The Spermatozoon of Arthropoda. XXVII. Uncommon Axoneme Patterns in Different Species of the Cecidomyid Flies. J Ultrastruct Res 55(1976)50-69

Bass, N.R.; Brafield, A.E.: The Life Cycle of the Polychaete *Nereis virens.* J Marine Biol Assoc 52(1972)701-726

Bertout, M.: Spermatogenèse de *Nereis diversicolor* O.F. Müller (Annélide, Polychète). 1. Évolution du Cytoplasme et Élaboration de l'Acrosome. J Micr Biol Cell 25(1976)87-94

Cavanaugh, C.M.: Observations on Mating Behavior in *Limulus polyphemus.* Biol Bull 149(1975)422

Chia, F.-S.; Atwood, D.; Crawford, B.: Comparative Morphology of Echinoderm Sperm and Possible Phylogenetic Implications. Am Zool 15(1975)533-565

Defretin, R.; Wissocq, J.-C.: Le Spermatozoïde de *Nereis irrorata* Malmgren (Annélide, Polychète). J Ultrastruct Res 47(1974)196-213

Fahrenbach, W.H.: Spermiogenesis in the Horseshoe Crab, *Limulus polyphemus.* J Morphol 140(1973)31-52

Fallon, J.F.; Austin, C.R.: Fine Structure of Gametes of *Nereis limbata* (Annelida) before and after Interaction. J Exp Zool 166(1967)225-242

Flood, P.R.; Afzelius, B.A.: The Spermatozoon of *Oikopleura dioica.* Cell Tissue Res, 191(1978)27-37

Fontaine, A.R.; Lambert, P.: The Fine Structure of the Sperm of a Holothurian and an Ophiuroid. J Morphol 148(1976)209-226

Franc, J.-M.: Étude Ultrastructurale de la Spermatogenèse du Cténaire *Beroe ovata.* J Ultrastruct Res 42(1973)255-267

Franzén, Å.: On Spermiogenesis, Morphology of the Spermatozoon, and Biology of Fertilization among Invertebrates. Zool Bidr Uppsala 31(1956)355-482

Gibbons, J.R.: The Relationship between the Fine Structure and Direction of Beat in Gill Cilia of a Lamellibranch Mollusc. J Biophys Biochem Cytol 11(1961)179-205

Hinsch, G.W.; Clark, W.H., Jr.: Comparative Fine Structure of Cnidaria Spermatozoa. Biol Reprod 8(1973)62-73

Hyman, L.H.: The Invertebrates. McGraw-Hill, New York, 1940.

Kubo, M.; Sawada, N.: Electron Microscope Study on Sperm Differentiation in *Perinereis brevicirris* (Polychaeta). Cell Struct Funct 2(1977)135-144

Longo, F.J.; Anderson, E.: Sperm Differentiation in the Sea Urchins, *Arbacia punctulata* and *Strongylocentrotus purpuratus.* J Ultrastruct Res 27(1969)486-509

Marcus, E.: On the Evolution of the Animal Phyla. Q Rev Biol 33(1958)24-58

Popham, J.D.: Comparative Morphometrics of the Acrosomes of the Sperms of "Externally" and "Internally" Fertilizing Sperms of the Shipworms (*Teredinidae, Bivalvia, Mollusca*) Cell Tissue Res 150(1974)291-297

Retzius, G.: Zur Kenntnis der Spermien der Evertebraten I. Biologische Untersuchungen. NF 11(1904)1-32

Retzius, G.: Zur Kenntnis der Spermien der Evertebraten II. Biologische Untersuchungen, NF, 12(1905)79-102

Sawada, N.; Ochi, O.; Kubo, M.: Electron Microscope Studies of Sperm Differentiation in Marine Annelid Worms. I. Sperm Formation in *Ikedosoma gogoshimense.* Dev Growth Diff 17(1975)77-87

Summers, R.G.; Hylander, B.L.; Colwin, L.H.; Colwin, A.L.: The Functional Anatomy of the Echinoderm Spermatozoon and Its Interaction with the Egg at Fertilization. Am Zool 15(1975)523-551

Valentine, J.W.: General Patterns of Metazoan Evolution. In: Patterns of Evolution as Illustrated by the Fossil Record, pp. 27-57, ed. by A. Hallam. Elsevier, Amsterdam, 1977

Woollacott, R.M.: Spermatozoa of *Ciona intestinalis* and Analysis of Ascidian Fertilization. J Morphol 152(1977)77-88

AN OVERVIEW OF ATYPICAL SPERMATOZOA IN INSECTS

R. Dallai

Institute of Zoology, University of Siena, Italy

The most representative sperm model of insects is a long cell, well adapted to internal fertilization, with elongated head, an acrosomal complex located at the anterior extremity, an extraordinarily long and thin tail with a flagellum showing the familiar $9+9+2$ array of tubules, flanked by two mitochondrial derivatives usually filled with a particular proteinaceous crystalline material (Baccetti et al., 1977) and by two accessory bodies rising from the Golgi apparatus (Baccetti, 1975).

During the past 10 years several aberrant sperm models with specific structural and physiological characteristics have been described in the different orders. These models usually have been regarded as cytological curiosities, even though very important in some instances for the evaluation of the incidence of different morphological structures in sperm motility (Baccetti, 1972; Phillips, 1974). The author is convinced, instead, that from the standpoint of the evolutionary history of an animal group, the deviations from the classical sperm model occurring in this group might be considered as the result of the several attempts to accomplish or improve internal fertilization.

Atypical spermatozoa may be discussed from different points of view, but perhaps the most interesting aspect is the phylogenetic because such spermatozoa provide useful elements to study the relation between different insect orders.

Insects have long been adapted to land life and consequently have completely achieved internal fertilization. But to reach this goal they have attempted different solutions.

The first solution has been to encyst their sperm. In insects we find this peculiar sperm arrangement only in Collembola (Fig. 1, 2), an ancient group still strictly bound to damp habitats. It is to be remembered that in Collembola no mating occurs and fertilization is carried out by means of spermatophores produced (Hale, 1965; Bretfeld, 1970, 1971; Dallai, 1975) and deposited by the male on the substrate sometimes after a long, quaint courtship. According to Davey (1960) spermatophores probably just happened to be the particular method of internal fertilization employed by the group while they were making the transition to terrestrial life. The spermatophore, in fact, increases the efficiency of sperm transfer in animals with internal fertilization but lacking copulating organs. Collembola sperm, provided with acrosome, maintain a $9+2$ conventional and functioning axoneme pattern, but encysted conditions often lead either to aberrant sperm flagella or to aflagellarity. This is evident in the Arachnida encysted sperm: in Pseudoscorpions the axoneme is still of the $9+2$ type (Boissin, 1970; Legg, 1973), in Uropygi and Araneida, instead it is $9+3$ (Osaki, 1969; Baccetti et al., 1970; Reger, 1970; Phillips, 1976); Opilions, the most primitive species, exhibit the $9+2$ axoneme model, even though not functional, while the more evolved species lack axoneme (Reger, 1969; Baccetti, 1970; Juberthie et al., 1976).

The second possibility used by insect sperm during the evolution of fertilization is to make the flagellum longer and to provide the axoneme with a supplementary set of nine microtubules external to the $9+2$. It is the most common model of insect spermatozoa and all the orders that are well adapted to terrestrial life share it. The need to acquire a row of nine single microtubules, as an adaptation to progression of the sperm in a viscous medium, is already evident among Apterygota Diplura: the Campodeids, in fact, possess nine accessory tubules. These tubules originate, as in the most evolved orders, from a B-subfiber projection of each doublet (Fig. 3) (Cameron, 1965; Warner, 1971) but successively during spermiogenesis they become disordered and migrate toward two opposite points of the axoneme (Fig. 4) (Baccetti and Dallai, 1973b). A similar feature also occurs in the sperm of the most primitive Thysanura, the Machilids (Dallai, 1972; Wingstrand, 1973) which also show the striking peculiarity of being bent about the middle, with the two halves closely opposite surrounded by a common membrane. This gives the erroneous impression that the functional unit consists of joined spermatozoa.

The Paurometabolic orders Blattaria, Orthoptera, and Dermaptera as well as Embioptera, Plecoptera, Odonata, Neuroptera, Heteroptera, Coleoptera, Strepsiptera, Hymenoptera, and Diptera (with the exception

---

© 1979 Urban & Schwarzenberg, Inc. Baltimore-Munich *The Spermatozoon*, edited by D.W. Fawcett and J.M. Bedford

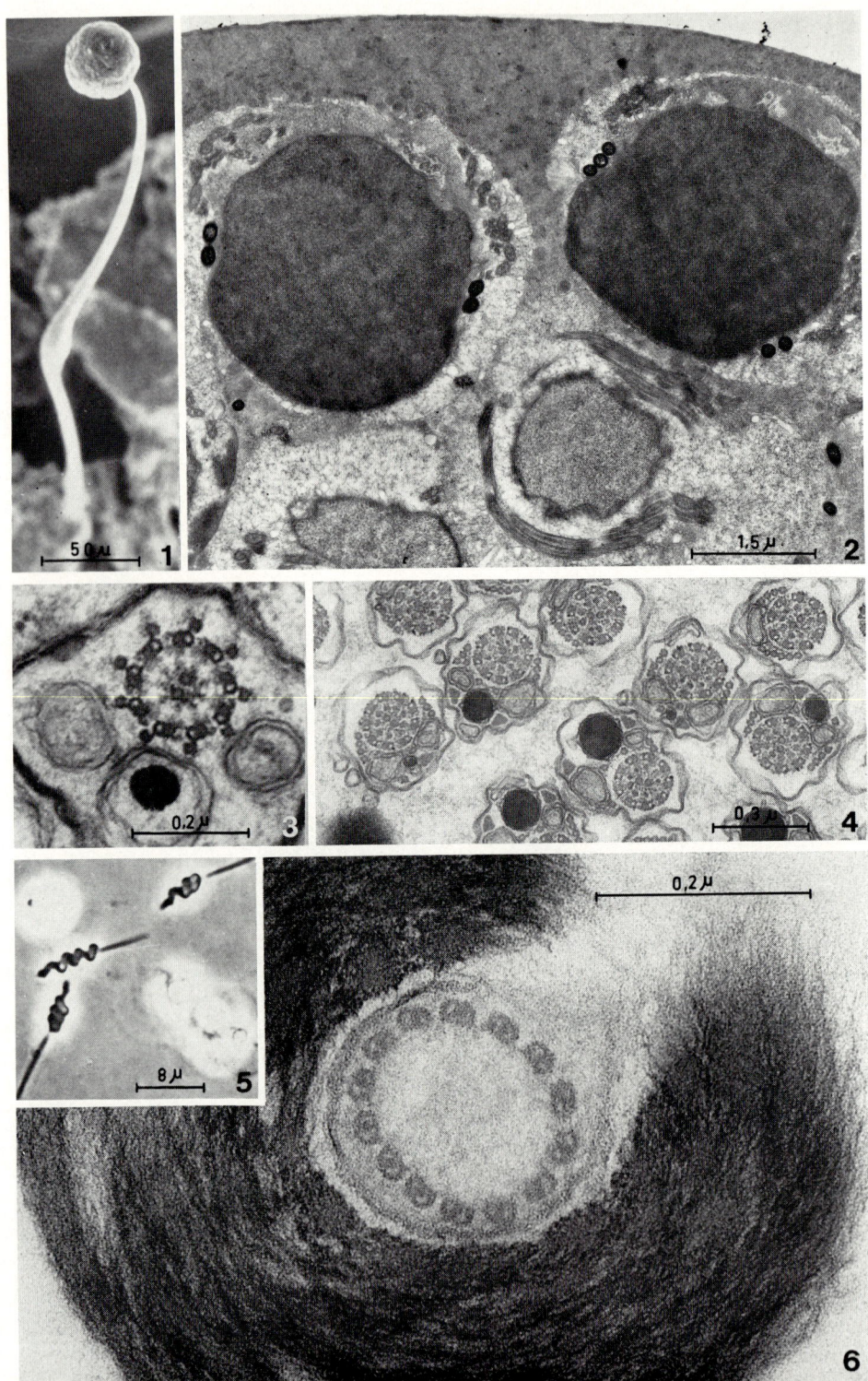

Figure 1. A spermatophore of Collembolan *Dicyrtoma ornata*. The sperm droplet is on top of the long stem. X300
Figure 2. Sperm droplet cross section showing a few encysted rolled-up spermatozoa. X12,000 (from Dallai, 1974)
Figures 3 and 4. Cross section of a *Campodea* spermatid: accessory tubules are visible around the 9+2 axoneme. X90,000 (from Dallai, 1974)
Figures 5 and 6. *Acerentomon* sperm viewed in contrast phase (Fig. 5) and in cross section (Fig. 6). The axoneme is of the 14+0 model and the doublets are devoid of arms. Figure 5, X1300; Figure 6, X160,000 (from Dallai, 1974)

of many Nematocera) have conventional sperm (Phillips, 1970; Baccetti, 1972). Nevertheless, in some of them uncommon features are detectable. In Phasmid insects early mitochondrial degeneration takes place and the mitochondria are replaced by peculiar large bodies, rich in adenosine triphosphatase (ATPase) and uridine triphosphatase (UTPase), consisting of periodically arranged proteinaceous laminae (Baccetti *et al.*, 1973a); whereas in the Coleopteran order *Divales* (Mazzini, 1975) and in the Heteroptera *Notonecta* (Afzelius *et al.*, 1976), the development of the mitochondrial derivatives is enormous.

As to the acrosome, the situation is variable in the different orders (Baccetti, 1972).

Variations concerning the typical axoneme structures, the nine accessory outer tubules or the two central ones, are also eventually evident. Both the sister groups, Mecaptera and Siphonaptera, which exhibit significant similarities (Hinton, 1958; Kristensen, 1975), have flagella without the outer row of single microtubules, thus the axoneme belongs to the simple 9+2 pattern (Baccetti, 1968; Phillips, 1969). This might suggest that an inverse mutation has occurred.

Tricoptera and Lepidoptera are also closely related groups. Their accessory tubules thicker than usual (more than 300 Å in diameter) are filled with glycoprotein material and push out the cell membrane (Phillips, 1969; Baccetti *et al.*, 1969b). It is to be emphasized that a similar configuration has been found in the Micetophilidae *Exechia* (Fig. 7), thus providing new evidence for the close relationship between Diptera and Trichoptera. A very unusual feature has been noticed in this fungus gnat: the accessory tubules are only seven in all because tubules 7 and 8 are missing. It would be interesting to follow the formation of the single mitochondrial derivative during spermiogenesis to see whether it blocks the B-subfiber projection on these two doublets. Variations in the number of the central tubules are frequently encountered. Phillips (1969) has already beautifully illustrated many examples. In two caddis-fly species each axoneme shows seven central tubules; in Simuliid (Baccetti *et al.*, 1974a) and Mycetophilid flies there are three central tubules, while only one is present in culicid diptera. A thick central cylinder replacing central tubules is present in Bibionid diptera sperm (Trimble and Thompson, 1974;[1]) (Fig. 8) and a rod-like structure in those of Psocids; finally, mature mayfly sperm lack central tubules (Phillips, 1969; Baccetti *et al.*, 1969a). In many of the above-mentioned examples sperm are nevertheless able to beat actively indicating that the mutation-induced loss of central tubules does not prevent sperm movement. The same conclusion is true for axonemes with aberrant doublet numbers such as in Sciarids and Cecidomyids. A peculiar doublet modification has been found in *Gryllotalpa* where the doublets in the posterior end of the tail are invaded by tanned glycoprotein material that makes this region stiff (Baccetti *et al.*, 1971).

We shall now consider the attempt to improve sperm motility presented by axonemes arising from both centrioles, which are present in the young spermatid. Two groups illustrate this event well: Phthiraptera (Mallophaga + Anoplura) and Isoptera.

As is well known, there is a controversy whether one or two centrioles are present in insect spermatids (Friedländer and Wahrman, 1966; Anderson, 1967; Breland *et al.*, 1968; Phillips, 1970). According to Friedländer and Wahrman's work (1971), insect spermatid in general seem to have a single centriole because of failure of its replication after the first meiotic division. Nevertheless in other examples, two orthogonally arranged centrioles are formed but one of them, namely the proximal, disappears during spermiogenesis and only the distal centriole remains and is responsible for the production of the axonemal microtubules. However in abnormal insect spermatids, derived from a usual cell division, such as those of Mallophaga and Anoplura, two parallel centrioles are present and give rise to two axonemes in the same flagellum (Ito, 1966; Baccetti *et al.*, 1969c).

A similar situation may be found in Thysanoptera (Baccetti *et al.*, 1969c), but in this group, of which two species have recently been studied (*Aeolothrips* sp. and *Thrips* sp.[1]), the two 9+2 axonemes have become dissociated and the ninefold symmetry is lost.

The centrioles in the Isopteran *Mastotermes* have a different fate. As recently described (Baccetti and Dallai, 1978) the early spermatids have two centrioles albeit aberrant owing to the presence of doublet microtubules instead of triplets in their wall (Fig. 10), but as spemiogenesis proceeds, the number of centrioles increases many times up to 100. Very soon, they become parallel and migrate toward the posterior pole of the nucleus and each of them originates a long axoneme surrounded by a membrane. Consequently the mature sperm is a multiflagellate cell (Fig. 9 and 11) characterized by feeble motility.

Now we shall discuss the tendency of insect sperm to reach aflagellarity as the final stage of evolution in each order. Protura, Isoptera, Homoptera, and Cecidomyid flies are good examples of this tendency. Protura is a very odd group of Apterygota. The 9+2 model probably present in the sperm of the unknown ancestral form is completely lost and new axoneme patterns have been

---

[1] Author's unpublished results.

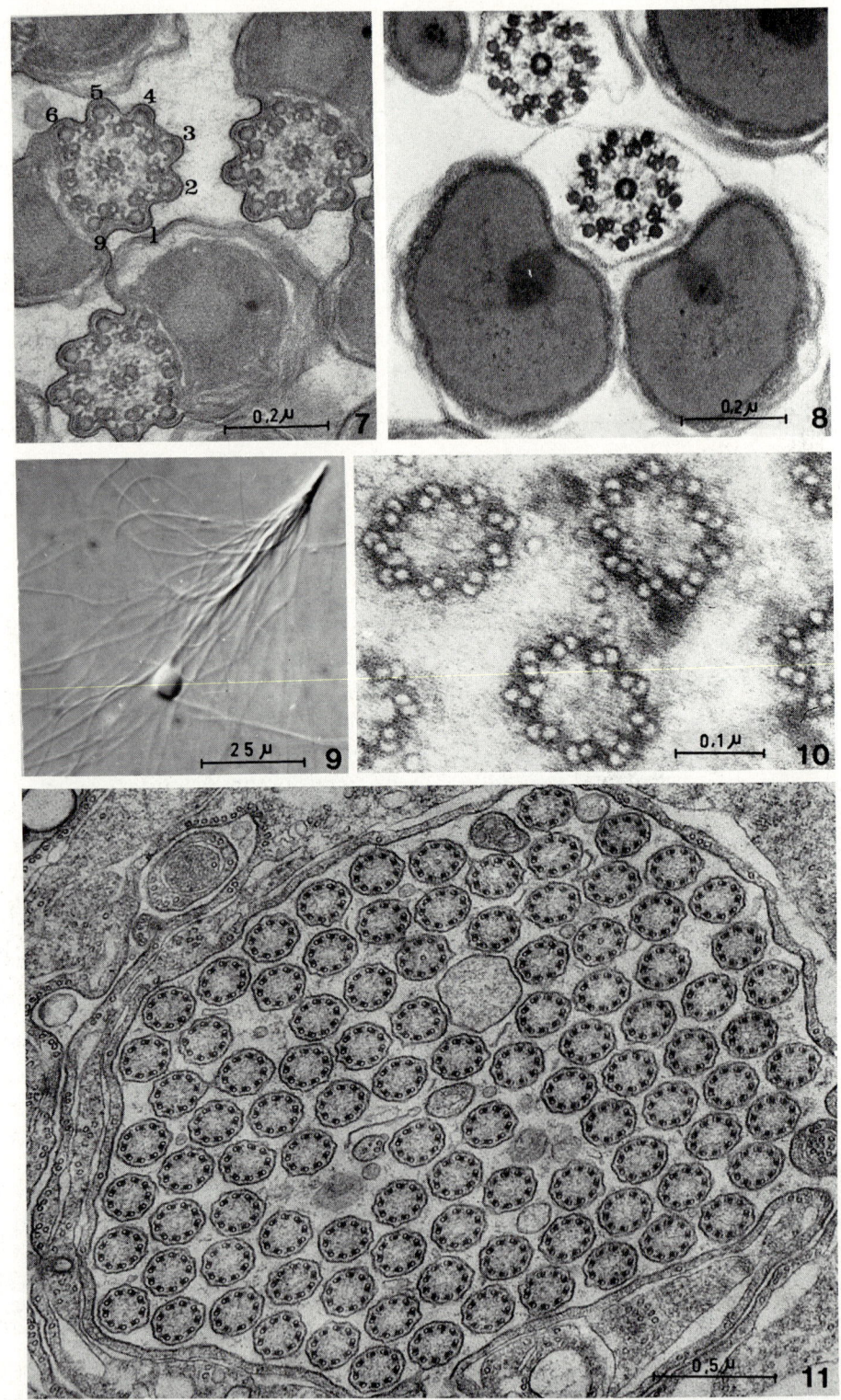

Figure 7. *Exechia* sperm cross section. Accessory tubules are numbered; No. 7 and 8 are missing. X75,000
Figure 8. *Bibio* sperm cross section. A cylinder is in the center of the axoneme. X75,000
Figure 9. *Mastotermes* multiflagellate sperm viewed in interference contrast. X600 (from Baccetti and Dallai, 1978)
Figures 10 and 11. Cross section of centrioles (Fig. 10, X125,000) and flagella (Fig. 11, X35,000) in *Mastotermes* sperm. (from Baccetti and Dallai, 1978)

256 / The Spermatozoon

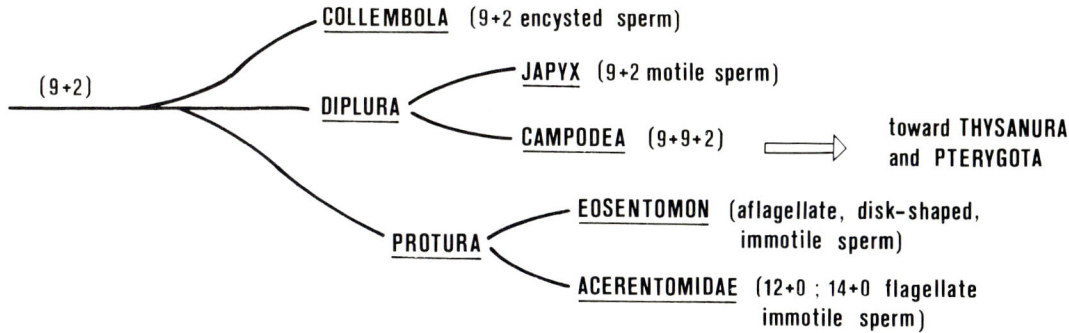

Figure 12. Scheme of Apterygotan sperm evolution.

developed (Fig. 5, 6, and 12). In *Acerentulus* the axoneme model is $12+0$ and in *Acerentomon* $14+0$ (Fig. 5 and 6). In both of these species the doublets are devoid of dynein arms (Fig. 6) and the flagellum is nonmotile. It is obvious that at this point the step toward the disappearance of the axoneme is short. This final stage occurs in *Eosentomon* where we find a sperm like a red blood cell, devoid of axoneme and acrosome (Baccetti et al., 1973d).

On the basis of light microscopic investigations it has been affirmed that primitive Isoptera, a group closely related to Blattariae (Kristensen, 1975), have conventional flagellate sperm like their ancestors. In the separate family (Mastotermitidae), as we have already seen, there is an aberrant multiflagellate sperm, but in *Reticulitermes* and *Calotermes* (Baccetti et al., 1974b), which belong to different and more evolved families, the sperm lack flagella. The sperm of the former species is a roundish cell containing a spherical nucleus, two mitochondria, and two orthogonally arranged centrioles; the sperm of the latter, instead, is elongated and has a peripheral "manchette" of microtubules forming many festoons.

As to Homoptera, many of the Auchenorrhyncha (Fig. 13) still have a classical sperm with a conventional axonemal pattern (Herold and Munz, 1967; Phillips, 1969, 1974; Mazzini, 1970; Folliot and Maillet, 1970). Nevertheless some tree-hopper membracidae show a very odd branched flagellum, each "tail" containing some of the axonemal elements. According to Phillips (1974) the sperm is still able to swim. In Sternorrhyncha, starting from Aphydoidea toward Coccoidea, there is evidence of a progressive involution of the axoneme (Fig. 13). In the anterior region of the Psyllids sperm, in fact, the axoneme is quite normal; in the posterior region, on the other hand it becomes progressively flat (Fig. 14). Nevertheless this sperm is still able to beat. *Aleyrodids*, still more advanced, shows during spermiogenesis a gradual degeneration of the axonemal elements. In fact, the spermatid of *Aleyrodids* is almost normal having two mitochondria and a conventional axoneme but, as spermiogenesis proceeds, the axonemal elements become dense and compact (Fig. 15). At the same time the acrosome starts forming many projections (Fig. 15 and 16). At maturity the sperm is aflagellate and nonmotile with a thin rod along the length of the sperm in place of the axoneme (Baccetti and Dallai, 1977) (Fig. 17). Coccoidea, the most evolved Auchenorrhyncha, have lost sperm flagella but the sperm show a large helix of longitudinal microtubules surrounding the nucleus (Robison, 1966, 1972). ATPase activity has been detected in the microtubules, and these sperm arranged in a bundle are motile (Moses, 1966).

Finally in a group of Diptera Nematocera, the gall-midge Cecidomyids, we find the most unusual and variable axonemal pattern so far discovered in an insect family (Baccetti and Dallai, 1976;[1]) (Fig. 18). Two main evolutionary trends have been identified: species with motile spermatozoa belong to the first; those with nonmotile spermatozoa to the second. The author and colleagues have termed the first trend "*Sciara*-like" because of the superficial resemblance to this better-

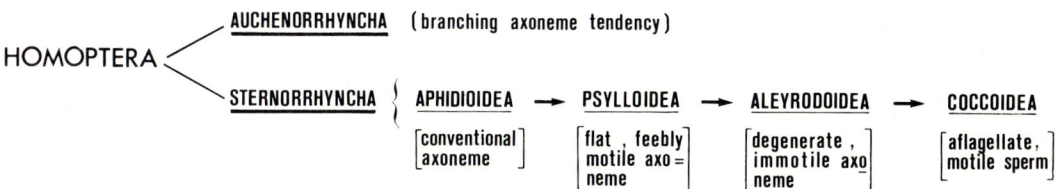

Figure 13. Scheme of Homoptera sperm evolution.

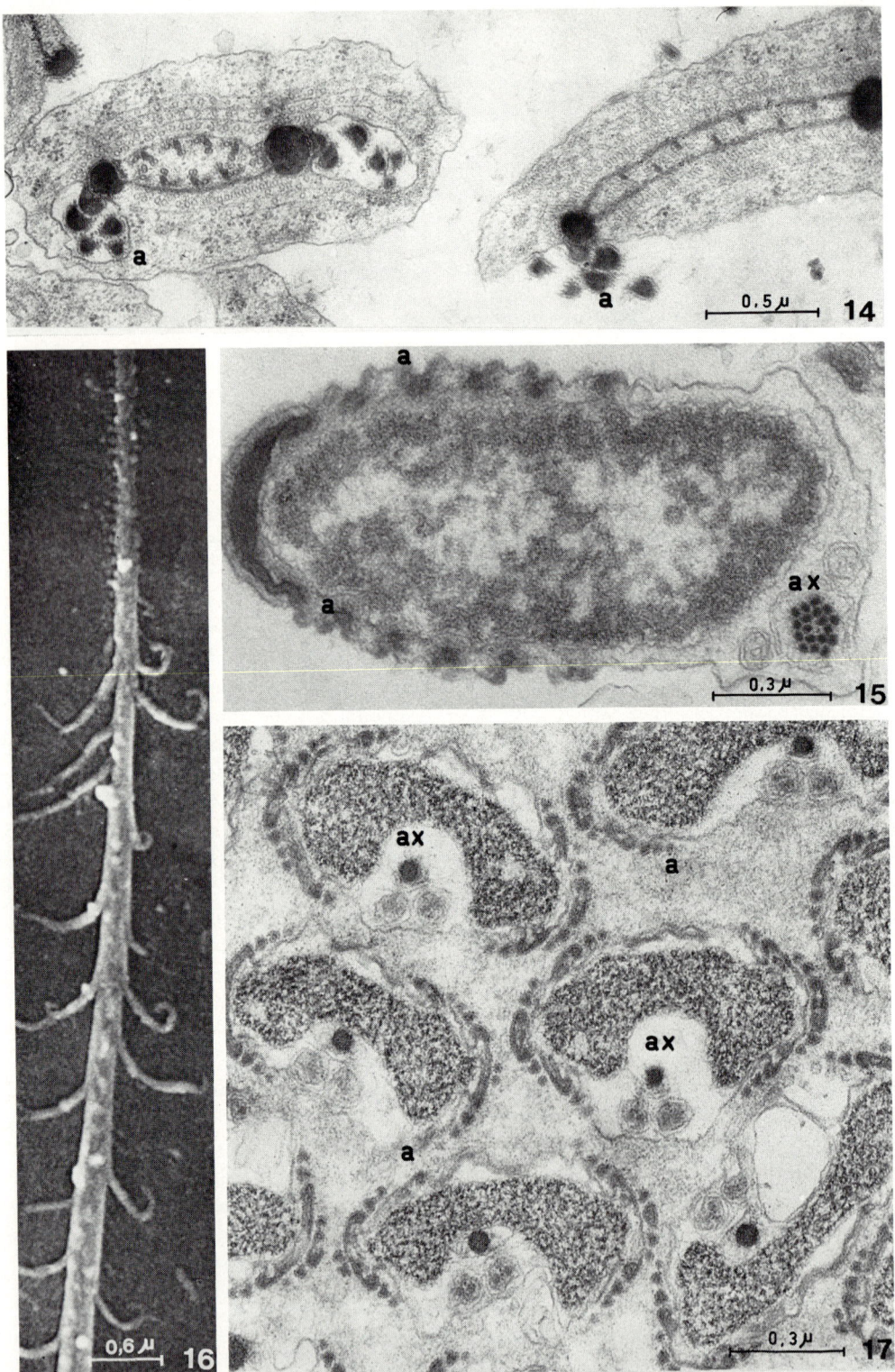

Figure 14. Cross section of the posterior part of Psyllid spermatids showing flattened axonemes. The acrosome originates many appendages (a). X33,000

Figures 15 and 17. Cross sections of Aleyrodid spermatid (Fig. 15) and spermatozoa (Fig. 17) showing progressive axoneme (ax) degeneration. The acrosome forms many projections (a). X57,000 (from Baccetti and Dallai, 1977)

Figure 16. Scanning electron microscope view of Aleyrodid sperm with acrosome projections. X17,500 (from Baccetti and Dallai, 1977)

known aberrant insect sperm (Phillips, 1966). The sperm that belong to this line show, as *Sciara*, a great number of longitudinal doublets. Nevertheless some differences from *Sciara* have been pointed out and can be summarized as follows:

1. Absence of acrosome, a characteristic shared with all Cecidomyids.
2. Absence of accessory tubules.
3. Doublets with outer arms only (Fig. 19). In negative staining these arms appear tilted and with a normal repeat of about 22 nm along the length of each doublet (Fig. 20).
4. Normal mitochondria instead of a mitochondrial derivative (Fig. 21 and 22). Only in the genus *Lestremia*, belonging to a different subfamily, it has recently been possible to find a beginning of crystallization within the mitochondria (Fig. 23). In longitudinal section the resulting paracrystalline body shows a fishbone pattern with a periodicity of 45 nm as in many insect orders.

The evolutional tendency in this line is toward a progressive increase in number of doublets starting from *Asphondilia* toward *Diplolaboncus*. In fact *Asphondilia* has from 30-70 doublets (Fig. 21) whereas *Diplolaboncus* shows the highest number of doublets reported till now in a sperm flagellum; its giant axoneme has about 1000 doublets (Fig. 22). As in *Sciaridae* spermatozoa become motile only when they reach the female spermatheca; when they leave it, they very soon stop moving. It is to be emphasized that a reduction of sperm motility is connected with the greater number of doublets.

Considering the increasing number of doublets in flagella of the sperm belonging to the *Sciara*-like model, from *Asphondilia* to *Diplolaboncus*, one is led to believe that orthogenesis occurs. In fact such a characteristic progressively changes into a straight line irrespective of selective pressure until a breaking point is reached (Austin, 1976). Nevertheless, one cannot exclude the possibility that in some respect this odd axonemal structure is more efficient than one with the ninefold symmetry, or that it may be connected with other advantageous characteristics. In fact it is to be remembered that the visible phenotype is merely the incidental by-product of a pleiotropic genotype selected for its overall fitness (Mayr, 1963).

The second evolutionary trend contains the species whose spermatozoa are nonmotile. The general shape of the sperm here is more variable (Fig. 18). In the sperm flagella, doublets are still evident but they lack dynein arms. Moreover, some spermatozoa have more or fewer microtubules (Fig. 24). In some instances the cytoplasm is filled with microtubules among which it is very difficult to recognize the axonemal doublets (Fig. 25 and 26). At present only *Semudobia* spermatozoa have two axonemes, which in cross section show disordered doublets. All the other species show only one $9+0$ axoneme. A peculiar characteristic of many species, such as *Dryomyia*, *Oligotrophus*, *Cystiphora*, and *Rabdophaga*, is the presence of numerous and long cell membrane expansions containing microtubules (Fig. 25 and 26). These expansions are often visible with the light microscope but sometimes they are not distinguishable at all.

In a separate line of this evolutionary trend each doublet, always without dynein arms, is contained in a separate plasma membrane evagination (Fig. 18). To this sperm model belong the genera *Contarinia* with one disordered $9+0$ axoneme (Fig. 27), *Lestodiplosis* with two $9+0$ axonemes (Fig. 28), and *Myricomyia* which has an unusual axoneme with 14 doublets. As in other insect groups, Protura for example, the mutation resulting in the lack of dynein arms on the doublets probably leads first to the appearance of odd axonemal patterns and then to complete loss of the axoneme. This latter condition has been found in a second species of *Lestodiplosis* sp. b, which is to be considered aflagellate, though it has many of the features characteristic of the genus such as a special type of chromatin condensation, and the presence of outpocketings along the cell membrane (Fig. 18). This is also a good example of selective pressure against a character that is no longer useful.

When insect sperm have lost axonemes and have become nonmotile two possibilities remain for the sperm to reach the egg. The first is to recover motility but, being unable to produce a new axoneme, motility is achieved through a different microtubular system, such as the "manchette" of Coccoidea. Other animal classes with aflagellate spermatozoa have developed a similar condition. For example turbellarians, trematodes, and cestodes as well as a Gnathostomulid species (Graebner and Adams, 1970) have, beneath their limiting membrane, a layer of microtubules that is considered to be responsible for amoeboid sperm movement.

The second possibility is to reduce the sperm length and to form appendages that somehow facilitate passive transport of the sperm. Thin expansions extending from the cell profile and containing microtubules, which are observed in many gall-midges, evidently subserve this function. The same also applies to the acrosomal expansions in Aleyrodid spermatozoa. But parallel adaptation of the female genital apparatus might also be suggested. In the psichodid family, Diptera with elongated aflagellate nonmotile sperm (Baccetti et al., 1973e), a peculiar morphological situation permits the fortuitous meeting of sperm and egg. In this family, in fact, no spermatheca exists and at mating sperm are

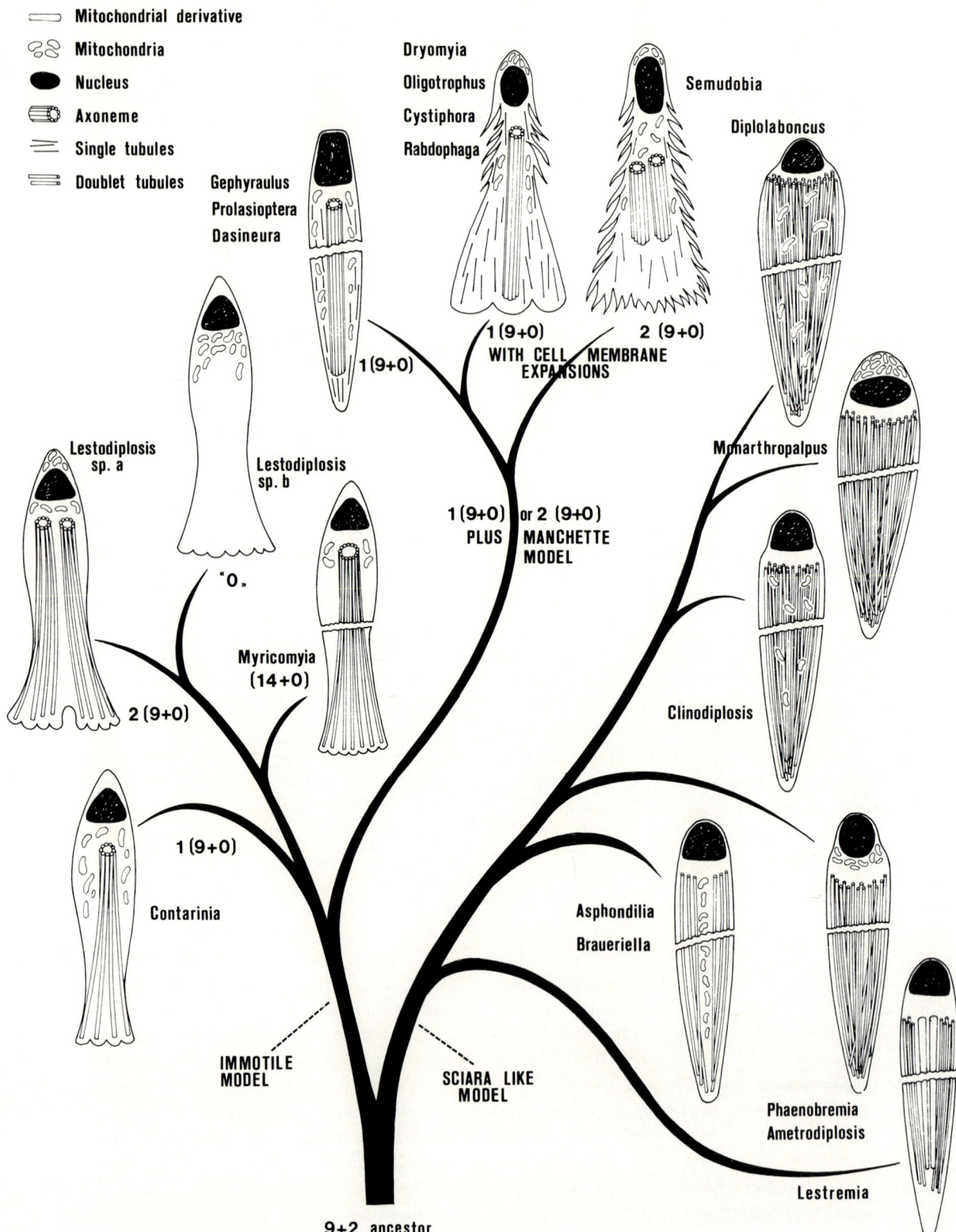

Figure 18. Schematic drawing of Cecidomyid sperm evolution.

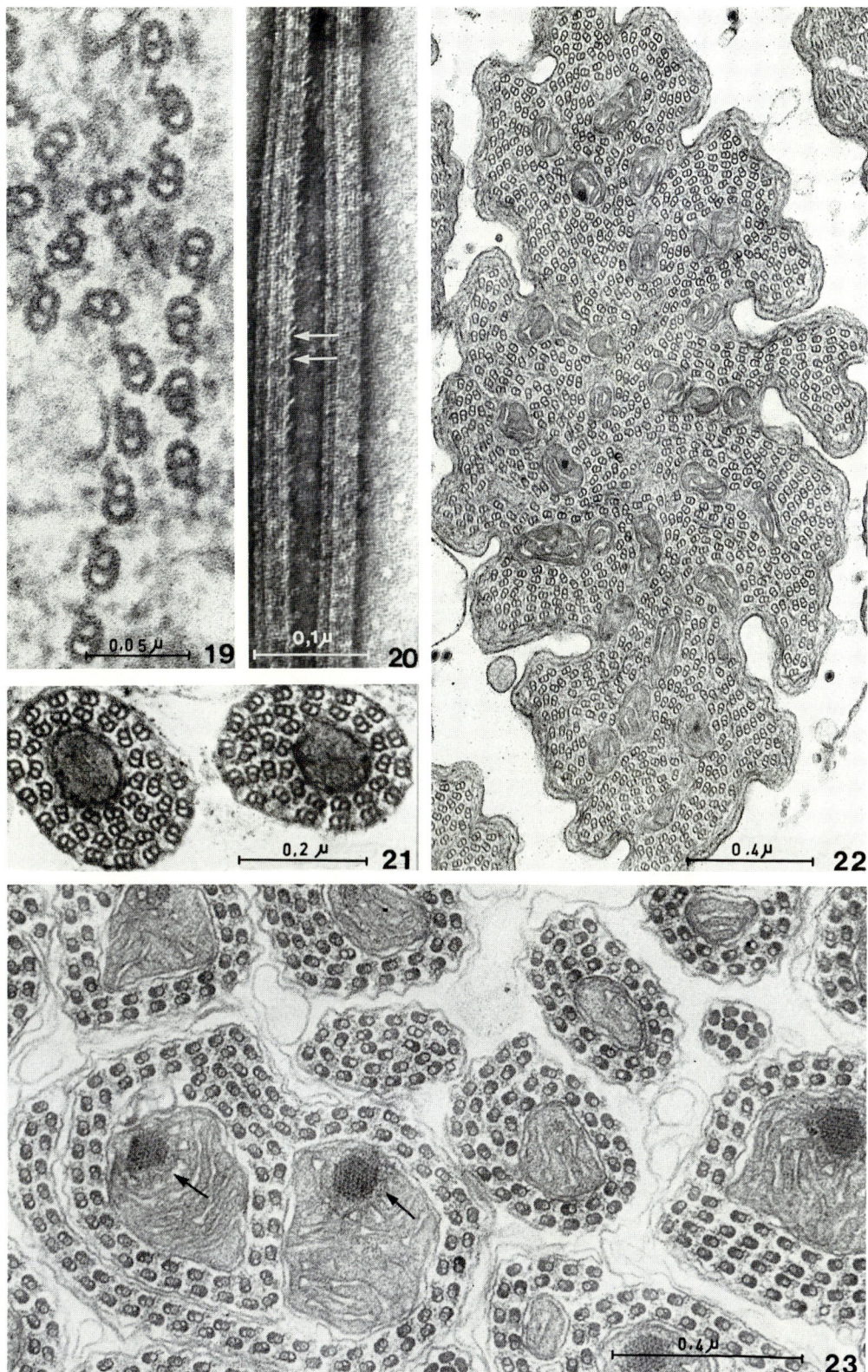

Figure 19. Cross sections of *Diplolaboncus* axoneme doublets. Only outer arms are visible. X210,000 (from Baccetti and Dallai, 1976)

Figure 20. Negative staining of *Diplolaboncus* axoneme doublets showing tilted outer arms with 22 nm repeat (arrows). X175,000

Figures 21 and 22. Cross sections of *Asphondilia* (Fig. 21, X100,000) and *Diplolaboncus* (Fig. 22, X49,000) spermatozoa. (Fig. 22 from Baccetti and Dallai, 1976).

Figure 23. Cross sections of *Lestremia* sperm. Crystallization is starting in the mitochondrial derivatives in the anterior part of the sperm (arrows). X75,000

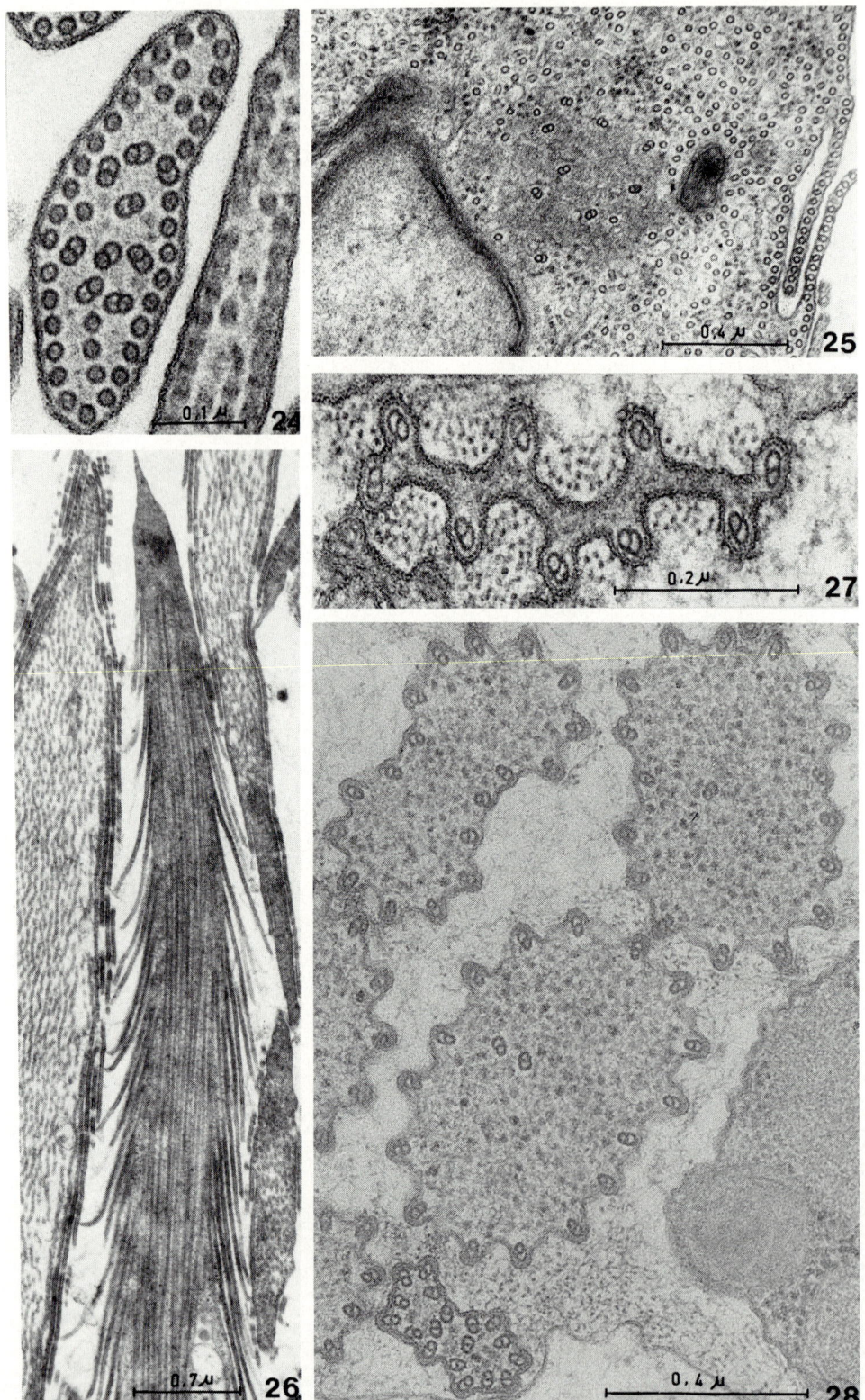

Figure 24. Cross section of *Gephyraulus* sperm showing a "manchette" of microtubules and nine doublets devoid of arms. X130,000 (from Baccetti and Dallai, 1976)
Figure 25. Cross section of *Rabdophaga* sperm. Nine doublets and many microtubules are in the cytoplasm. X45,700
Figure 26. Longitudinal section of *Oligotrophus* sperm showing many expansions from the cell. X23,000
Figures 27 and 28. Cross sections of *Contarinia* (Fig. 27, X140,000) and *Lestodiplosis* (Fig. 28, X75,000) spermatozoa. Doublets devoid of arms are in the outpockets of the cell membrane. (Fig. 27 from Baccetti and Dallai, 1976)

deposited in the female genital ducts from which they reach the ovary by contraction of the duct wall. As the egg micropyle is oriented toward the ovariole peduncle, the meeting between gametes is easily accomplished (Burrini and Dallai, 1975).

In conclusion, three main points should be made:

1. A general tendency toward aflagellarity in the more specialized groups. This tendency, already stressed by Baccetti (1979), is widespread among the higher representatives of all Arthropod classes (for instance Opilions and Acarina among Arachnida; Ostracoda, Peracarida, and Eucarida among Crustacea; Diplopods among Myriapoda).

2. Flagellar movement is dependent on the presence of dynein arms but it is independent of the ninefold pattern of symmetry in the axoneme. The motility in axonemes with $3+0$ or $6+0$ patterns having doublet arms, found in the male gametes of two gregarines (Prensier, 1973; Schrével and Besse, 1973, 1975), and the observation that human, Proturan, and gall-midge sperm, devoid of dynein arms are nonmotile (Baccetti et al., 1973d; Pedersen and Rebbe, 1975; Afzelius et al., 1975) seems to support this view. In addition, the recent data on Cecidomyids (Baccetti and Dallai, 1976) as well as unpublished observations on mayfly Chloeon suggest that only one arm is sufficient for sperm motility, namely either the outer arm, as in the many Cecidomyids studied so far, or the inner arm, as in mayfly sperm.

3. An aflagellate sperm never regains an axoneme. When nonmotile, it can develop peculiar accessory structures, such as festoons of membrane to facilitate passive sperm transport; in other cases there appear to be adaptations at mating to insure that the sperm are placed in contact with the egg. On the other hand, when the sperm regains motility it utilizes a new microtubular system, probably arising as a transformation of the manchette of the spermatid (Baccetti, 1977).

SUMMARY

The many aberrant sperm found in insects very often provide evidence of the relationship between the different orders. Three main points are made from this general view of atypical sperm: 1) tendency to aflagellarity in the more specialized groups; 2) the flagellar movement depends on the presence of dynein arms but is independent of the sperm tail ninefold symmetry pattern; and 3) immotile sperm produce cell expansions to facilitate passive transport, or they regain motility later in evolution through a new microtubular system.

ACKNOWLEDGMENT

Research performed under C.N.R. "Biology of Reproduction" project.

REFERENCES

Afzelius, B.A.; Eliason, R.; Johnsen, O.; Lindholmer, C.: Lack of Dynein Arms in Immotile Human Spermatozoa. J Cell Biol 66(1975)225-232

Afzelius, B.A.; Baccetti, B.; Dallai, R.: The Giant Spermatozoon of Notonecta. J Submicros Cytol 8(1976)149-161

Anderson, W.A.: Cytodifferentiation of Spermatozoa in Drosophila melanogaster: The Effect of Elevated Temperature on Spermiogenesis. Mol Gen Genet 99(1967)257-273

Austin, C.R.: Specialization of Gametes. In: The Evolution of Reproduction, pp. 149-182, ed. by C.R. Austin and R.V. Short, Cambridge University Press, Cambridge, 1976

Baccetti, B.: Lo Spermatozoo Degli Artropodi. V. Aphaniptera. Redia 51(1968)153-158

Baccetti, B.: The Spermatozoon of Arthropoda. IX. The Sperm Cell as an Index of Arthropoda Phylogenesis. In: Comparative Spermatology, pp. 169-181, ed. by B. Baccetti. Academic Press, New York, 1970

Baccetti, B.: Insect Sperm Cells. Adv Insect Physiol 9(1972)315-397

Baccetti, B.: The Role of the Golgi Complex during Spermiogenesis. Curr Top Dev Biol 10(1975)103-122

Baccetti, B.: Unusual Features of Insect Spermiogenesis. In: International Cell Biology, pp. 580-587, ed. by B.R. Brinkley and K.R. Porter. The Rockefeller University Press, Boston, 1976-1977

Baccetti, B.: Ultrastructure of Sperm and Its Bearing on Arthropod Phylogeny. In: Arthropod Phylogeny, pp 609-644, ed. by A.P. Gupta. Van Nostrand Reinhold Company, New York, 1979

Baccetti, B.; Dallai, R.; Giusti, F.: The Spermatozoon of Arthropoda. IV. Ephemeroptera. J Ultrastruct Res 29(1969a)343-349

Baccetti, B.; Dallai, R.; Rosati, F.: The Spermatozoon of Arthropoda. III. The Lowest Holometabolic Insects. J Microsc 8(1969b)233-248

Baccetti, B.; Dallai, R.; Rosati, F.: The Spermatozoon of Arthropoda. IV. Corrodentia, Mallophaga and Thysanoptera. J Microsc 8(1969c)249-262

Baccetti, B.; Dallai, R.; Rosati, F: The Spermatozoon of Arthropoda. VIII. The $9+3$ Flagellum of Spider Sperm Cells. J Cell Biol 44(1970)681-682

Baccetti, B.; Rosati, F.; Selmi, G.: The Spermatozoon of Arthropoda. XV. An Unmotile $9+2$ Pattern. J Microsc 11(1971)133-142

Baccetti, B.; Burrini, A.G.; Dallai, R.; Pallini, V., Periti, P.; Piantelli, F.; Rosati, F.; Selmi, G.: Structure and Function in the Spermatozoon of Bacillus rossius. The Spermatozoon of Arthropoda. XIX. J Ultrastruct Res 44(1973a)1-73

Baccetti, B.; Dallai, R.: The Spermatozoon of Arthropoda. XXI. New Accessory Tubule Patterns in the Sperm Tail of Diplura. J Microsc 16(1973b)341-344

Baccetti, B.; Dallai, R.; Burrini, A.G.: The Spermatozoon of Arthropoda. XVIII. The Non-motile Bifurcated Sperm of Psycodidae Flies. J Cell Sci 12(1973c)287-311

Baccetti, B.; Dallai, R.; Fratello, B.: The Spermatozoon of Arthropoda. XXII. The $9+0$, $14+0$ or Aflagellate Sperm of Protura. J Cell Sci 13(1973d)321-335

Baccetti, B.; Dallai, R.; Giusti, F.; Bernini, F.: The Spermatozoon of Arthropoda. XXIII. The "9 + 9 + 3" Spermatozoon of Simuliid Diptera. J Ultrasstruct Res 46(1974a)427-440

Baccetti, B.; Dallai, R.; Rosati, F.; Giusti, F.; Bernini, F.; Selmi, G.: The Spermatozoon of Arthropoda. XXVI. The Spermatozoon of Isoptera, Embioptera and Dermaptera. J Microsc 21(1974b)159-172

Baccetti, B.; Dallai, R.: The Spermatozoon of Arthropoda. XXVII. Uncommon Axoneme Patterns in Different Species of the Cecidomyid Flies. J Ultrastruct Res 55(1976)50-69

Baccetti, B.; Dallai, R.: The Spermatozoon of Arthropoda. XXIX. The Degenerated Axoneme and Branched Acrosome of Aleyrodids. J Ultrastruct Res 61(1977)260-270

Baccetti, B.; Dallai, R.; Pallini, V.; Rosati, F.; Afzelius, B.A.: Protein of Insect Sperm Mitochondrial Crystals. Crystallomitin. J Cell Biol 73(1977)594-600

Baccetti, B.; Dallai, R.: The First Multiflagellate Animal Spermatozoon in *Mastotermes darwiniensis* (The Spermatozoon of Arthropoda XXX). J Cell Biol 76(1978)569-576

Boissin, L.: Gametogenèse au Cours du Développement Postembryonnaire et Biologie de la Reproduction chez *Histerochelifer meridianus* (L. Koch) (Arachnides, Pseudoscorpions). Thèse, Université Montpellier, 1970

Breland, O.P.; Barker, K.R.; Eddleman, C.D.; Biesele, J.J.: Centrioles in the Spermatids of Insects. Ann Ent Soc Am 61(1968)1037-1039

Bretfeld, G.: Grundzüge des Paarungsverhaltens Europäischer *Bourletiellini* (Collembola, Sminthuridae) und daraus Abgeleitete Taxonomischnomenklatorische Folgerungen. Sond Z Zool Syst Evol 8(1970)259-273

Bretfeld, G.: Der Paarungsverhalten Europäischer *Bourletiellini* (Sminthuridae). Rev Ecol Biol Sol 8(1971)145-153

Burrini, A.G.; Dallai, R.: Preliminary Electron Microscope Studies of Fertilization in *Telmatoscopus albipunctatus* (Williston) (Diptera, Psychodidae). Mon Zool Ital 9(1975)137-152

Cameron, M.L.: Some Details of Ultrastructure in the Development of Flagellar Fibers of the *Tenebrio* Sperm. Can J Zool 43(1965)1005-1010

Dallai, R.: The Arthropod Spermatozoon. XXVII. *Machilis distincta* (Insecta, Thysanura). Mon Zool Ital 6(1972)37-61

Dallai, R.: Spermatozoa and Phylogenesis. A few Data on Insecta Apterygota. Pedobiologia 14(1974)148-156

Dallai, R.: Ultrastructural and Polarizing Light Microscope Studies on Spermatophores of *Dicyrtoma ornata* (Insecta, Collembola). J Ultrastruct Res 50(1975)355-361

Davey, K.G.: The Evolution of Spermatophores in Insects. Proc R Ent Soc Lond 35(1960)107-113

Folliot, R.; Maillet, P.L.: Ultrastructure dè la Spermiogenèse et du Spermatozoide de Divers Insectes Homoptères. In: Comparative Spermatology, pp. 289-300, ed. by B. Baccetti. Academic Press, New York, 1970

Friedländer, M.; Wahrman, J.: Giant Centrioles in Neuropteran Meiosis. J Cell Sci 1(1966)129-144

Friedländer, M.; Wahrman, J.: The Number of Centrioles in Insect Sperm. A Study in Two Kinds of Differentiating Silkworm Spermatids. J Morphol 4(1971)383-397

Graebner, I.; Adam, H.: Electron Microscopical Study of Spermiogenesis and Sperm Morphology in Gnathostomulids. In: Comparative Spermatology, pp. 375-382, ed. by B. Baccetti. Academic Press, New York, 1970

Hale, W.G.: Observations on the Breeding Biology of Collembola (I). Pedobiologia, 5(1965)146-152

Herold, F.; Munz, K.: Ultrastructure of Spermatozoa of *Peregrinus maidis* (Homoptera, Delphacidae). Z Mikrosk Anat Forsch 83(1967)364-374

Hinton, H.E.: The Phylogeny of the Panorpoid Orders. Ann Rev Ent 3(1958)181-206

Ito, S.: Movement and Structure of Louse Spermatozoa. J Cell Biol 31(1966)128A

Juberthie, C.; Manier, J.F.; Boissin, L.: Étude Ultrastructurale de la Double Spermiogenèse chez l'Opilion Cyphophthalme *Siro rubens* Latreille. J Microsc Biol Cell 25(1976)137-148

Kristensen, N.P.: The Phylogeny of Hexapod "Orders." A Critical Review of Recent Accounts. Zool Syst Evolutforsch 13(1975)1-44

Legg, G.: The Structure of Encysted Sperm of some British Pseudoscorpions (Arachnida). J Zool 171(1973)420-440

Mayr, E.: Animal Species and Evolution. The Balknap Press of Harvard University Press, Cambridge, Mass., 1963

Mazzini, M.: Lo Spermatozoo di un Afide: *Megoura viciae* Kalt. Atti Accad Fisiocritici 14(1970)1-6

Mazzini, M.: Giant Spermatozoa in *Divales bipustulatus* F. (Coleoptera, Cleridae). J Insect Morphol Embryol 5(1975)107-115

Moses, M.J.: Cytoplasmic and Intranuclear Microtubules in Relation to Development, Chromosome Morphology and Motility of an Aflagellate Spermatozoon. Science, New York, 154(1966)424

Osaki, H.: Electron Microscope Study on the Spermatozoon of the Liphistid Spider, *Heptatela kimurai*. Acta Arachnol Tokyo 22(1969)1-12

Pedersen, H.; Rebbe, H.: Absence of Arms in the Axoneme of Immobile Human Spermatozoa. Biol Reprod 12(1975)541-544

Phillips, D.M.: Fine Structure of *Sciara coprophila* Sperm. J Cell Biol 30(1966)499-517

Phillips, D.M.: Exceptions to the Prevailing Pattern of Tubules (9+9+2) in the Sperm Flagella of Certain Insect Species. J Cell Biol 40(1969)28-43

Phillips, D.M.: Insect Sperm: Their Structure and Morphogenesis. J Cell Biol 44(1970)243-277

Phillips, D.M.: Structural Variants in Invertebrate Sperm Flagella and Their Relationship to Motility. In: Cilia and Flagella, pp. 379-402, ed. by M. Sleigh. Academic Press, London, 1974

Phillips, D.M.: Nuclear Shaping during Spermiogenesis in the Whip Scorpion. J Ultrastruct Res 54(1976)397-405

Prensier, G.: Formation d'un Flagelle Atypique, sans Structure Centriolaire Basale, au Cours de la Gamétogenèse chez *Diplauxis hatti*. J Microsc 17(1973)88-99

Reger, J.F.: A Fine Structure Study on Spermiogenesis in the Arachnid *Leiobunum* sp. (Phalangida, Harvestmen). J Ultrastruct Res 28(1969)422-434

Reger, J.F.: Spermiogenesis in the Spider, *Pisaurina* sp.: a Fine Structure Study. J Morphol 130(1970)421-434

Robison, W.G.: Microtubules in Relation to the Motility of a Sperm Syncytium in Armored Scale Insect *Parlatoria oleae* (Homoptera, Coccoidea). J Cell Biol 29(1966)251-265

Robison, W.G.: Microtubular Patterns in Spermatozoa of Coccid Insects in Relation to Bending. J Cell Biol 52(1972)66-83

Schrével, J.; Besse, C.: Ultrastructure d'un Flagelle à base 6 chez les Gamètes Mâles de *Lecudina tuzetae* (Protozoaire Parasite). J Microsc 17(1973)93a

Schrével, J.; Besse, C.: Un Type Flagellaire Fonctionel de Base 6+0. J Cell Biol 66(1975)492-507

Trimble, J.J.; Thompson, S.A.: Fine Structure of the Lovebug, *Plecia neartica* Hardy (Diptera, Bibionidae). J Insect Morphol Embryol 3(1974)425-432

Warner, F.D.: Spermatid Differentiation in the Blowfly *Sarcophaga bullata* with Particular Reference to Flagellar Morphogenesis. J Ultrastruct Res 35(1971)210-232

Wingstrand, K.G.: The Spermatozoon of the Thysanuran Insects *Petrobius brevistylis* Carp. and *Lepisma saccharina* L. Acta Zool Stockholm 54(1973)31-52

STRUCTURAL, COMPARATIVE, AND FUNCTIONAL ASPECTS OF SPERMATOZOA IN URODELES

B. Picheral

Faculty of Biological Sciences, Laboratory of Cellular Biology, University of Rennes, France

The sperm cell of the Urodeles exhibits a very complex structure: the acrosome, the nucleus, and the tail are different from those that we know in most of the other vertebrate sperm. In fact the sperm of the Urodeles differ from all other vertebrate sperm[1] by having a lateral flagellum held to an axial fiber with a thin undulating membrane (Fig. 1 and 2).

The first known observation of a Urodele sperm was Pouchet's (1847), and around the turn of this century many very precise descriptions were made. Ballowitz (1890), Champy (1913), Czermak (1879), Eimer (1874), McGregor (1899), Janssens (1901), Meves (1897), Retzius (1906). With the use of the electron microscope, new very detailed descriptions of two newt sperm appeared (Picheral, 1967; Fawcett, 1970), in addition to a number of partial descriptions (Furieri, 1960, 1962; Fawcett and Hilfer, 1961; Fawcett, 1962; Baker, 1966; Barker and Biesele, 1967; Pankratz, 1967. Today, new analyses of Urodele sperm structure might be undertaken in view of its chemical composition or in view of its function, that is, in reference to the particular conditions of fertilization (Picheral, 1977a, b).

GENERAL DESCRIPTION OF THE SPERMATOZOON

All the urodele spermatozoa are built on the same general model, the only differences being in lesser details. The sperm of the Salamandridae (the newts and the salamanders) is the best known and it will be used as a general model (Fig. 3). The following description will refer to mature sperm from the spermiduct or spermatophore, while most of the data previously published refer to testis sperm.

The spermatozoa are very long and thin in all species. The sperm cell of *Pleurodeles waltl* (Fig. 3 and 4) is one of the smallest (250 μm), while in the very common European *Triturus palmatus* the sperm is about 650 μm long. The longest sperm seems to be that of *Necturus maculosus* which is nearly 1 mm long. The tail is two to three times longer than the head.

In the sperm of *Pleurodeles waltl*, the head (Fig. 4) is nearly cylindrical and lightly conical, tapering gradually from its base to its foremost tip. The nucleus is, in most of the species, laterally bordered by a linear nuclear ridge. The acrosome, which is often provided with a lateral recurving barb, ends with a knob or with a more or less sharp point. At the base of the nucleus, a neck piece is prolongated by the axial fiber which is the main part of the tail. The undulating membrane is attached to one side of the axial fiber. The flagellum, bordered by the marginal filament, lies along the edge of the undulating membrane. A semicylindrical sheath of mitochondria covers the axial fiber along the midpiece which is a little longer than two-fifths of the tail in the sperm of *Pleurodeles* (Fig. 37). In other species, the sheath of mitochondria may extend from half to two-thirds of the tail. The part of the tail without mitochondria is the principal piece. In some species, the axial fiber ends abruptly before the end of the undulating membrane (Fig. 4 and 6), but in others, the size of the axial fiber and the undulating membrane progressively decrease together (Fig. 5), in which case there is no terminal piece.

The Acrosome

The organization of the acrosome is the most complex among the vertebrate sperm acrosomes. The small diameter of this organelle renders it difficult to study. Under a long acrosomal cap, an elongated conical subacrosomal space contains the perforatorium (Fig. 7-10). This acrosomal cap displays at least two or three components: the terminal part (the knob or the point), the dense lateral recurving barb, and the main part of the cap which appears more dense under the transmission electron microscope (Fig. 10 and 15). The plasma membrane shows local differentiation. Some particles may be observed outside the plasma membrane (Fig. 15), and others may be viewed in freeze-fracture replicas (Fig. 13 and 14). The barb may or may not be present among the Salamandridae, *e.g.*, the sperm of *Plethodon cinereus* (Plethontidae) has one. The outline of the acrosomal cap in transverse sections is usually circular, but

---

© 1979 Urban & Schwarzenberg, Inc. Baltimore-Munich *The Spermatozoon*, edited by D.W. Fawcett and J.M. Bedford

[1] The sperm of the Anuran amphibian *Bombina variegata* is the only one exception, (Furieri, 1975; Folliot, 1979).

that of the sperm *Hynobius nebulosus* (Hynobidae) is trifoliate (Fig. 41 and 42).

The acrosome contains lytic enzymes. Some hydrolases (proteinase, DNase, RNase, and β-glucuronidase) might be present according to Buongiorno-Nardelli and Bertolini (1967). These authors have demonstrated an acid phosphatase activity localized on the external and internal sides of the acrosomal cap of the sperm from *Triturus cristatus cristatus*. The same result has been obtained with the Pleurodele sperm. Furthermore, when spermatozoa are applied on gelatin, the characteristic digestion of substrate appeared. This "halo reaction" demonstrates an acrosomal protease content (Fig. 11 and 12). The characteristic aspect of the canal, pierced by the acrosome through the vitelline layer, indicates a protease activity (Fig. 47 and 48). The perforatorium, so named in view of its function during the fertilization process (Picheral, 1977a, b) is a fine sharp point made of three different concentric parts (Fig. 9 and 10). The inner one is an axial rod which extends down into the nucleus. A very thin hexagonal network may be seen in the transverse sections of this axial rod and corresponds to a longitudinal fiber organization. Two superimposed periodical structures may be observed by means of special techniques, at the level of the more peripheral sheath (Fig. 8). The transitional level between the acrosome and the nucleus is complex, as the posterior part of the peripheral acrosomal sheath covers the tip of the nucleus (Fig. 10).

The Nucleus

Two different parts constitute the nucleus: the chromatin area and the nuclear ridge (Fig. 4 and 18). In the center of the main dense chromatin area is an endonuclear canal limited by the nuclear envelope. This canal contains the rod which extends from the anterior part of the perforatorium to the first third of the nucleus (Pleurodele sperm).

The Nuclear Ridge

Anteriorly, the nuclear ridge usually forms a short peripheral ring around the chromatin, then it decreases in size and appears as a lateral ridge more caudally (Fig. 4). It ends with, or just anterior to, the nucleus (Pleurodeles). The important feature is that this nonchromatin nuclear structure is surrounded by the nuclear envelope and localized within the nucleus (Fig. 19 and 20) (Picheral *et al.*, 1966). In mature sperm, the nuclear envelope is intimately fused to the surface of the nuclear ridge, as well as to the surface of the chromatin area. The nuclear ridge is composed of minute tubular subunits closely packed together. The nuclear ridge from the Pleurodele sperm

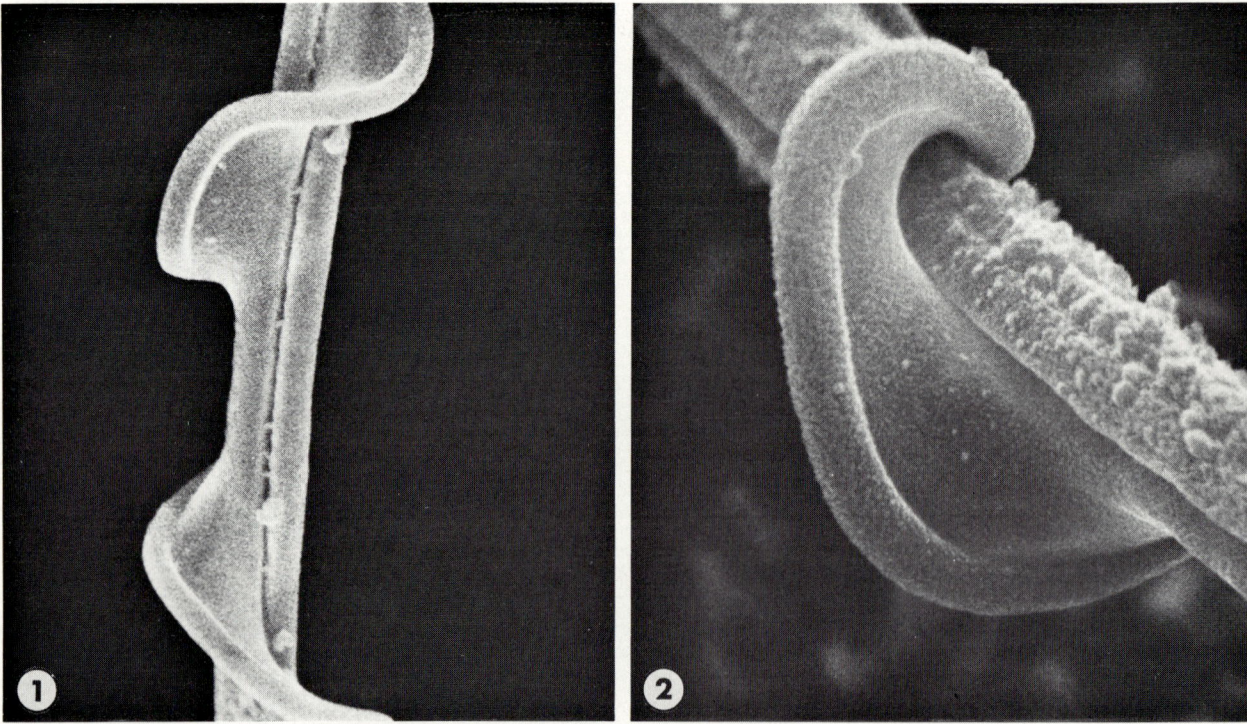

Figures 1 and 2. Scanning electron micrographs of the sperm tail of *Pleurodeles waltl*.

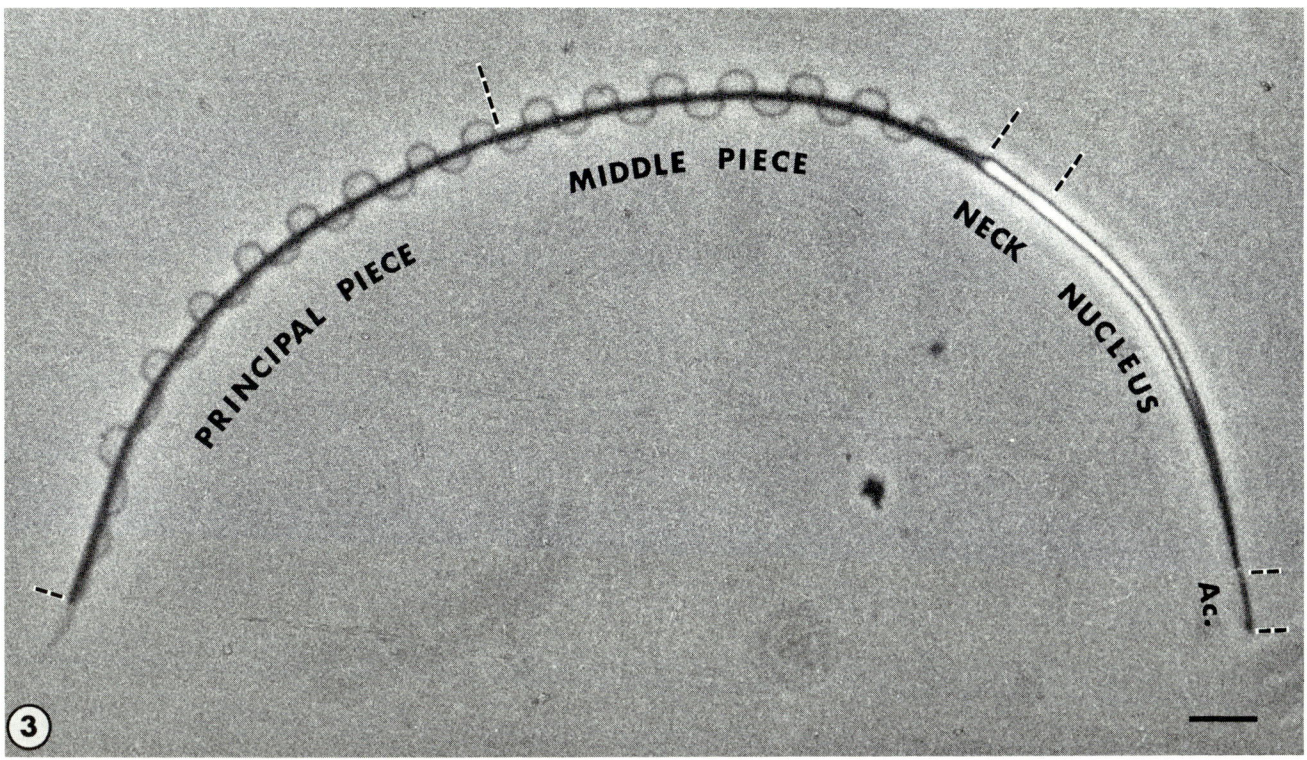

Figure 3. Phase contrast micrographs of a sperm of *Pleurodeles waltl*, with the different main parts. The terminal piece of the tail is distal to the principal piece. Scale bar = 10 μm.

is well developed compared with the chromatin area, but this is not the case for all species. Moreover this structure is usually made of only one bundle of tubules, but in *Euproctus asper* and *Salamandra salamandra* (Salamandridae) the nuclear ridge subdivides into several little bundles. This is also true of the sperm of *Hynobius nebulosus* (Fig. 43).

This unusual structural element is devoid of any DNA and basic proteins. The nuclear ridge which has been supposed to be composed of cystine- and cysteine-rich acid proteins, does not resist sodium dodecyl sulfate (SDS) or N-lauryl-sarcosine-sodium salt (Sarkosyl) treatments.[2] After treatment with these two detergents, the nuclear ridge still persists but the tubular substructure disappears (Fig. 24 and 25).

The integrity of the nuclear ridge is preserved with 2M NaCl while the basic proteins from the chromatin are extracted (Fig. 22 and 23). This, followed by DNase extraction, is a method useful to separate the nuclear ridge from the chromatin area in order to determine its chemical composition.

The Chromatin Area The chromatin area of the mature sperm from Pleurodeles is not homogeneous along the nucleus. Anterior sections of the nucleus (Fig. 18) or freeze-fractured nuclei (Fig. 19) show a concentric lamellar organization. Caudally these structures disappear, and the lamellae are progressively replaced by large granules (Picheral, 1971). In certain cases at the lamellar level, the chromatin may present a very unusual fiber disposition. After sodium chloride, SDS, or Sarkosyl extraction, transverse sections of fibers alternate with longitudinal fibers, as can be seen in both transverse and longitudinal sections. In addition, oblique and arced fibers may be seen in sperm nuclei when they enter the ovocyte, while an arc-like configuration already exists in some longitudinal sections of late spermatid nuclei. The pictures (Fig. 21) are similar to those of the Dinoflagellate chromosomes (Bouligand, 1972; Bouligand *et al.*, 1968), or to some bacterial nucleoids (Gourret, 1978). This special chromatin fiber organization in a cholesteric liquid crystal pattern, confirms the results obtained by physical, chemical, and theoretical means by Sipki and Wagner (1977) with regard to mammalian sperm which also show a lamellar organization (Koehler, 1970).

The anterior part of the pleurodele sperm nucleus is birefringent (Fig. 16) (Picheral, 1972). This property might be attributable to the nuclear ridge or to the

---

[2]Charbonneau M. and Picheral, B.: unpublished

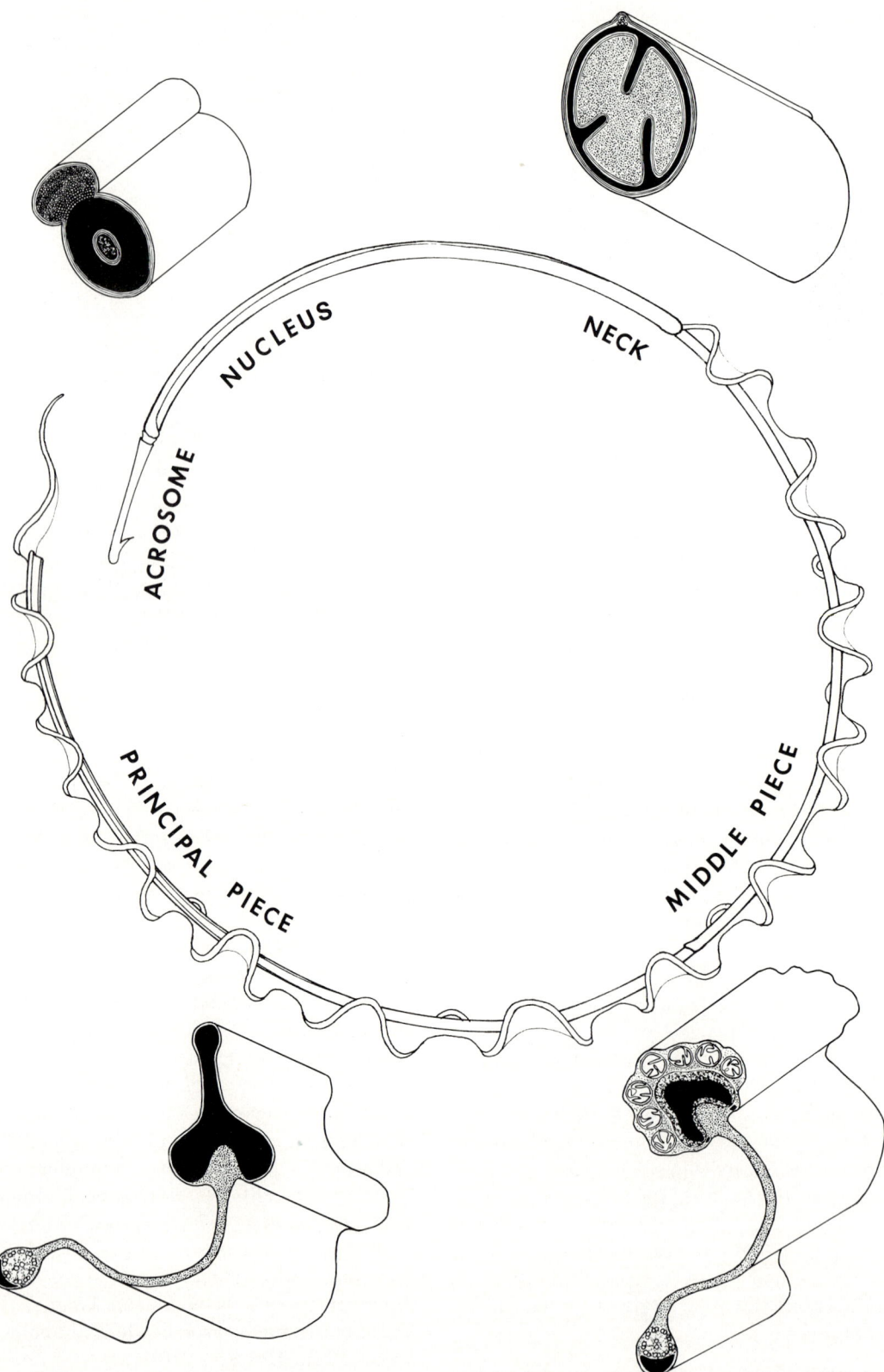

Figure 4. The spermatozoon of *Pleurodeles waltl*, with the reconstitution of the four main parts: the nucleus (upper left), the neck piece (upper right), the middle piece (lower right) and the principal piece (lower left). See the text for detailed interpretations.

chromatin part of the nucleus. After sodium chloride extraction of the basic proteins, this birefringence disappears (Fig. 17) while the DNA fibers aggregate and their spatial organization is disturbed (Fig. 22 and 23). In addition the birefringence of the nucleus is negative with respect to its length (Picheral, 1972) as are other anisotropic sperm nuclei. So it is now expected that this birefringence is due to the special structural organization of the nucleoprotein fibers.

Other data are known about the arrangement of the chromosomes in nuclei of Urodele sperm. In the sperm nuclei from *Plethodon cinereus* each chromosome is arranged in a *U* formation with its centromere at the base of the nucleus, and the chromosome arms extending forward along the length of the nucleus. The nucleolar organizer is always located at the rear half of the nucleus. Such is not the case with sperm nuclei from *Triturus cristatus cristatus* in which the position of the nucleolar organizer varies from sperm to sperm (McGregor and Walker, 1973).

The basic proteins from the Pleurodele sperm nucleus are very easily extracted with $2M$ NaCl. After migration on polyacrylamide gel, two bands characterize these nuclear basic proteins (Picheral and Thomas, 1977). They have an electrophoretic mobility intermediate between calf thymus histones and protamines from herring and salmon sperm (Fig. 26). All the basic proteins of the sperm of Salamandridae[3] including the sperm of *Nothophthalmus viridescens* analyzed by Bols et al., (1976), have the same properties (Fig. 27). In some species, polyacrylamide gel separates three bands. The basic proteins of the sperm of other families like Ambystomidae (Fig. 28) and the primitive Hynobidae are also similar.[4]

The Neck Piece In the salamandrid sperm cells the neck (also called "connecting piece") is a long cylinder that fits into a deep cavity at the basal end of the nucleus in such a way that the neck is surrounded by a thin shell of chromatin limited by two nuclear envelopes (Fig. 29). Its length varies from one-quarter to about one-sixth of the nucleus. At the caudal end of the neck a lateral semicircular knob has often been described. In fact, this structure is characteristic of testicular sperm, as it is still always present in the more mature testicular sperm, and is never observed in those of the spermiduct or spermatophore. This piece is the remnant of the annulus which begins to elongate along the midpiece very late in spermiogenesis (Fig. 30) as shown by Meves (1897) and Lommen (1970). At the caudal end of the neck, two centrioles are embedded in a pericentriolar granule; the more caudal corresponding to the basal body of the axoneme (Fig. 29).

The neck is proteinaceous and stains like basic proteins (Picheral, 1970). During spermiogenesis the neck strongly incorporates tritiated arginine and lysine (Picheral, 1972). In the sperm of *Triturus alpestris*, the central part of the neck is made of proteins in which arginine prevails (Werner, 1972).

The sperm of *Hynobius* (Fig. 44) and *Cryptobranchus* (Baker, 1963) has a very short neck piece which resembles the connecting piece of the mammalian sperm. An intermediate situation is observed with the spherical neck piece of the sperm from *Amphiuma* (Barker and Biesele, 1967; Pankratz, 1967).

The Tail Among the vertebrates, the sperm of the Urodele have, with the mammalian sperm, the more complex and voluminous additional components annexed to the axoneme. These additional components are the *axial fiber* (also named axial rod or supporting filament), the *marginal filament* and the *undulating membrane*. The first extends down the neck just in its axis while the second runs along the axoneme in the edge of the undulating membrane (Fig. 29 and 30). There are some differences between the neck, the axial fiber and the marginal filament which can be demonstrated with cytochemical (Picheral, 1970 and 1972c) and chemical technics (Werner, 1972).

The shape of the axial fiber of the Salamandridae changes all along the tail (Fig. 4). The outlines of the different levels of section were originally described with the light microscope, and recently, a second time with the electron microscope. Although there are some differences between species, the anterior sections near the neck are usually horseshoe or *U* shaped, while more caudally, at the level of the principal piece, the outline changes progressively into a trifoliate (Fig. 31) or a *Y*, or *I*-beam shaped cross section. The sections are circular all along the sperm tail of *Hynobius* (Fig. 45 and 46).

The axial fiber has a cortex and a medulla (Fig. 4, 25, and 30). Progressively, when the tail takes on a trifoliate or *Y* outline, the cortex becomes very thin and finally disappears; the medulla continuing alone to the end of the fiber. The two components of the axial fiber are different in their chemical constitution. After detergent treatments or enzymatic extractions (Picheral, 1972c), the cortex appears to be very resistant, while the medulla quickly disappears (Fig. 25, 33-35). The resistance of the medulla to these treatments varies along the tail. Moreover detergents may separate it into two parts at the level of the cortex, the smaller being located in the groove of the axial fiber, the other at the opposite side near the mitochondria (Fig. 33). These two parts are

---

[3]Thomas D., Charbonneau M., and Picheral, B.: unpublished.
[4]Thomas D. and Picheral, B.: unpublished.

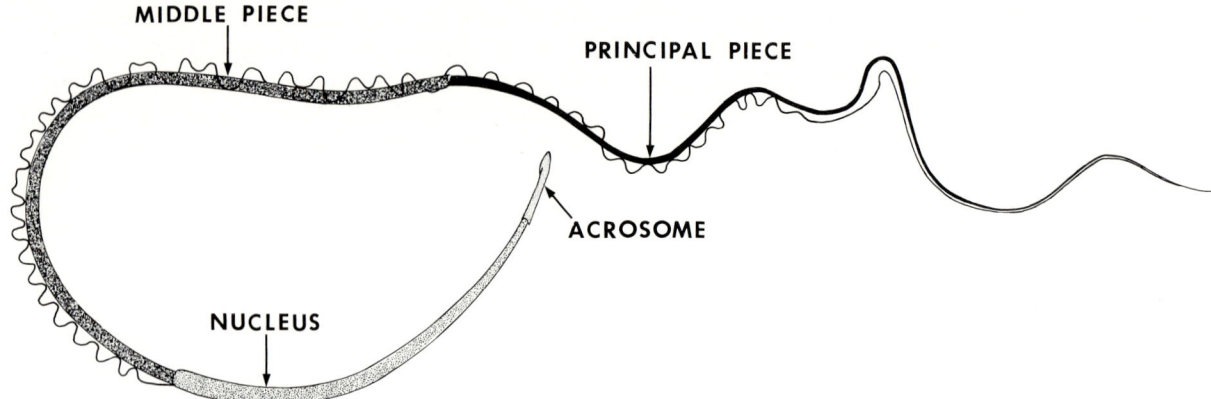

Figure 5. The mature sperm of *Euproctus asper* (Salamandridae) from a phase contrast micrograph.

fused together at the level of the two dense lines coming from the extended annulus, which is also the point where the two leaves of the plasma membrane are firmly attached to the axial fiber before converging to form the undulating membrane (Fig. 30). On the other side of the undulating membrane, between the convex part of the axial fiber and the sheath of mitochondria, is a thin layer of a special hyaloplasm which exhibits an ATPase activity (Fig. 38). In mature sperm there is no cytoplasm at the midpiece level; it disappears during the late spermatogenesis process. Mitochondria are, as in mammalian sperm, obliquely disposed, but it is not clear whether every arc of mitochondria is a part of a sectioned helix. The sperm tail of Cryptobranchidae (Baker, 1963) and Hynobidae (Fig. 44, 45, 46) do not display any mitochondria, and in addition there is no remnant of annulus along the round axial fiber. The mitochondria seem to be located in a protoplasmic bead observed around the nucleus (Fig. 6 and 43), even in the mature sperm.

The undulating membrane consists of the two parallel leaves of the plasma membrane enclosing a dense cytoplasmic matrix (Fig. 31) which appears to be stabilized by —S—S— bonds (Bedford and Calvin, 1974).

The axonemal complex is typical. Doublets 3 and 4 lie next to the undulating membrane, while No. 7, 8, and 9 lie adjacent to the marginal filament. In section the marginal filament is crescentic and bissected by a lamina (Fig. 31 and 32) which is very resistant to protease digestion or detergent treatments (Fig. 33-35). This lamina displays a periodic structure (150 Å) (Fig. 36) and is always in close relation to microtubule A of doublet No. 8 (Fig. 32). On each side of the marginal fiber a dense area of hyaloplasm also exhibits an ATPase activity (Fig. 38).

Picheral (1967) and Fawcett (1970) have attempted to homologize the major components of the Urodele sperm tail with those of the mammalian sperm tail. It has been suggested that the axial fiber would correspond to the outer dense fiber in No. 3: the two structures both appear in close connection with the doublet 3 during the spermiogenesis process (Picheral, 1972c) and they have the same behavior during fertilization (Picheral, 1977b).

The marginal fiber, which displays a periodic fine structure and which has no cortex, may correspond to one of the longitudinal columns of the fibrous sheath of the mammalian sperm tail.

Symmetry

The sperm of Pleurodeles show a bilaterally symmetrical structure (Picheral, 1972c). The barb of the acrosomal cap, the nuclear ridge, and the elongated ridge of the axial fiber near its end, lay in the same plane of symmetry (Fig. 4). The undulating membrane may correspond to this plane during its beat. According to the terminology, given by Folliot and Maillet (1970) using axoneme disposition for orientation, the acrosomal barb projects ventrally while the nuclear ridge and the undulating membrane lie on the opposite or dorsal side. Thus it may be useful to refer to the dorsal and ventral sides of the sperm, for describing certain details. Referring to this data, it has been possible to analyze on which side the sperm contacts the plasma membrane during the fertilization process (Picheral, 1977b).

Motility

Some observations have been made with dark and light phase-contrast microscopy. When sperm cells of Pleurodeles are observed in physiological solutions, they are almost semicircular and then swirl around in the same plane with their dorsum outside (Fig. 4 and 39). The sperm that are swimming in the viscous external, and more-resistant middle jelly coat of the egg become straight, and their trajectory is linear (Fig. 40) without any helical motility. After penetrating the internal jelly coat which is liquid, the shape and the trajectory of the sperm become circular again. This change affects both the nucleus and the tail, and seems to be a physical reaction to the medium. The flagellum executes short sinusoidal movements which become slower and easy to observe when the sperm swims in the external jelly coat of the egg. This sinusoidal movement consists of three dimensional waves inscribed in a cylinder. The waves appear to originate at the base of the head and progress caudally, and give the sperm tails an endless screw aspect when they are observed sideways.

The sperm of Pleurodeles never reverse their motility, which according to Baker (1962) seems to be the case for the sperm of *Amphiuma* and *Triturus*. The motility is restricted to the flagellum. Baker (1966) has suggested that the undulating membrane moves while the flagellum is nonmotile and Fawcett (1970) also discusses the potential motility of the axial fiber. The close relationship between the mitochondria, the axial fiber, and the undulating membrane, does not seem to be an argument for the potential motility of these two parts of the tail; but the large distance between the mitochondria and the axoneme remains an unsolved problem. This same distance is even longer in the Hynobidae (Fig. 6).

Unlike the Pleurodele sperm, in some species such as *Amphiuma tridactylum* the sperm exhibit a slightly helical shape that causes the sperm to rotate as it moves forward (Baker, 1962). The sperm of *Necturus* (Proteidae) has a very prominent helical form, and when in motion the sperm quickly rotates but has a straight trajectory (Baker 1963)[5]. The undulating membrane is narrow

[5]Picheral, B.: unpublished

and in contrast with the other species, the flagellum winds tightly around the axial fiber which is itself twisted. The wave movements of the flagellum are of very short amplitude like slight vibrations. The twisted sperms do not have a plane of symmetry.

DISCUSSION

This general review of the sperm structure of Urodeles allows us to see the complexity of this vertebrate sperm cell. The more detailed the investigation into structure and function of the sperm of Urodeles, the more complicated the problems seem to become.

It would be of particular interest to know the functional significance of the three different parts of the acrosomal cap: do they correspond to different proteases acting sequentially during transit through the several and various envelopes of the Urodele eggs? The first study of the fertilization process does not permit us to answer the question (Picheral, 1977a). New analyses and observations have to be done concerning the different proteases of the acrosome, and the exact time and mechanism of the acrosomal cap disappearance.

The nucleus of the sperm of Urodeles seems to be a good material to study nucleoprotein fiber organization, and the nuclear ridge provides a unique model of a proteinaceous inclusion. It is of particular interest to study the sperm nucleus with the aim of understanding its modifications during the pronucleus formation and related phenomena.

Comparative study of the urodele sperm tail and the mammalian sperm tail suggests some homologies. It would be of particular interest to compare the chemical properties of the sperm tail components of these two groups. In addition, the tail of the sperm from Urodeles offers a fortunate opportunity to study the direction of

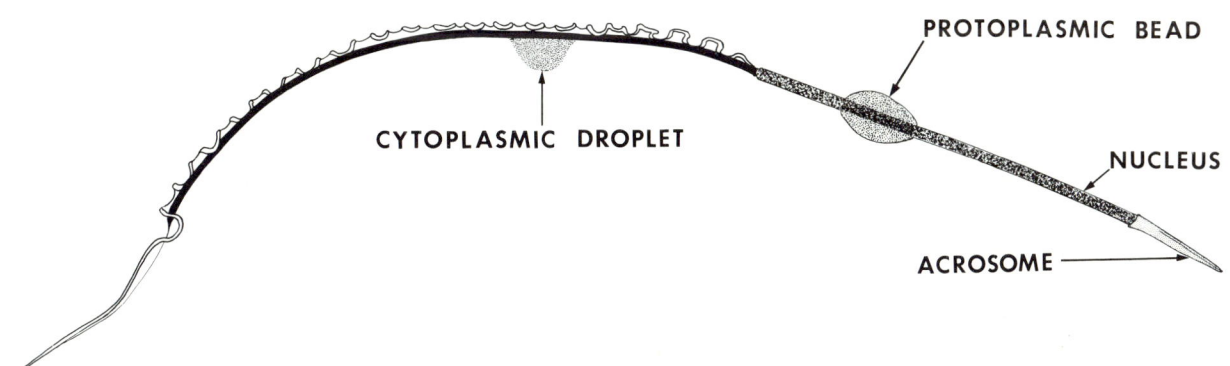

Figure 6. The mature sperm of *Hynobius nebulosus* (Hynobiidae). This sperm has no mitochondria along its tail, but a protoplasmic bead around its nucleus (see the text and Fig. 41-46).

flagellar movements, owing to its planar symmetry which corresponds to that of the axial fiber. Thus, using an adequate fixation procedure, it might be possible to study the direction of the beat in relation to the orientation of the two central microtubules (Fig. 4).

Finally, even though the purpose of this chapter is not zoological, some observations suggest that the fine morphology of the Urodele sperm may be used as a tool for phylogenic studies. For instance, the sperm of the two closely related primitive families Cryptobranchidae and Hynobidae have the same unique characteristics that set them apart from the other families. In addition, the sperm of Pseudobranchus from the Sirenidae family seem to be very different (see the only picture published, Barker and Baker, 1970) from all other sperm of Urodeles; and in fact the exact place of these amphibians is in dispute. Thus, after one century of cytological investigations, the sperm of Urodeles, as always, offers attractive new perspectives.

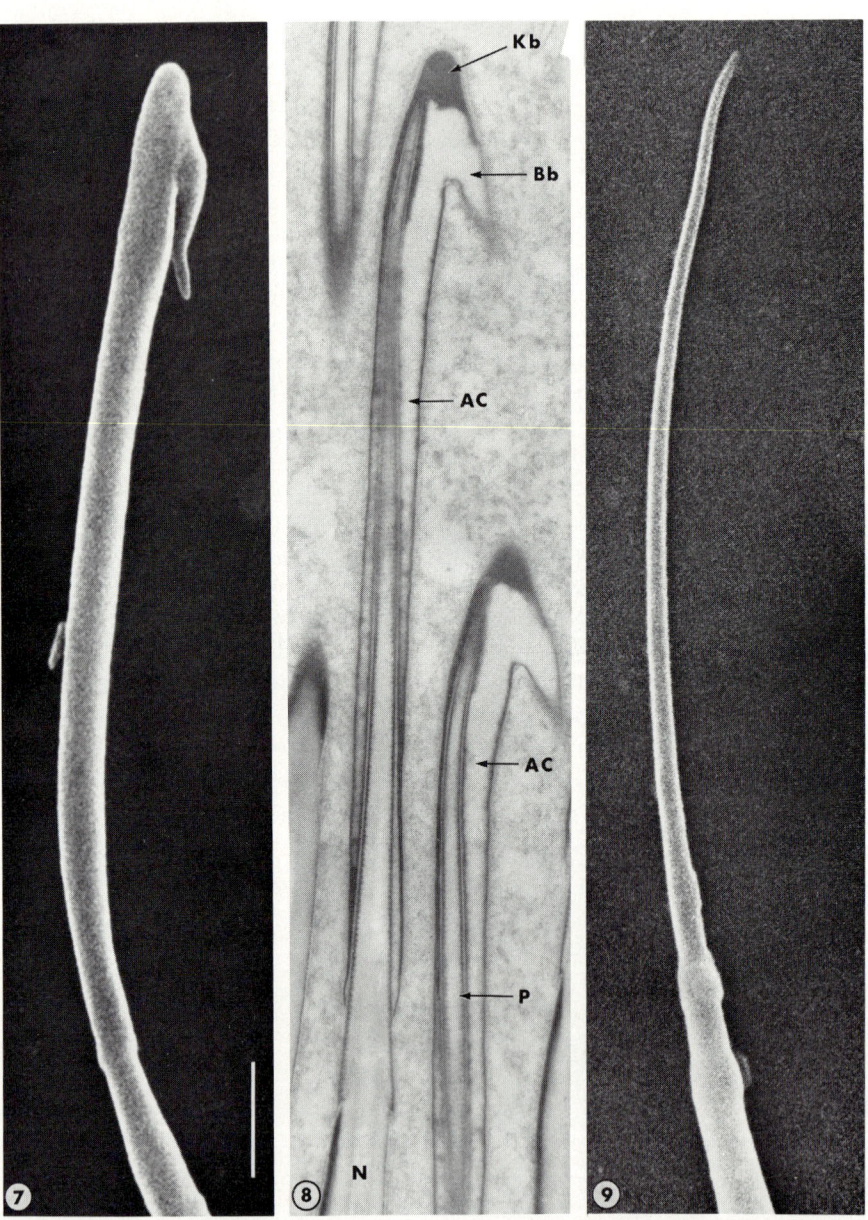

Figures 7-9. Acrosomes of the sperm of *Pleurodeles*. Scale bar: 1 μm. Figure 7. Scanning electron micrograph of an intact acrosome. Figure 8. Longitudinal section of acrosomes from the nucleus (N), to the anterior knob (Kb) which is, with the barb (Bb), a part of the acrosomal cap (AC), perforatorium (P). The peripheral sheath of the perforatorium shows a periodical organization. (Phosphotungstic acid treatment on block, GMA embedded). Figure 9. Scanning electron micrograph of a denuded acrosome. The acrosomal cap has been cleared off and the perforatorium persists.

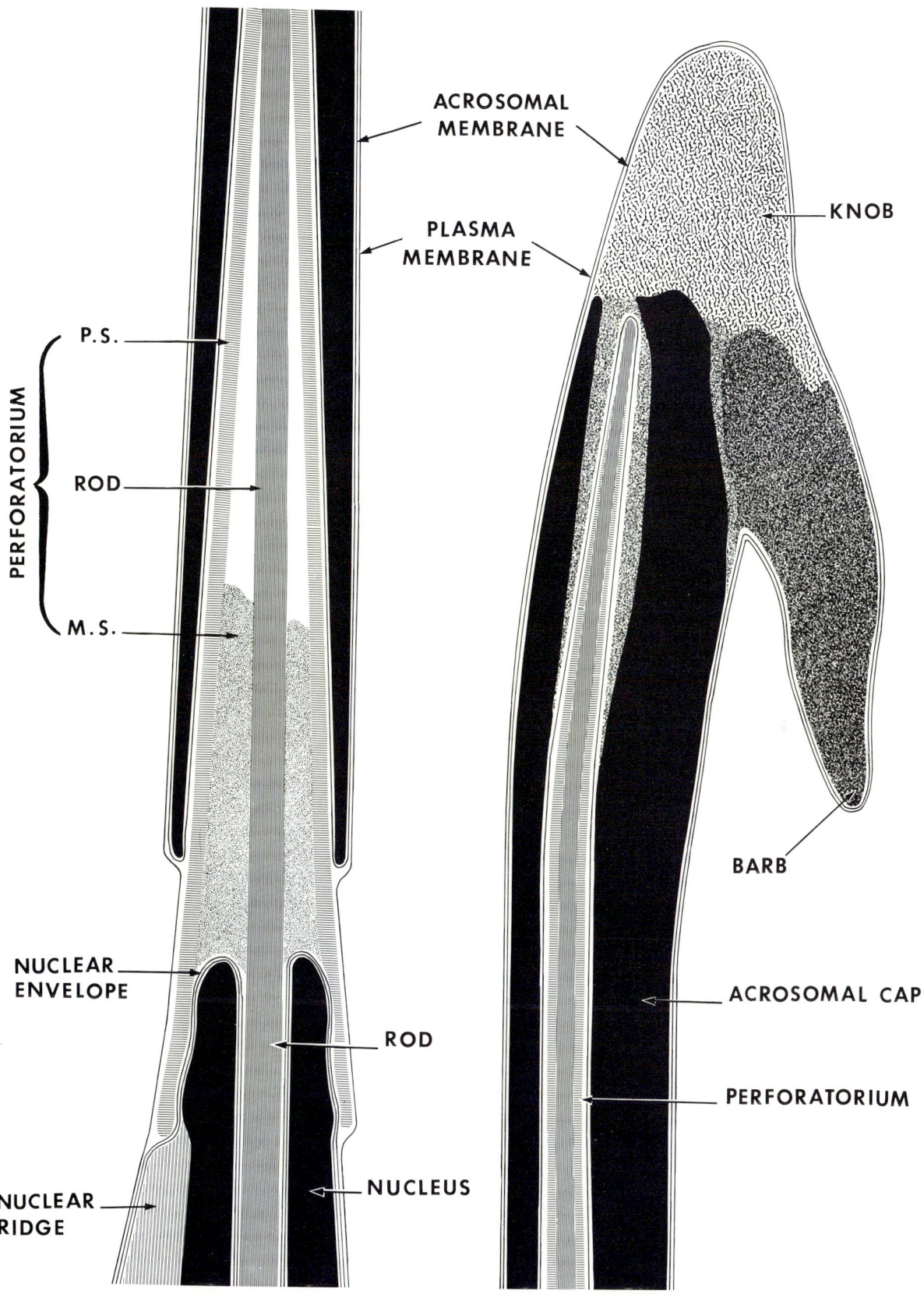

Figure 10. Diagrammatic reconstruction of the acrosomal region of a pleurodele sperm. (See the text for explanations).

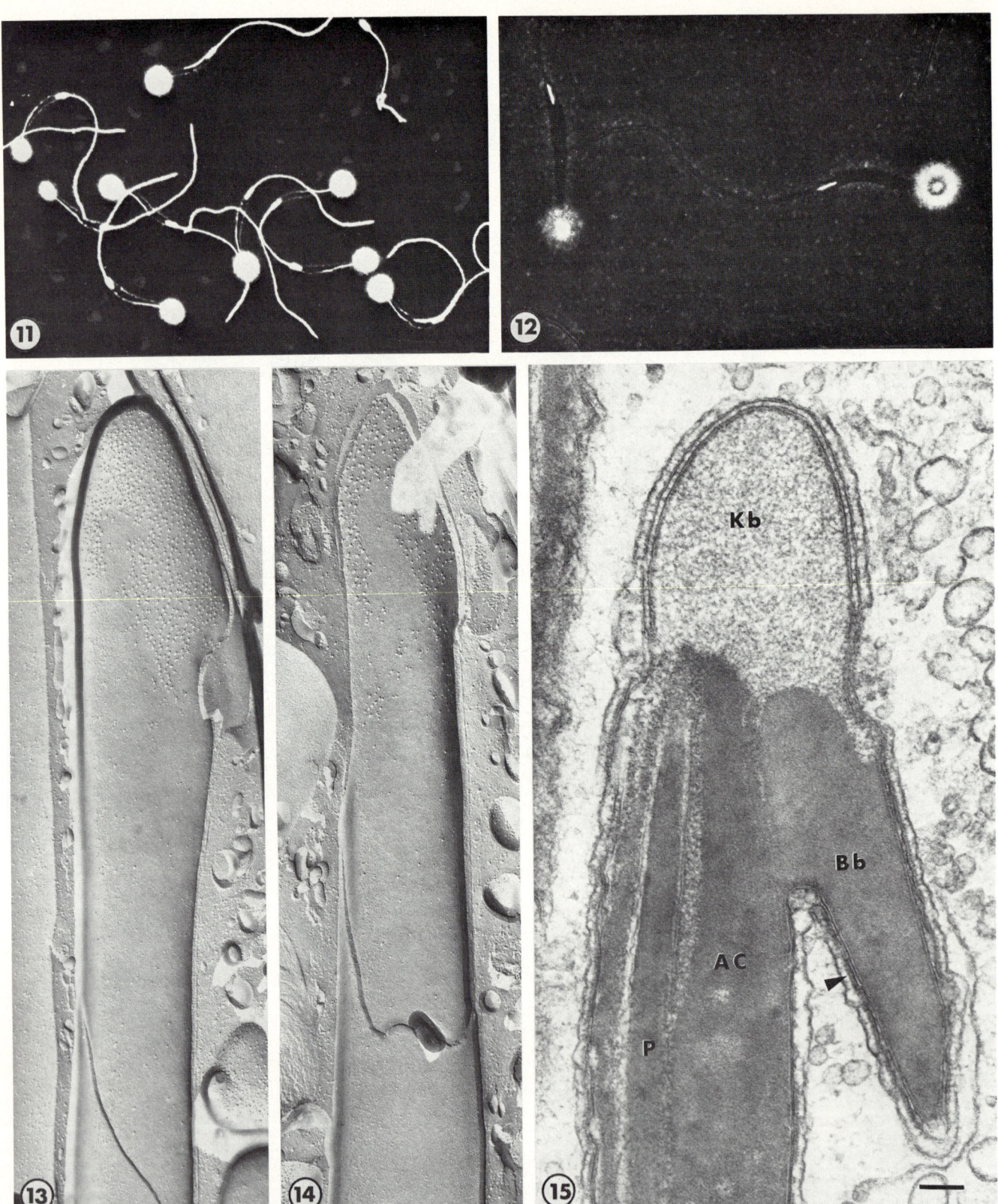

Figures 11 and 12. Dark phase-contrast micrographs of pleurodele sperm applied to a gelatin membrane (Kodak AR 10 autoradiographic plate previously exposed to light). The "halo reaction" is localized at the acrosomal level and centered at the tip of the acrosome.
Figures 13 and 14. Electron micrographs of replicas of two freeze-fractured surfaces of acrosomes (testis sperm cells of *Pleurodeles*).
Figure 15. The apical part of the acrosome of a testis sperm cell. The arrow indicates granules on the plasma membrane. Ac, acrosomal cap; Bb, barb; Kb, anterior knob; P, perforatorium.

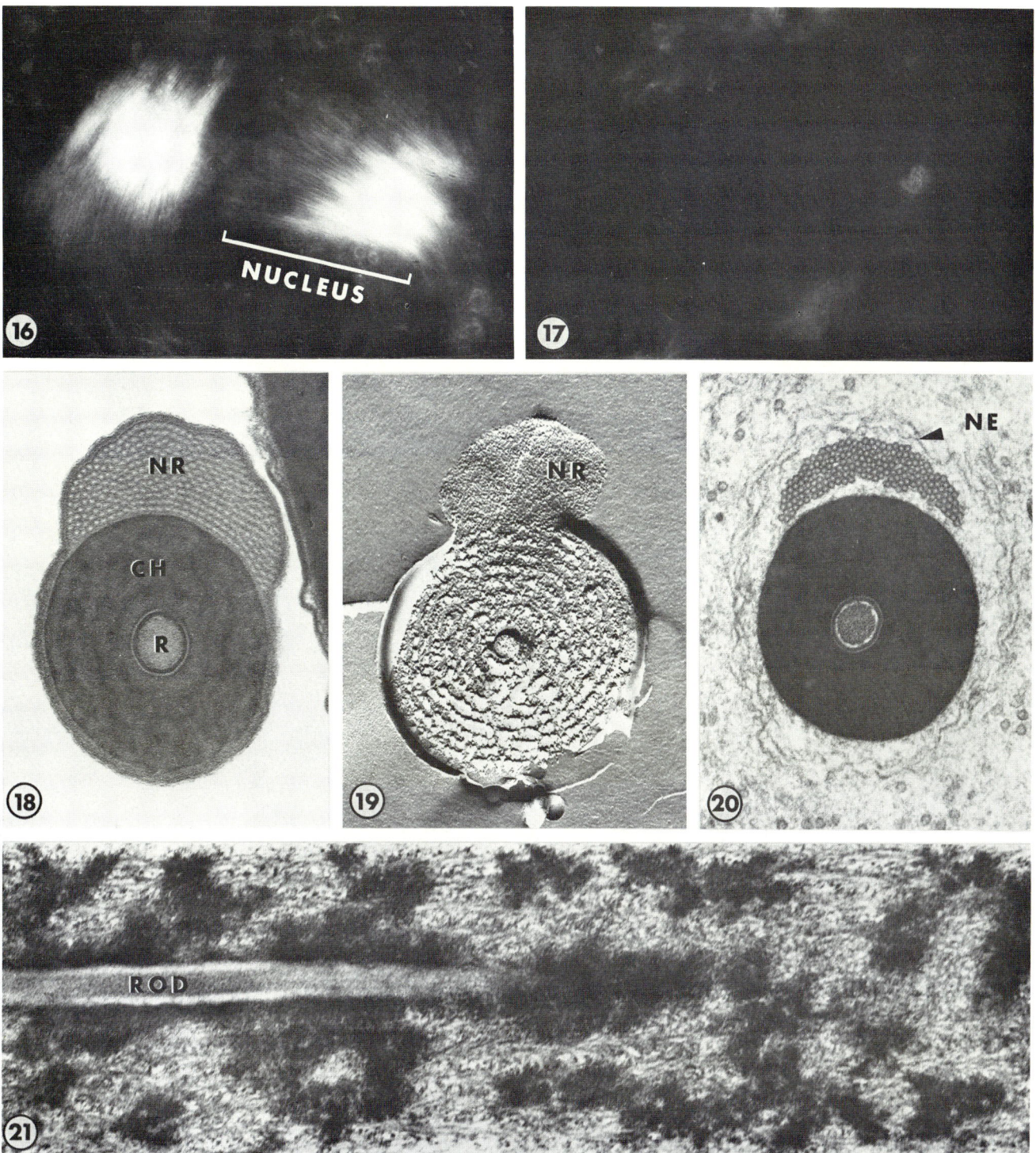

Figures 16 and 17. Polarizing-microscope micrographs of two bundles of testis sperm (frozen sectioned with cryostat). The birefringence observed along the anterior part of the nuclei (Fig. 16) disappears after treatment of the same section with 2M NaCl solution (Fig. 17).

Figures 18 and 19. Comparable areas of mature pleurodele sperm showing in thin section (Fig. 18) and in a freeze-fracture preparation (Fig. 19), the two parts of the nucleus: the lamellar chromatin area (CH), the endonuclear canal with its rod in the center (R), and the nuclear ridge (NR).

Figure 20. Section of late spermatid nucleus. The minute tubules that will form the nuclear ridge, are localized within the nuclear envelope (NE).

Figure 21. Longitudinal section of spermatid nucleus showing the arced pattern organization of the fibrils between the dense area.

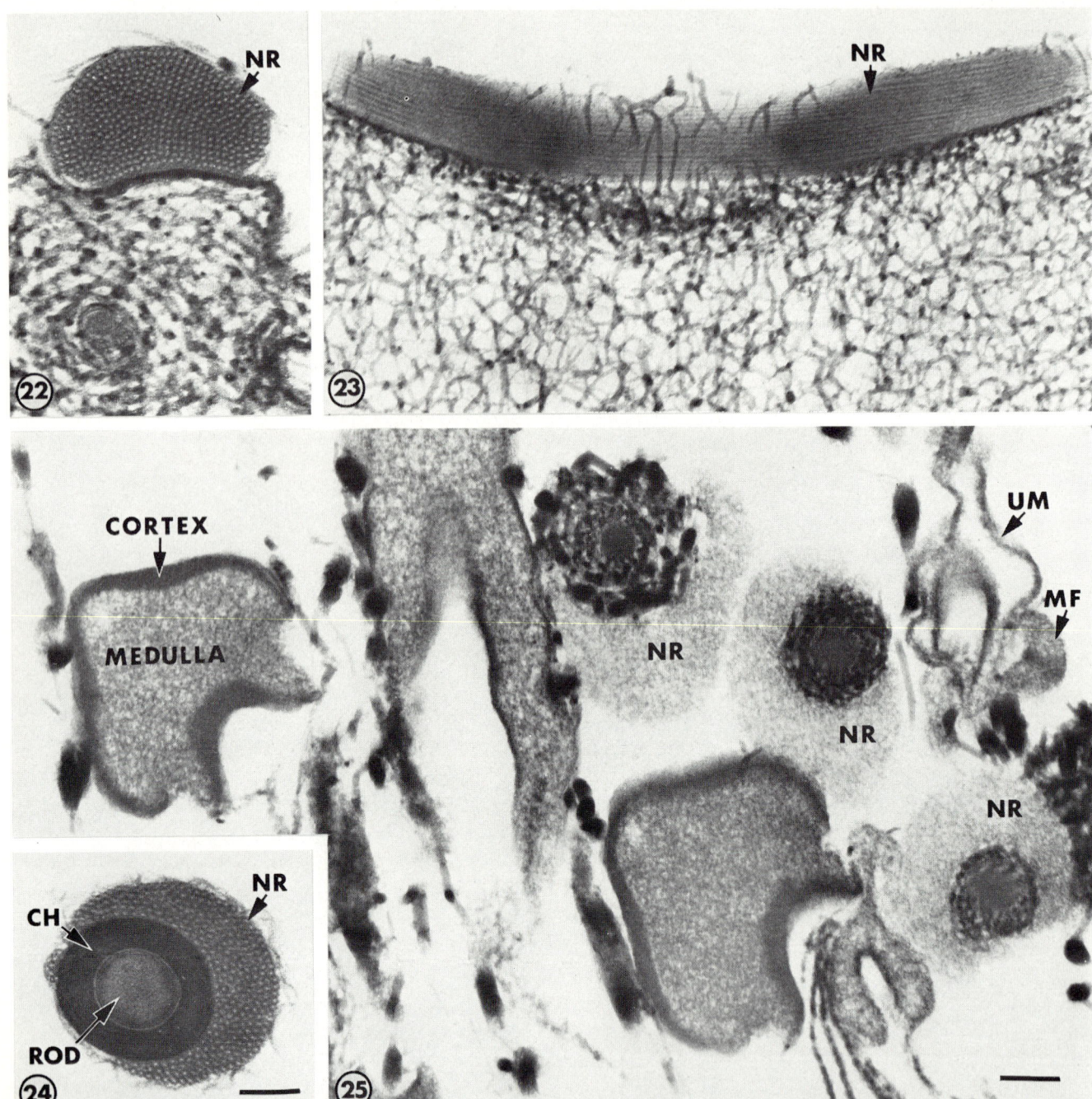

Figures 22 and 23. Transverse and longitudinal section of nuclei extracted with a 2M NaCl solution. The nuclear ridges (NR) are well preserved while the fibers of DNA agglutinate after the basic protein extraction (Pleurodeles).

Figure 24. Transverse section of the anterior part of a nucleus (*Triturus palmatus*). Scale bar = 0.1 μm. At this level the nuclear ridge (NR) is more developed than the chromatin area (CH).

Figure 25. Sperms of *Triturus palmatus*, after treatment with 0.5% SDS for 15 min. The minute tubular organization of the nuclear ridge (NR) is no longer observed. The cortex of the axial fiber and the undulating membrane (UM) are well preserved, while the medulla and the marginal filament (MF) are less dense. Scale bar = 0.1 μm.

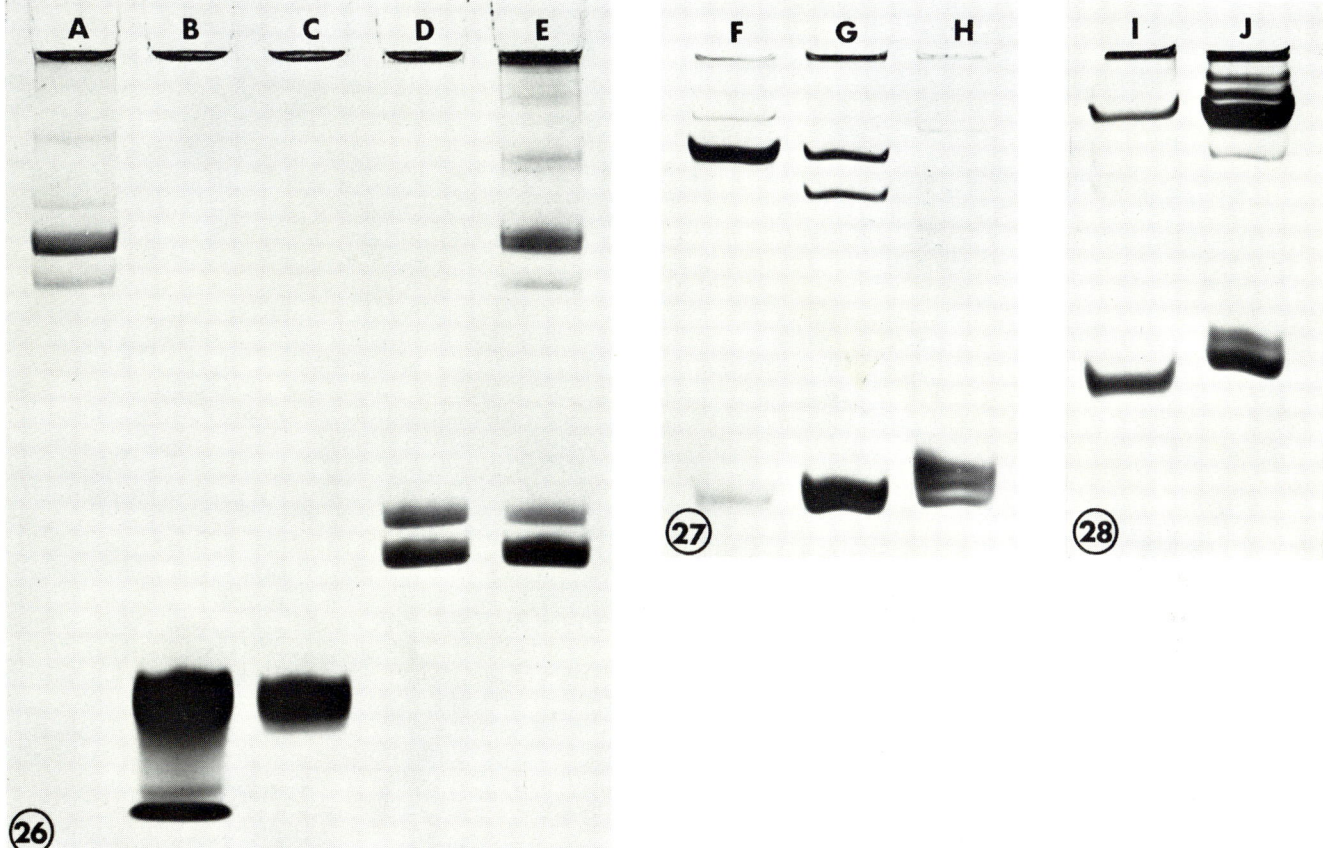

Figure 26. Polyacrylamide gel electrophoresis of the nuclear basic protein fractions extracted from spermiductal sperm (D) and whole testis (E) of *Pleurodeles waltl*. Calf thymus (A), Clupeine (B) and Salmine (C) were run as standards.

Figures 27 and 28. Comparison between nuclear basic proteins from *Pleurodeles* (F and I), *Ambystoma* (G), *Salamandra* (H), and *Euproctus* (J).

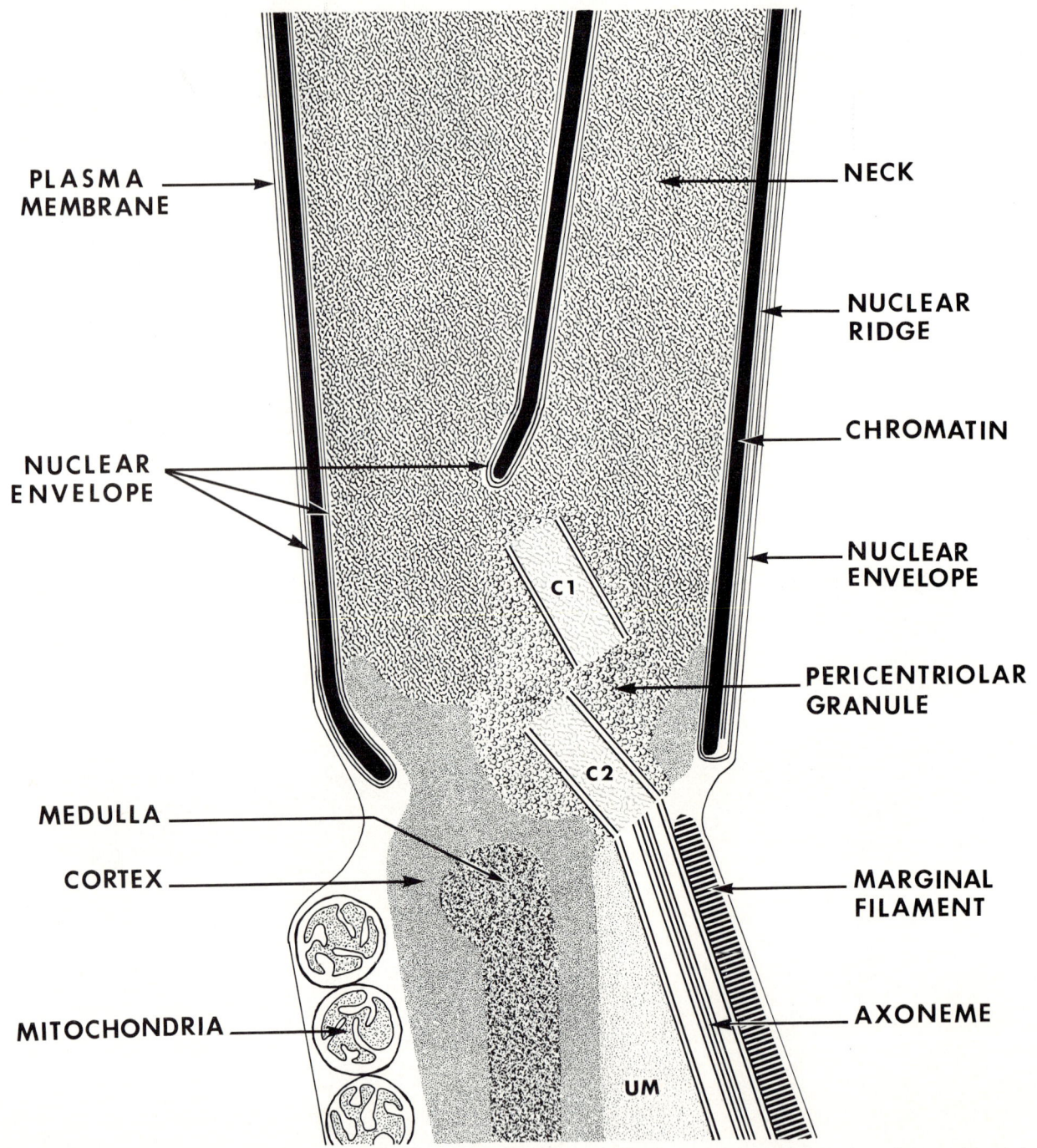

Figure 29. Diagrammatic representation of the transition level between the head (nucleus and neck piece) and the tail. See the text for explanations.

Figure 31. Transverse sections throughout the principal piece. At this level, the axial fiber corresponds to the medulla.
Figure 32. Enlargement of the edge part of the undulating membrane. The close connection between the A tubule of doublet 8 with the transversally sectioned lamina of the marginal filament is indicated by the arrow.

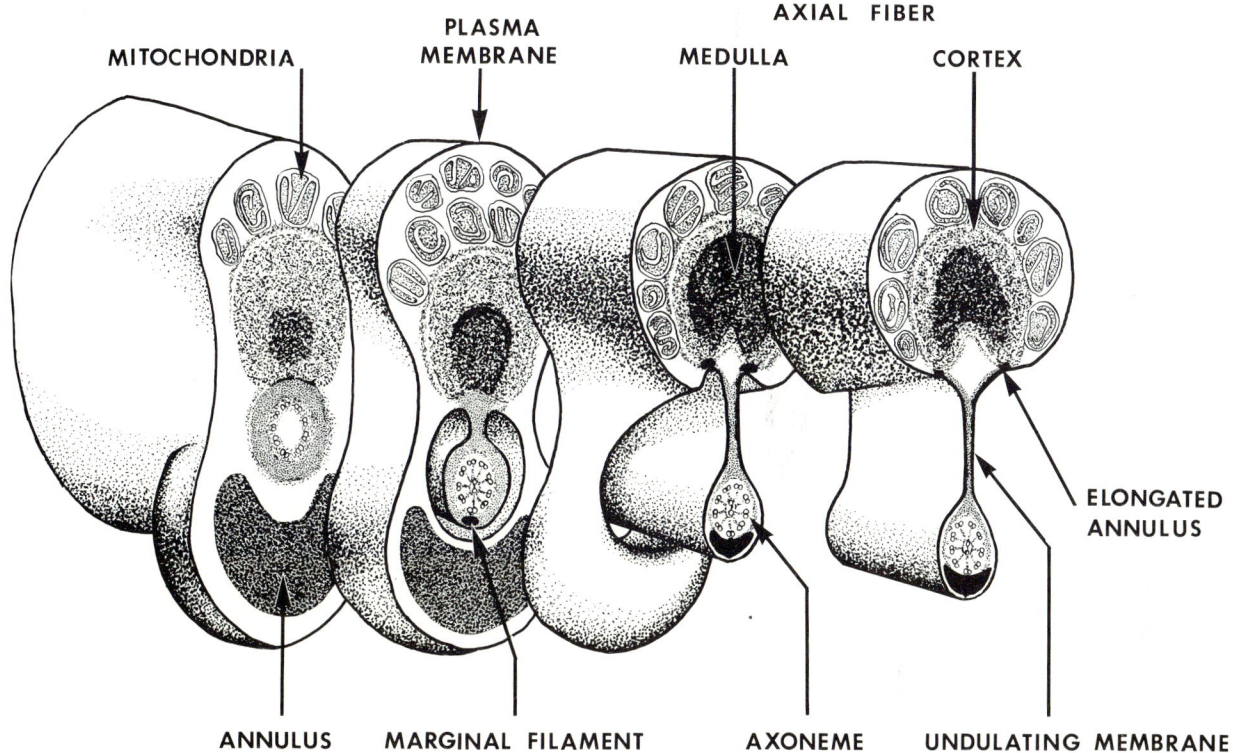

Figure 30. Diagrammatic representation of the foremost part of the tail (near the neck piece) of a testicular pleurodeles sperm. The two dense lines along the axial fiber correspond to the partially elongated annulus still forming a lateral knob.

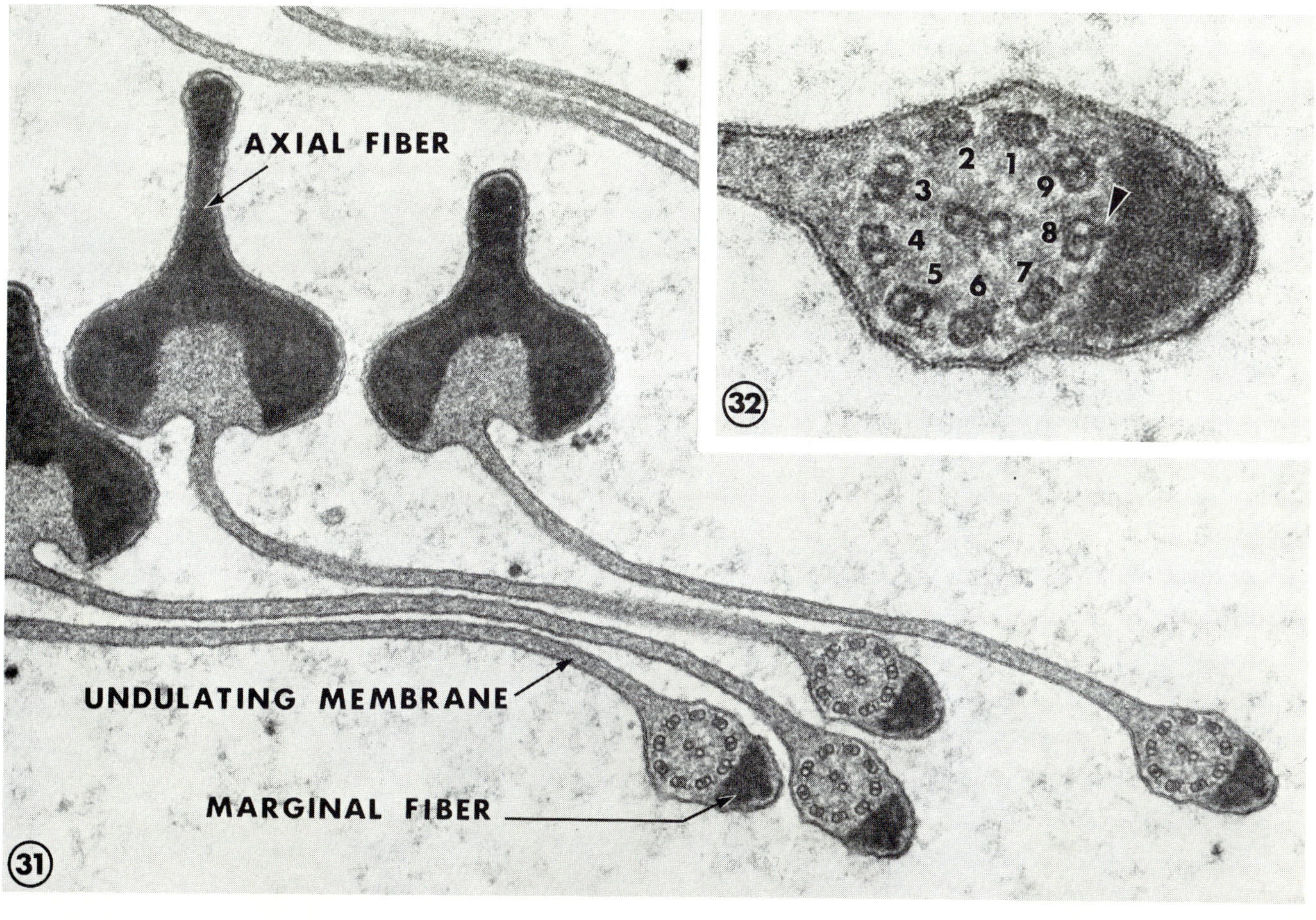

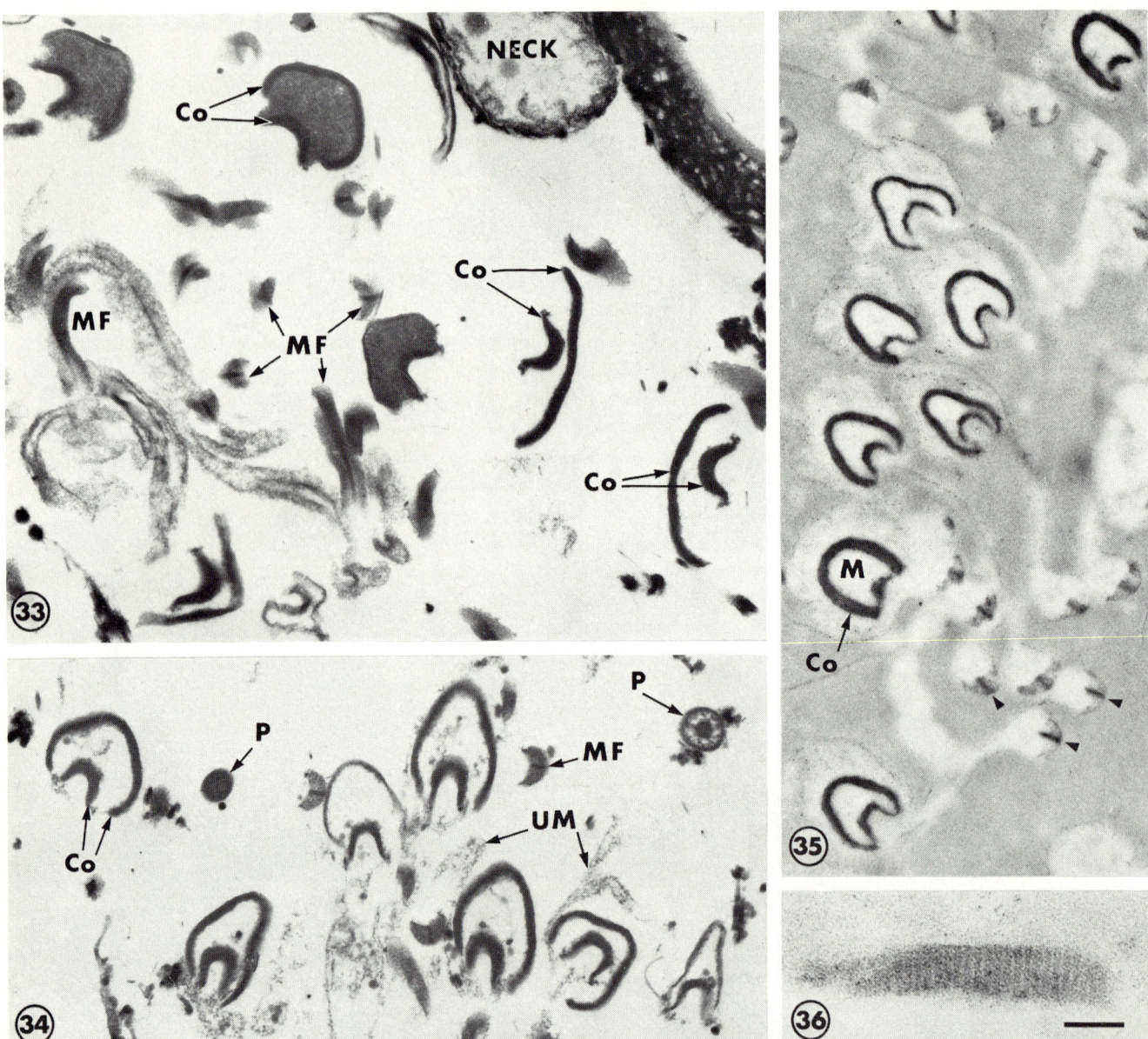

Figure 33. Sperm of *Triturus palmatus* treated with 0.5% SDS for 1 h. The medulla of the axial fiber is more or less extracted, the two sections on the right are fully extracted and the two parts of the cortex (Co) are separated. The marginal filament (MF) is resistant, especially the transverse dense lamina.

Figure 34. Sperm of *Triturus palmatus* treated with 0.5% N-lauroyl-sarcosine-sodium-salt for 15 min. The medulla is extracted while the transverse dense lamina of the marginal filament (MF) is well preserved. The matrix of the undulating membrane remains resistant as does the perforation (P) of the acrosome. UM, undulating membrane.

Figure 35. Ultra-thin pleurodele sperm tail section floated on a trypsine solution. The cortex (Co) and the dense lamina (arrow) of the marginal filament are well preserved, while the medulla (M) is extracted.

Figure 36. Same treatment as in Figure 35. Longitudinal section of the lamina showing the periodical structure. Scale bar = 0.1 μm.

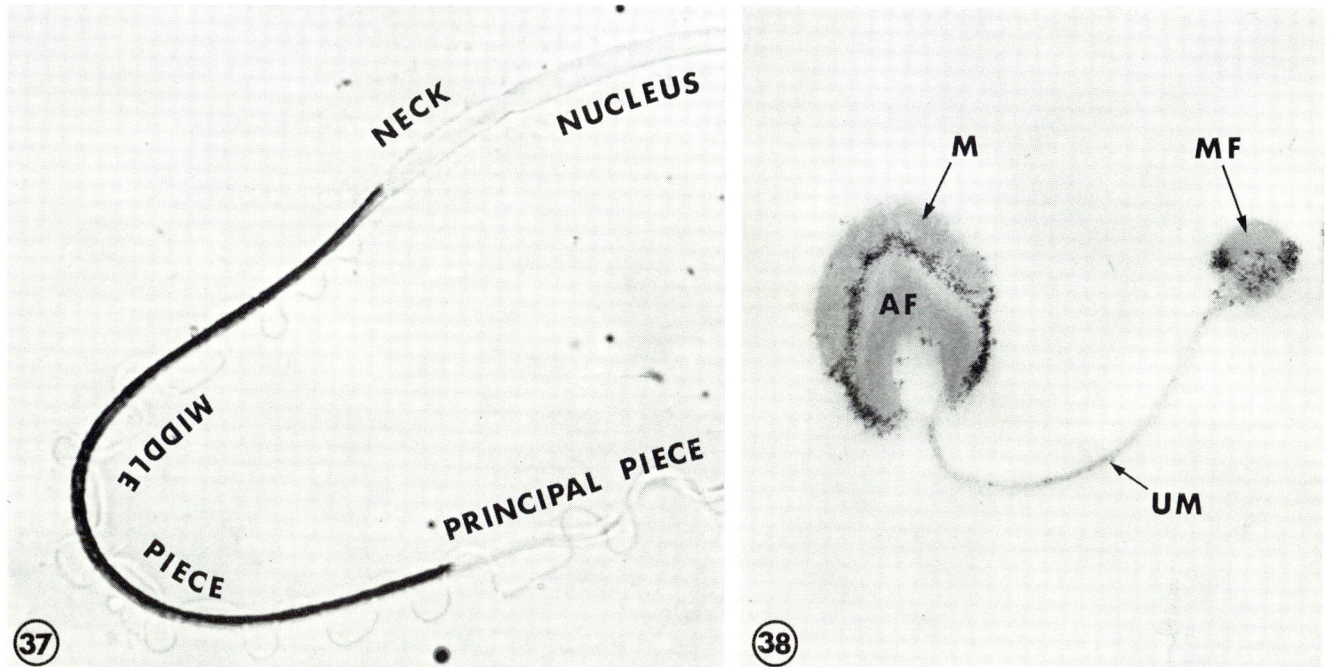

Figure 37. Sperm of *Pleurodeles*. Mitochondria of the middle piece visualized by means of a diaminobenzidine reaction. The sheath of mitochondria terminates abruptly.
Figure 38. Sperm of *Pleurodeles*. ATPase activity on a transverse section through the middle piece. AF, axial fiber M, mitochondria; MF, marginal filament; UM, undulating membrane.

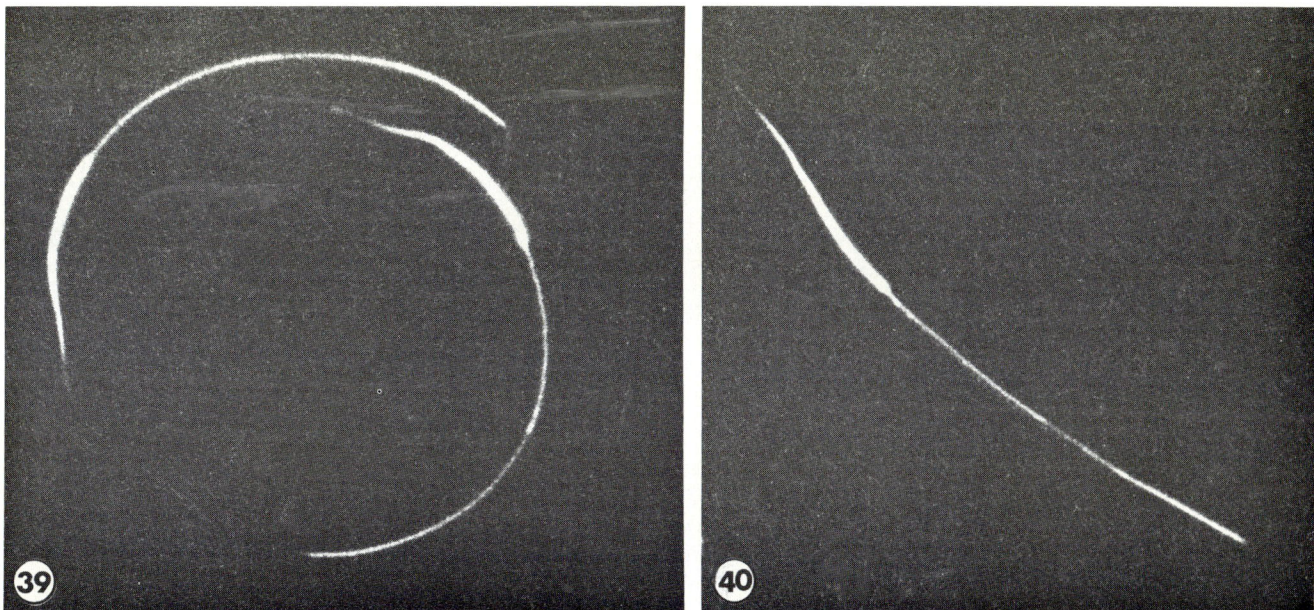

Figure 39. Curved spermatozoa of *Pleurodeles* swimming in a salt solution.
Figure 40. Straight spermatozoon of *Pleurodeles* swimming in the external jelly envelope of the egg.

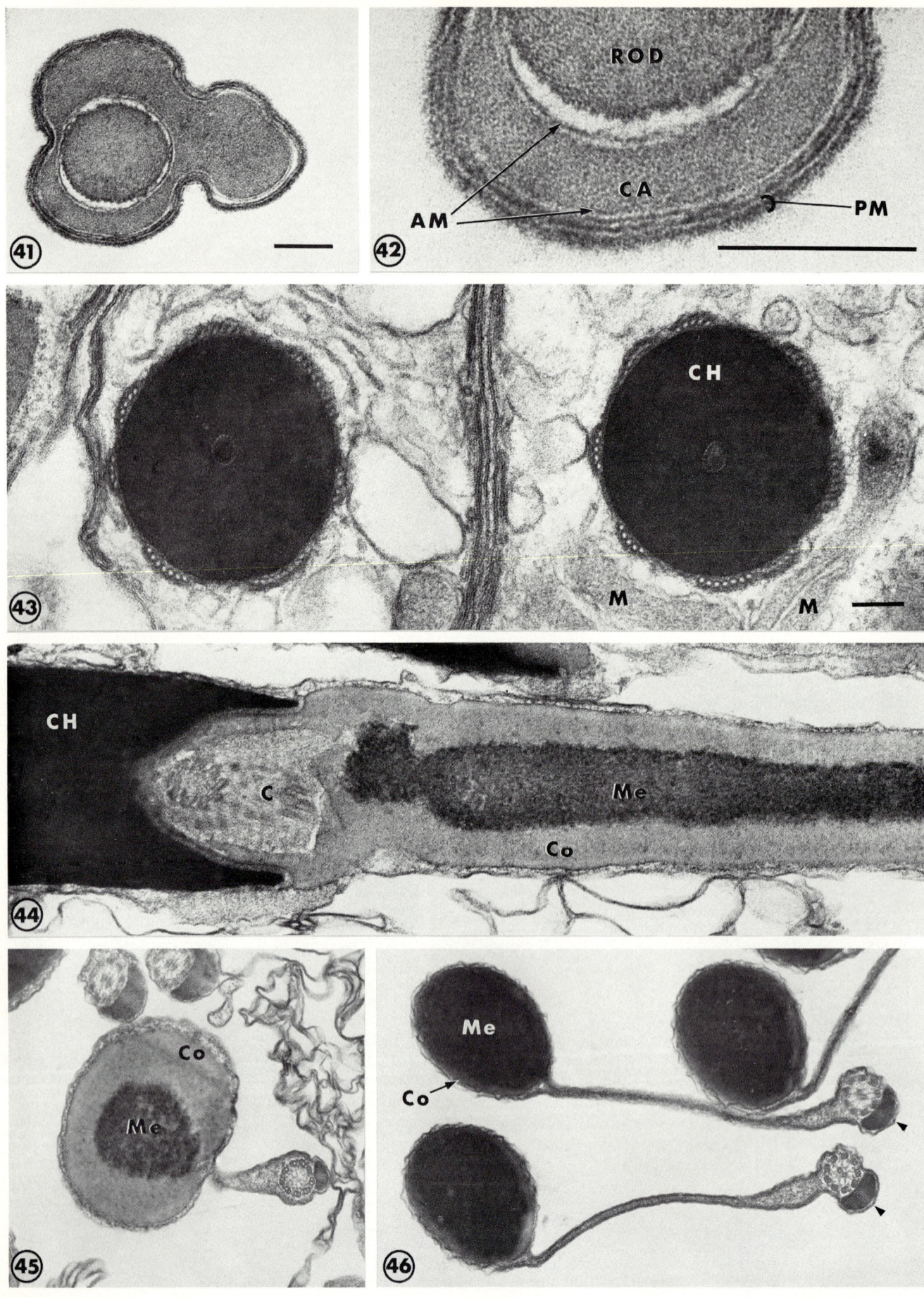

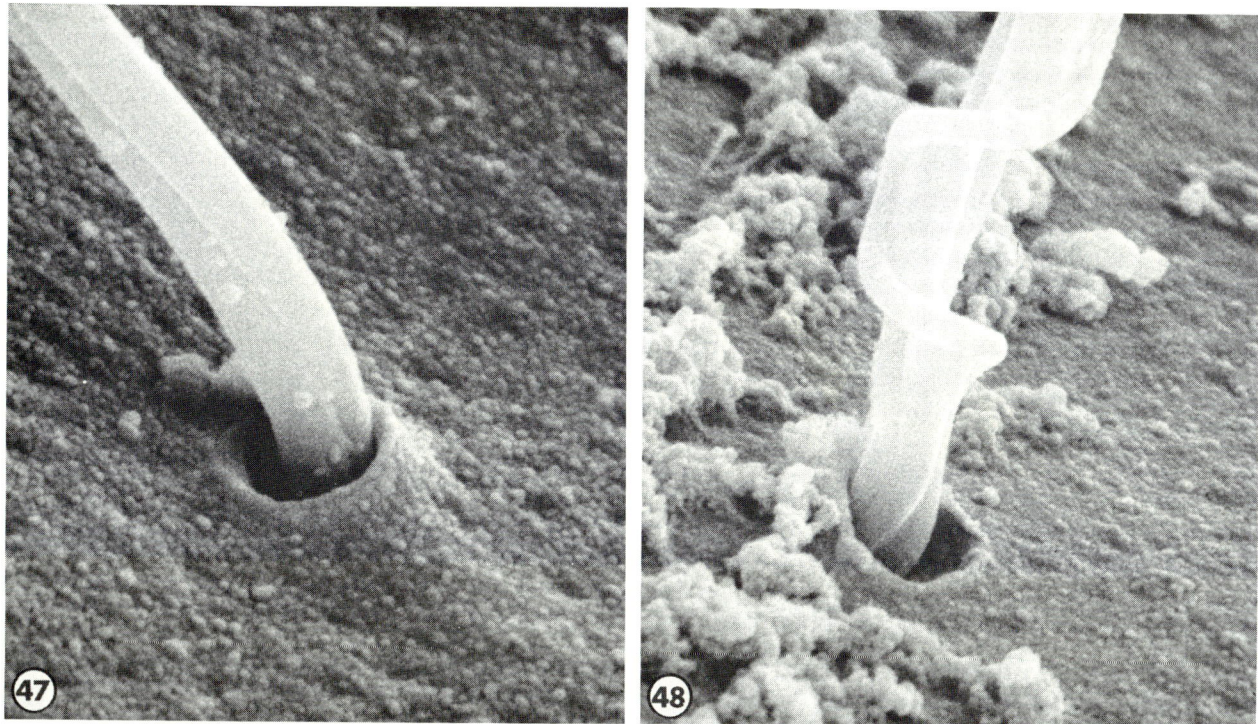

Figures 47 and 48. Scanning electron micrographs of the sperm penetration through the vitelline layer of the egg (*Pleurodeles*). Figure 47 shows the initial process (at the nucleus level, note the nuclear ridge), while Figure 48 shows a more advanced stage at the principal piece level of the tail. In both cases there is a lip around the aperture, indicating the previous protease activity of the acrosome.

Figures 41-46. Sections of sperm of *Hynobius nebulosus*. Figure 41. Transverse section of the acrosome. The acrosomal cap is trifoliated. Scale bar = 0.1 μm. Figure 42. Enlargement of Figure 41. Transverse sections of fibrils appear at the rod level, the plasma membrane (PM) is coated with a thick mantle of dense material. AM, membrane of the acrosomal cap. Scale bar = 0.1 μm. CA, acrosomal cap. Figure 43. Two transverse sections of nuclei (CH) with their several bundles of minute tubules. M, mitochondria. Scale bar = 0.1 μm. Figure 44. Longitudinal section at the transitional level between the head and the tail. The connected piece is reduced to a transversally striated pericentriolar granule (C, centriole.). The axial fiber, with its two parts, the cortex (Co) and the medulla (Me), has no sheath of mitochondria. Figure 45. Section of the tail close to the nucleus, there is no sheath of mitochondria. The axoneme has only peripheral doublets. Figure 46. More basal section. The two parts of the cylindrical axial fiber are still present. The lamina (arrows) is less electron dense than the marginal filament as a whole.

REFERENCES

Baker, C.L.: Spermatozoa of Amphiumae: Spermateleosis, Helical Motility and Reversibility. J Tennessee Acad Sci 37(1962)23-37

Baker, C.L.: Spermatozoa and Spermateleosis in *Cryptobranchus* and *Necturus*. J Tennessee Acad Sci 38(1963)1-11

Baker, C.L.: Spermatozoa and Spermateleosis in the Salamandridae with Electron Microscopy of *Diemictylus*. J Tennessee Acad Sci 41(1966)1-25

Ballowitz, E.: Untersuchungen über die Struktur der Spermatozoen zugleich ein Beitrag zur Lehre vom feineren Bau der kontraktilen Elemente. Z Wiss Zool 50(1890)317-407

Barker, K.R.; Baker, C.L.: Urodele Spermateleosis: A Comparative Electron Microscope Study. In: Spermatologia Comparata, pp. 81-84, ed. by B. Baccetti. Academic Press, New York, 1970

Barker, K.R.; Biesele, J.: Spermateleosis of a Salamander *Amphiuma tridactylum* Cuvier. Cellule 67(1967)91-118

Bedford, J.M.; Calvin, H.I.: Changes in —S—S-linked Structures of the Sperm Tail during Epididymal Maturation, with Comparative Observations in Submammalian Species. J Exp Zool 187(1974)181-203

Bols, N.C.; Byrd, E.W.; Kasinsky, J. & H.E.: On the Diversity of Sperm Histones in Vertebrates. I Changes in Basic Protein during Spermiogenesis in the Newt *Notophthalmus viridescens*. Differentiation 7(1976)31-38

Bouligand, Y.: Twisted Fibrous Arrangements in Biological Materials and Cholesteric Mesophases. Tissue Cell 4(1972)189-217

Bouligand, Y.; Soyer, M.O.; Puiseux-Dao, S.: La Structure Fibrillaire et l'Orientation des Chromosomes chez les Dinoflagellés. Chromosoma 24(1968)251-287

Buongiorno-Nardelli, M.; Bertolini, B.: Subcellular Localization of some Acid Hydrolases in *Triturus cristatus* Spermatozoa. Histochemie 8(1967)34-44

Champy, C.: Recherches sur la Spermatogenèse des Batraciens. Arch Zool Exp 52(1913)13-304

Czermak, J.N.: Ueber die Spermatozoiden von *Salamandra atra*. Ein Beitrag zur Kenntniss der festen Formbestandteile im Sämen der Molche. Gesammelte Schriften I (1879)

Eimer, T.: Untersuchungen über den Bau und die Bewegung der Samenfäden. Verh Physik-Med Ges Würzl 6(1874)93-160

Fawcett, D.W.; Hilfer, S.R.: The Fine Structure of the Spermatozoa of *Triturus viridescens*. Ant Rec 193(1961)329

Fawcett, D.W.: Cilia and Flagella. In: The Cell, pp. 218-292, ed. by J. Brachet and A.E. Mirsky. Academic Press, New York, 1961.

Fawcett, D.W.: Sperm Tail Structure in Relation to the Mechanism of Movement. In: Spermatozoon Motility, pp. 147-169, ed. by D. Bishop. A.A.A.S., Washington, 1962.

Fawcett, D.W.: A Comparative View of Sperm Ultrastructure. Biol Reprod 2 (1970) 90-127

Folliot, R.: Ultrastructural Study of Spermiogenesis of the Anuran Amphibian *Bombina variegata*. In: The Spermatozoon, pp. 333–339, ed. by D.W. Fawcett and J.M. Bedford. Urban and Schwarzenberg, Baltimore, 1979

Folliot, R.; Maillet, P.-L.: Ultrastructure de la Spermiogenèse et du Spermatozoïde de divers Insectes Homoptères. In: Comparative Spermatology, pp. 289-300, ed. by B. Baccetti. Academic Press, New York, 1970

Furieri, P.: Prime Osservazioni al Microscopio Elettronico sullo Spermatozoo di *Trituros cristatus carnifex* (Laurenti). Boll Soc Ital Biol Sper 36(1960)1006-1009

Furieri, P.: Osservazioni sullo Spermatozoo di *Triturus cristatus carnifex*. Studio al Microscope Elettronico. Monit Zool Ital 68(1962)90-106

Furieri, P.: The Peculiar Morphology of the Spermatozoon of *Bombina variegata* L. Monit Zool Ital 9(1975)185-201

Gourret J.-P.: Description et Interprétation des Nucléoïdes Structurés Observés dans des Bactéroïdes de Rhizobium. Biol Cell 32(1978)301-308

Janssens, F.A.: La Spermatogenèse chez les Tritons. Cellule 19(1901)7-116

Koehler, J.K.: A Freeze-etching Study of Rabbit Spermatozoa with Particular Reference to Head Structures. J Ultrastruct Res 33(1970)598-614

Lommen, M.A.J.: Development of the Ring during Spermiogenesis of a Salamander. J Microsc 9(1970)785-800

McGregor, J.H.: The Spermatogenesis of *Amphiuma*. J Morphol 15(1899)57-104

McGregor, J.H.; Walker, M.H.: The Arrangement of Chromosomes in Nuclei of Sperm from Plethodontid Salamanders. Chromosoma 40(1973)243-262

Meves, F.: Ueber Struktur und Histogenese der Samenfäden von *Salamandra maculosa*. Arch Mikr Anat 50 (1897) 110-414

Nicander L.: Comparative Studies on the Fine Structure of Vertebrate Spermatozoa. In: Spermatologia Comparata, pp. 47-56, ed. by B. Baccetti. Academic Press, New York and London, 1970.

Pankratz, H.S.: The Sperm Cell of *Amphiuma*; with Special References to the Connecting Piece and Associated Redundant Envelope. J Cell Biol 35(1967)155A

Picheral, B.: Structure et Organisation du Spermatozoïde de *Pleurodeles waltlii* Michah. (Amphibien, Urodèle). Arch Biol 78(1967)193-221

Picheral, B.: Nature et Evolution des Protéines Basiques au Cours de la Spermiogenèse chez *Pleurodeles waltlii* Michah., Amphibien, Urodèle. Histochemie 23(1970)189-206

Picheral, B.: Ultrastructure du Noyau en Rapport avec l'Évolution des Protéines Basiques Nucléaires au Cours de la Spermiogenèse du Triton *Pleurodeles waltlii* Michah. J Microsc 12(1971)107-132

Picheral, B.: Les Éléments Cytoplasmiques au Cours de la Spermiogenèse du Triton *Pleurodeles waltlii* Michah. I La Genèse de l'Acrosome. Z Zellforsch 13(1972a)347-370

Picheral, B.: Les Éléments Cytoplasmiques au Cours de la Spermiogenèse du Triton *Pleurodeles waltlii* Michah. II La Formation du Cou et l'Évolution des Organites Cytoplasmiques non Intégrés dans le Spermatozoïde. Z Zellforsch 131(1972b)371-398

Picheral, B.: Les Éléments Cytoplasmiques au Cours de la Spermiogenèse du Triton *Pleurodeles waltlii* Michah. III L'évolution des Formations Caudales. Z Zellforsch 131(1972c)399-416

Picheral, B.: Etude Cytophysiologique des Cellules Somatiques et Germinales du Testicule des Amphibiens Urodèles. Thèse de Doctorat d'Etat, Université de Rennes, C.N.R.S. N° AO 7452(1972d)

Picheral, B.: La Fécondation chez le Triton Pleurodèle. I La Traversée des Enveloppes de l'Oeuf par les Spermatozoïdes. J Ultrastruct Res 60(1977a)181-202

Picheral, B.: La Fécondation chez le Triton Pleurodèle. II La

Pénétration des Spermatozoïdes et la Réaction Locale de l'Oeuf. J Ultrastruct Res 60(1977b)106-120

Picheral, B.; Folliot, R.; Maillet, P.-L.: Sur la Structure du Noyau du Spermatozoïde de *Pleurodeles waltlii* Michah. (Amphibien, Urodèle). C R Acad Sci [D] (Paris) 262(1966)1579-1582

Picheral, B.; Thomas, D.: La Chromatine du Noyau du Spermatozoïde du Pleurodèle et son comportement lors de la Fécondation. Biol Cell 29(1977)33A

Pouchet,: 1847. Cited by Retzius, 1906

Retzius, G.: Die Spermien der Amphibiens. Biol Untersuch 13(1906)49-70

Sipski, M.L.; Wagner, T.E.: The Total Structure and Organization of Chromosomal Fibers in Eutherian Sperm Nuclei. Biol Reprod 16(1977)428-440

Werner, G.; Hubers, H.; Hubers, E.; Morgenstern, E.: Beziehungen zwischen Struktur und chemischer Zusammensetzung der Spermien vom Bergmolch, *Triturus alpestris* Laur. Histochemie 30(1972)345-358

SPECIAL FEATURES OF SPERM STRUCTURE AND FUNCTION IN MARSUPIALS

H.R. Harding, F.N. Carrick, and C.D. Shorey

Department of General Studies, University of New South Wales, Australia; School of Veterinary Anatomy, University of Queensland, Australia; and Department of Histology and Embryology, University of Sydney, Australia

The Marsupialia is a major mammalian group of some 220 species whose diversity approaches that found within the Eutheria, but whose distribution is limited to the Americas, Australia, and Papua-New Guinea and nearby islands. The two major mammalian groups (the Marsupialia and the Eutheria) are thought to have diverged from a common ancestor in the Early Cretaceous period (Clemens, 1968; Lilliegraven, 1976), and thus they have had a long evolutionary separation. Consequently, marsupials and eutherians may be expected to exhibit divergent structural and physiological solutions to common mammalian functional problems, and thus study of marsupial sperm may contribute comparative data of value for our overall understanding of mammalian sperm structure and function.

A good deal of information has accumulated on eutherian sperm as a result of wide use of the range of available ultrastructural techniques, but in contrast observations for the Marsupialia are limited to relatively few species and almost entirely to use of standard transmission electron microscopy. To date a comprehensive ultrastructural description of the mature spermatozoon has not been published for any marsupial species. Very detailed studies have been made on spermiogenesis in the Australian long-nosed bandicoot (*Perameles nasuta*) (Sapsford and Rae, 1969; Sapsford et al., 1966, 1967, 1969a, b, 1970). Much briefer descriptions of various aspects of spermiogenesis or mature sperm structure have been published for the Australian species: *Perameles nasuta* (Cleland and Rothschild, 1959; Cleland, 1965); *Trichosurus vulpecula* (Olson, 1975; Harding et al., 1976a, b, c); *Phascolarctos cinereus* (Hughes, 1977); *Sarcophilus harrisii* (Hughes, 1976); other Australian species (Harding et al., 1976c, 1977); and for the American species: *Didelphis virginiana* (Holstein, 1965;

Rattner, 1972; Olson et al., 1977); *Caluromys philander* (Phillips, 1970a, b), and *Marmosa mitis* (Rattner, 1972). In addition there has been recent interest in aspects of epididymal sperm maturation in *Trichosurus vulpecula* (Harding et al., 1975, 1976a, c; Cummins, 1976, 1977; Temple-Smith and Bedford, 1976); *Phascolarctos cinereus* (Hughes, 1977); *Sarcophilus harrisii* (Hughes, 1976); a number of other Australian species (Harding et al., 1977); and the American species: *Caluromys philander* (Olson and Hamilton, 1976) and *Didelphis virginiana* (Olson et al., 1977).

Despite their emphasis on maturation changes, papers published on sperm of the Australian brush-tailed possum *Trichosurus vulpecula* (Olson, 1975; Harding et al., 1975, 1976a, b, c; Temple-Smith and Bedford, 1976) provide the most comprehensive picture of mature sperm structure and epididymal sperm maturation in marsupials to date. The purpose of this chapter is to give a preliminary assessment of the extent to which this picture is characteristic of the Marsupialia as a group. To this end, mature sperm ultrastructure and morphological sperm maturation changes have been examined for 16 additional species from five Australian marsupial families (Table 1) using methods previously described (Harding et al., 1975, 1976a). This information is compared with published descriptions for American species.

Since most of the authors' work has been concerned with the morphological changes occurring during epididymal sperm maturation, emphasis will be placed on this aspect. In addition, it has been suggested (Harding et al., 1976a) that some of the maturation changes are a continuation or rectification of processes which started during spermiogenesis, and thus it is necessary to consider briefly those aspects of spermiogenesis which are particularly relevant to the later maturation changes.

OBSERVATIONS AND DISCUSSION

Family Phalangeridae: *Trichosurus vulpecula*

Detailed descriptions of certain aspects of sperm maturation and ultrastructure in *Trichosurus vulpecula* are

---

The authors would like to thank Dr. D.J.H. Cockayne, Director of the Electron Microscope Unit, University of Sydney, and Dr. M.R. Dickson, Electron Microscopist in charge, Biomedical Electron Microscope Unit, University of New South Wales, for the provision of electron microscope and photographic facilities. They also particularly thank Dr. P. Woolley of La Trobe University who collected and fixed sperm samples from three of the dasyurid species examined.

© 1979 Urban & Schwarzenberg, Inc. Baltimore-Munich *The Spermatozoon*, edited by D.W. Fawcett and J.M. Bedford

Table 1. Species Investigated for This Study: Arranged to Show Evolutionary Relationships of Australian Marsupial Families[1]

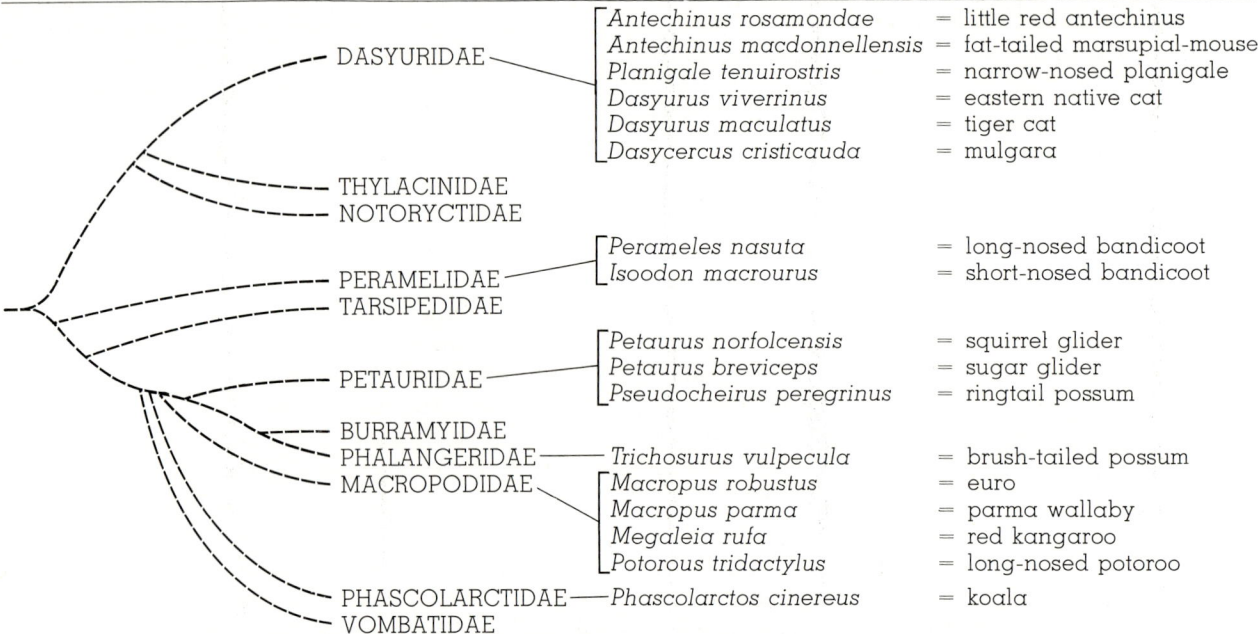

[1] *The evolutionary relationships indicated by the branching broken lines are modified from Keast (1977).*

available in the literature (Olson, 1975; Harding et al., 1975, 1976a, b, c; Cummins, 1976, 1977; Temple-Smith and Bedford, 1976) and it is appropriate here to give only a brief review of this body of data and to add the authors' relevant unpublished observations, in order to provide a basis for comparison with other species.

Sperm of *Trichosurus vulpecula* conform to the generalized mammalian pattern that has emerged from eutherian sperm morphology studies, but with two major exceptional features. The first concerns the location and form of the acrosome, and the second, the location of the neck insertion into the nucleus.

The location and form of the acrosome in *Trichosurus* serves to distinguish sperm of this species, and indeed all marsupials examined so far, from those of eutherians. As previously described (Harding *et al.*, 1976a), the acrosome in *Trichosurus* forms a convex ovate body lying on the anterior third of the dorsal nuclear surface. It thus covers only a small proportion of the latter and does not form a cap surrounding the anterior portion of the nucleus as does the eutherian acrosome (Fawcett, 1975). In addition, the acrosome in *Trichosurus* and other marsupials shows no differentiation into the regions (apical, principal, and equatorial segments) recognized in eutherian sperm (Fawcett, 1975). *Trichosurus* also differs from eutherians in early acrosomal development, since in this species (Harding *et al.*, 1976b) and in other marsupials (Sapsford *et al.*, 1967, 1969a; Harding *et al.*, 1976d; Harding, Carrick, and Shorey, unpublished observations), the presence of a proacrosomal granule in the development of the acrosomal granular component as it does in eutherians (Burgos, 1974).

It is interesting to speculate whether these differences in acrosomal development, location, and form between marsupials and eutherians, may reflect differences in function. There is no information at present on fertilization in marsupials, but it may be of interest to note that ovulated marsupial eggs lack the cumulus that surrounds eutherian eggs (Hughes, 1974; Hughes and Harding, unpublished observations). The major part of the acrosome in eutherian sperm disappears during the dispersal of the egg cumulus, leaving only the inner membranes and equatorial segments for penetration of the zona pellucida (Bedford, 1970). This raises the question of whether the marsupial acrosome may perform a similar function to the inner membrane and equatorial segment of the eutherian acrosome. Clearly, fertilization studies for marsupials would be of great interest.

The second feature under consideration here is the location of the neck insertion. The nucleus in *Trichosurus* is flattened in what has come to be described as the dorso-ventral plane, and the neck is inserted into the central region of the long ventral axis, while the acrosome lies on the anterior dorsal surface (see Harding et al., 1976a for the origins of this axial naming). In contrast, the neck in eutherian sperm is inserted into the short caudal surface of the nucleus (Fawcett, 1970). This difference in the location of neck insertion is a consequence of events occurring during spermiogenesis; namely, the plane in which nuclear flattening takes place with respect to the long axis of the flagellum. In *Trichosurus* nuclear flattening occurs in a plane perpendicular to the long axis of the sperm flagellum (Harding et al., 1976a), and as previously reported for the marsupials *Perameles nasuta* (Sapsford et al., 1969a) and *Caluromys philander* (Phillips, 1970a), this differs from the eutherian process of flattening, which is in a plane parallel to that of the flagellar long axis. All other marsupials examined so far, except the koala *Phascolarctos cinereus* (see below), have a similar neck insertion location to *Trichosurus*, and in each case this appears to result from a perpendicular mode of nuclear flattening during spermiogenesis. A further consequence of this nuclear flattening process and the manner of neck insertion in *Trichosurus* is that the nucleus must undergo a rotation about its axis with the neck in order to bring the long axis of the sperm head close to the parallel with the long axis of the flagellum, and thus achieve the streamlined form of the mature spermatozoon (Harding et al., 1976a). This streamlined form is further enhanced by the presence of a groove in the ventral nuclear surface distal to the neck insertion, which allows for accommodation of the neck and proximal midpiece when the distal nucleus overlies these regions following rotation. In *Trichosurus* two such rotations of the nucleus occur; the first following shaping of the nucleus during spermiogenesis (Harding et al., 1976b), and the second during epididymal transit (Harding et al., 1976a). A similar rotation process occurs in all marsupials having a similar neck insertion to *Trichosurus*; that is, in all species examined so far except for the koala and wombat (*Vombatus ursinus*) (Hughes, 1965). However, in many species only a single rotation occurs, rather than the double rotation observed in *Trichosurus* (Harding, Carrick and Shorey, unpublished observations).

The above discussion has drawn attention to two aspects of sperm structure in *Trichosurus* that are widely shared throughout the Marsupialia. There are however other unusual features of mature sperm and the sperm maturation process in this species that are not such common features among members of this group.

Of particular interest are the pronounced changes in sperm morphology which occur during epididymal transit (Table 2). These have been described in some detail previously (Cummins, 1976, 1977; Harding et al., 1975, 1976a, c, 1977; Temple-Smith and Bedford, 1976) and shown to include: the development of a helically arranged fibrous network that immediately underlies the plasma membrane and surrounds the distal two-thirds of the midpiece; the development of randomly arranged flask-like invaginations of the plasma membrane between the parallel bands of the fiber network; the anteriorly directed contraction and eccentric displacement of the cytoplasmic droplet, followed by its shedding from the proximal region of the midpiece (this contrasts with the distal movement before shedding of the droplet in eutherians); a pronounced reorganization of the acrosomal material that converts the acrosome from an attenuated cup-like structure into its definitive ovate form; the appearance in many cauda epididymidal sperm of stacks of membranes (membranous whorls) that emanate from the neck region and project anteriorly and posteriorly to surround the distal region of the nucleus and the proximal mitochondria of the midpiece; an increase in the electron density of the mitochondrial matrix material. In addition, modification of the sperm surface over the head and tail occurs during epididymal transit (Temple-Smith and Bedford, 1976) as does the development of progressive motility (Cummins, 1976; Temple-Smith and Bedford, 1976). The latter is accompanied by an enhanced stability of the dense outer fibers, midpiece fiber network and principal piece fibrous sheath, as evidenced by their greater resistance to disruption by sodium dodecyl sulfate (SDS) and dithiothreitol (DTT) (Temple-Smith and Bedford, 1976). A fibrous network is also present in the principal piece of *Trichosurus* sperm, but this is already developed in newly released testicular spermatozoa, and is far less regular in its organization than the midpiece network (Harding et al., 1975).

The functional significance of these unusual features of *Trichosurus* sperm is not clear. It has been suggested previously that the midpiece fiber network may have a supportive function (Harding et al., 1975) and others have correlated its development with the onset of progressive motility (Temple-Smith and Bedford, 1976), while some role in the transport of materials between the spermatozoon and its environment has been suggested for the midpiece plasma membrane invaginations (Harding et al., 1975; Temple-Smith and Bedford, 1976).

The reason for the acrosomal changes in *Trichosurus* seems more obvious. In describing the development of the acrosome in this species (Harding et al., 1976b) it was noted that contraction of the nuclear ring during the later stages of spermiogenesis appeared to effect the containment of the acrosome to its final reduced area on the dorsal nuclear surface, but in so doing caused folding, and projection away from the nucleus of atten-

Table 2. Epididymal Sperm Maturation Changes

Family / Species	Midpiece Fiber Network	Midpiece Invagination	Acrosomal Compaction	Rotation of Head	Membranous Whorls	Pairing
PHALANGERIDAE						
Trichosurus vulpecula	x	x	x	xx	x	—
MACROPODIDAE						
Macropus robustus	x	—	x	xx	?	—
Macropus parma	x	—	x	xx	x	—
Megaleia rufa	x	—	x	xx	x	—
Potorous tridactylus	x	—	x	xx	x	—
PETAURIDAE						
Petaurus breviceps	x	x	—	x	—	—
Petaurus norfolcensis	x	x	—	?	—	—
Pseudocheirus peregrinus	x	x	x	—	—	—
PHASCOLARCTIDAE						
Phascolarctos cinereus	?	—	—?	—	—	—
DASYURIDAE						
Dasyurus viverrinus	x	—	—	x	—	—
Dasyurus maculatus	x	—	—	x	—	—
Dasycercus cristicauda	x	—	—	x	—	—
Antechinus rosamondae	x	—	—	x	—	—
Antechinus macdonnellensis	x	—	—	x	—	—
Planigale tenuirostris	x	—	—	x	—	—
PERAMELIDAE						
Perameles nasuta	?	—	—	x	—	—
Isoodon macrourus	?	—	—	x	—	—
DIDELPHIDAE						
Didelphis virginiana	x?	—	—	x	—?	x
Caluromys philander	x?	—	—	x	—?	x

x = structure present or process occurs.
— = structure absent or process does not occur.

uated extensions of acrosomal material. Therefore it was suggested (Harding et al., 1976a) that the unusual acrosomal modifications seen during epididymal transit, are necessary in order to effect the compaction of the acrosomal material into its definitive ovate form within the reduced acrosomal area on the nuclear surface. Thus they may be regarded as completing and rectifying events which occurred during spermiogenesis.

Family Petauridae

On the basis of sperm structure, the petaurid species studied here are clearly separated into their two subfamilies: Petaurinae (*Petaurus breviceps; P. norfolcensis*) and Pseudocheirinae (*Pseudocheirus peregrinus*).

Sperm of the two *Petaurus* species are very similar to one another and also closely resemble those of *Trichosurus* in general flagellar structure and in the morphological changes that take place in the flagellum during epididymal transit. As indicated in Table 2, both the midpiece fiber network (Fig. 1a) and midpiece plasma membrane invaginations develop during this maturation process, while the principal piece fiber network is already developed in newly released testicular sperm.

However, there are marked differences between *Petaurus* and *Trichosurus* in relation to the sperm head. In contrast to *Trichosurus*, the acrosome in *Petaurus* forms a thin layer covering the greater part of the dorsal nuclear surface, but excluding its peripheral regions (Fig. 1a). The acrosome has a similar appearance in caput and cauda epididymal sperm and thus does not undergo the maturation changes that are so pronounced in *Trichosurus*. In addition, the membranous whorls that surround the distal nucleus and proximal midpiece of some cauda epididymal sperm in *Trichosurus* do not develop in *Petaurus* or *Pseudocheirus* sperm.

Sperm of *Pseudocheirus peregrinus* display a number of unusual features, not only in comparison with the related *Petaurus* group, but also with all other marsupials examined to date. They are characterised by a very broad (2.9 ± 0.18 μm) and fairly short (7.7 ± 0.25 μm) midpiece (for *Trichosurus* the comparative midpiece dimensions are: length 12.4 ± 0.57 μm; width 1.2 ± 0.04 μm). In transverse sections (Fig. 1c) it is notable that this large midpiece diameter is due to extreme development of mitochondria which have a most unusual form, while the dense outer fibers are relatively

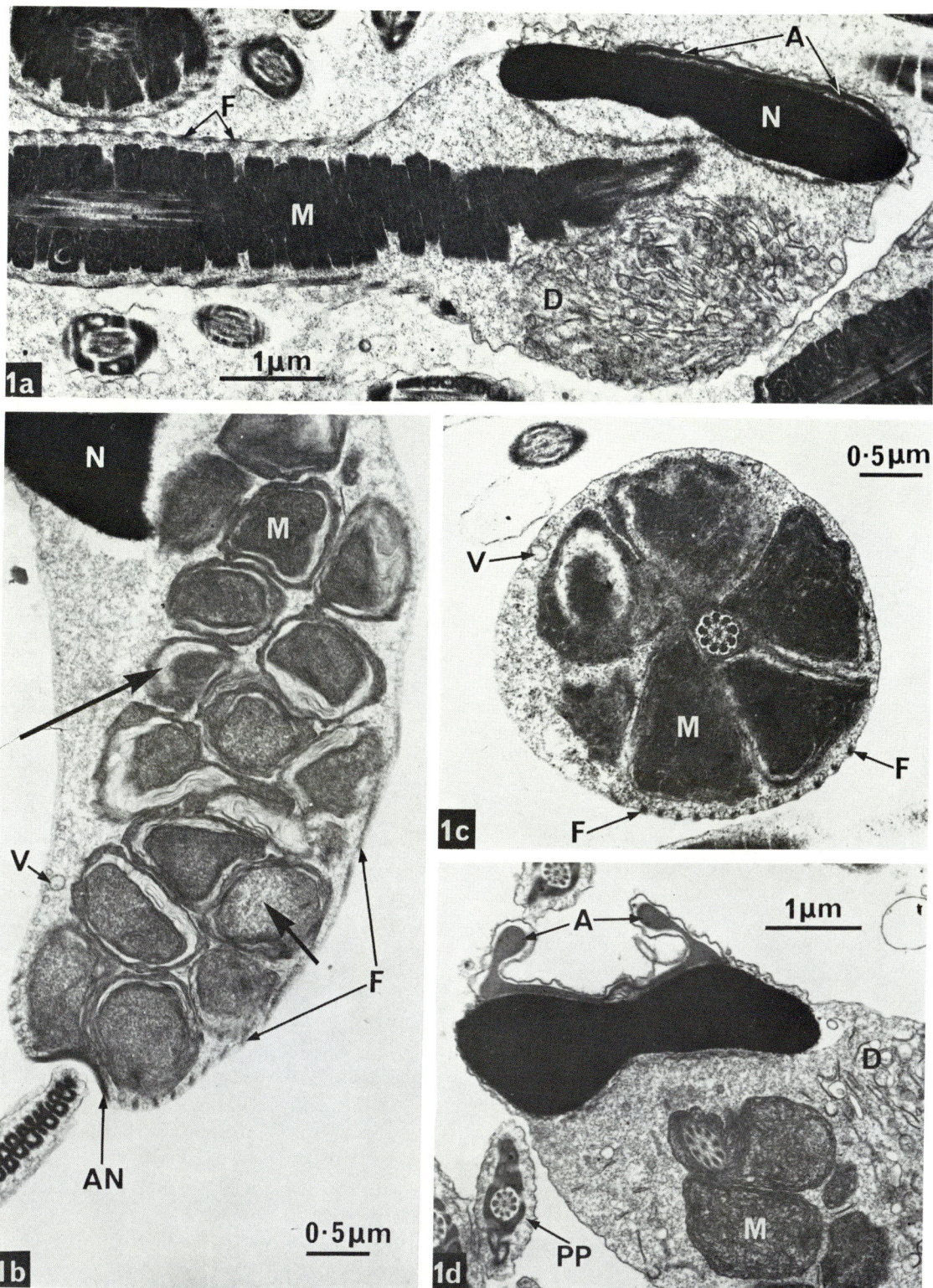

Figure 1. a: Longitudinal section through the head and proximal midpiece of a caput epididymidal sperm of *Petaurus norfolcensis*. Acrosome (A) is fully compacted in caput sperm. Cytoplasmic droplet (D) is eccentrically placed and has retracted toward the anterior midpiece. F, midpiece fiber network; M, mitochondria; N, nucleus. b: Longitudinal section through cauda epididymidal sperm of *Pseudocheirus peregrinus*. Note the electron-lucent patches (arrows) within the mitochondria (M). AN, annulus; F, midpiece fiber network; N, nucleus; V, invaginations of midpiece plasma membrane. c: Transverse section through the midpiece of a cauda epididymidal sperm of *Pseudocheirus peregrinus*. Mitochondria (M) are of very large diameter compared with axoneme-dense outer fiber complex. Profiles of the midpiece fiber network (F) cover only one-quarter of the circumference of the midpiece. V, invaginations of midpiece plasma membrane. d: Transverse section through the head of a caput epididymidal sperm of *Pseudocheirus peregrinus*, showing acrosomal projections (A). D, Cytoplasmic droplet; M, mitochondria. Note also the flattened form of the principal piece (PP) seen in transverse section.

poorly developed and closely overlie the axoneme doublets. There is a marked constriction at the annulus (Fig. 1b), and the much narrower principal piece is seen in transverse sections to be extremely flattened in comparison with that of other marsupials (Fig. 1d). The mitochondria, as in *Trichosurus*, undergo morphological maturation changes including an increase in the electron density of the matrix material, but the resulting mitochondria in cauda epididymidal sperm of *P. peregrinus* have a unique appearance. To a large extent this is due to the development of electron-lucent areas within the mitochondria, which appear to be due to extreme dilatation of some of the electron-lucent cristae, and also to the development of electron-lucent regions within the otherwise electron-dense matrix material (Fig. 1b).

A midpiece fiber network and invaginations of the midpiece plasma membrane develop during epididymal transit in *P. peregrinus* (Fig. 1b, c), but the fiber network is highly unusual in that it does not completely surround the midpiece as in *Trichosurus*. In longitudinal sections, the electron-dense profiles of the fiber network are apparent on either side of the midpiece in its distal region near the annulus, and these profiles extend proximally up only one side of the sectioned midpiece (Fig. 1b). In transverse sections, the electron-dense profiles of the network are evenly spaced, but located over only one-quarter of the midpiece circumference (Fig. 1c). Their location is consistent with respect to the orientation of the axoneme and is always centralized on the plane perpendicular to a line joining the central axoneme pair, and always on the plane lying closest to dense outer fiber No. 8 rather than No. 3. Scanning electron microscopy will be required to reconcile these sectional views of the fiber network in *Pseudocheirus*, and all that can be noted at present is that this network is incomplete compared with that in other marsupial species, but that it is incomplete in a consistent and highly ordered fashion. Since the functions of the midpiece fiber network are not clear, comment on the possible significance of its unusual form in *P. peregrinus* would not be meaningful at this stage. However, the earlier suggestion of a supportive function for the network and consequently of a possible modifying role in sperm motility indicates that comparative sperm motility studies using *P. peregrinus* and species with a "complete" fiber network, may be worthwhile.

The acrosome in *P. peregrinus* sperm covers a similar proportion of the dorsal nuclear surface to that in *Petaurus*, but is slightly thicker dorsoventrally than in the latter species. Unlike *Petaurus*, it undergoes similar epididymal maturation changes to those seen in *Trichosurus* (Fig. 1d).

Family Macropodidae

In overall shape, in acrosomal form and location, and in the morphological changes occurring during epididymal transit (Table 2), there is a fairly close resemblance between the sperm heads of the four macropod species examined here and that of *Trichosurus* (Fig. 2a). The major differentiating feature between macropod and *Trichosurus* sperm is the lack of development of the invaginations of the midpiece plasma membrane in the former group (*cf* Fig. 2b and c). In all other respects the sperm flagella in these macropods (Fig. 2a, c, d) are fairly similar in appearance to that in *Trichosurus* (Fig. 2c) and undergo similar maturation changes (Table 2). However, minor variations in both head and flagellar shape and size enable these macropod species to be distinguished from one another on the basis of sperm morphology.

Family Phascolarctidae

In a comparative light-microscope study, Hughes (1965) found sperm of the koala (*Phascolarctos cinereus*) and wombat (*Vombatus ursinus*) to be similar to one another, but markedly different from other Australian marsupial species in sperm head form and location of the neck insertion.

Wombat sperm have not been examined as part of the present study, but in view of Hughes' findings it seems very likely that the general comments given here for koala sperm are applicable to the entire superfamily Vombatoidea, which comprises the wombat species (family Vombatidae) and koala (family Phascolarctidae).

As mentioned above, koala sperm stand apart from those of other marsupial species in that the neck is inserted into a short rather than a long axis of the nucleus, and the long axis of the nucleus is parallel with the long axis of the flagellum at all stages (Fig. 3a). Thus superficially at least, koala and eutherian sperm are similar in these respects. However, the koala conforms with other marsupials in that although its acrosome is fairly extensive it covers only one surface of the nucleus and does not form a "cap" as in eutherians (Fig. 3a).

In view of the earlier discussion in this chapter, the unusual and somewhat "eutherian" placement of the neck insertion in the koala raises the question of whether the nucleus is flattened perpendicular to the long axis of the flagellum as in other marsupials, or parallel to this axis as in eutherians and monotremes (Benda, 1906). Preliminary investigation of spermiogenesis in the koala suggests that the latter may occur (Fig. 3c). If this is shown to be the case, then this very

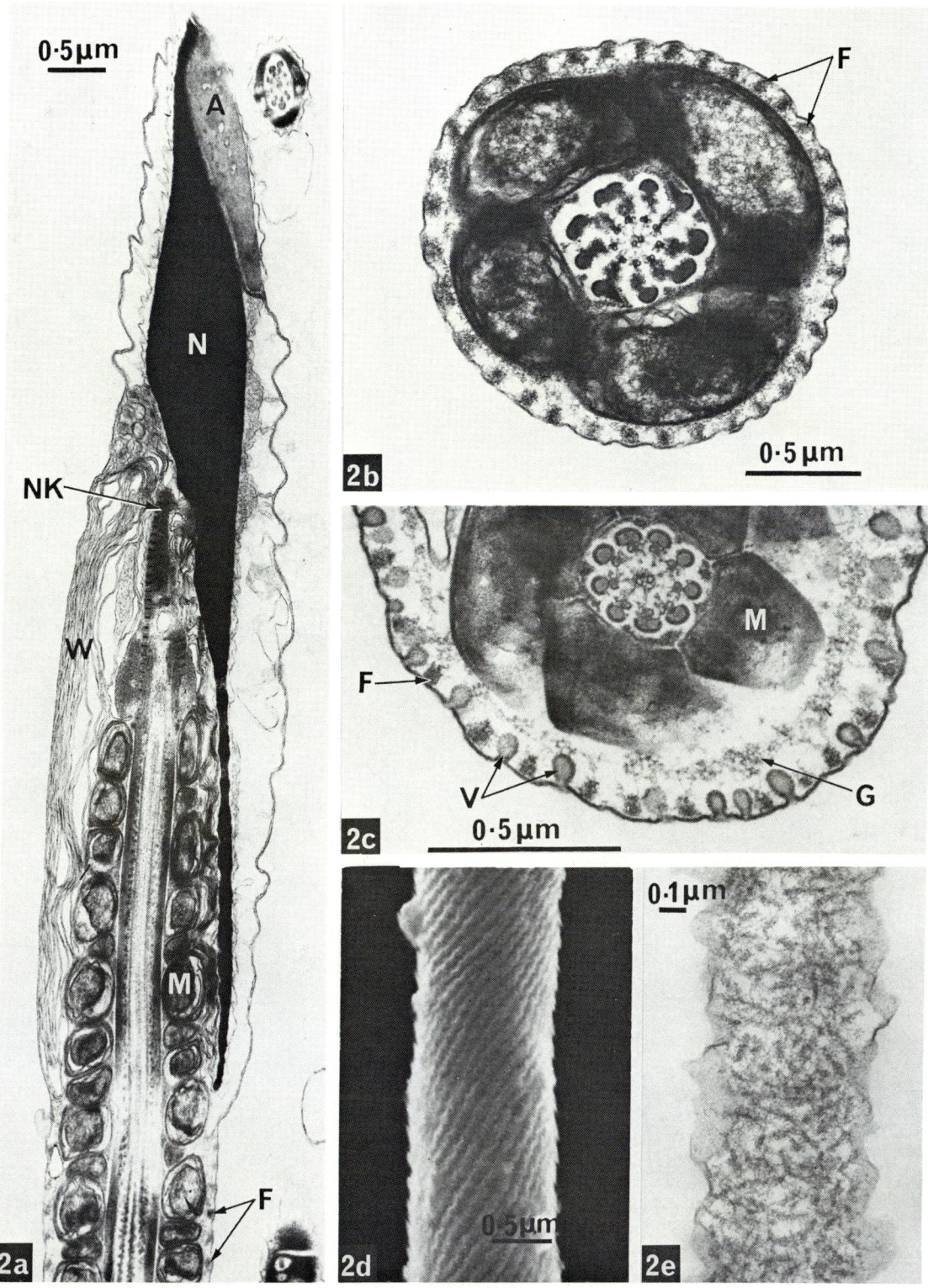

Figure 2. a: Longitudinal section of head and proximal midpiece of a cauda epididymidal sperm of *Potorous tridactylus*. A, acrosome; F, midpiece fiber network; M, mitochondria; N, nucleus; NK, neck of sperm; W, membranous whorls. b: Transverse section of the midpiece of a cauda epididymidal sperm of *Potorous tridactylus*. F, midpiece fiber network. Note that invaginations of the midpiece plasma membrane as seen in Figure 2c are not present. c: Transverse section of the midpiece of a sperm from the vas deferens of *Trichosurus vulpecula*. F, midpiece fiber network; G, granular layer underlying fiber network; M, mitochondria; V, invaginations of midpiece plasma membrane. d: Scanning electron micrograph of the midpiece of a sperm from the distal regions of the epididymis in *Macropus parma*. The helically wound fibers of the midpiece fiber network are obvious. e: Superficial longitudinal section of a cauda epididymidal sperm of *Macropus parma*. The irregularly arranged fibers of the principal piece fiber network are obvious.

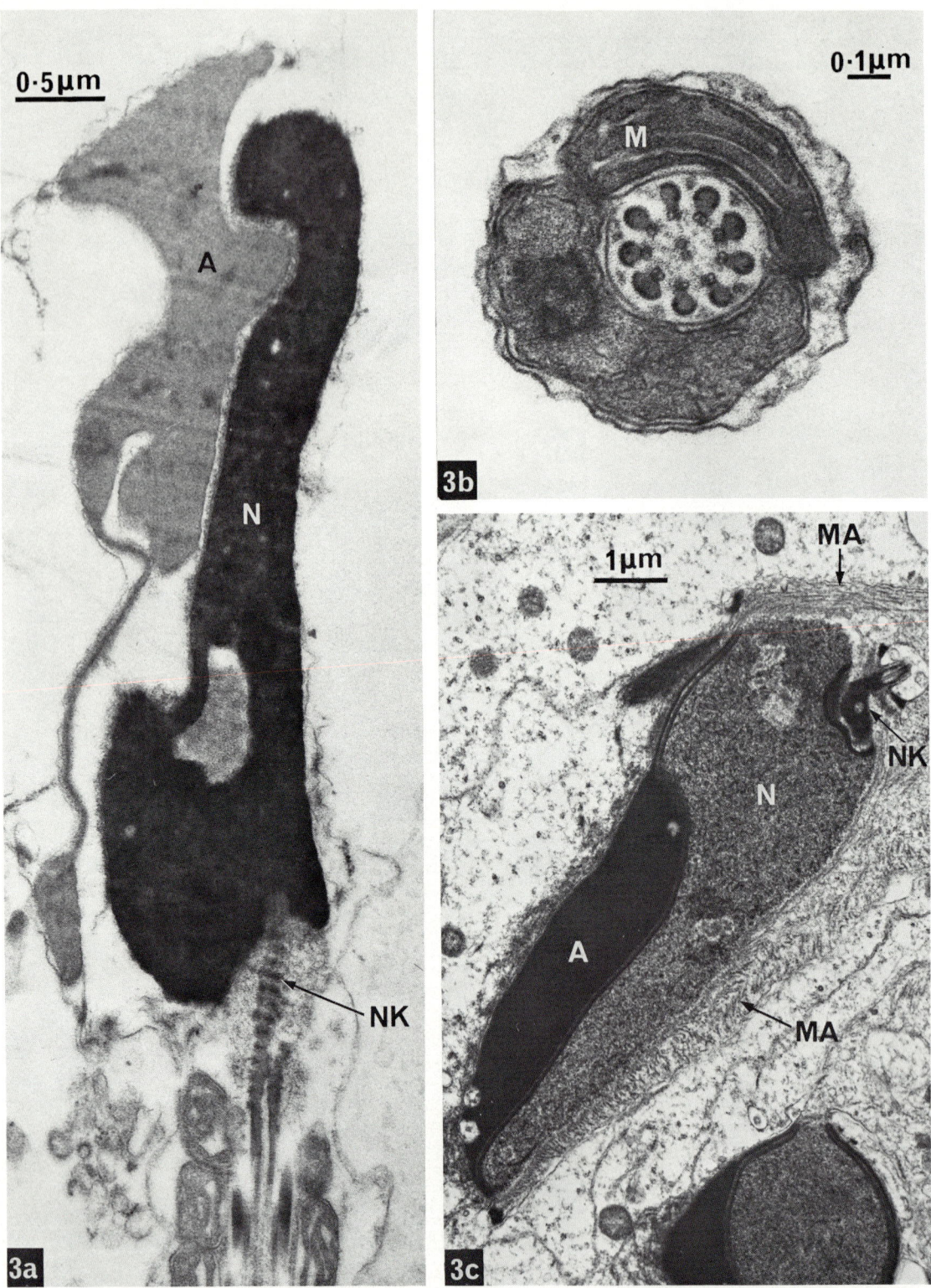

Figure 3. a: Longitudinal section of the head and proximal midpiece of a cauda epididymidal sperm of *Phascolarctos cinereus*. Note that the neck (NK) is inserted into a short rather than a long axis of the nucleus (N). A, acrosome. b: Transverse section of the midpiece of a cauda epididymidal sperm of *Phascolarctos cinereus*. Note the unspecialized nature of the midpiece and the absence of a fiber network or invaginations of the plasma membrane. M mitochondria. c: Longitudinal section of the head region of a late spermatid of *Phascolarctos cinereus*. The nucleus (N) appears to be flattening in a plane parallel to the long axis of the flagellum (indicated by the long axis of the manchette (MA)) rather than perpendicular to the latter as in other marsupials. A, acrosome; NK, developing neck of spermatid.

basic developmental difference between the koala and the other marsupials would support suggestions of a very long evolutionary separation of the Vombatoidea from other marsupial groups. Moreover, similarity in this respect with the eutherians and monotremes could raise interesting questions for speculation in the wider evolutionary context. For example, does the vombatoid sperm form represent a highly specialized product of a long evolutionary separation from other marsupials? Or, are many of its features primitive or conservative, and is this sperm type close to that of the ancestral marsupial? Attempts to answer such questions must clearly be highly speculative, but with this in mind it is perhaps worth commenting that in many respects koala sperm appear to be rather unspecialized in form, indicating that the latter of the above suggestions may have some merit. The form of the flagellum in particular, is very unspecialized, and the appearance of the midpiece in transverse section (Fig. 3b) is not unlike that of the platypus (Hughes and Carrick, unpublished observations).

Invaginations of the midpiece plasma membrane are not formed during epididymal maturation in koala sperm, but it is uncertain as to whether a rudimentary fiber network forms. Certainly, a well developed network as seen in transverse and longitudinal sections of *Trichosurus* sperm never develops in *Phascolarctos*, but in occasional superficial longitudinal sections of the flagellum there are indications of the presence of helically arranged electron-dense fibers in both the mid- and principal piece.

Families Peramelidae and Dasyuridae

On dental criteria the final two Australian families under consideration here (the Peramelidae and Dasyuridae) are grouped with the American Didelphidae as the Polyprotodonta, while the other Australian families discussed above are grouped as the Diprotodonta. This link between the peramelids and dasyurids and their separation from the other Australian families is certainly reflected in their sperm ultrastructure, but the same is not true of their grouping with the American didelphids.

Peramelid and dasyurid sperm are most strikingly distinguished from those of other Australian marsupials by an extreme displacement of their dense outer fibers from the corresponding axoneme doublets (Fig. 4c, 5d). The dense outer fibers closely overlie the doublets in proximal regions of the midpiece but the two are widely separated over most of the length of the latter and of the proximal principal piece, with the displacement narrowing in more distal regions of the latter. A characteristic feature of dasyurid sperm is a precocious displacement of dense outer fiber No. 1 in the proximal midpiece where the other fibers still closely overlie the doublets (Fig. 5c). Narrow fibrous bands or connecting laminae, which are single in the dasyurids (Fig. 5d) and double in the peramelids (Fig. 4c), join the dense outer fibers to their corresponding doublets. Further common features include: the almost identical diameter of the mid- and principal piece at the annulus, such that the plasma membrane smoothly covers the latter and is not inturned in this region as in other species; an unusual "sculpted" form of the inner surface of the mitochondria that serves to accommodate the displaced dense outer fibers. The latter is most pronounced in the dasyurids (Fig. 4c, 5d).

Peramelid and dasyurid sperm are also notable for their large size. Hughes (1965) reported total sperm length of up to $250 \mu m$ in some dasyurids and around $200 \mu m$ in *Perameles*, making dasyurid sperm among the largest of mammalian sperm. The nucleus in dasyurid sperm is similarly very long ($\simeq 10 \mu m$) and thus after nuclear rotation the extent to which it overlies the proximal mitochondria is greater than in other marsupials (Fig. 5a). In order to accommodate the mitochondria and achieve a streamlined form for the mature sperm, the distal nucleus comprises only a very thin curved dorsal plate that closely covers the underlying mitochondria (Fig. 5c).

As previously described by Hughes (1965) and Sapsford *et al.* (1969a) head shape in the peramelids differs somewhat from that in other marsupials, in that the lateral margins of the nucleus are concave when viewed dorsally rather than convex as in the other species examined here, and the neck is particularly deeply inserted into the nucleus (Fig. 4a). The acrosome in the peramelids covers a similar proportion of the dorsal nuclear surface as that in *Trichosurus* but differs from the latter in forming a rudimentary "cap" over the rostral tip of the nucleus (Fig. 4a), and in that it is already fully compacted in caput epididymidal sperm and thus is not modified during epididymal transit. In contrast, the dasyurid acrosome more closely resembles that of *Petaurus*, and forms a thin layer covering approximately the anterior four-fifths of the length of the dorsal nuclear surface (Fig. 5a). Although acrosomal maturation changes as found in *Trichosurus* do not occur in the dasyurids, occasional small vacuities are seen in the acrosomal material (Fig. 5e) of some caput epididymidal sperm, indicating that the acrosome may undergo minor compaction during epididymal transit.

Unusual modification of certain regions of the nu-

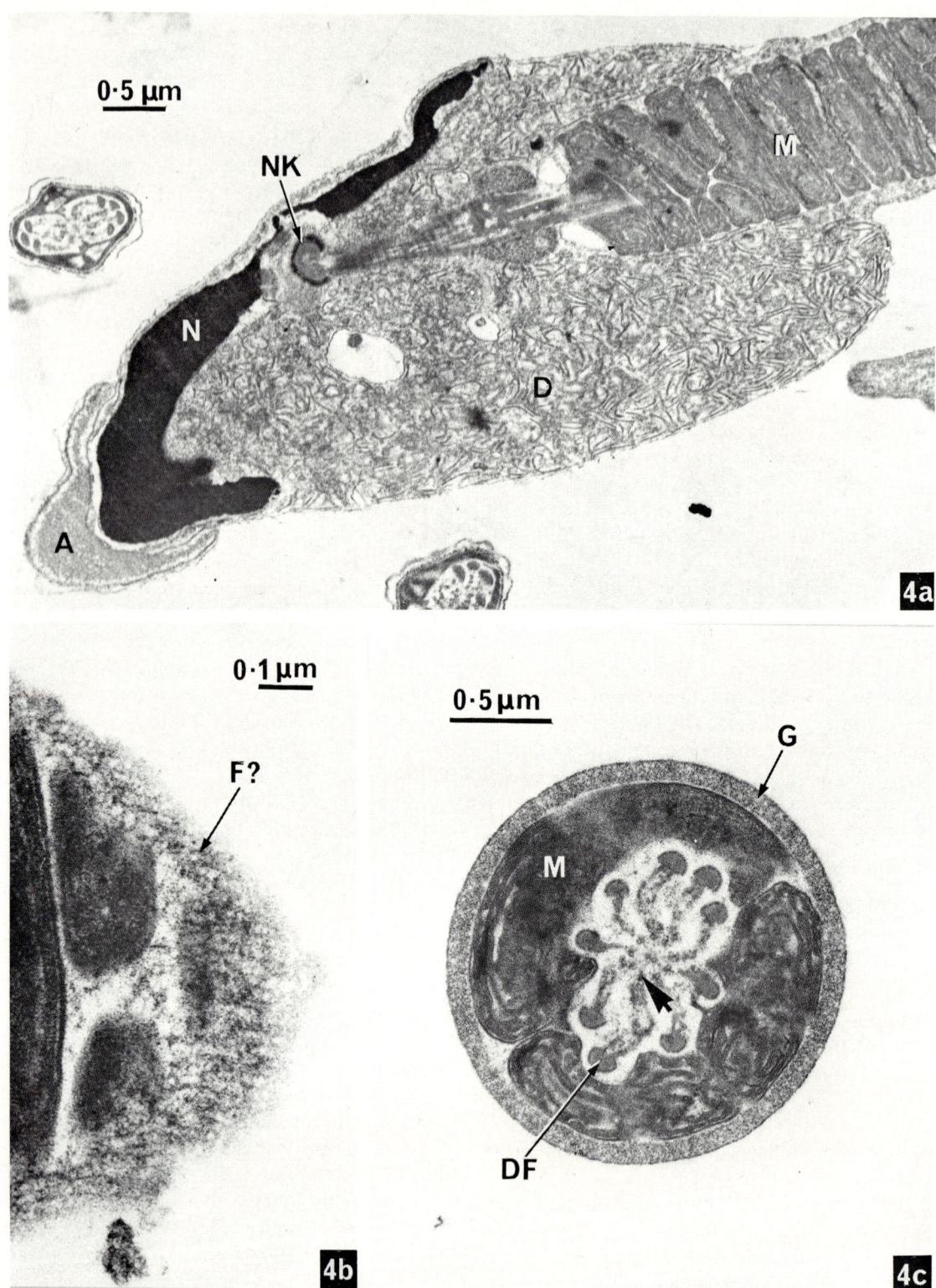

Figure 4. a: Longitudinal section through the head and proximal midpiece of corpus epididymal sperm of *Isoodon macrourus*. Note the deep insertion of the neck (NK) into the ventral surface of the nucleus (N). Cytoplasmic droplet (D) has retracted toward the anterior of the midpiece. A, acrosome; M, mitochondria. b: Superficial longitudinal section of the midpiece of a corpus epididymal sperm of *Isoodon macrourus*. Note that the granular layer surrounding the mitochondria has a faint fibrous substructure (F?) reminiscent of the fiber network of other marsupials. c: Transverse section of the midpiece of a cauda epididymal sperm of *Perameles nasuta*. A granular layer (G) surrounds the mitochondria (M) and the dense outer fibers (DF) are widely displaced from the axoneme (arrow).

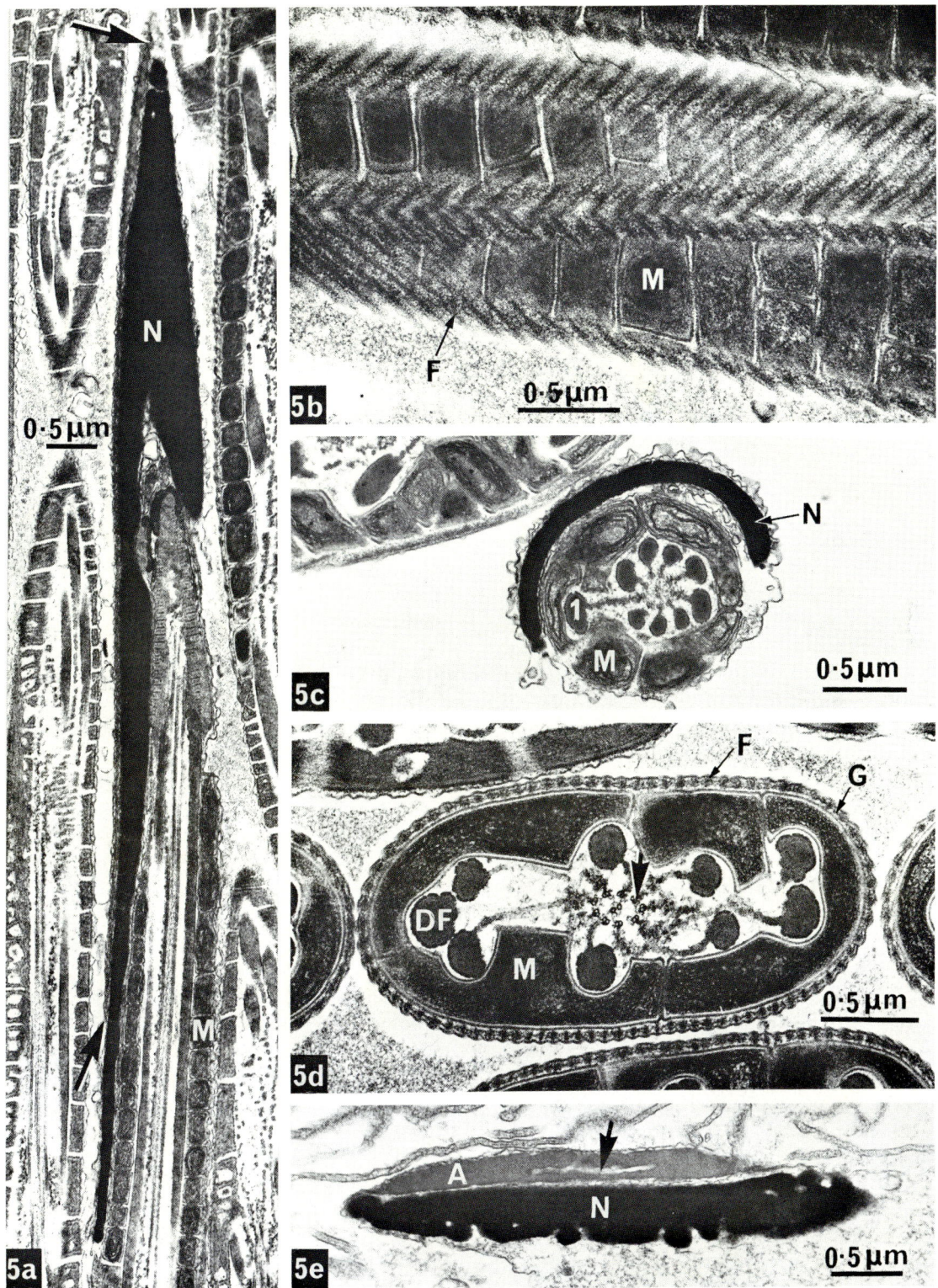

Figure 5. a: Longitudinal section through the head and proximal midpiece of a corpus-cauda epididymal sperm of *Dasyurus viverrinus*. Arrows indicate the anterior and posterior margins of the elongated acrosome. M, mitochondria; N, nucleus. b: Superficial longitudinal sections through the midpiece of corpus-cauda epididymal sperm of *Dasyurus viverrinus* showing the regular helical arrangement of the midpiece fiber network (F) and its opposite angle of orientation to the mitochondrial helices. The mitochondria (M) fit together very compactly. c: Transverse section through the proximal midpiece and overlying distal nucleus (N) of a corpus-cauda epididymal sperm of *Antechinus rosamondae*. Note the precocious displacement of dense outer fiber number 1(1). M, mitochondria. d: Transverse section through the midpiece of a cauda epididymal sperm of *Dasyurus viverrinus*. Note the sculpted form of the inner surface of the mitochondria (M) and the marked displacement of the dense outer fibers (DF) from the axoneme (arrow). F, midpiece fiber network; G, granular material between fibers of the network. e: Oblique section through the head of a caput-corpus epididymal sperm of *Dasyurus viverrinus* to show the indentations of the surface of the nucleus (N). The indented nuclear material is seen to be slightly more electron dense than the main body of the nucleus. The acrosome (A) has a small vacuity (arrow) within it, indicating that it is not fully compacted at this stage.

clear periphery is a further feature shared by peramelid and dasyurid sperm which has not been reported in other mammalian species. This is most pronounced in the dasyurids in which peripheral regions of the nucleus (particularly on the ventral surface) may appear as a demarcated layer of differing electron density to the main body of this structure. Most commonly, this layer is also indented such that the nuclear surface appears in sections as a series of globular projections (Fig. 5e). In the peramelids the ventral flanges of the nucleus frequently contain electron-lucent areas giving a pitted or vesiculated appearance. These however constitute a rather minor modification compared with that seen in the dasyurids. It is difficult to imagine what function these modifications might serve. The deep indentations observed in dasyurids in particular, must enormously increase the area of nuclear surface exposed to the environment, but in epididymal sperm, protection of the nuclear contents would seem likely to be more advantageous than would increased exposure. Perhaps the completion of nuclear condensation and removal of excess nuclear material is delayed in these species, and the peripheral modifications may represent a method of disposal of such excess material. This seems unlikely however, since no changes are observed in these peripheral modifications during epididymal transit.

Epididymal sperm maturation changes for these two groups are summarized in Table 2. The invaginations of the midpiece plasma membrane as found in *Trichosurus* and the petaurid species do not develop in either the dasyurids or peramelids, and the principal piece fiber network is similarly lacking. A well formed midpiece fiber network develops in dasyurid (Fig. 5b,d), but not in peramelid sperm (Fig. 4c). Instead, a layer of granular material surrounds the mitochondrial sheath in caput epididymidal sperm of the peramelids and increases in thickness during epididymal transit (Fig. 4c). It is notable however, that certain superficial longitudinal sections of the peramelid sperm midpiece show a faint fibrous substructure in this granular layer which is reminiscent of the fiber network (Fig. 4b).

Although the midpiece fiber network in the dasyurids generally resembles that of *Trichosurus, Petaurus,* and the macropods, a few differences are apparent and may form a useful comparative base for attempts at correlating structure and function. The midpiece plasma membrane in the dasyurids overlies the mitochondrial sheath more closely and evenly than in these diprotodont species, leaving space only for the fibrous helices (Fig. 5d). An underlying granular layer as seen in the latter species (Fig. 2c) is therefore not found although granular material is apparent between the fibers in transverse sections (Fig. 5d). In addition, the separation between the fibers is narrower among the dasyurids than the other species, varying from 0.06-0.08 μm between centers of the fibers in the dasyurids to 0.1-0.13 μm among the diprotodonts (*cf* Fig. 2b and 5d). It is perhaps noteworthy that the narrower spacing and extreme regularity of the fiber network in the dasyurids is matched by a mitochondrial sheath in sperm of this group, in which the mitochondria are more regularly arranged, narrowly spaced, and compact than in the diprotodonts (Fig. 5b). In addition, it is also notable that in all species possessing a midpiece fiber network, the angle of winding of this helical network is always counter to that of the underlying mitochondrial helix (Fig. 1a, 5b). The possibility of a supportive function for the network, with a modifying role in flagellar bending was outlined earlier. The above observations make it plausible to further suggest that the network may provide some counterbalancing force to the mitochondrial sheath. This idea seems particularly interesting in view of Harris' (1976) suggestion that the mitochondria may act as accessory motor organelles in mammalian sperm flagella. However, an immediate objection to the mitochondria as accessory motor elements, may be that their outer membranes have been shown to be stabilized by —S—S— bonding (Bedford and Calvin, 1974) as is the cortical layer of the dense outer fibers, and the latter observation has been used to support the argument for a passive stiffening role for the latter structures (Bedford and Calvin, 1974).

A final point of interest with regard to the dasyurids and peramelids is the extreme consistency in sperm form found among species within each of these groups. As mentioned above, it is possible to differentiate the various macropod species examined here by minor differences in sperm form. Other than by subtle quantitative differences, it is not possible to do the same for the dasyurids examined, even though these comprise six species representing four different genera.

American Marsupial Families

Recent evidence from the fields of plate tectonics and continental drift supports the view that marsupials reached Australia from South America via Antarctica at a time when these continents were joined (Jardine and Mackenzie, 1972; Raven and Axelrod, 1972). Australian fossil evidence indicates that the Australian and American marsupial branches have been separated since at least the Oligocene period (Tedford et al., 1975) and thus for at least 25 million years, and some authors suggest since the end of the Cretaceous (Lilliegraven, 1969), meaning a separation of 70 million years or more.

Although certain features such as acrosome form and location, mode of nuclear flattening during spermiogenesis, and location of neck insertion, enable sperm from marsupials of both geographic groups to be readily identified as marsupial sperm, the wide spatial and temporal dichotomy of the two groups is clearly reflected by a major difference in the sperm maturation process. Sperm from all American species examined to date (including representatives from the two extant American families, Didelphidae and Caenolestidae) undergo a pairing of spermatozoa over their acrosomal regions during epididymal transit (Biggers et al., 1963; Biggers and DeLamater 1965). This unusual phenomenon has not been observed in any Australian marsupial species so far, and among the vertebrates seems to be unique to the American marsupials; a similar process has been reported only for sperm of a water beetle, gastropod mollusc, and lepismatid insect. The functional significance of pairing remains to be determined.

The scant available ultrastructural information on maturation changes in American marsupial sperm is summarized in Table 2. The acrosome in American species is involved in the pairing process during epididymal sperm transit, and thus as might be expected, acrosomal maturation changes as described for some Australian species do not occur. Invaginations of the midpiece plasma membrane are similarly not found in the two American species (*Didelphis virginiana* and *Caluromys philander*) for which ultrastructural descriptions are available (Holstein, 1965; Phillips, 1970b; Olson and Hamilton, 1976; Olson et al., 1977). On the other hand morphological maturation changes do occur in the sperm midpiece of these species during epididymal transit (Olson and Hamilton, 1976; Olson et al., 1977), and these show some similarity with the development of the midpiece fiber network in Australian species. The midpiece structures that develop in these American marsupials are however, more closely associated with the plasma membrane than in the latter species. In addition, freeze-fracture studies for cauda sperm of *D. virginiana* have demonstrated the presence of parallel rows of regularly aggregated intramembranous particles over the same length of the midpiece as the modifications observed by transmission and scanning electron microscopy (Olson et al., 1977). Freeze-fracture observations have not been made for any Australian marsupial to date.

The principal piece in both *Caluromys* (Phillips, 1970b; Olson and Hamilton, 1976) and *Didelphis* sperm (Olson et al., 1977) also resembles that in many Australian marsupials in having an irregular fiber network in the region between the fibrous sheath and plasma membrane, at least in the anterior regions of the principal piece.

CONCLUDING REMARKS

The relative lack of interest in marsupials during the early ultrastructural studies of spermatozoa has meant that our image of the mammalian sperm has resulted from examination of eutherian sperm ultrastructure. Although marsupial sperm display a number of unusual features when compared with those of eutherians, they are nevertheless recognizable via this image as mammalian sperm.

This chapter has attempted to assess the extent to which the unusual features of sperm ultrastructure and maturation found in the Australian brush-tailed possum *Trichosurus vulpecula* characterize marsupial sperm in general. Ultrastructural observations have been made on sperm from an additional 16 Australian marsupial species and these are included with those available in the literature for two American species. Since these species represent seven of the 12 families of extant marsupials, this seems a reasonable sample on which to base such a preliminary assessment.

The only reliable distinguishing characteristic of marsupial sperm appears to be the location and form of the acrosome. In monotreme (Hughes, cited by Griffiths, 1968; Hughes and Carrick, unpublished observations) and eutherian sperm (Fawcett, 1975), the acrosome forms a "cap" which surrounds at least the proximal region of the nucleus and projects varying distances beyond its rostral tip. In contrast, the acrosome in all marsupials examined to date, covers in varying degrees, only one surface of the flattened nucleus.

Flattening of the nucleus in a plane perpendicular to the long axis of the flagellum during spermiogenesis, and the consequent positioning of the neck insertion and rotation of the nucleus described above, typify sperm of most marsupials, but cannot be regarded as diagnostic characters of marsupial sperm because of the exception provided by the koala and presumably also the wombats.

Perhaps the most interesting aspects of marsupial sperm concern the pronounced morphological changes that occur in the acrosome and midpiece of sperm of a number of species during epididymal transit. These add up to a far more drastic and readily visible sperm maturation process than is common in eutherians. Thus sperm appear to be less mature when released into the testis tubules in marsupials than in eutherians, and this raises the question of whether the epididymis may play a greater role in the sperm maturation process in marsupials than in eutherians.

The full range of morphological maturation changes seen in *Trichosurus* sperm do not occur in all marsupials. Development of a helical midpiece fiber network as described for *Trichosurus,* or of other somewhat similar modifications of the midpiece plasma membrane or underlying cytoplasm, are most common and it seems likely that they may be found to occur in varying degrees in all marsupials. Formation of the invaginations of the midpiece plasma membrane is far less common, and of the species examined to date only occurs among some members of the superfamily Phalangeroidea (the phalangerid and petaurid, but not the macropodid species). Likewise, pronounced acrosomal modifications of the type seen in *Trichosurus* occur only in some species of the Petauridae, Phalangeridae, and Macropodidae. Such acrosomal modifications most commonly occur in species in which the acrosome covers a relatively small proportion of the dorsal nuclear surface, and in which containment of the acrosome within this reduced area during spermiogenesis leads to folding and projection of the acrosomal material away from the nuclear surface. The main exceptions to this generalization are the peramelids and *Pseudochirus peregrinus*. In the peramelids the acrosome covers only a relatively small proportion of the dorsal nuclear surface, but pronounced acrosomal maturation changes do not occur. The reverse situation is true of *Pseudocheirus* since acrosomal maturation changes are pronounced, but the acrosome covers a relatively large proportion of the dorsal nuclear surface. Examination of the possible reasons for these exceptions is beyond the scope of this chapter and will form the subject of a future paper (Harding, Carrick, and Shorey, in preparation).

This brief survey has demonstrated that marsupial sperm studies are still at a very rudimentary and descriptive level in comparison with eutherian sperm research. However, the many unusual features of marsupial sperm ultrastructure and maturation suggest that rewarding comparative information may result from examination of marsupial sperm alongside those of eutherians using the many ultrastructural techniques now available. Moreover, the very obvious nature of the sperm maturation changes observed in some marsupials and their rather rigid correlation with certain regions of the epididymis, suggests that marsupials such as *Trichosurus vulpecula* may be valuable in studying the interaction between the sperm and the epididymis in the sperm maturation process.

REFERENCES

Bedford, J.M.: Sperm Capacitation and Fertilization in Mammals. Biol Reprod 2(1970)128-158S

Bedford, J.M.; Calvin, H.I.: Changes in —S—S—linked Structures of the Sperm Tail during Epididymal Maturation with Comparative Observations in Sub-mammalian Species. J Exp Zool 187(1974)181-205

Benda, C.: Die Spermiogenese der Monotremen. Denkschr med-naturwiss gesamte Jena 6(1906)413-438

Biggers, J.D.; Creed, R.F.S.; DeLamater, E.D.: Conjugated Spermatozoa in American Marsupials. J Reprod Fertil 6(1963)324

Biggers, J.D.; DeLamater, E.D.: Marsupial Spermatozoa Pairing in the Epididymis of American Forms. Nature 208(1965)402-404

Burgos, M.H.: Ultrastructure of the Mammalian Sperm Head during Differentiation and Maturation. In: Physiology and Genetics of Reproduction. Part A, pp. 209-225, ed. by E.M. Couthino and F. Fuchs. Plenum Press, New York, 1974

Cleland, K.W.: Electron Microscope Structure of the Dasyuroid Sperm. J Anat 99(1965)953

Cleland, K.W.; Rothschild, Lord: The Bandicoot Spermatozoon: An Electron Microscope Study of the Tail. Proc R Soc Lond (Biol) 150(1959)24-42

Clemens, W.A.: Origin and Early Evolution of Marsupials. Evolution 22(1968)1-18

Cummins, J.M.: Epididymal Maturation of Spermatozoa in the Marsupial *Trichosurus vulpecula:* Changes in Motility and Gross Morphology. Aust J Zool 24(1976)499-512

Cummins, J.M.: Sperm Maturation in the Phalanger, *Trichosurus vulpecula.* In: Fourth International Symposium on Comparative Biology of Reproduction. pp. 153-154. Australian Academy of Science, Canberra, 1977

Fawcett, D.W.: A Comparative View of Sperm Ultrastructure. Biol Reprod 2(1970)90-127S

Fawcett, D.W.: The Mammalian Spermatozoon. Dev Biol 44(1975)394-436

Griffiths, M.: Echidnas. Pergamon Press, Oxford, 1968

Harding, H.R.; Carrick, F.N.; Shorey, C.D.: Ultrastructural Changes in Spermatozoa of the Brush-tailed Possum, *Trichosurus vulpecula* (Marsupialia) during Epididymal Transit. Part I: The Flagellum. Cell Tissue Res 164(1975)121-132

Harding, H.R.; Carrick, F.N.; Shorey, C.D.: Ultrastructural Changes in Spermatozoa of the Brush-tailed Possum, *Trichosurus vulpecula* (Marsupialia). Part II: The Acrosome. Cell Tissue Res 171(1976a)61-73

Harding, H.R.; Carrick, F.N.; Shorey, C.D.: Spermiogenesis in the Brush-tailed Possum, *Trichosurus vulpecula* (Marsupialia). The Development of the Acrosome. Cell Tissue Res 171(1976b)75-90

Harding, H.R.; Carrick, F.N.; Shorey, C.D.: Ultrastructure of the Midpiece of the Spermatozoon in the Marsupial, *Trichosurus vulpecula.* J Reprod Fertil 46(1976c)501

Harding, H.R.; Carrick, F.N.; Shorey, C.D.: Acrosome Development during Spermiogenesis in some Australian Marsupials: an Ultrastructural Study. Theriogenology 6(1976d)657

Harding, H.R.; Carrick, F.N.; Shorey, C.D.: Spermatozoa of Australian Marsupials: Ultrastructure and Epididymal

Development. In: Fourth International Symposium on Comparative Biology of Reproduction, pp. 151-152. Australian Academy of Science, Canberra, 1977

Harris, W.F.: Motility of Mammalian Spermatozoa, Dislocations in the Mitochondrial Sheath, and a Possible Active Role for the Sheath in Motility. S Afr J Sci 72(1976)82-84

Holstein, A.F.: Elektronenmikroskopische Untersuchungen am Spermatozoon des Opossum (*Didelphys virginiana* Kerr). Z Zellforsch 65(1965)904-914

Hughes, R.L.: Comparative Morphology of Spermatozoa from Five Marsupial Families. Aust J Zool 13(1965)533-543

Hughes, R.L.: The Tertiary Egg Membranes of the Marsupial, *Trichosurus vulpecula*. Ph.D. Thesis, University of New South Wales, 1974

Hughes, R.L.: Reproduction in the Male Marsupial Devil *Sarcophilus harrisii* with Particular Reference to the Ultrastructure of Epididymal Spermatozoa. In: Proceedings VIIIth International Congress of Animal Reproduction and Artificial Insemination Vol. 4, Pathology of Reproduction and Artificial Insemination, pp 908-910. Krakow, 1976.

Hughes, R.L.: Light and Electron Microscope Studies on the Spermatozoa of the Koala, *Phascolarctos cinereus* (Marsupialia). J Anat 124(1977)513

Jardine, N.; McKenzie, D.: Continental Drift and the Dispersal and Evolution of Organisms. Nature 235(1972)20-24

Keast, A.: Historical Biogeography of the Marsupials. In: Biology of Marsupials, pp. 69-95, ed. by B. Stonehouse and D. Gilmore. Macmillan, London, 1977

Lilliegraven, J.A.: Latest Cretaceous Mammals from the Upper Part of the Edmonton Formation of Alberta, Canada, and Review of Marsupial Placental Dichotomy in Mammalian Evolution. Univ Kansas Publ Paleont Contr Art 50 (Vertebrate 12) (1969)1-122

Lilligraven, J.A.: Biological Considerations of the Marsupial-Placental Dichotomy. Evolution 29(1976)707-722

Olson, G.: Observations on the Ultrastructure of a Fiber Network in the Flagellum of Sperm of the Brush-tailed Phalanger, *Trichosurus vulpecula*. J Ultrastruct Res 50(1975)193-198

Olson, G.E.; Hamilton, D.W.: Morphological Changes in the Midpiece of Wooly Opossum Spermatozoa during Epididymal Transit. Anat Rec 186(1976)387-404

Olson, G.E.; Lifsics, M.; Fawcett, D.W.; Hamilton, D.W.: Structural Specializations in the Flagellar Plasma Membrane of Opossum Spermatozoa. J Ultrastruct Res 59(1977)207-221

Phillips, D.M.: Development of Spermatozoa in the Wooly Opossum with Special Reference to the Shaping of the Sperm Head. J Ultrastruct Res 33(1970a)369-380

Phillips, D.M.: Ultrastructure of Spermatozoa of the Wooly Opossum *Caluromys philander*. J Ultrastruct Res 33(1970b)381-397

Rattner, J.B.: Nuclear Shaping in Marsupial Spermatids. J Ultrastruct Res 40(1972)498-512

Raven, P.H.; Axelrod, D.I.: Plate Tectonics and Australian Paleogeography. Science 176(1972)1379-1386

Sapsford, C.S.; Rae, C.A.: Ultrastructural Studies on Sertoli Cells and Spermatids in the Bandicoot and Ram during the Movement of Mature Spermatids into the Lumen of the Seminiferous Tubule. Aust J Zool 17(1969)415-445

Sapsford, C.S.; Rae, C.A.; Cleland, K.W.: The Development of the Principal Piece Sheath of the Bandicoot Spermatozoon: An Electron Microscope Study. J Anat 100(1966)950

Sapsford, C.S.; Rae, C.A.; Cleland, K.W.: Ultrastructural Studies on Spermatids and Sertoli Cells during Early Spermiogenesis in the Bandicoot *Perameles nasuta* Geoffroy (Marsupialia). Aust J Zool 15(1967)881-909

Sapsford, C.S.; Rae, C.A.; Cleland, K.W.: Ultrastructural Studies on Maturing Spermatids and on Sertoli Cells in the Bandicoot *Perameles nasuta* Geoffroy (Marsupialia). Aust J Zool 17(1969a)195-292

Sapsford, C.S.; Rae, C.A.; Cleland, K.W.: The Fate of the Residual Bodies and Degenerating Germ Cells in the Bandicoot *Perameles nasuta* (Marsupialia). Aust J Zool 17(1969b)729-753

Sapsford, C.S.; Rae, C.A.; Cleland, K.W.: Ultrastructural Studies on the Development and Form of the Principal Piece Sheath of the Bandicoot Spermatozoon. Aust J Zool 18(1970)21-48

Tedford, R.H.; Banks, M.R.; Kemp, N.R.; McDougall, I.; Sutherland, F.L.: Recognition of the Oldest Known Fossil Marsupials from Australia. Nature 255(1975)141-142

Temple-Smith, P.; Bedford, J.M.: The Features of Sperm Maturation in the Epididymis of a Marsupial, the Brush-tailed Possum, *Trichosurus vulpecula*. Am J Anat 147(1976)471-500

THE EVOLUTION OF THE ACROSOMAL COMPLEX

B. Baccetti

Institute of Zoology, University of Siena, Italy

> In parte anteriore corporis, multorum ex his animalculis detexi plagam pellucidam rotundam...
>
> Leeuwenhoek, Epistola 142, 1701

THE ACROSOME AS ANIMAL ORGANELLE

Apical organelles, located close to the nucleus, have been depicted in animal spermatozoa (Fig. 1) from the beginning of microscopical cytology (Leeuwenhoek, 1677, 1678, 1684, 1701) but not until a century ago were the acrosomal structures recognized and interpreted. Retzius (1881) gave the organelle the name "Spiess," imitated by Herrmann (1882) with "pointe cephalique," and by Waldeyer (1887) who used the name "Zugespitze." Sometime later Benda (1887) demonstrated that the "spitzen Kappe," presumably the whole acrosomal complex, originates from the Golgi complex, and contemporaneously Jensen (1887) applied to rat sperm the name "Hakenstäbchen" to the organelle destined later to be called perforatorium, which is located close to the "Hakenspitze" (Fig. 2). Ballowitz (1891) continued to call the complex "Spitzenstück." Lenhossek (1898) introduced the term "Akrosoma" (Fig. 3). Waldeyer (1906) introduced the term "perforatorium" (Fig. 4) used for the first time in an amphibian, and for the mammalian acrosome the term "galea capitis." Due to this confusion, the terms acrosome and perforatorium were long regarded as synonyms, and other names were introduced such as "head cap" for the former; "inner cone," "rod," "fibrous core" for the latter, mainly in invertebrates. With electron microscopy, Fawcett and Burgos (1955) demonstrated that acrosome and galea capitis or head cap are the same organelle; Clermont et al. (1955) observed that the perforatorium in the rat is a separate structure, which later Burgos and Fawcett (1956) recognized also in toad sperm. Definitive clarification on the confused nomenclature in vertebrates was provided by Fawcett (1958). Kaye (1962), Colwin and Colwin (1963), and Dan (1967) recognized the homology of the vertebrate perforatorium to the equivalent structure of invertebrates. This view was accepted by Baccetti and Afzelius (1976) who distinguish in the acrosomal complex of any kind of sperm only acrosome and perforatorium.

It is apparent that the primitive spermatozoon lacks an acrosome. The acrosome is not only lacking in the primitive aflagellate spermatozoa of mesozoa (Bresciani and Fenchel, 1965, 1967), red algae (Manton and Friedman, 1960; Christensen, 1962; Manton, 1970), and in the male gamete of protozoa (Aikawa et al., 1970; Cavalier-Smith, 1975) but also in all plant male germ cells. The manner of penetration of the spermatozoid has been followed in the cycad, Zamia (Norstog, 1975) and in the fern *Pteridium* (Duckett and Bell, 1972) where the anterior rim of a microtubular band affects flexing movements and acts as a rigid girder which breaks the egg membrane. The egg surface is generally reached through a hole of the overlying cell wall (Myles, 1975).

The acrosome is acquired only through animal evolution. Sperm of Porifera (Tuzet et al., 1970) and of the fresh water cnidarian *Hydra* (Schincariol et al., 1967; Weissman et al., 1969; Stagni and Lucchi, 1970; Moore and Dixon, 1972) have no apical structures located on the nucleus. Several marine cnidarians have a few lateral vesicles arising in association with the Golgi complex, both in hydrozoans (*Tubularia:* Afzelius, 1971a; *Eudendrium:* Summers, 1972) and anthozoans (*Metridium:* Hinsch and Clark, 1973; *Bunodosoma*, Dewel and Clark, 1972). Finally, the majority of hydrozoans and all the scyphozoans studied to date have many vesicles filled with electron-dense material, capping the anterior end of the nucleus (Summers, 1970; Afzelius and Franzen, 1971; O'Rand, 1972; Lunger, 1971; Hinsch and Clark, 1973; O'Rand and Miller, 1974; Hinsch, 1974; Lyke and Robson, 1975). All these authors assume that the vesicles subserve the function of rudimentary acrosomes. In fact those species that lack them have eggs with micropyles or indentations (Hinsch, 1974). Moreover, the vesicles are lost after the penetration into the egg (O'Rand and Miller, 1974).

The question can be raised whether the absence of vesicles in fresh water hydroids is a regressive character

---

This research has been carried out under the auspices of the Consiglio Nazionale delle Ricerche project "Biology of Reproduction."

© 1979 Urban & Schwarzenberg, Inc. Baltimore-Munich *The Spermatozoon*, edited by D.W. Fawcett and J.M. Bedford

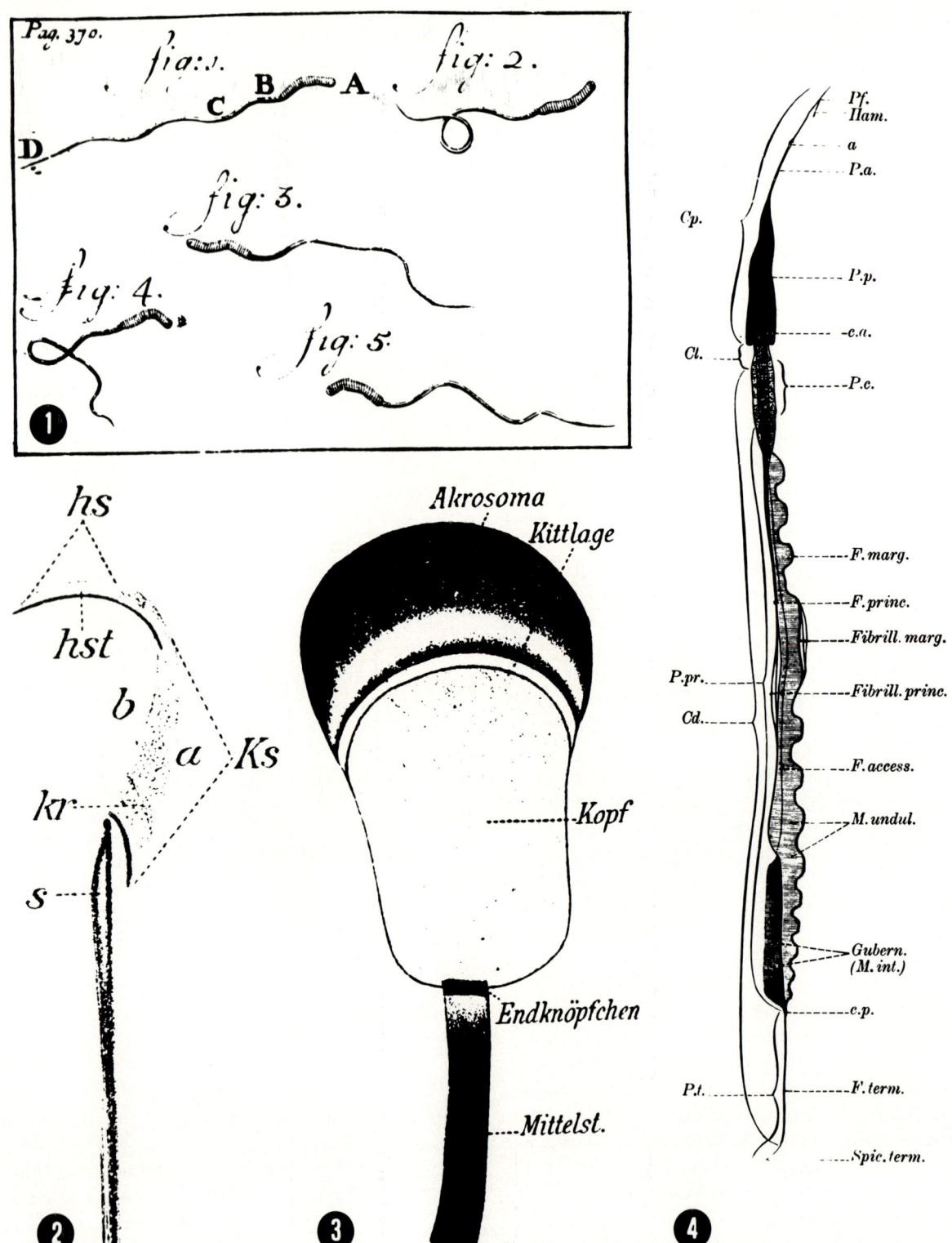

Figure 1. Leeuwenhoek (1701) was able to recognize in the anterior part of chicken spermatozoa a "plaga pellucida rotunda."
Figure 2. Jensen (1887) in the optical region of rat spermatozoon distinguished between "Hakenstabchen (hst)" and "Hakenspitze" (hs).
Figure 3. Lenhossek (1898) introduces the term "Akrosoma" for the rat sperm.
Figure 4. Waldeyer (1906) introduces the "Perforatorium" (Pf) in an amphibian.

acquired after their passage from marine to fresh water environment (Afzelius, 1971a) or a more primitive condition closer to that of Porifera. In either case, the presence of vesicles in the whole phylum Cnidaria clearly represents a preliminary step to the acquisition of a typical acrosome.

THE CONVENTIONAL MARINE ACROSOMAL COMPLEX

The metazoan phyla immediately above cnidarians show a classical acrosomal complex (Fig. 5) made up of a convex acrosome and a subjacent bundle of filamen-

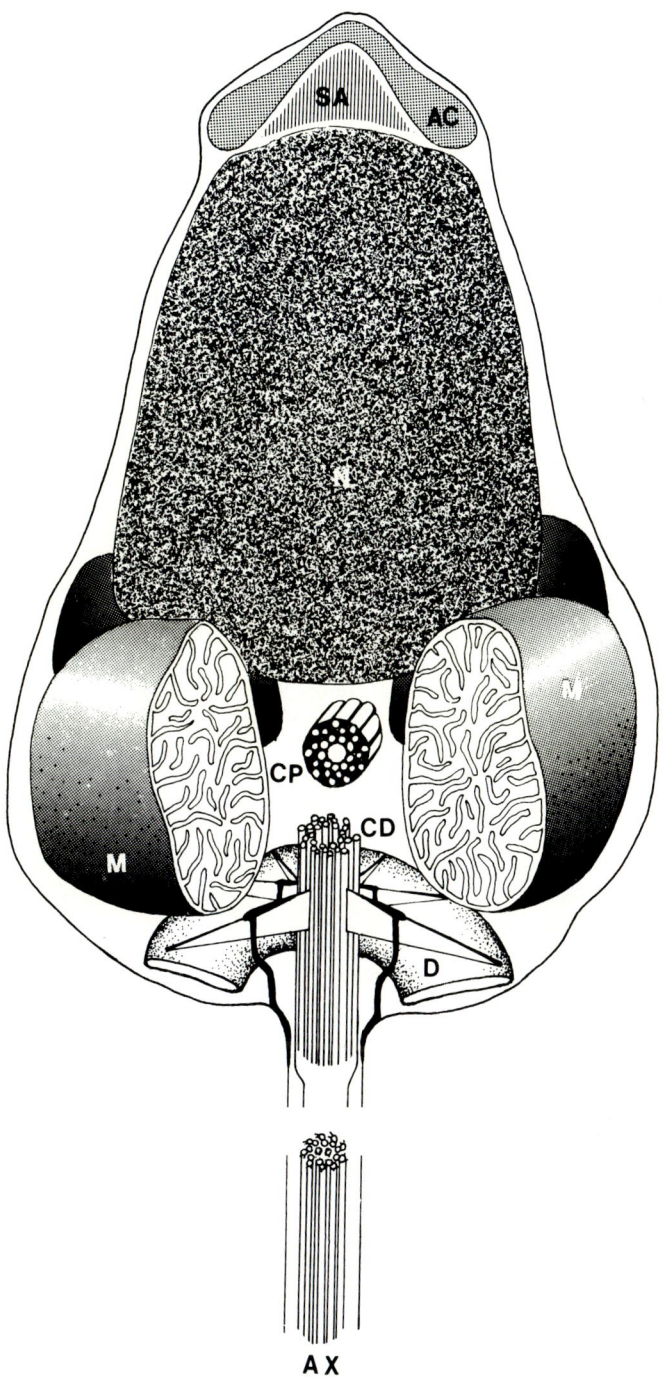

Figure 5. The classical aquatic sperm model (*Sipunculida*, from Baccetti, 1977). AC, acrosome; AX, axoneme, CD, distal centriole; CP, proximal centriole; D, dense laminae; M, mitochondria; N, nucleus; SA, subacrosomal material, or perforatorium.

tous material or granules more or less concentrated to form a rod-like perforatorium. The lower examples described (Fig. 6) are the Ctenarian *Beroe* (Franc, 1973) and the Nemertea, *Cerebratulus, Emplectonema, Micrura,* and *Malacobdella* (Clark and Hinsch, 1969; Whitfield, 1972; Afzelius, 1971 a, b, 1972). Other lower phyla (Fig. 6) such as Rotifera (Koehler, 1965), Platyhelmintha (see Hendelberg, 1977), Ectoprocta (Reger, 1971), Bryozoa (Franzen, 1976), Kinorhyncha (Nyholm, 1976), and Acanthocephala (Marchand and Mattei, 1976), completely lack acrosomes, and it is difficult to say whether this is due to an involution, or the conservation of primitive characteristics. In the majority of them, the author favors the first hypothesis (Baccetti and Afzelius, 1976). Mature sperm of some nematoda bear plurilocular vesicles of Golgi origin that Clark *et al.* (1967) assume to be proacrosomal granules serving an acrosomal function. They are probably the so-called "spongy chambers" present in many other kinds of aflagellate spermatozoa that also have an acrosome (Baccetti and Afzelius, 1976) and they probably have nothing to do with an acrosomal function. Nematoda must therefore be regarded as devoid of an acrosome, as claimed by Jamuar (1966). At higher levels (Fig. 6), a more or less classical marine acrosome has been found in Gastrotricha (Teuchert, 1976), in Sipunculida (Baccetti, 1977), Priapulida (Afzelius and Ferraguti, 1978), Nematomorpha (Lora Lamia Donin and Cotelli, 1977), Brachiopoda (Afzelius and Ferraguti, 1978). This structure is conserved, with a few variations, in all the major aquatic phyla. It is found in aquatic Annelida (Colwin and Colwin, 1961; Fallon and Austin, 1967; Cotelli and Lora Lamia Donin, 1975; Malecha, 1975; Bertout, 1976), Pogonophora (Franzen, 1973), Enteropneusta (Colwin and Colwin, 1963), and Echinodermata, where the most penetrating research has been conducted (from

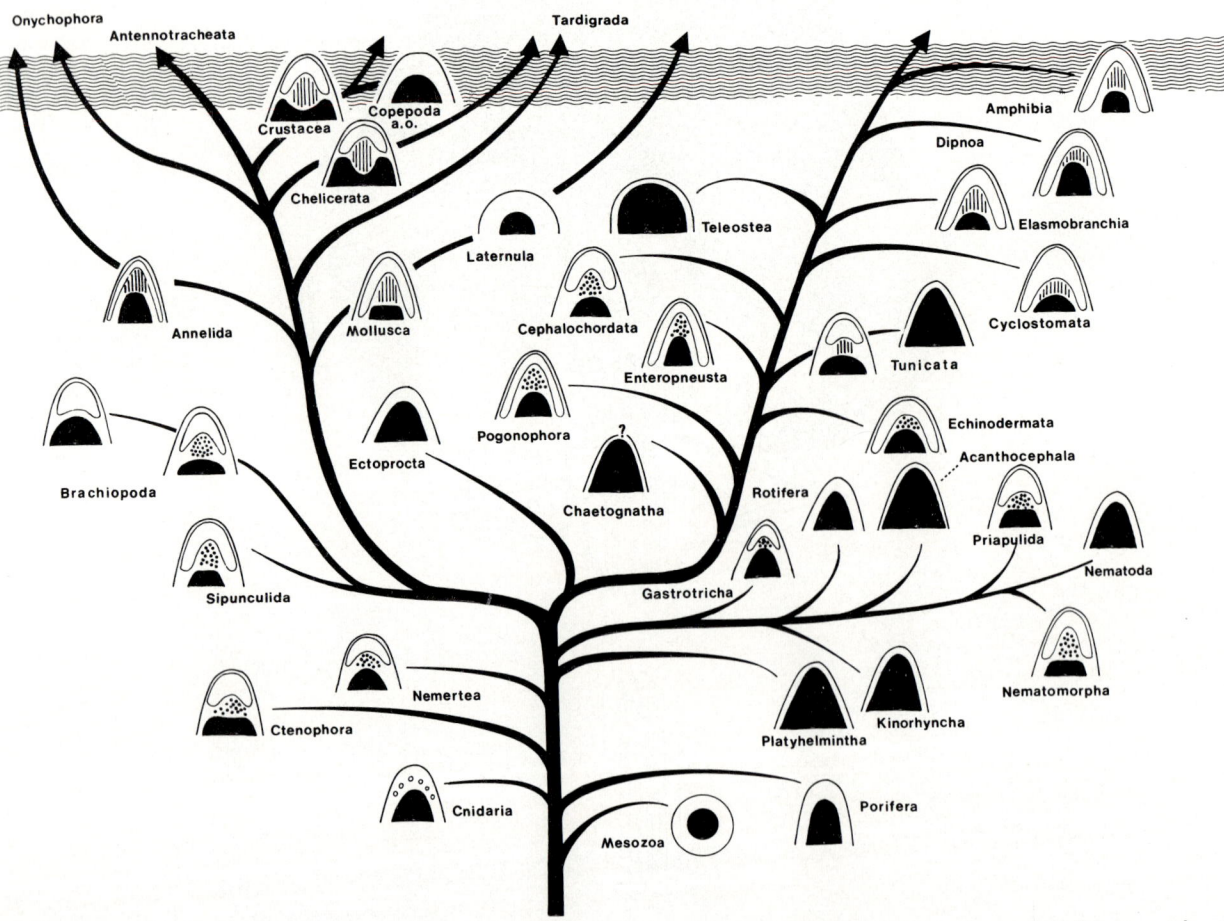

Figure 6. Phylogenetic tree of aquatic acrosome evolution. The acrosome is depicted as a hollow vesicle, the subacrosomal substance or perforatorium as a group of spots or lines (according to the "profilactin" or "filamentous actin" models), the nucleus as a black body, the plasma membrane as a peripheral line.

Afzelius, 1955, to Tilney, 1975), in most aquatic Mollusca, from Bivalvia to Gastropoda, Prosobranchia and Cephalopoda (Niijima and Dan, 1965, a, b; Walker and MacGregor, 1968; Giusti, 1969; Longo and Anderson, 1969; Buckland-Nicks, 1973; Hylander and Summers, 1977); also in the primitive arthropodan *Limulus* (André, 1963), most Crustacea, from Cephalocarida (Brown and Metz, 1967) to Decapoda (Brown, 1966); the aquatic Chordata *Amphioxus* (Baccetti et al., 1972), some lower Tunicata (Flood and Afzelius, 1978), Cyclostomata (Nicander and Sjöden, 1971), Elasmobranchia (Stanley, 1971), dipneustan fish (Jespersen, 1971); and Amphibia (from Burgos and Fawcett, 1956, to Furieri, 1975). Only a few lines that have arisen from the above have lost the whole acrosome complex: some Crustacea, few Mollusca, some Tunicata, and all of the teleost fishes. Chaetognatha need to be further investigated because presence and function of the acrosome are still uncertain (Van Deurs, 1972).

It can be concluded that structure and function of the acrosome complex remained basically unchanged in the aquatic environment, even though studies on acrosomal proteins have been carried out on only a few of them: horseshoe crab, mussel, starfish, and sea urchin.

The Acrosome

In the aquatic sperm model the acrosome is usually cap shaped, with an inner central concavity holding the perforatorium. Usually the lateral regions of the acrosome are thicker, while the apex is quite thin. The acrosome is a Golgi derivative, and it is therefore enveloped by a Golgi membrane. A few studies have been carried out on this subject in Mollusca and Echinodermata (Fig. 7). The outer acrosomal membrane examined by freeze-fracture methods in both *Mytilus* and in sea urchin shows 7-9-nm particles, spaced about 10 nm from one another, arranged without a precise geometry and the particles are more abundant in a small apical area[1] (Fig. 7). This area, where the acrosomal membrane is in close contact with the plasma membrane, triggers the acrosomal reaction which involves a fusion between acrosomal membrane and plasma membrane (Dan, 1967, 1970; Dan et al., 1972, 1975) which in this area lacks intramembrane particles (Fig. 7). The inner acrosomal membrane which has very sparse particles[1] covers the emerging perforatorium after the acrosomal reaction. It is interesting to note that although the perforatorium elongates for a long distance, ample new membrane to cover it is synthesized in a short time from material stored in the mature acrosome (Dan, 1970). This membrane seems to be responsible for the adhesion of the sperm to the egg (Collins, 1976). The acrosomal membranes of starfish and *Mytilus* contain a Ca^{2+}-activated adenosine triphosphatase (ATPase) (Mabuchi and Mabuchi, 1973). Collins and Epel (1977) have recently reviewed the role of Ca in triggering the acrosomal reaction in sea urchin sperm. From results of application of the ionophore A23187, which transports Ca^{2+} across membranes (Talbot et al., 1976; Decker et al., 1976), it is suggested that Ca represents the initial step of the acrosome reaction. Probably other ions, completing the acrosome reaction, cross the sperm membrane at this time, *e.g.*, a loss of acid from sea urchin sperm undergoing the acrosome reaction has been observed (Collins and Epel, 1977).

The content of the acrosome of aquatic sperm shows a PAS positive reaction (Turquier and Pochon-Masson, 1969; Langreth, 1969; Picheral, 1972; Sandoz, 1970a, b). Its main function is lysis of the egg jelly coat. Discovered in an amphibian *Discoglossus* (Hibbard, 1928), "lysin" was later extracted from the acrosomes of some bivalve molluscs (Tyler, 1939, 1949). It seems to be a trypsin-like protein, sedimenting at 3 S (Hauschka, 1963), similar to the better known acrosin of the mammalian acrosome (Levine et al., 1978). Wada et al. (1956) and Niijima and Dan (1965a, b) believed that it is located apically, and in a basal ring of the *Mytilus* acrosome; while Endo (1976) partially modifies this view, demonstrating by PTA staining and pronase digestion, an axial distribution along the whole length of the acrosome. The more peripheral region of the *Mytilus* acrosome closer to the membranes is, according to Endo (1976) occupied by another protein, stained by silver methenamine and not affected by pronase digestion. In another bivalve *Spisula*, Hylander and Summers (1977) also find two different acrosomal materials. Indeed, in the last year, Vacquier has demonstrated in a series of papers (Vacquier and Moy, 1977; Bellet et al., 1977;[2]) that the major component of sea urchin acrosome is an insoluble 35,000 M_r protein which bonds the sperm to the vitelline layer covering the egg plasma membrane. This protein has been named "bindin" and is probably a carbohydrate-binding protein, specific for galactose and lactose, that has affinity for a glycoprotein located on the vitelline layer. Studied in two species of sea urchin, the bindins show considerable homology in the terminal amino acid sequences. It may well be a class of proteins responsible for the attachment of sperm to eggs, that is of broad occurrence in animals. In Vacquier's laboratory, the isolation of bindin from acro-

---

[1]Author's unpublished observation

[2]Vacquier, V.D.; Moy, G.W.: in preparation

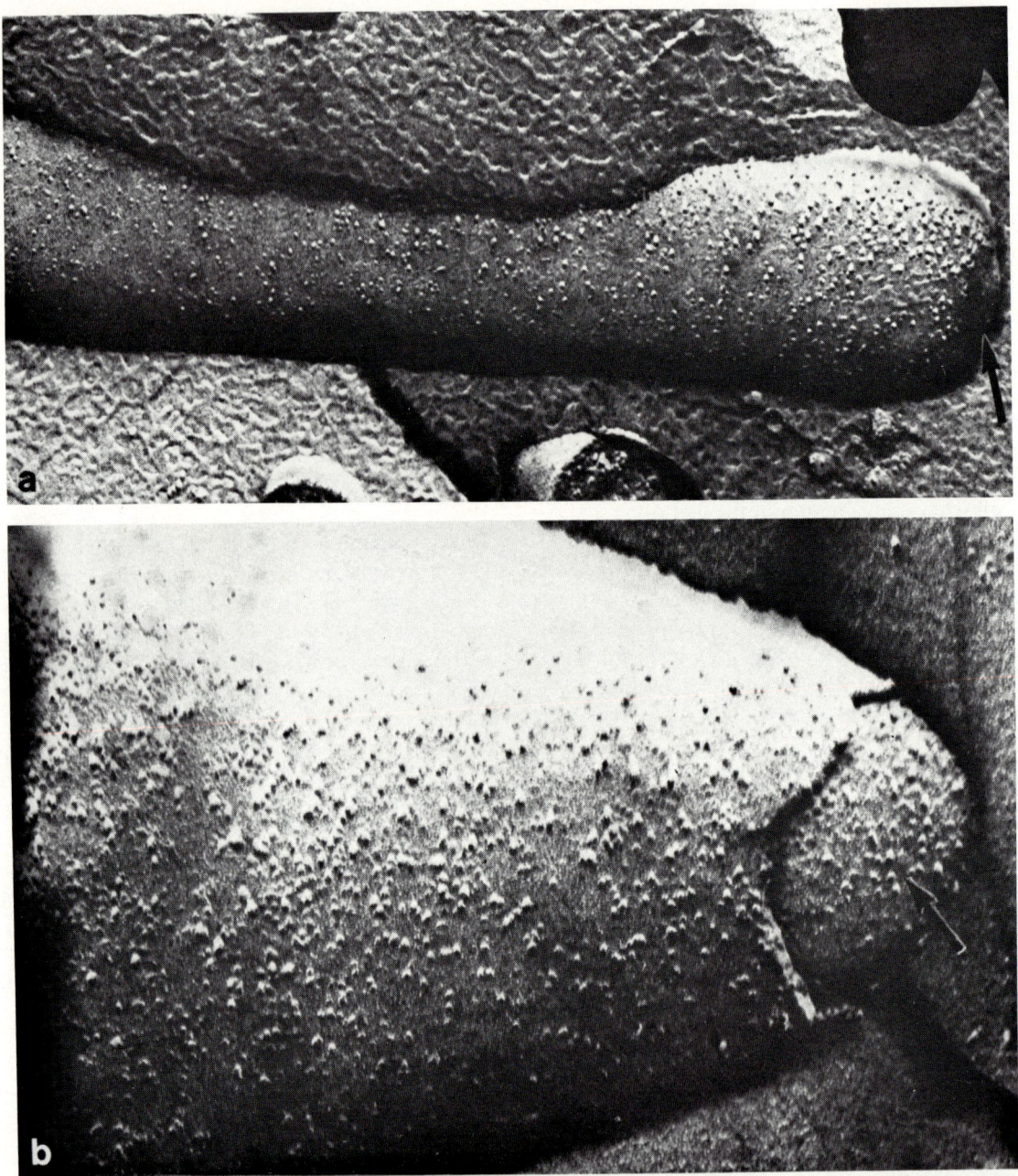

Figure 7. The sperm tip in the mussel *Mytilus* spermatozoon, after freeze-fracture. In (a) the plasma membrane is intact showing regular rows of particles absent from the "trigger" region (arrow). (X47,500) In (b) the plasma membrane is broken, and the particles of the outer acrosomal membrane (arrow) can be seen. (X85,000)

somes of Mollusca and Polychaeta is under investigation (personal communications).

In some aquatic Arthropoda the acrosomal architecture seems to be different. A fibrous perforatorium is demonstrated; but in Decapod crustaceans Chevallier (1967) described, with histochemical methods, a new basic protein called "decapodin" axially located around the perforatorium, in the same position where lysins are detected in the classic aquatic sperm. More information on acrosome evolution in terrestrial Arthropods is needed.

The Perforatorium

All aquatic sperm possessing an acrosome have sub-acrosomal material that projects outward at the time of the acrosomal reaction. As mentioned in the introduction, it may be useful to extend the term perforatorium to this structure.

A number of electron microscopic investigations give information on the shape, structure, and position of the perforatorium. First of all, the perforatorium usually is more or less deeply recessed in an anterior nuclear indentation; in extreme cases it may traverse the whole nucleus in a complete axial canal (*Limulus,* Cephalocarid crustaceans, *Petromyzon*). However, in other cases (Nemertea, Gastrotricha, Nematomorpha, Pogonophora, Annelida, and Mollusca Prosobranchia) the material is completely extranuclear. Moreover, several instances have been described in which no fibrous material can be discerned in the subacrosomal space but only a more or less dense mass of granules (Fig. 8): *e.g.,* in Ctenophora (Franc, 1973), Nemertea (Afzelius, 1971, 1972), Gastrotricha (Teuchert, 1976), Priapulida (Afzelius and Ferraguti, 1978), Nematomorpha (Lora Lamia Donin and Cotelli, 1977), and from Sipunculida (Baccetti, 1977) up to Pogonorphora (Franzen, 1973), Echinodermata (Tilney, 1975b), Enteropneusta (Colwin and Colwin, 1963), some Tunicata (Flood and Afzelius, 1978), and Cephalochordata (Baccetti *et al.*, 1972). There are the more primitive groups in the two main metazoan evolutionary branches. In fact at higher levels (Fig. 9) Annelida, Mollusca, and Arthropoda show obvious fibrous perforatoria, as do also Cyclostomata, Elasmobranchia, and Dipnoa (Fig. 14), all these groups approaching terrestrial life. We can thus interpret the fibrous perforatorium as a more advanced step, possibly related to internal fertilization and departure from an aquatic environment (Fig. 6). The two perforatorium models have been studied biochemically only in a few instances, and clearly appear to be different in protein composition.

After a preliminary investigation by Jessen *et al.* (1973)

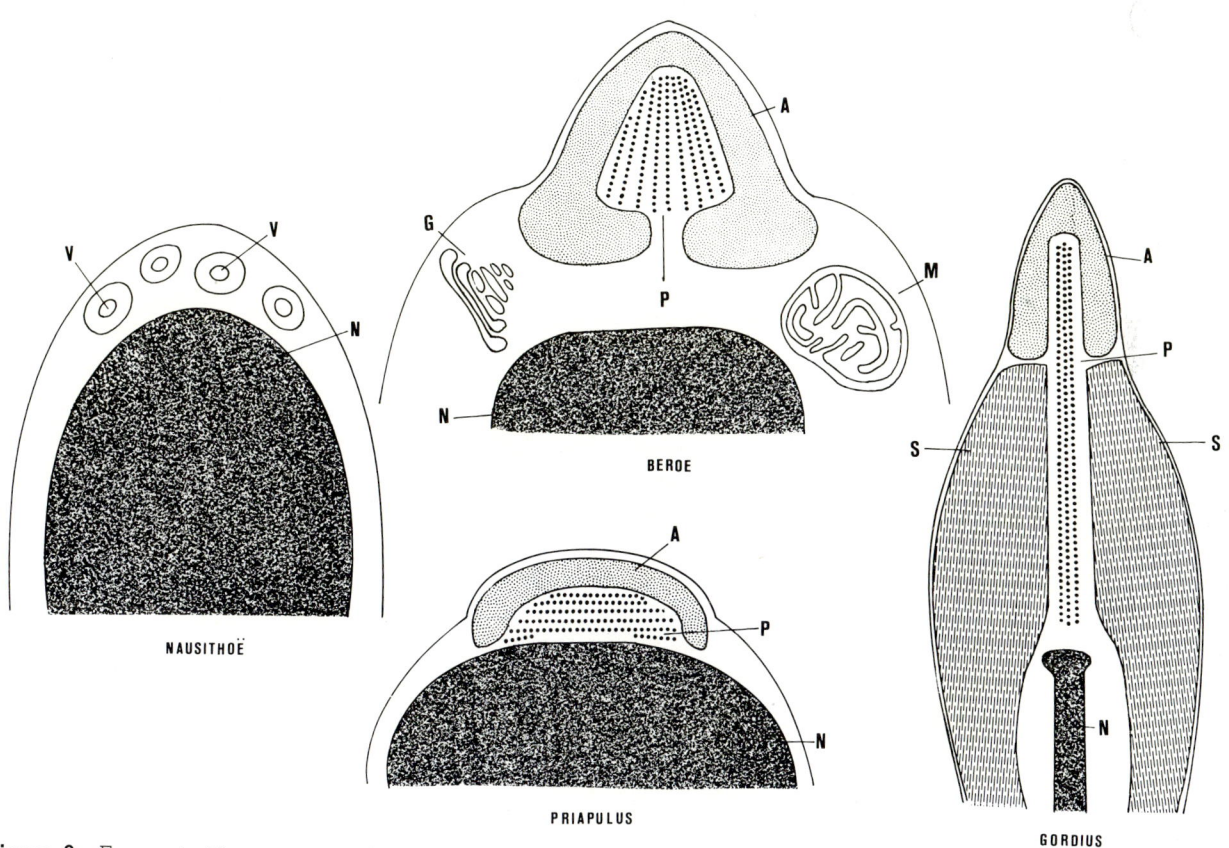

Figure 8. Four primitive sperm models. In the Cnidarian *Nausithoë* (according to Afzelius and Franzen, 1971), near the nucleus (N), the acrosomal material is represented by a few vesicles (V). In the Ctenarian *Beroe* (according to Franc, 1973) the acrosome (A) lies on a stratus of granular material interpreted here as perforatorium (P), located on the nucleus (N). Golgi complex (G) and mitochondria (M) are also present. In the Priapulid *Priapulus* (according to Afzelius and Ferraguti, 1978) a stratus of granular perforatorium material is also present between nucleus (N) and acrosome (A). In the nematomorph *Gordius* (according to Lora Lamia Donin and Cotelli, 1977) a granular perforatorium material (P) is also interposed between nucleus (N) and acrosome (A), partially surrounded by an asymmetrical sheath (S).

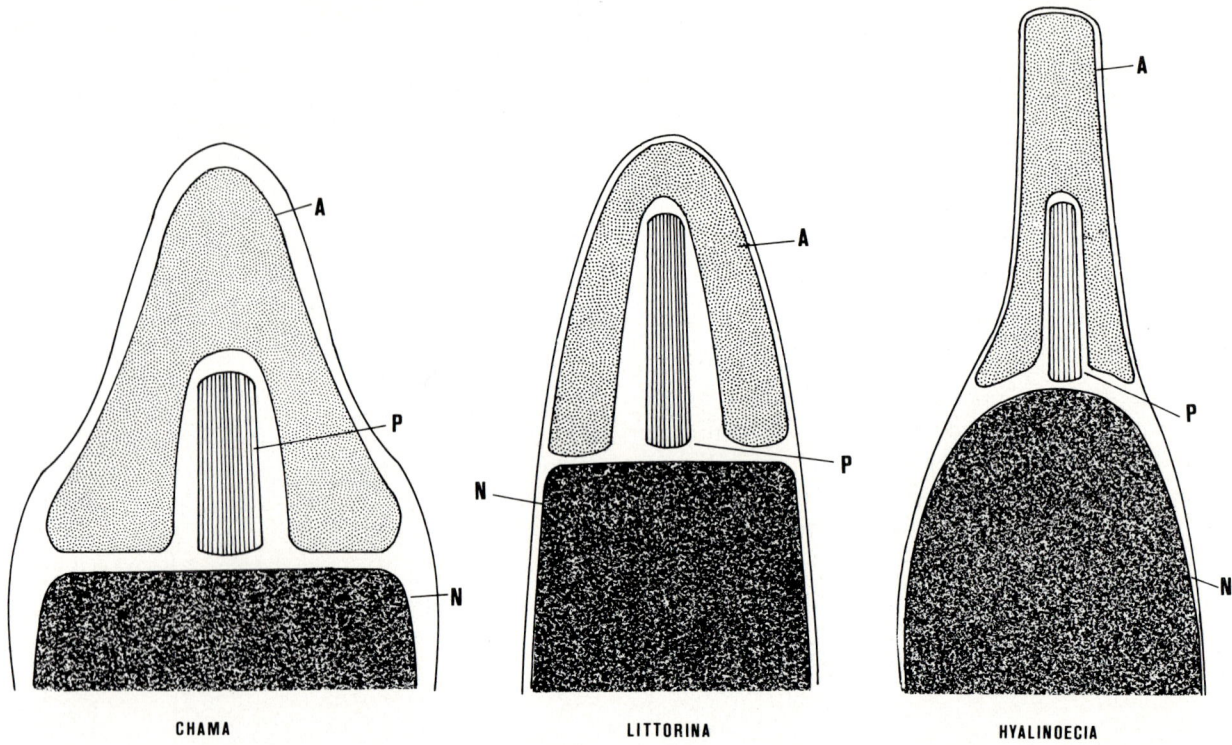

Figure 9. Three models of higher aquatic acrosomal complexes. In the bivalve mollusc *Chama* (according to Hylander and Summers, 1977) as in the Prosobranch *Littorina* (according to Buckland-Nicks, 1973) and the Annelid *Hyalinoecia* (according to Cotelli and Lora Lamia Donin, 1975), a filamentous perforatorium (P) is interposed between nucleus (N) and acrosome (A).

on sea urchin, Tilney (1975a, b; 1976a, b; Tilney et al., 1973) has clarified the problem in a series of papers: actin is always present in the subacrosomal space, but can be stored in different conditions. In the starfish *Thyone* or *Asterias*, where the unreacted perforatorium is amorphous, actin is in a peculiar "storage form," neither globular, nor filamentous. In *Mytilus*, and for the most part in *Limulus*, the perforatorium before its reaction is instead a bundle of hexagonally arranged filaments, the actin being stored in a filamentous form. Therefore perforatorium elongation in the first case is due to polymerization, in the second to a changement in packing of the already polymerized actin. In such a scheme the role of the other proteins detected in the perforatorium is important. In the case of amorphous perforatoria, actin is maintained in the "storage form" ("profilactin," according to Tilney, 1976a), it being associated with the common spectrins (250-230,000 M_r) and with another low molecular weight protein (16,000 M_r) named "profilin" by Carlsson et al. (1976a, b; 1977) and which was found in a number of nonmuscular cells, including echinoderm sperm, where actin is monomeric. Heggeness et al. (1977) and Davies et al. (1977) describe "filamin," a 240,000-M_r protein which, in cultured fibroblasts, interacts with F-actin filaments to form bundles and inhibits the actin activation of heavy meromyosin ATPase. Possibly a band in the spectrin region may be due to filamin. Moreover Mabuchi (1976) isolates myosin from starfish sperm heads, and proposes that it becomes attached to the actin filaments during the polymerization, which is consequently accelerated. Quite recently Tilney (1978) demonstrated that the assembly of actin filaments in *Thyone* sperm initiates from a nucleating body, the "actomere," composed of 20-25 filaments embedded in a dense matrix.

In the case of filamentous perforatoria, actin filaments in *Limulus* are arranged in a supercoil (Tilney, 1975a, b; De Rosier et al., 1977) which at the time of perforatorium elongation becomes a parallel bundle. The proteins gluing actin filaments in the coiled form are the so-called "scruin" (55,000) and α-actinin (95,000). The latter could be involved in determining polarity of the actin filaments (which is consistent and directed toward the cell base in *Mytilus*) and may be concentrated near the tip of the perforatorium. The perforatorium tip may be comparable to the muscle Z-line, as is the case for the tips of the microvilli of the intestine (Tilney, 1975b). Scruin, on the contrary, is associated with every actin molecule in the unreacted *Limulus* perforatorium (De Rosier *et al.*, 1977). The *Mytilus* perforatorium has not yet been studied in this respect.

In conclusion, the structure of aquatic perforatoria has become clear in recent years. Actin appears to be the universal, basic protein, whether associated with spectrins, profilin, myosin, and possibly filamin in the unreacted amorphous type that can be called a "profilactin model" typical of lower groups; or whether associated with scruin and α-actinin in the "filamentous model" typical of higher groups. The reacted perforatorium may contain only actin, but the possible participation of myosin in the process needs to be clarified. It will be interesting to see what the situation will prove to be in the internal fertilization of terrestrial animals, and to determine whether the models in aquatic phyla are really unique in their possession of two actin binding proteins. The strange model of Gastrotricha, where the perforatorium is organized in a longitudinal series of granular cubic blocks (Teuchert, 1976), would be promising to study.

The Extra-acrosomal Layer

The space between acrosomal and plasma membrane may be occupied in some animals by a layer of granular filaments or amorphous material. This layer is more common in several terrestrial sperm models (see below), but it has also been described occasionally in primitive aquatic forms. André (1963), Fahrenbach (1973), and Tilney (unpublished) find it in *Limulus*, Franc (1973) in the ctenophoran *Beroe*. Although no information is available on it, it can be assumed the material is involved in the acrosomal reaction.

The Postacrosomal Ring

A ring of dense material, embedded in the subacrosomal substance, has been described by Afzelius (1971b) in a Nemertean and by Nicander and Sjöden (1971) in a lamprey (Fig. 14). The perforatorium runs through the ring at the time of the acrosomal reaction. The nature and role of the ring are unclear; it may be mechanical.

The Disappearance of the Acrosomal Complex and the Pseudo-acrosome

At the beginning of this chapter, several phyla lacking an acrosome were mentioned, but it is difficult to establish whether this lack is original or secondary. For the following animals, the acrosome seems to have disappeared during evolution: Copepod, Branchiopod, and Branchiuran crustaceans (Brown, 1970; Wingstrand, 1972) and Pycnogonida (Van Deurs, 1974); the bivalve molluscs *Laternula* (Kubo, 1977), and *Lyonsia* (Kubo and Ishikawa, 1978) some of the Ascidians (Georges, 1969; Tuzet *et al.*, 1972; Villa, 1975; Woolacott, 1977) and all teleosts (Mattei and Mattei, 1973; Mattei, 1970; Ginsburg, 1963; Porte and Follenius, 1960; Stanley, 1969). In some of these, both acrosome and perforatorium begin to differentiate, but disappear late in spermiogenesis, as in *Laternula* and *Lyonsia* (Kubo, 1977; Kubo and Ishikawa, 1978) and in Branchiura and Pentastomida (Wingstrand, 1972). In these latter groups Wingstrand (1972) describes the formation of a newly appearing acrosome-like organelle, in place of the disappeared acrosome. It is of unknown function, is called the pseudo-acrosome, and is formed from the pericentriolar structures. In Ostracodans, a true acrosome is lacking (Gupta, 1968; Zissler, 1969) but there is a membranous organelle which is possibly a transformed acrosome (Reger and Florendo, 1969a, b) and needs to be studied further.

EVOLUTION OF THE ACROSOME IN TERRESTRIAL INVERTEBRATES

Terrestrial invertebrates show a great variety of acrosomal devices, apparently arising from the basic aquatic model which is conserved in some of them. In general, the perforatorium is reduced, often unable to extend and frequently has disappeared altogether. The acrosome, too, is involuted in many instances, and in several higher groups is completely absent.

Conservative Features in Oligochaeta, Gastropoda, Tardigrada

All these groups belonging to phyla that are definitely adapted to land and exhibiting internal fertilization, have acrosomes that retain the most typical characteristics of the aquatic models. Moreover, the extra-acrosomal layer is present in oligochaets (Reger, 1967; Anderson and Ellis, 1968; Shay, 1972) as it is in gastropods (Starke, 1971; Walker, 1970; Buckland-Nicks, 1973). The acrosome has an elongated shape, associated with the acuminate profile of the sperm head, and is sustained by an inner perforatorium that is partially located in a nuclear canal and clearly belongs to the "filamentous model" of the aquatic ancestors (see mainly Lanzavecchia and Lora Lamia Donin, 1972, for Oligochaeta, and Giusti, 1969; Giusti and Mazzini, 1973, Walker and MacGregor, 1968 for Gastropoda; Baccetti *et al.*, 1971b, for Tardigrada). No information is available on the enzyme content of the acrosome, nor on the presence of actin and other proteins in the perforatorium which elongates during the acrosomal reaction (Henley, 1970). In some gastropods microtubules have been described in the mature acrosome (Walker and MacGregor, 1968; Giusti and Mazzini, 1973).

Acrosomal Evolution in Terrestrial Arthropoda

As is well known, the evolution of Arthropoda toward terrestrial life is more advanced than in Mollusca and Annelida, and the reproductive biology more specialized in having unusual forms of internal fertilization. The acrosomal complex undergoes changes of function and shape; usually it becomes reduced and frequently disappears (Fig. 10). Unfortunately its structural components and the proteins involved in the acrosome reaction have been investigated in only a very few phyla, and then not completely. In general it can be stated that the more conservative aquatic-like organization is present only in the lowest Arachnida, in the few Crustacea adapted to terrestrial life and in some insect orders, whereas in the highest Arachnida, in Myriapoda, in most Insecta as well as in Onychophorans the evolutionary trend is toward the early loss of the perforatorium, and later of the whole acrosomal complex. The course of this involution is traced later.

Arachnida (Fig. 10) begin with forms that maintain

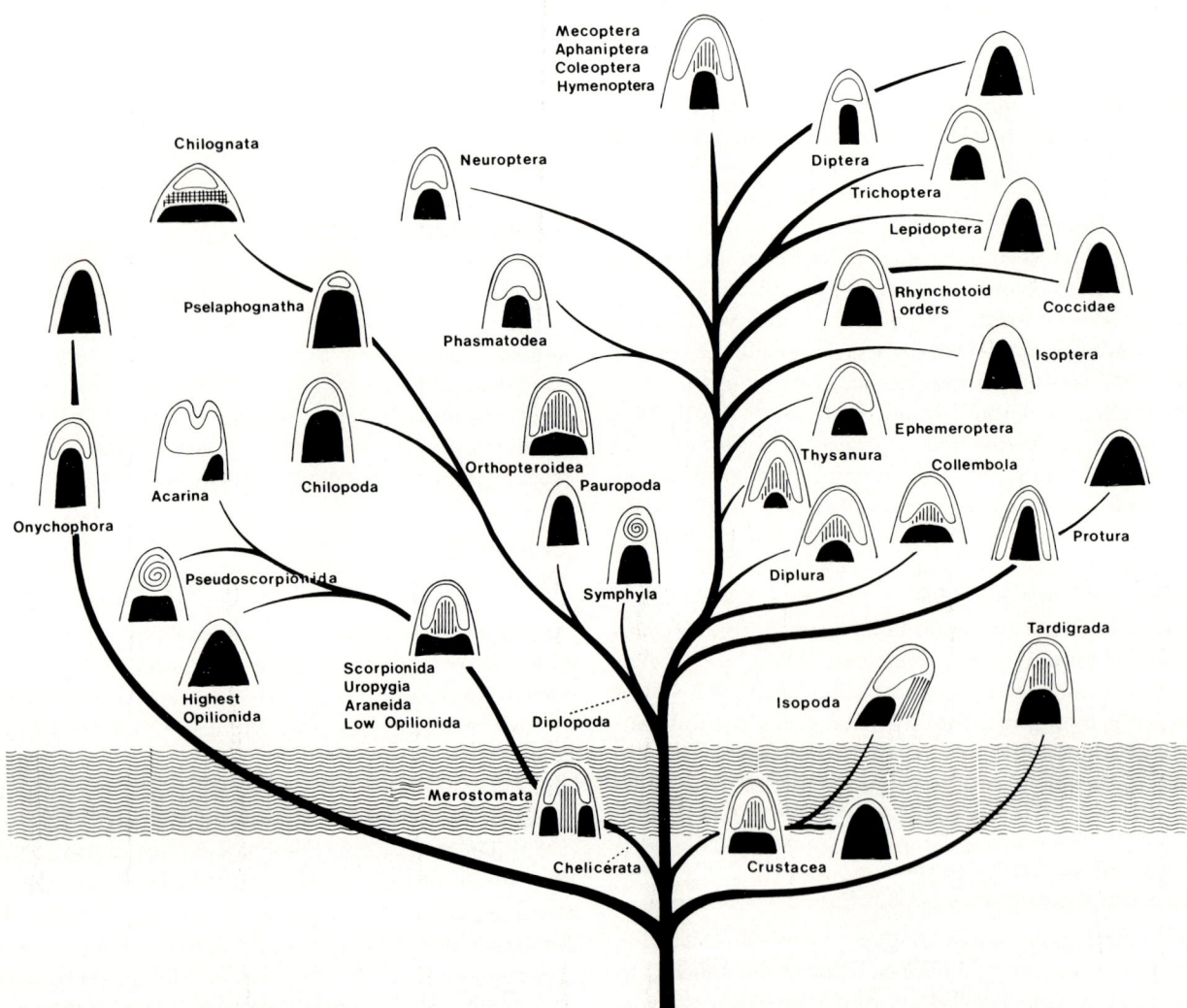

Figure 10. The evolutionary tree of the acrosomal complex structure in terrestrial Arthropoda and related phyla. The organelles are represented by the same symbols as in Figure 6; only the "filamentous actin" model of the perforatorium is present; the grid picture in the subacrosomal region indicates the presence of a pseudoperforatorium.

the classical aquatic acrosome even though reduced in comparison with that of their ancestor *Limulus*. Scorpions (Jespersen and Hartwick, 1973), Uropygi (Phillips, 1976), spiders (Reger, 1970), and the most primitive Opilionid (Juberthie *et al.*, 1976) show a cup-like acrosome, superimposed on a short fibrous perforatorium which seems not to elongate at the time of the acrosome reaction. At higher levels, the involution is dramatic. Highest opilionids (Reger, 1969), pseudoscorpions (Legg, 1973), and mites (Reger, 1963) lack a perforatorium and have a very reduced or absent acrosome.

Insects (Fig. 10) generally show an elongate, conical, sometimes arrow-like acrosome, capping a long, fibrous, rod-like perforatorium. This condition has been found in many different orders, from Collembola, Diplura Thysanura, Orthopteroidea, Mecoptera, to Aphaniptera, Coleoptera, Hymenoptera. Some of them have a perforatorium partially located in the nucleus (see Baccetti, 1972). Although the situation seems to be similar to the classical aquatic one, little information is available. An amorphous extra-acrosomal layer has been detected in Phasmatodea, Rhynchota, and Coleoptera (Baccetti *et al.*, 1973a, b; Tandler and Moriber, 1966). The acrosome clearly shows a crystalline organization with a 95-Å vertical and 25-Å horizontal period in Diptera and Coleoptera (Warner, 1971; Baccetti *et al.*, 1973a). In Notonecta, Afzelius *et al.* (1976) are able to distinguish three strata having different texture, only one of which is reminiscent of transformed microtubules. The presence of at least two proteins is suspected but the actual substances contained in the insect acrosome are completely unknown. A general PAS-positive reaction has been detected by Tandler and Moriber (1966) and Baccetti *et al.* (1971a). With regard to the perforatorium, it seems to retain the major characteristics of the primitive model: the bundle of filaments could contain actin, but so far as it is known, it does not elongate at the time of acrosomal reaction, and probably plays only a skeletal role. In fact, most of the insect orders lack a perforatorium, even though they conserve an active acrosome. Such is the case in some Proturans, Ephemeroptera, Plecoptera, Phasmatodea, Embioptera, all Rhynchotoid orders (from Psochoptera to Rhynchota), Lepidoptera, and all Diptera (see Baccetti, 1979). In several Rhynchotans the acrosome, devoid of perforatorium, is supported by a bundle of microtubules (Payne, 1966; Tandler and Moriber, 1966; Folliot and Maillet, 1970).

As in arachnids, the general acrosomal involution in insects (Fig. 10) culminates in the complete absence of acrosomal complex (Baccetti, 1979). This absence characterizes one high Proturan, all Isopterans (Fig. 11), the highest Homopterans, Coccids, most Neuroptera, Tri-

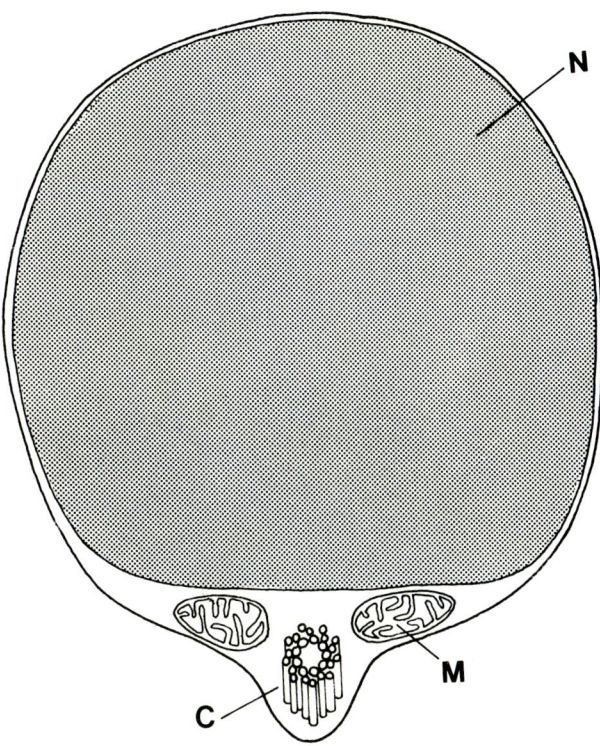

Figure 11. Spermatozoon of the Isopteran *Reticulitermes*, lacking an acrosome and where only centriole (C), mitochondria (M), and nucleus (N) are present.

choptera, and Cecydomyid Diptera. No devices substitute for perforatoria or for the whole acrosomal complex after these have been lost. This involution is concurrent with the evolution of a thick chorion around the egg, which has micropyles that permit sperm penetration.

The situation seems to be quite different in Myriapoda (Fig. 10), treated at the end of this section. First of all, the aquatic acrosome model is completely lacking and from the reproductive point of view myriapods seem to be a more specialized group. Two separate classes have evolved toward the lack of the perforatorium, and have therefore only an acrosome which is compact and conical in Chilopoda,[3] membranous and ovoid in Symphyla (Fig. 11 and 12) where it surrounds the unique mitochondrion (Rosati *et al.*, 1970). In Pauropoda the acrosomal complex is completely lacking. In Diplopoda, which are the richest class among myriapods, the acrosomal evolution is quite peculiar. In the most primitive group, Pselaphognatha (Baccetti *et al.*, 1974), the ribbon-like sperm retains an acrosome that flanks the long nucleus, lacks a perforatorium, and

---

[3]Camatini, M.; Franchi, E.: Morphology of the Spermatozoon in *Scolopendromorpha* (Chilopoda), in preparation

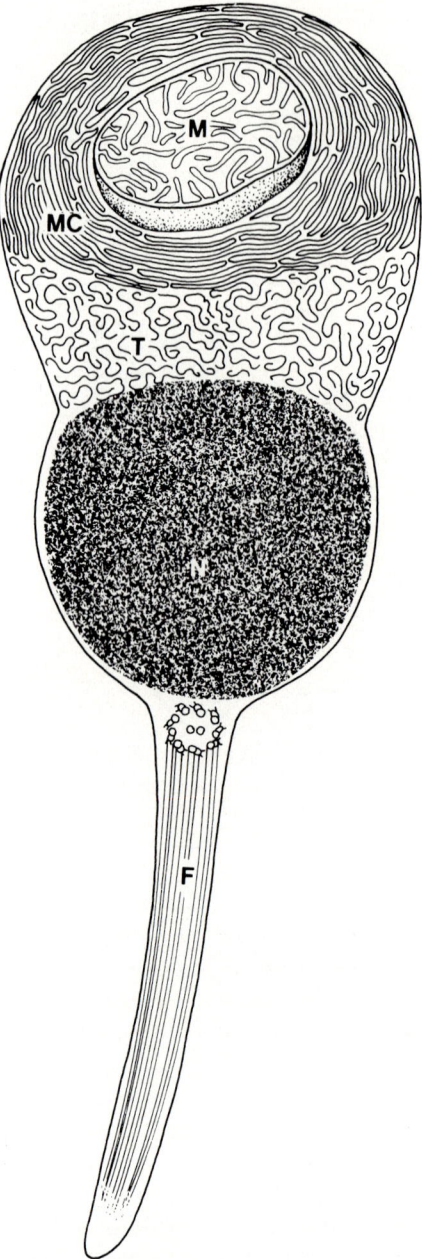

Figure 12. The spermatozoon of the low Myriapod *Symphylella*, where the acrosome is represented by complex of membranes (MC) and tubules (T) surrounding the unique mitochondrion (M). N, nucleus; F, flagellum.

has an uncertain function. In the completely separate group Colobognatha, the quite simple sperm has completely lost the acrosome (Baccetti et al., 1979), but in the others, e.g., Chilognatha, a progressive evolution occurs. In the lowest group Glomeroidea, the acrosomal complex is made up only of the acrosome and is very poorly developed (Boissin et al., 1972). In Polydesmoidea (Manier and Boissin, 1975), the complex is made up of an aspheroidal acrosomal vesicle, lying on a thin layer of dense material. In Juliformia this material shows a crystalline structure as it does in Spirostreptoidea and Spiroboloidea (Horstmann and Breucker, 1969; Manier et al., 1974; Manier and Boissin, 1976). Juloidea complicates the situation and the subacrosomal crystal becomes extremely large, occupying most of the sperm body (Fig. 13). Unlike the other terrestrial invertebrates, an enormous acrosome reaction occurs in these millipeds, culminating in the production of a long filament that suddenly protrudes from one of the aflagellate sperm bodies, and which was thought for a long time to be a flagellum. This filament is made up of both acrosomal and subacrosomal material (Baccetti et al., 1977a), and shows a very obvious filamentous substructure. But the proteins involved are unusual, and quite different from those of the classical aquatic perforatoria. Analyses carried out by gel electrophoresis, heavy meromyosin decoration, and fluorescent antibody staining have consistently given negative results for actin and tubulin, positive results for myosin, and for some other polypeptides between 40,000 and 90,000 M_r, the most abundant of which was 60,000 M_r. The milliped acrosomal reaction therefore cannot be related to the classic reaction of aquatic invertebrates, including the primitive arthropodan Limulus. Nor can the subacrosomal crystal be considered a perforatorium. This structure in fact has already been lost by the primitive myriapodans. In the author's opinion it is an alternative device that has evolved near the top of the myriapodan line, using distinctive proteins not usually found in the perforatorium. It might appropriately be called a pseudoperforatorium, being an organelle secondarily evolved to replace the lost perforatorium.

Another terrestrial group closely related to Arthropoda follows the same course of involution. In Onychophorans, in fact, the spermatozoon which is well adapted for internal fertilization like that of the Insecta (Baccetti et al., 1976; Baccetti and Dallai, 1977) conserves a simple, helicoidal acrosome in some species, but lacks an acrosome completely in others. Onychophora being vivaparous, oviparous or ovoviviparous animals, the eggs are correspondingly different, and acrosomal involution seems to parallel the simplification of egg envelopes in viviparous species (Baccetti and Dallai, 1977).

In the acrosome-lacking Onychophorans (Baccetti et al., 1976) as well as in the acrosome-lacking insects Termites (Baccetti et al., 1974), total involution seems quite recent; the spermatid stage, in fact, shows the presence of a transient acrosome of Golgi origin which is destroyed during late spermiogenesis.

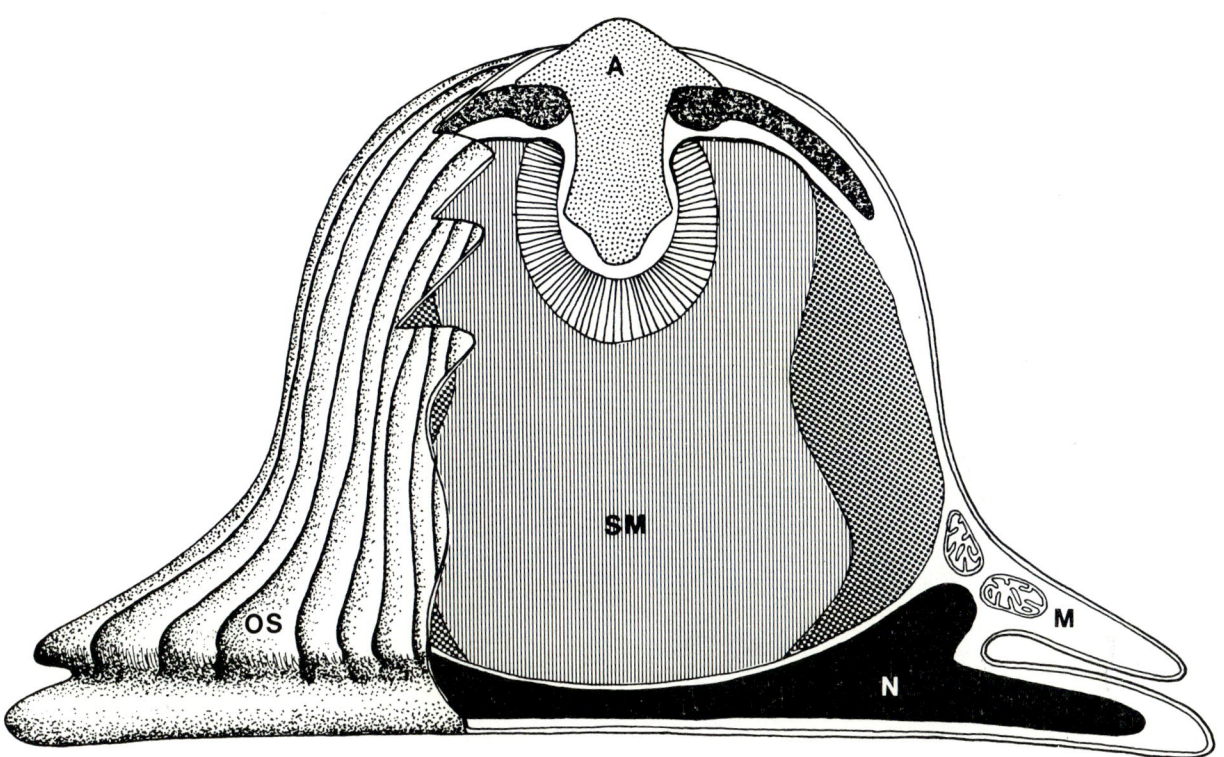

Figure 13. The spermatozoon of the high Diplopod *Pachyjulus*. The acrosomal complex includes an apical acrosome (A), surrounded by an amorphous layer of crystalline subacrosomal material (SM). M, mitochondria; N, nucleus; OS, outer surface.

THE ACROSOMAL EVOLUTION IN TERRESTRIAL VERTEBRATES

Vertebrates are the only terrestrial group in which a true evolution of the acrosomal complex from the primitive aquatic model is occurring. The acrosome in fact becomes more and more rich in enzymatic proteins while the perforatorium conserved in the first classes disappears in mammals, and in some of them substitutive devices develop. Moreover the whole acrosomal complex is present in every group, no instances of acrosome lack have been observed so far.

Conservative Organization in Reptiles and Birds

The general shape of the acrosomal complex in reptiles and birds closely recalls that of amphibians, Dipnoi, Selachians, Cyclostomata, and so on (Fig. 14). In reptiles (Hamilton and Fawcett, 1968; Furieri, 1970; 1974; Da Cruz-Landim and Da Cruz-Höfling, 1977) and in birds (Humphreys, 1972; Tingari, 1973; Okamura and Nishiyama, 1976) the acrosome is a compact cone (helically shaped in passerine birds; Mattei *et al.*, 1972) containing a fibrous perforatorium made up of a parallel bundle of filaments (Fig. 15) which remain unchanged during the acrosome reaction (Okamura and Nishiyama, 1978). To evaluate the situation, the laboratory of the author and colleagues, in collaboration with the Institute of General Pathology of the University of Geneva, carried out some determinations with gel electrophoresis and with immunofluorescent antibodies. The results show that the perforatorium is made up of actin; myosin seems to be absent. It seems likely, therefore, that the perforatorium remained unchanged from aquatic ancestors to Sauropsida. Little is known about the acrosomal proteins. Ho and Meizel (1970), and Allen *et al.* (1974), using various approaches, detect a trypsin-like activity in the chicken acrosome. The former authors are able to distinguish electrophoretically four bands inhibited by trypsin-inhibitors which have a mobility similar to that of bull acrosomal proteases. Yanagimachi and Teichman (1972) demonstrated hyaluronidase in bird acrosome. Both enzymes have been studied carefully in mammals (see below). While the proteinase, acrosin, is similar to the invertebrate lysin (Levine et al., 1978), hyaluronidase seems to have appeared in acrosomes at the vertebrate level. Baccetti *et al.* (1971a) have demonstrated that it is absent from insect acrosomes.

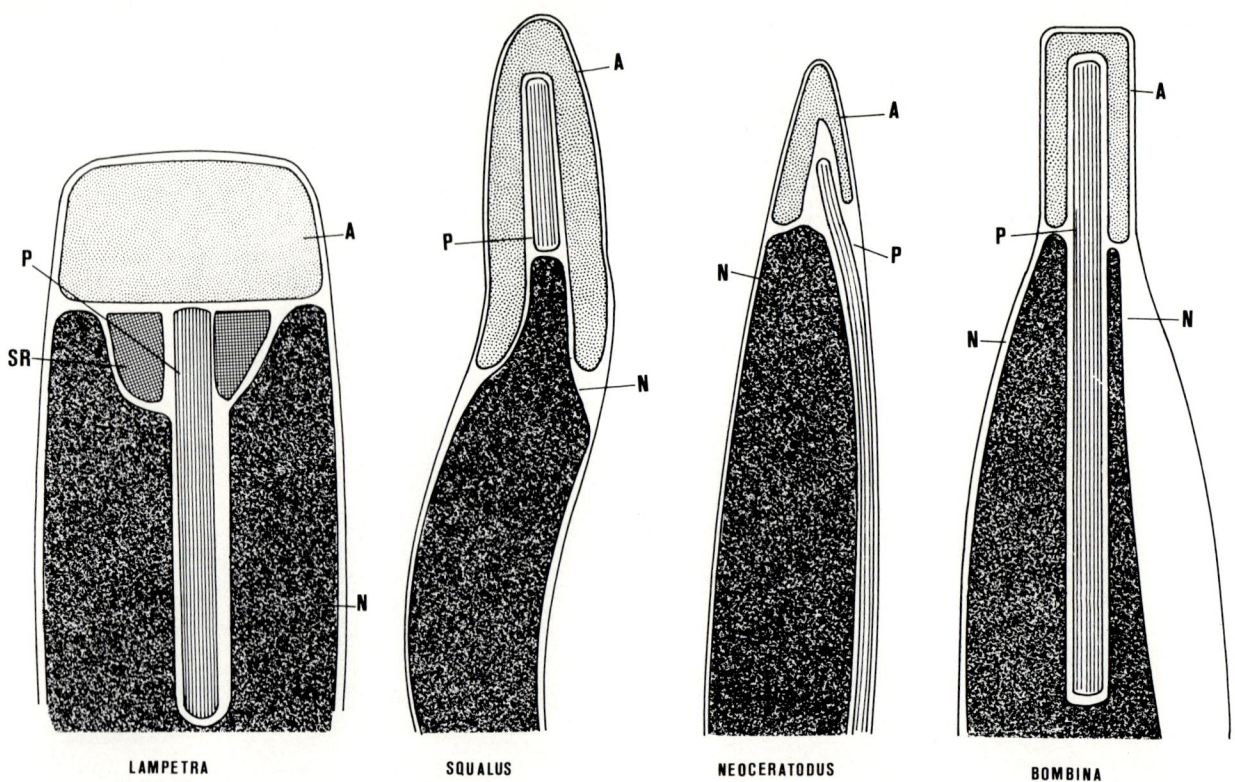

Figure 14. The aquatic vertebrate spermatozoon, according to Nicander and Sjöden (1971); Stanley (1971); Jespersen (1971); Furieri (1975). Between acrosome (A) and nucleus (N) a filamentous perforatorium (P) is located. In *Lampetra* the subacrosomal ring (SR) is also evident.

Mammalian Evolution

Mammals show a greater variety of shapes in the acrosomal complex than do other animal groups (Fawcett, 1970). The basic structure however is very stable in all orders, except in Rodentia where it acquires a very peculiar configuration. From Echnidnas (Griffiths, 1968) to Marsupials (Hughes, 1965; Phillips, 1970), to Chiroptera (Fawcett and Ito, 1965), Primates (Fawcett, 1970); Edentata (Nagy and Edmons, 1973), Lagomorpha (Nicander and Bane, 1966), Carnivora (Nicander and Bane, 1966), Proboscidea (Jones *et al.*, 1974), Perissodactyla (Nicander and Bane, 1966), and Artiodactyla (Nicander and Bane, 1966), the acrosome is a thick layer capping the nucleus, and separated from the nuclear envelope by a narrow space wherein a small amount of filamentous material can be discerned especially near the apex. In Rodentia the material occupying the subacrosomal space becomes more and more abundant from the guinea pig and the chinchilla until it reaches an enormous size in the myomorph rodents (Fawcett and Phillips, 1970; Fawcett, 1970).

The Acrosome The shape of the acrosome in mammals is usually that of a cap-like structure, capping the anterior region of the nucleus. Its thickness is quite uniform over the whole acrosome, except in Rodentia where the apical portion of the acrosome profile is more prominent and variously shaped (see Fawcett, 1970). The acrosomal membranes in rodents have been carefully studied. Phillips (1975) finds in their surface an ultrastructural appearance of hexagonally packed 90-Å particles, but Koehler (1972) in man finds particles of 200-Å diameter. According to Pedersen (1972) the acrosomal membrane in the posterior area (equatorial segment) is pentalaminar. Phillips (1977) in *Rhesus* and other mammals is able to resolve in this region a system of regular rows of hexagonally packed particles, with a center-to-center spacing of 170 Å, while in the postacrosomal region the material is arranged in parallel ridges with a center-to-center spacing of 150 Å. As far as enzymes are concerned, only an ATPase, active at pH 9 in the presence of Ca^{2+}, has been found in the acrosomal membranes of rodents and man (Gordon and Barnett, 1967; Gordon, 1973). In fact the outer membrane, in the human acrosome, selectively binds Ca (Roomans, 1975). The situation seems to be similar to that of aquatic sperm, where Ca has been demonstrated to trigger the acrosomal reaction. In fact, Yanagimachi and Usui (1974) demonstrate a Ca^{2+} dependence in the guinea pig acrosome reaction that can be induced, as in sea urchin by Ca^{2+} ionophore (Talbot and Franklin, 1976; Talbot et al., 1976; Summers et al., 1976). Gonzales and Meizel (1973) found in the rabbit acrosomal membrane two phosphatases, one of them stimulated by Zn^{2+}. On the other hand, the more specific enzymatic activities appropriate to the acrosome (trypsin-like enzyme and hyaluronidase) are bound to the membranes only in small amounts (Zahler and Dak, 1975). The outer acrosomal membrane undergoes several changes during capacitation and the acrosome reaction. Those changes are limited to the vertebrate acrosomal reaction, in contrast to what happens in the aquatic invertebrates, where the perforatorium plays an important role. According to Talbot and Franklin (1976) the

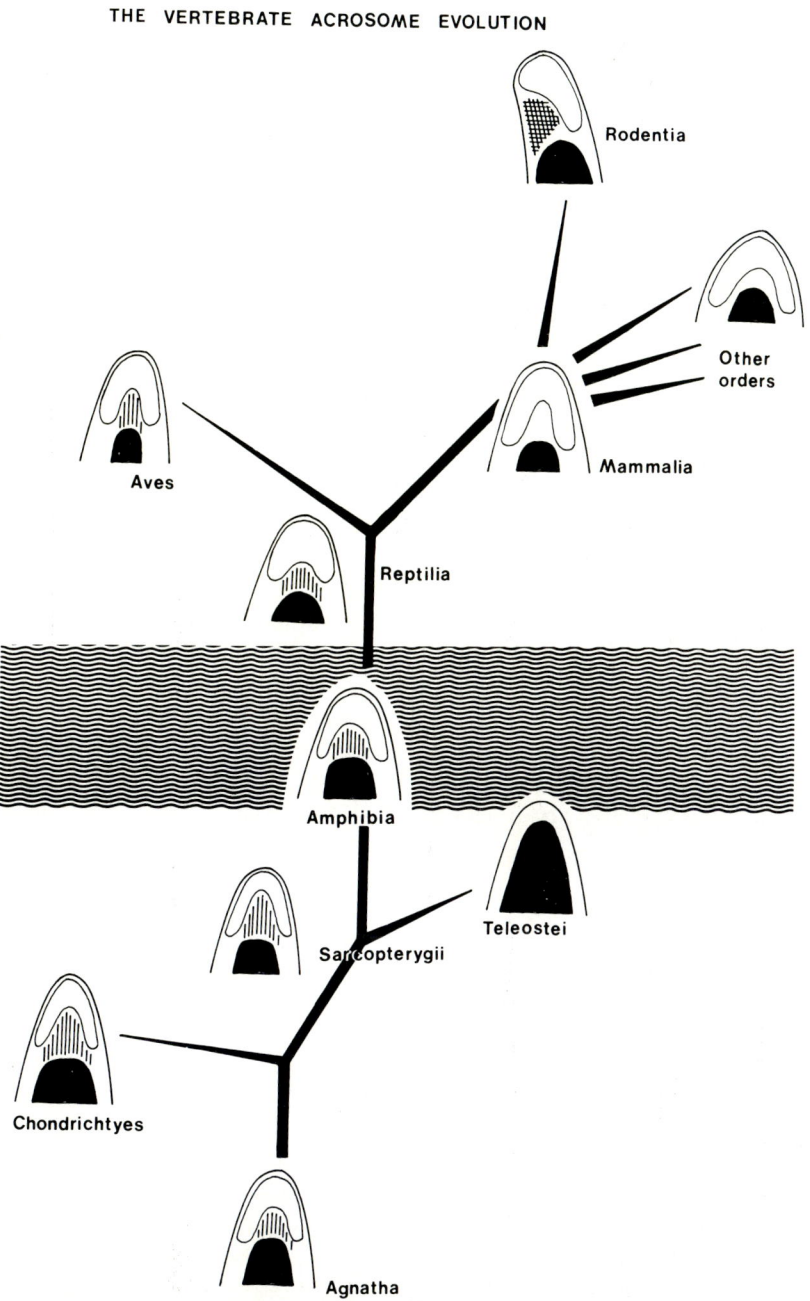

Figure 15. The evolutionary tree of the acrosome structure in vertebrates. Symbols are the same as in Figures 6 and 10.

acrosome becomes swollen, crenulated, and fragmented during acrosome reaction and many other authors describe fusion between the outer acrosomal membrane and the plasma lamina and formation of multiple openings (Bedford, 1970; Roomans and Afzelius, 1975). Freeze-fracture, in fact, reveals disintegration of the geometric pattern of the intramembrane particles (Friend and Rudolf, 1974).

The material enclosed in the acrosomal membranes in mammals has been the object of intensive study. With regard to its structure, few data are available from cryofixation or freeze-fracture. Phillips (1972) demonstrated a 42-Å periodicity in the cortical outer region of the rat acrosome; Plattner (1971) and Fléchon (1974) describe a "cobblestone-like" fracture pattern. But it is difficult to relate this organization to the chemical content. The mammalian acrosome like that of Arthropoda exhibits a PAS-positive and amylase insensitive reaction for polysaccharide (Clermont and Leblond, 1955; Onuma and Nishikawa, 1963; Dan, 1970), probably attributable in part to a glycoprotein enzyme. This polysaccharide was named "acrosomin" by Clermont and Leblond (1955) but the term was abandoned. Several enzymatic activities are present that seem to be quite similar in all species. It has been noted in fact that the most important of them are already present at Sauropsid level.

The first enzyme to be released in the acrosome reaction is hyaluronidase, which emerges from the acrosome of capacitated sperm through the holes formed by membrane fusion during the early stages of the acrosomal reaction (Rogers and Morton, 1973; Rogers and Yanagimachi, 1975); and is responsible for the penetration of spermatozoa through the cumulus oophorus. There are some doubts concerning the molecular weight of this enzyme. According to McRorie and Williams (1974), it is likely that it consists of four subunits, each of them with 14,000 M_r (Khorlin et al., 1973); this datum is consistent with the weight of 62,000 found by Yang and Srivastava (1974) for bovine sperm. The optimum pH is 3.8 for bull, 4.3 for ram (Yang, 1972) and is different from lysosomal hyaluronidase present in organs other than the testis (Zaneveld et al., 1973). As far as the localization of hyaluronidase is concerned, Gould and Bernstein (1973) in the bull, and Morton (1975) in the ram, localize the enzyme immunocytochemically in the central acrosomal zone, far from the inner acrosomal membrane. Fléchon (1975) in the same and other farm species finds it closer to the outer acrosomal membrane in the anterior acrosome region. Therefore, it can be released early when the acrosome reacts.

A second enzyme released is the so-called "corona radiata-penetrating enzyme" (C.P.E.), a hydrolase discovered and studied by the Williams group (Zaneveld and Williams, 1970; Tillman, 1972). The enzyme dissolves the intercellular material of the corona radiata, and is active at pH 7.7 (McRorie and Williams, 1974). More information is needed on this enzyme.

The third and most important enzyme released by the mammalian acrosome is the "zona pellucida proteolytic enzyme." This enzyme was compared with trypsin by Yamane (1930) and its similarity definitely demonstrated by Zaneveld et al. (1970) who stressed also certain differences suggesting that it is a distinct enzyme. The name "acrosin" was therefore proposed. The enzyme was purified by Zaneveld et al. (1972a), Polakoski et al. (1972, 1973a, b) and Fink et al. (1972). In rabbits it is a dimer of two units 27,300 M_r, active at an optimum pH 8.0. In boars it seems to occur as a monomer 30,000, without a dimeric form, with optimum pH 8.5. Human acrosin seems to be quite similar to that of the boar (Zaneveld et al., 1972b). For bull the situation seems to be similar to that of rabbit, but needs to be clarified (McRorie and Williams, 1974). Garner and Easton (1977) find no differences between acrosin of various mammals from an immunological point of view. Some differences in response to inhibitors are known, and have been summarized by McRorie and Williams (1974). This enzyme seems to be localized closer to the inner acrosomal membrane than hyaluronidase, and is apparently not bound to the outer membrane because after membrane isolation, more than 70% of the activity remains associated with the sperm pellet with which the inner membrane is still associated. Acrosin is also extracted differently from the inner and the outer membrane (Multamaki and Suominen, 1976). Stambaugh et al. (1975) find in the rabbit a complex distribution consisting of six linear loops of evenly spaced granules, running diagonally across the flat side of the sperm head in a criss-cross pattern with the two most anterior loops. In general acrosin is detected only in the rostral portion of the acrosome (Garner et al., 1977; Fléchon et al., 1977). Distribution and chemical properties to the degree that they are known suggest that mammalian acrosin is very similar to aquatic invertebrate lysin (Levine et al., 1978). If this is confirmed, it would suggest that this family of enzymes has been conserved throughout the whole of animal evolution.

According to Polakoski et al. (1977), at the time of ejaculation 95% of the total acrosin present is in the form of an inactive precursor, proacrosin, described by Meizel (1972), and it is later activated during the capacitation process when the "acrostatin" previously bound to the enzyme is removed (Bhattacharyya and

Zaneveld, 1978). This sequence of events has been demonstrated in the boar system. The newly formed acrosin seems to play a role in stimulating the acrosomal reaction (Meizel and Lui, 1976; Battacharyya and Zanevehd, 1976), which is in fact suppressed by inhibitors of trypsin-like enzymes. Acrosin leaves the acrosome somewhat later than hyaluronidase (Thibault, 1964).

A second acrosomal peptidase, which seems to be peculiar to mammalian sperm, is a collagenase with optimum pH 7.5, and M_r about 110,000 (Koren and Milkovic, 1973). Its natural substrate in the reproductive process is still unknown. Other peptidases, and some phosphatases, generally defined as "lysosomal enzymes" have also been obtained in mammalian acrosome studies: viz. acid phosphatase, β-glucuronidase, arylaminidase, arylsulfatase, β-N-acetylglucosaminidase, phospholipase A, nonspecific esterases, β-aspartyl-N-acetylglucosamine-amino-hydrolase, acid proteinases (Couchie and Mann, 1957; Dott and Dingle, 1968; Allison and Hartree, 1970; Meizel and Colham, 1972; Bernstein and Teichman, 1973; Bryan and Unnithan, 1973; Bhalla et al., 1973). Finally the enzyme most exclusively bound to the inner membrane is neuraminidase (Srivastava et al., 1970). McRorie and Williams (1974) suspect that this enzyme is active at the level of the zona pellucida since neuraminic acid is a component of this layer.

It is of interest to know how the enzymatic activities are stored in the acrosomal space. In a recent paper, Stambaugh and Smith (1978) and Stambaugh (1978) using immunofluorescence and electron microscopy, detect tubulin in the rabbit and Rhesus acrosome and find that microtubules polymerize after in vitro incubation in a silver-proteinate solution. Acrosin and tubulin have the same distribution in the acrosome and these authors suggest that tubulin is the binding structure for the proteinase.

Except for tubulin, no other structural components have been detected so far in the mammalian acrosome, which is basically a storage site for enzymes. An important open question is whether the mammalian acrosome contains bindin, a protein until now isolated only from aquatic sperm.

The Subacrosomal Space and the Perforatorium Problem As already pointed out, the space between the nuclear envelope and inner acrosomal membrane is very narrow and contains very little material in sperm of any order, except Rodentia. Also in the most primitive form, Echidna (Griffiths, 1968), this space is quite small and no traces of the sauropsid fibrillar actin perforatorium can be found. In most mammals only a small apical region sometimes shows an electron-dense appearance, and is called a perforatorium by Jones (1970). This density is absent from human sperm and very poorly developed generally in primates (Fawcett, 1970; 1975b). According to Nicander and Bane (1966) and Courtens et al. (1976), the subacrosomal space contains a proteinaceous substance lacking sugar residues. It is claimed that lysine concentrates in this substance during spermiogenesis, as a result of protein turnover in the nucleus (Courtens et al., 1976) and at the same time —S—S— cross (Calvin and Bedford, 1970; Bedford and Calvin, 1974). In a study in cooperation with the Institute of General Pathology of the University of Geneva (Prof. G. Gabbiani), it has been found by immunofluorescent staining that the whole perinuclear space in human sperm contains actin and myosin, mainly concentrated in an apical region. It is difficult to detect the exact localization of these proteins, but assuming that they are absent from the acrosome, and that there is so little space between the outer acrosomal membrane and plasma membrane, the only possible localization would seem to be between the acrosome and nucleus. In the immature spermatozoon, one can see that this space contains the same material that underlies the plasma membrane. As a general view, it can be assumed that in the typical mammalian sperm the acrosome lies in a matrix containing actin and myosin and also proteins that can be stabilized by S—S bonds. It can be assumed that all these proteins play a role in release of enzymes at the time of the acrosomal reaction. Rodents' sperm show a situation that has clearly evolved from the more generalized case just described. The subacrosomal material acquires a pyramidal shape that is progressively larger in the various species, reaching maximal dimensions in the rat (Clermont et al., 1955; Hadek, 1963; Bane and Nicander, 1963; Hancock, 1966; Fawcett, 1970, 1975b). Calvin and Bedford (1970) observe an increasing content in S—S groups in this region during epididymal migration. Olson et al. (1976) are able to demonstrate that it is composed of a single polypeptide, 13,000 Mr with a content of 6.5% cystein. The author and colleagues carried out both immunofluorescent stainings, HMM decorations, and electrophoretic analyses on testicular and epididymal material, and found that myosin is consistently lacking. Actin is very abundant around the nucleus in testicular material, but absent in epididymal spermatozoa. The 13,000-Mr protein appears only in the sperm from the epididymis. It was concluded that this subacrosomal region changes role during sperm maturation. Actin probably plays only a morphogenetic role during the molding of the head region, and the newly appeared 13,000-Mr protein endows the region with a skeletal role. Whether actin is conserved in an undetectable form or is eliminated is unknown. Talbot and Kleve (1977) in fact detect actin by immunological means along the concave margin of the acrosome in the hamster. In conclusion, the subacrosomal material of mammals starts (Fig. 15) from a very involuted situation where a true perforatorium is lacking, and is represented only by a thin layer of actin and myosin, in the superficial region of the sperm head cytoplasm. In rodents a perforatorium-like organelle is newly acquired, consisting only of a cystein-rich cytoskeletal protein characteristic of these sperm. (It has in fact been observed that it is lacking in human spermatozoa.) This organelle is not a true perforatorium, as already pointed out by Fawcett and Phillips (1970) and Fawcett (1970), because not only does it play a different role, but it appears *de novo* in evolution when the true perforatorium is lost. It is a case similar to that in millipeds, and the author proposes to call it a "pseudoperforatorium."

CONCLUSION

After this overview of acrosomal evolution, the author proposes certain conclusions even though some obscure points obviously need further investigation. The main points are:

1. The acrosome is an animal organelle, first appearing at the beginning of metazoan status. Among the actual phyla, only Cnidarians conserve the evolutionary steps of incipient acrosomal organization.
2. The primitive acrosomal model is the one present in almost all the aquatic groups of every phylum. This model includes two structures: an acrosome containing lysin and bindin, and a perforatorium, almost always present and necessary for the acrosomal reaction. This perforatorium is able to elongate, and is made up mainly of actin in one of two forms: the "profilactin model" which is more primitive, and the "filamentous actin model" typical of the higher aquatic animal groups.
3. Some invertebrate aquatic or endoparasitic groups (Nematods, Platyhelminths a.o.) completely lack an acrosomal complex. Steps of involution are not conserved, and one cannot distinguish between an involution and the conservation of a primitive characteristic. In some cases, as in teleosts, the lack of an acrosome is certainly an involutional adaptation, possibly associated with an environmental change from sea water to fresh water.
4. The evolution to terrestrial life in all the invertebrate phyla is usually followed by acrosomal involution, mainly in groups having eggs with a thick chorion and correspondingly large micropyles. The acrosome reaction frequently occurs without a significant elongation of the perforatorium, which is merely a thin bundle of actin filaments inherited from the "filamentous actin model" of aquatic ancestors, and probably playing only a marginal role in the process. In many groups it disappers completely. The acrosome seems to be quite simple, sometimes functioning in the absence of a perforatorium, and frequently it too disappears. No information is available concerning acrosomal enzymes or the presence of bindin.
5. The evolution to terrestrial life in vertebrates parallels that of invertebrate major phyla only insofar as the perforatorium is concerned. The acrosome, in fact, is always present and acquires a rich repertoire of new enzymatic activities. Among these only acrosin seems to be related to the lysin of aquatic ancestors; the presence of bindin is yet to be investigated. The perforatorium retains characteristics of a filamentous actin model but without any important participation in the acrosomal reaction in Sauropsida (elongation has not been described) and later disappears in all mammalia where only a thin layer of diffuse actomyosin is present around the nucleus.
6. At the top of the evolutionary tree in groups where acrosome and perforatorium have been lost, newly formed alternative devices have sometimes been described. In the two related aquatic arthropodan groups, Branchiura and Pentastomida, a pseudoacrosome appears to have evolved in place of the lost acrosome, but no information is available on its composition and function. With respect to the perforatorium, two cases of reacquisition of perforatoria (pseudoperforatoria) are known in groups where the original perforatorium seems to have been lost. The first in millipeds, where the reacting filament is made up of myosin and other unusual protein chains, not including actin. The second, in rodents, where there also appears a structure made up of a new protein (the 13,000-M_r protein) that was absent in ancestral forms.

REFERENCES

Afzelius, B.A.: The Fine Structure of the Sea Urchin Spermatozoa as Revealed by the Electron Microscope. Z Mikrosk Anat Forsch 42(1955)134-148

Afzelius, B.A.: Fine Structure of the Spermatozoon of Tubularia Larynx (Hydrozoa, Coelenterata). J Ultrastruct Res 37(1971a)679-689

Afzelius, B.A.: The Spermatozoon of the Nemertine *Malacobdella grossa*. J Submicrosc Cytol 3(1971b)181-192

Afzelius, B.A.: Sperm Morphology and Fertilization Biology.

In: The Genetics of the Spermatozoon, pp. 131-143, ed. by R.A. Beatty and Gluecksohn-Waelsch. Edinburgh and New York, 1972

Afzelius, B.A.; Baccetti, B.; Dallai, R.: The Giant Spermatozoon of Notonecta. J Submicrosc Cytol 8(1976)149-161

Afzelius, B.A.; Ferraguti, M.: The Spermatozoon of *Priapulus caudatus* Lamarck. J Submicrosc Cytol 10(1978)71-79

Afzelius, B.A.; Ferraguti, M.: Fine Structure of Brachiopod Spermatozoa. J Ultrastruct Res 63(1978)308-315

Afzelius, B.A.; Franzen, Å.: The Spermatozoon of the Jellyfish *Nausithoë*. J Ultrastruct Res 37(1971)186-199

Aikawa, M.; Huff, C.G.; Strome, C.P.A.: Morphological Study of Microgametogenesis of *Leucocytozoon simondi*. J Ultrastruct Res 32(1970)43-68

Allen, G.J.; Bishop, M.W.H.; Thompson, T.E.: Lysis of Photographic Emulsions by Mammalian and Chicken Spermatozoa. J Reprod Fertil 36(1974)249-252

Allison, A.C.; Hartree, E.F.: Lysosomal Enzymes in the Acrosome and Their Possible Role in Fertilization. J Reprod Fertil 21(1970)501

Anderson, W.A.; Ellis R.A.: Acrosome Morphogenesis in *Lumbricus terrestris*. Z Mikrosk Anat Forsch 85(1968)398-407

Andre, J.: A Propos d'une Leçon sur la Limule. Ann Fac Sci 26(1963)27-38

Baccetti, B.: Insect Sperm Cells. Advances Insect Physiol 9(1972)315-397

Baccetti, B.: Lo Spermatozoo dei Sipunculidi. Accad Naz dei Lincei Rendiconti della Classe di Scienze Fisiche Matematiche e Naturali 62(1977)89-93

Baccetti, B.: L'Evoluzione dello Spermatozoo. In: IV Seminario sulla "Evoluzione Biologica" pp. 95-126. Accademia Nazionale dei Lincei, Roma, 1978

Baccetti, B.: Ultrastructure of Sperm and Its Bearing on Arthropod Phylogeny. In: Arthropod Phylogeny, pp. 609-644, ed. by A.P. Gupta. Van Nostrand Reinhold Co., N. York, 1979.

Baccetti, B.; Afzelius, B.A.: The Biology of the Sperm Cell. Monographs in Developmental Biology, Vol. 10. S. Karger AG, Basel, 1976

Baccetti, B.; Burrini, A.G.; Dallai, R.: The Spermatozoon of *Branchiostoma lanceolatum* L. J Morphol 136(1972)211-226

Baccetti, B.; Burrini, A.G.; Dallai, R.; Giusti, F.; Mazzini, M.; Renieri, T.; Rosati, F.; Selmi, G.: Structure and Function in the Spermatozoon of *Tenebrio molitor*. XX. The Spermatozoon of Arthropoda. J Mechenochem Cell Motil 2(1973a)149-161

Baccetti, B.; Burrini, A.G.; Dallai, R.; Pallini, V.; Periti, P.; Piantelli, F.; Rosati, F.; Selmi, G.: Structure and Function in the Spermatozoon of *Bacillus rossius*. The Spermatozoon of Arthropoda. XIX. J Ultrastruct Res 44 12(1973b)1-73S

Baccetti, B.; Burrini, A.G.; Dallai, R.; Pallini, V,: News in Myriapod Biology, ed. by M. Camatini. Academic Press, N. York, 1979 (in press).

Baccetti, B.; Burrini, A.G.; Dallai, R.; Pallini, V.; Camatini, M.; Franchi, E.; Paoletti, L.: The "Delayed Flagellum" of Milliped Sperm is a Reacted Acrosome. XXVIII. The Spermatozoon of Arthropoda. J Submicrosc Cytol 9(1977a)187-219

Baccetti, B.; Dallai, R.: The Spermatozoon of Onychophorans. II. *Peripatoides leuckarti*. Tissue Cell 9(1977)563-566

Baccetti, B.; Dallai, R.; Burrini, A.G.; Selmi, G.: Fine Structure of the Spermatozoon of an Onychophoran, *Peripatopsis*. Tissue Cell 8(1976)659-672

Baccetti, B.; Dallai, R.; Rosati, F.; Giusti, F.; Bernini, F.; Selmi, G.: The Spermatozoon of Arthropoda. XXVI. The Spermatozoon of Isoptera, Embioptera, Dermaptera. J Microsc 21(1974)159-172

Baccetti, B.; Rosati, F.; Selmi, G.: The Spermatozoon of Arthropoda. XVI. The Acrosome of Orthoptera. J Submicrosc Cytol 3(1971a)319-337

Baccetti, B.; Rosati, F.; Selmi, G.: Electron Microscopy of Tardigrades. IV. The Spermatozoon. Monit Zool Ital 5(1971b)231-240

Ballowitz, E.: Weitere Beobachtungen über den feineren Bau der Säugetier Spermatozoen. Z Wiss Zool 52(1891)217

Bane, A.; Nicander, L.: The Structure and Formation of the Perforatorium in Mammalian Sperm. Int J Fertil 8(1963)865-866

Bedford, J.M.: Sperm Capacitation and Fertilization in Mammals. Biol Reprod 2(1970)128-158S

Bedford, J.M.; Calvin, H.I.: The Occurrence and Possible Functional Significance of —S—S— Crosslinks in Sperm Heads, with Particular Reference to Eutherian Mammals. J Exp Zool 188(1974)137-156

Bellet, N.F.; Vacquier, J.P.; Vacquier, V.D.: Characterization and Comparison of "Bindin" Isolated from Sperm of Two Species of Sea Urchin. Biochem Biophys Res Commun 79(1977)159-165

Benda, C.: Untersuchungen uber den Bau des functionirenden Samenkanälschens einiger Saügetiere und Folgerungen für die Spermatogenese dieser Wirbelthierklasse. Arch Mikrosk Anat 30(1887)49

Bernstein, M.H.; Teichman, R.J.: A Chemical Procedure for Extraction of the Acrosomes of Mammalian Spermatozoa. J Reprod Fertil 33(1973)239-244

Bertout, M.: Spermatogenèse de *Nereis diversicolor* O.F. Müller (Annélide, Polychète). I. Evolution du Citoplasme et Elaboration de l'Acrosome. J Microsc Biol Cell 25(1976)87-94

Bhalla, V.K.; Tillman, W.L.; Williams, W.L.: Presence of 2-Aspartyl-*N*-acetyl Glucosamine Amino Hydrolase in Mammalian Spermatozoa. J Reprod Fertil 34(1973)137-139

Bhattacharyya, A.K.; Zaneveld, L.J.D.: Kinetic Studies on the Interaction and Specificity of Synthetic Proteinase Inhibitors towards Human Acrosin. Andrologia 8(1976)1-119S

Bhattacharyya, A.K.; Zaneveld, L.J.D.: Release of Acrosin Inhibitor from Human Spermatozoa. Fertil Ster 30(1978)70-78

Boissin, L.; Manier, J.F.; Tuzet, O.: Étude Ultrastructurale de la Spermatogenèse de Glomeris Marginata Villers (Myriapods, Diplopode). Ann Sci Nat Zool 12e Sér. 14(1972)221-239

Bresciani, J.; Fenchel T.: Studies on Dicyemid Mesozoa. I. The Fine Structure of the Adult (the Nematogen and Rhombogen Stage). Vidensk Meddr Dansk Naturh Foren 128(1965)85-92

Bresciani, J.; Fenchel, T.: Studies on Dicyemid Mesozoa. II. The Fine Structure of the Infusoriform Larva. Ophelia 4(1967)1-18

Brown, G.G.: Ultrastructural Studies of Sperm Morphology and Sperm-Egg Interaction in the Decapod *Callinectes sapidus*. J Ultrastruct Res 14(1966)425-440

Brown, G.G.: Some Comparative Aspects of Selected Crustacean Spermatozoa and Crustacean Phylogeny. In: Comparative Spermatology, pp. 183-205, ed. by B. Baccetti. Academic Press, New York, 1970

Brown, G.G.; Metz, C.B.: Ultrastructural Studies on the Spermatozoa of Two Primitive Crustaceans, *Hutchinsoniella macracantha* and *Derocheilocaris typicus*. Z Mikrosk Anat Forsch 80(1967)78-92

Bryan, J.H.D.; Unnithan, R.R.: Cytochemical Localization of Non-specific Esterase and Acid Phosphatase in Sperma tozoa of the Mouse (*Mus musculus*). Histochemic 33(1973) 169-180.

Buckland-Nicks, J.A.: The Fine Structure of the Spermatozoon of *Littorina* (Gastropoda, Prosobranchia) with Special Reference to Sperm Motility. Z Mikrosk Anat Forsch 144(1973)11-29

Burgos, M.H.; Fawcett, D.W.: An Electron Microscope Study of Spermatid Differentiation in the Toad, *Bufo arenarum* Hensel. J Biophys Biochem Cytol 2(1956)223-240

Calvin, H.I.; Bedford, J.M.: Maturation of the Sperm Nucleus after Spermiation in Mammals. In: Morphological Aspects of Andrology, pp. 77-80, ed. by Holstein and Horstmann. Grosse, Berlin 1970

Carlsson, L.; Nyström, L.E.; Sundkvist I.; Markey, F.; Lindberg, U.: Profilin, a Low-Molecular Weight Protein Controlling Actin Polymerizability. In: Contractile Systems in Non-muscle Tissues, pp. 39-49, ed. by Perry, *et al*. Elsevier/North Holland Biomedical Press, Amsterdam, 1976a

Carlsson, L.; Nystrom, L.E.; Lindberg, U.; Kannan, K.K.; Cid-Dresdner, H.; Lovgren, S.; Jornvall, H.: Crystallization of a Non-muscle Actin. J Mol Biol (1976b)356-366

Carlsson, L.; Nystrom, L.E.; Sundkvist, I.; Markey, F.; Lindberg, U.: Actin Polymerizability is Influenced by Profilin, a Low Molecular Weight Protein in Non-muscle Cells. J Mol Biol (1977)465-483

Cavalier-Smith, T.: Electron and Light Microscopy of Gametogenesis and Gamete Fusion in *Chlamydomonas reinhardii*. Protoplasma 86(1975)1-18

Chevallier, P.: Mise en Évidence et Étude Cytochimique d'une Protéine Basique Extranucléaire dans les Spermatozoides des Crustacés Décapodes. J Cell Biol 32(1967)547-556

Christensen, T.: Alger. In: Botanik, Vol. 2, ed. by Bocher, Lange and Sørensen. Munksgaard, Kobenhavn, 1962

Clark, W.H., Jr.; Hinsch, G.W.: Some Aspects of Sperm-egg Interaction in *Cerebratulus lacteus*. Biol Bull Marine Biol Lab Woods Hole 137(1969)395

Clark, W.H.; Moretti, R.L.; Thompson, W.W.: Electron Microscopic Evidence for the Presence of an Acrosomal Reaction in *Ascaris lumbricoides* var. *suum*. Exp Cell Res 47(1967)643-647

Clermont, Y.; Einberg, E.; Leblond, C.P.; Wagner, S.: The Perforatorium—an Extension of the Nuclear Membrane of the Rat Spermatozoon. Anat Rec 121(1955)1-12

Clermont, Y., Clegg, R.E.; Leblond, C.P.: Presence of Carbohydrates in the Acrosome of the Guinea Pig Spermatozoa. Exp Cell Res 8(1955)453-458

Clermont, Y.; Leblond, C.P.: Spermiogenesis of Man, Monkey, Ram and Other Mammals as Shown by the "Periodic-Acid Schiff" Technique. Am J Anat 96(1955)229-253

Collins, F.; Epel, D.: The Role of Calcium Ions in the Acrosome Reaction of Sea Urchin Sperm. Exp Cell Res 106(1977)211-222

Collins, F.: A Re-evaluation of the Fertilizin Hypothesis of Sperm Agglutination and the Description of a Novel Form of Sperm Adhesion. Dev Biol 49(1976)381-394

Colwin, A.L.; Colwin, L.H.: Fine Structure of the Spermatozoon of *Hydroides hexagonus* (Annelida) with Special Reference to the Acrosomal Region. J Biophys Biochem Cytol 10(1961)211-230

Colwin, A.L.; Colwin, L.H.: Role of the Gamete Membranes in Fertilization in *Saccoglossus kowalevskii* (Enteropneusta). I. The Acrosomal Region and its Changes in Early Stages of Fertilization. J Cell Biol 19(1963)477-500

Cotelli, F.; Lora Lamia Donin, C.: Ultrastructural Analysis of Mature Spermatozoa of *Hyalinoecia tubicola* (O.F. Müller) (Annelida, Polychaeta). Monit Zool Ital 9(1975)51-66

Couchie, J.; Mann, T.: Glycosidases in Mammalian Sperm and Seminal Plasma. Nature 179(1957)1190

Courtens, J.L.; Courot, M.; Flechon, J.E.: The Perinuclear Substance of Boar, Bull, Ram and Rabbit Spermatozoa. J Ultrastruct Res 57(1976)54-64

Da Cruz-Landim, C.; Da Cruz-Hofling, M.A.: Electron Microscope Study of Lizard Spermiogenesis in *Tropidurus torquatus* (Lacertilia). Caryologia 30(1977)151-162

Dan, J.C.; Kakizawa, Y.; Kushida, H.; Fujita, K.: Acrosomal Triggers. Exp Cell Res 72(1972)60-68

Dan, J.C.: Acrosome Reaction and Lysins. In: Fertilization, pp. 237-293, ed. by Metz and Monroy. Academic Press, New York, 1967

Dan, J.C.: The Acrosomal Process Membrane. In: Comparative Spermatology, pp. 487-497, ed. by B. Baccetti. Academic Press, New York, 1970

Dan, J.C.; Hashimoto, S.; Kubo, M.; Yonehara, K.: The Fine Structure of the Acrosomal Trigger. In: The Functional Anatomy of the Spermatozoon, pp. 39-45, ed. by B. Afzelius. Pergamon Press, Oxford, 1975

Davies, P.; Bechtel, P.; Pastan, I.: Filamin Inhibits Actin Activation of Heavy Meromyosin ATPase. FEBS Lett 77(1977)228-232

Decker, G.L.; Joseph, D.B.; Lennerz, W.J.: A Study of Factors Involved in Induction of the Acrosomal Reaction in Sperm of the Sea Urchin *Arbacia punctulata*. Dev Biol 53(1976)115-125

De Rosier, D.; Mandelkow, E.; Silliman, A.; Tilney, L.; Kane, B.: Structure of Actin Containing Filaments from Two Types of Nonmuscle Cells. J Mol Biol 113(1977)679-695

Dewel, W.C.; Clark, W.H., Jr.: An Ultrastructural Investigation of Spermiogenesis and the Mature Sperm in the Anthozoan *Bunodosoma cavernata* (Cnidaria). J Ultrastruct Res 40(1972)417-431

Dott, H.M.; Dingle, J.T.: Distribution of Lysosomal Enzymes in the Spermatozoa and Cytoplasmic Droplets of Bull and Ram. Exp Cell Res 52(1968)523-540

Duckett, J.G.; Bell, P.R.: Studies on Fertilization in Archegoniate Plants. II. Egg Penetration in *Pteridium aquilinum* (L.) Kuhn. Cryobiology 6(1972)35-50

Endo, S.: Silver Methenamine and Phosphotungstic Acid Staining of the Acrosome of *Mytilus edulis*. Exp Cell Res 100(1976)71-78

Fahrenbach, W.H.: Spermiogenesis in the Horseshoe Crab, *Limulus polyphemus*. J Morphol 140(1973)31-52

Fallon, J.F.; Austin, C.R.: Fine Structure of Gametes of *Nereis limbata* (Annelida) before and after Interaction. J Exp Zool 166(1967)225-242

Fawcett, D.W.: The Structure of the Mammalian Spermatozoon. Int Rev Cytol 7(1958)195-234

Fawcett, D.W.: A Comparative View of Sperm Ultrastructure. Biol Reprod Suppl 2 2(1970)90-127

Fawcett, D.W.: Morphogenesis of the Mammalian Sperm Acrosome in New Perspective. In: The Functional Anat-

Fawcett, D.W.: omy of the Spermatozoon, pp. 199-210, ed. by B. Afzelius. Pergamon Press, Oxford, 1975a

Fawcett, D.W.: The Mammalian Spermatozoon. Dev Biol 44(1975b)394-436

Fawcett, D.W.; Burgos, V.M.H. Observations on the Cytomorphosis of the Germinal and Interstitial Cells of Human Testis. Ciba Foundation Symposium on Aging of Transient Structures, 1955

Fawcett, D.W.; Ito, S.: The Fine Structure of Bat Spermatozoa. Am J Anat 116(1965)567-610

Fawcett, D.W.; Burgos, M.H.: Observations on the Ultrastructure and Development of the Mammalian Spermatozoon. In: Comparative Spermatology, pp. 13-28, ed. by B. Baccetti. Academic Press, New York, 1970

Fink, E.; Schiebler, H.; Arnhold, M.; Fritz, H.: Isolation of a Trypsin-like Enzyme (Acrosin) from Boar Spermatozoa. Hoppe-Seylers Z Physiol Chem 353(1972)1633-1637

Fléchon, J.E.: Freeze-fracturing of Rabbit Spermatozoa. J Microsc 19(1974)59-64

Fléchon, J.E.: Immunocytochemical Localization of Hyaluronidase in the Sperm Acrosome of Farm Mammals. 3rd Int Symp Immunol Reprod Varna (1975), in press

Fléchon, J.E.; Huneau, D.; Brown, C.R.; Harrison, R.A.P.: Immunocytochemical Localization of Acrosin in the Anterior Segment of the Acrosomes of Ram, Boar and Bull Spermatozoa. Ann Biol Anim Bioch Biophys 17(1977)749-758

Flood, P.R.; Afzelius, B.A.: The Spermatozoon of *Oikopleura dioica* Fol (Larvacea, Tunicata). Cell Tiss Res 191(1978)27-37

Folliot, R.; Maillet, P.L.: Ultrastructure de la Spermiogenèse et du Spermatozoide de Divers Insectes Homoptères. In: Comparative Spermatology, pp. 289-300, ed. by B. Baccetti. Academic Press, New York, 1970

Franc, J.M.: Étude Ultrastructurale de la Spermatogénèse du Cténaire *Beroë ovata*. J Ultrastruct Res 42(1973)255-267

Franzen, Å.: The Spermatozoon of *Siboglinum* (Pogonophora). Acta Zool Stockholm 54(1973)179-192

Franzen, Å.: On the Ultrastructure of Spermiogenesis of *Flustra foliacea* (L.) and *Triticella korenii* G.O. Sars (Bryozoa). Zoon 4(1976)19-29

Friend, D.S.; Rudolf, I.: Acrosomal Disruption in Sperm. Freeze-fracture of Altered Membranes. J Cell Biol 63(1974)466-479

Furieri, P.: Sperm Morphology in Some Reptiles. In: Comparative Spermatology, pp. 115-131, ed. by B. Baccetti. Academic Press, New York, 1970

Furieri, P.: Sperms and Spermatogenesis in Certain Argentinian Iguanids. Riv Biol 67(1974)233-300

Furieri, P.: The Peculiar Morphology of the Spermatozoon of *Bombina variegata* (L.). Monit Zool Ital 9(1975)185-201

Garner, D.L.; Reamer, S.A.; Johnson, L.A.; Lessley, B.A.: Failure of Immunoperoxidase Staining to Detect Acrosin in the Equatorial Segment of Spermatozoa. J Exp Zool 201(1977)309-315

Garner, D.L.; Easton, M.P.: Immunofluorescent Localization of Acrosin in Mammalian Spermatozoa. J Exp Zool 200(1977)157-162

Georges, D.: Spermatogenèse et Spermiogenèse de *Ciona intestinalis* L. observées au Microscope Electronique. J Microsc 8(1969)391-400

Ginsburg, A.S.: Sperm-egg Association and its Relationship to the Activation of the Egg in Salmoid Fishes. J Embryol Exp Morphol 11(1963)13-33

Giusti, F.: The Spermatozoon of a Fresh-water Prosobranch Mollusc. J Submicrosc Cytol 1(1969)263-273

Giusti, F.; Mazzini, M.: The Spermatozoon of *Truncatella (s.str.) subcylindrica* (L.) (Gastropoda, Prosobranchia). Monit Zool Ital 7(1973)181-201

Gonzales, L.W.; Meizel, S.: Acid Phosphatases of Rabbit Spermatozoa. I. Electrophoretic Characterization of Multiple Forms of Acid Phosphatase in Rabbit Spermatozoa and other Semen Constituents. Biochim Biophys Acta 320(1973)166-175

Gordon, M.: Localization of Phosphatase Activity on the Membranes of the Mammalian Sperm Head. J Exp Zool 185(1973)111-120

Gordon, M.; Barnett, R.J.: Fine Structural Cytochemical Localizations of Phosphatase Activities of Rat and Guinea Pig. Exp Cell Res 48(1967)395-412

Gould, S.F.; Bernstein, M.H.: Localization of Bull Sperm Hyaluronidase. J Cell Biol 59(1973)119a

Griffiths, M.E.: Echidnas. Pergamon Press, London, 1968.

Gupta, B.L.: Aspects of Motility in the Non-flagellate Spermatozoa of Freshwater Ostracods. Symp Soc Exp Biol 22(1968)117-129

Hadek, R.: Study on the Fine Structure of Rabbit Sperm Head. J Ultrastruct Res 9(1963)110-122

Hamilton, D.W.; Fawcett, D.W.: Unusual Features of the Neck and Middle-piece of Snake Spermatozoa. J Ultrastruct Res 23(1968)81-97

Hancock, J.L.: The Ultrastructure of Mammalian Spermatozoa. Adv Reprod Physiol 1(1966)125-154

Hauschka, S.D.: Purification and Characterization of *Mytilus* Egg Membrane Lysin from Sperm. Biol Bull 125(1963)363

Heggeness, M.H.; Wang, K.; Singer, S.J.: Intracellular Distributions of Mechanochemical Proteins in Cultured Fibroblasts. Proc Natl Acad Sci USA 74(1977)3883-3887

Hendelberg, J.: Comparative Morphology of Turbellarian Spermatozoa Studied by Electron Microscopy. Acta Zool Fennica (1977)149-162

Henley, C.: Changes in Microtubules of Cilia and Flagella following Negative Staining with Phosphotungstic Acid. Biol Bull Marine Biol Lab Woods Hole 139(1970)265-276

Herrmann, F.: Quoted by Waldeyer, 1906

Hibbard, H.: Contribution à l'Étude de l'Ovogenèse de la Fécondation et de l'Histogenèse chez *Discoglossus pictus* Otth. Arch Biol 38(1928)251

Hinsch, G.W.: Comparative Ultrastructure of Cnidarian Sperm. Am Zool 14(1974)457-465

Hinsch, G.W.; Clark, W.H.: Comparative Fine Structure of Cnidaria Spermatozoa. Biol Reprod 8(1973)62-73

Ho, J.J.L.; Meizel, S.: Electrophoretic Detection of Multiple Forms of Trypsin-like Activity in Spermatozoa of the Domestic Fowl. J Reprod Fertil 23(1970)177-179

Horstmann, E.; Breucker, H.: Spermatozoen und Spermiohistogenese von *Graphidostreptus* spec. (Myriapoda, Diplopoda). I. Die reifen Spermatozoen. Z Mikrosk Anat Forsch 96(1969)505-520

Hylander, B.L.; Summers, R.G.: An Ultrastructural Analysis of the Gametes and Early Fertilization in Two Bivalve Molluscs, *Chama macerophylla* and *Spisula solidissima* with Special Reference to Gamete Binding. Cell Tiss Res 182(1977)469-489

Hughes, R.L.: Comparative Morphology of Spermatozoa from Five Marsupial Families. Aust J Zool 13(1965)533-543

Humphreys, P.N.: Brief Observations on the Semen and Spermatozoa of Certain Passerine and Non-passerine Birds. J Reprod Fertil 29(1972)327-336

Jamuar, M.P.: Studies of Spermiogenesis in a Nematode *Nippostrongylus brasiliensis*. J Cell Biol 31(1966)381-396

Jensen, O.S.: Untersuchungen über die Samenkörper der Saügetiere, Vögel un Amphibien. Arch Mikrosk Anat (1887)379-425

Jespersen, Å.: Fine Structure of the Spermatozoon of the Australian Lungfish *Neoceratodus forsteri* (Krefft). J Ultrastruct Res 37(1971)178-185

Jespersen, Å.; Hartwick, R.: Fine Structure of Spermiogenesis in Scorpions from the Family Vejovidae. J Ultrastruct Res 45(1973)366-383

Jessen, H.; Behnke, O.; Wingstrand, K.G.; Rostgaard, J.: Actin-like Filaments in the Acrosomal Apparatus of Spermatozoa of a Sea Urchin. Exp Cell Res 80(1973)47-54

Jones, R.C.: Studies of the Ultrastructure of the Head of some Mammalian Spermatozoa with Particular Reference to the Perforatorium. In: Proceedings of the 7th International Conference on Electron Microscopy, Grenoble. Vol. 3, pp. 641-642, 1970

Jones, R.C.; Rowlands, I.W.; Skinner, J.D.: Spermatozoa in the Genital Ducts of the African Elephant, *Loxodonta africana*. J Reprod Fert 41(1974)189-192.

Juberthie, C.; Manier, J.F.; Boissin, L.: Étude Ultrastructurale de la Double Spermiogenèse chez l'Opilion Cyphaphtalme *Siro rubens* Latreille. J Microsc Biol Cell 25(1976)137-148

Kaye, J.S.: Acrosome Formation in the House Cricket. J Cell Biol 12(1962)411-431

Khorlin, A.Y.; Vikha, I.V.; Milishnikov, A.N.: Subunit Structure of Testicular Hyaluronidase. FEBS Lett 31(1973)107-110

Koehler, J.K.: An Electron Microscope Study of the Dimorphic Spermatozoa of *Asplanchna* (Rotifera). I. The Adult Testis. Z Mikrosk Anat Forsch 67(1965)57-76

Koehler, J.K.: Human Sperm Head Ultrastructure: a Freeze-etching Study. J Ultrastruct Res 39(1972)520-539

Koren, E.; Milkovic, S.: Collagenase-like Peptidase in Human, Rat and Bull Spermatozoa. J Reprod Fertil 32(1973)349-356

Kubo, M.: The Formation of a Temporary Acrosome in the Spermatozoon of *Laternula limicola* (Bivalvia, Mollusca). J Ultrastruct Res 61(1977)140-148

Kubo, M.; Ishikawa, M.: Organizing Process of the Temporary-acrosome in Spermatogenesis of the Bivalve *Lyonsia ventricosa*. J Submicr Cytol 10(1978)411-421

Langreth, S.G.: Spermiogenesis in Cancer Crabs. J Cell Biol 43(1969)574-603

Lanzavecchia, G.; Lora Lamia Donin, C.: Morphogenetic Effects of Microtubules. II. Spermiogenesis in *Lumbricus terrestris*. J Submicrosc Cytol 4(1972)247-260

Leeuwenhoek, A.: Observationes de Natis e Semine Genitali Animalculis. Philos Trans R Soc Lond [Biol] 12(1677)1040-1042

Leeuwenhoek, A.: Observatoris Praemissis Literis Responsi. Philos Trans R Soc Lond [Biol] 13(1678)1044

Leeuwenhoek, A.: De Diuturna Vita Animalculorum in Semine Masculo, etc. (1684). Reprinted in Arcana Naturae, pp. 149-177. Lugduni Batavorum, Langerak, 1722

Leeuwenhoek, A.: Epistola 142 data ad Johannem Somerum, (1701). Reprinted in Arcana Naturae, pp. 367-374. Lugduni Batvorum, Langerak, 1719

Legg, G.: The Structure of Encysted Sperm of some British Pseudoscorpiones (Arachnida). J Zool 170(1973)429-440

Lenhossek, M.V.: Untersuchungen über Spermatogenese. Arch Mikrosk Anat 51(1898)215-318

Levine, A. E.; Walsh, K.A.; Fodor, E.J.B.: Evidence of an Acrosin-like Enzyme in Sea Urchin Sperm. Dev. Biol 63(1978)299-306

Longo, F.J.; Anderson, E.: Spermiogenesis in the Surf Clam *Spisula solidissima* with Special Reference to the Formation of the Acrosomal Vesicle. J Ultrastruct Res 27(1969)435-443

Lora Lamia Donin, C.; Cotelli, F.: The Rod-shaped Sperm of *Gordioidea* (Aschelminthes, Nematomorpha). J Ultrastruct Res 61(1977)193-200

Lunger, P.D.: Early Stages of Spermatozoan Development in the Colonial Hydroid *Campanularia flexuosa*. Z Mikrosk Anat Forsch 116(1971)37-51

Lyke, E.B.; Robson, E.A.: Spermatogenesis in Anthozoa: Differentiation of the Spermatid. Cell Tiss Res 157(1975)185-205

Mabuchi, I.: Isolation of Myosin from Starfish Sperm Heads. J Biochem 80(1976)413-415

Mabuchi, Y.; Mabuchi, I.: Acrosomal ATPase in Starfish and Bivalve Mollusc Spermatozoa. Exp Cell Res 82(1973)271-279

Malecha, J.: Étude Ultrastructurale de la Spermiogenèse de *Piscicola geometra* L. (Hirudinee, Rhynchobdelle). J Ultrastruct Res 51(1975)188-203

Manier, J.F.; Boissin, L.: Aspects Ultrastructuraux de la Spermiogenèse des Polydesmoidea (Myriapodes, Diplopodes). Ann Sci Nat Zool 17(1975)505-520

Manier, J.F.; Boissin, L.: Nouvelle Contribution à l'Étude Ultrastructurale de la Spermiogenèse des Diplopodes Spirobolides. Ann Sci Nat Zool 18(1976)437-448

Manier, J.F.; Boissin, L.; Tuzet, O.: Étude Ultrastructurale de la Spermiogenèse de *Plethocrossus acutiformis* Demage et *Isoporostreptus bouixi* Demange (Myriapodes, Diplopodes; Spirostreptoidea). Bull Biol 10(1974)169-183

Manton, I.: Plant Spermatozoids. In: Comparative Spermatology, pp. 143-158, ed. by B. Baccetti. Academic Press, New York, 1970

Manton, I.; Friedmann, I.: Gametes, Fertilization and Zygote Development in *Prasiola stipitata* Subr. II. Electron Microscopy. Nova Hedwigia 1(1960)443-462

Marchand, B.; Mattei, X.: La Spermatogenèse des Acanthocephales. I. L'Appareil Centriolaire et Flagellaire au Cours de la Spermiogenèse d'*Illiosentis furcatus* var. *africana* Golvan, 1956 (Paleacantocephala, *Rhadinorhynchidae*). J Ultrastruct Res 54(1976)347-358

Mattei, X.: Spermiogenèse Comparée des Poissons. In: Comparative Spermatology, pp. 57-69, ed. by B. Baccetti. Academic Press, New York, 1970

Mattei, C.; Mattei, X.: La Spermiogenèse d'*Albula vulpes* (L. 1758) (Poisson, Albulidae). Étude Ultrastructurale. Z Mikrosk Anat Forsch 142(1973)171-192

Mattei, C.; Mattei, X.; Manfredi, J.L.: Electron Microscope Study of the Spermiogenesis of *Streptopelia roseogrisea*. J Submicrosc Cytol 4(1972)57-73

McRorie, R.A.; Williams, W.L.: Biochemistry of Mammalian Fertilization. Ann Rev Biochem 43(1974)777-803

Meizel, S.: Biochemical Detection and Activation of an Inactive Form of a Trypsin-like Enzyme in Rabbit Testes. J Reprod Fertil 31(1972)459-462

Meizel, S.; Colham, J.: Partial Characterization of a New

Bull Sperm Arylaminidase. J Reprod Fertil 28(1972)303-307

Meizel, S.; Lui, C.W.: Evidence for the Role of a Trypsin-like Enzyme in the Hamster Sperm Acrosome Reaction. J Exp Zool 195(1976)137-144

Moore, G.P.M.; Dixon, K.E.: A Light and Electron Microscopical Study of Spermatogenesis in *Hydra cauliculata*. J Morphol 137(1972)483-502

Morton, D.B.: Acrosomal Enzymes: Immunochemical Localization of Acrosin and Hyaluronidase in Ram Spermatozoa. J Reprod Fertil 45(1975)375-378

Multamaki, S.; Suominen, J.: Distribution and Removal of the Acrosin of Bull Spermatozoa. Int J Fertil 21(1976)69-81

Myles, D.G.: Structural Changes in the Sperm of *Marsilea vestita* before and after Fertilization. In: The Biology of the Male Gamete, pp. 129-134, ed. by Duckett and Racey. Academic Press, London, 1975

Nagy, F.; Edmonds, R.H.: Some Observations on the Fine Structure of Armadillo Spermatozoa. J Reprod Fertil 34(1973)551-553

Nicander, L.; Bane, A.: Fine Structure of the Sperm Head in some Mammals, with Particular Reference to the Acrosome and the Subacrosomal Substance. Z Mikrosk Anat Forsch 72(1966)496-515

Nicander, L.; Sjöden, I.: An Electron Microscopical Study of the Acrosomal Complex and its Role in Fertilization in the River Lamprey, *Lampetra fluviatilis*. J Submicrosc Cytol 3(1971)309-317

Niijima, L.; Dan, J.C.: The Acrosome Reaction in *Mytilus edulis*. I. Fine Structure of the Intact Acrosome. J Cell Biol 25(1965a)243-248

Niijima, L.; Dan, J.C.: The Acrosome Reaction in *Mytilus edulis*. II. Stages in the Reaction, Observed in Supernumerary and Calcium-treated Spermatozoa. J Cell Biol (1965b)249-259

Norstog, K.: The Motility of Cycad Spermatozoa in Relation to Structure and Function. In: The Biology of the Male Gamete, ed. by Duckett and Racey. Academic Press, London, (1975)

Nyholm, K.G.: Ultrastructure of the Spermatozoa in *Homolorhagha kinorhyncha*. Zoon 4(1976)11-18

Okamura, F.; Nishiyama, H.: The Early Development of the Tail and the Transformation of the Shape of the Nucleus of the Spermatid of the Domestic Fowl, *Gallus gallus*. Cell Tiss Res 169(1976)345-359

Okamura, F.; Nishiyama, H.: The Passage of Spermatozoa Through the Vitelline Membrane in the Domestic Fowl, *Gallus gallus*. Cell Tiss Res 188(1978)497-508

Olson, G.E.; Hamilton, D.W.; Fawcett, D.W.: Isolation and Characterization of the Perforatorium of Rat Spermatozoa. J Reprod Fertil 47(1976)293-297

Onuma, H.; Nishikawa, Y.: Studies on the Acrosomic System of Spermatozoa of Domestic Animals. I. Cytochemical Nature of the PAS-positive Material in the Acrosomic System of Boar Spermatids. Bull Natl Inst Anim Husbandry 1(1963)125

O'Rand, M.G.: *In Vitro* Fertilization and Capacitation-like Interaction in the Hydroid, *Campanularia flexuosa*. J Exp Zool 182(1972)299-306

O'Rand, M.; Miller, R.L.: Spermatozoan Vesicle Loss during Penetration of the Female Gonangium in the Hydroid, *Campanularia flexuosa*. J Exp Zool 188(1974)179-195

Payne, F.: Some Observations on Spermatogenesis in *Gelastocoris oculatus* (Hemiptera) with the Aid of the Electron Microscope. J Morphol 119(1966)357-382

Pedersen, H.: The Postacrosomal Region of the Spermatozoa of Man and *Macaca arctoides*. J Ultrastruct Res 40(1972)366-377

Phillips, D.M.: Development of Spermatozoa in the Woolly Opossum with Special Reference to the Shaping of the Sperm Head. J Ultrastruct Res 33(1970)369-380

Phillips, D.M.: Substructure of the Mammalian Acrosome. J Ultrastruct Res 38(1972)591-604

Phillips, D.M.: Cell Surface Structure of Rodents Sperm Heads. J Exp Zool 191(1975)1-8

Phillips, D.M.: Nuclear Shaping during Spermiogenesis in the Whip Scorpion. J Ultrastruct Res 54(1976)397-405

Phillips, D.M.: Surface of the Equatorial Segment of the Mammalian Acrosome. Biol Reprod 16(1977)128-137

Picheral, B.: Les Éléments Cytoplasmiques au Cours de la Spermiogenèse du Triton *Pleurodeles waltlii* Michah. I. La Genèse de l'Acrosome. Z Mikrosk Anat Forsch 131(1972)347-370

Plattner, H.: Bull Spermatozoa: A Re-investigation by Freeze-etching Using Widely Different Cryofixation Procedures. J Submicrosc Cytol 3(1971)19-32

Polakoski, K.L.; McRorie, R.A.; Williams, W.L.: Boar Acrosin. I. Purification and Preliminary Characterization of a Proteinase from Boar Sperm. J Biol Chem 248(1973a)8178-8182

Polakoski, K.L.; McRorie, R.A.: Boar Acrosin. II. Classification, Inhibition, and Specificity Studies of a Proteinase from Sperm Acrosomes. J Biol Chem 248(1973b)8183-8188

Polakoski, K.L.; Zahler, W.L.; Paulson, J.D.: Demonstration of Proacrosin and Quantitation of Acrosin in Ejaculated Human Spermatozoa. Fertil and Steril 28(1977)668-670

Polakoski, K.L.; Zaneveld, L.J.D.; Williams, W.L.: Purification of a Proteolytic Enzyme from Rabbit Acrosomes. Biol Reprod 6(1972)23-29

Porte, A.; Follenius, F.: La Spermiogenèse chez *Lebistes Reticulatus*. Étude au Microscope Électronique. Bull Soc Zool Fr 85(1960)82-88

Reger, J.F.: Spermiogenesis in the Tick, *Amblyomma dissimili*, as Revealed by Electron Microscopy. J Ultrastruct Res 8(1963)607-621

Reger, J.F.: A Study on the Fine Structure of Developing Spermatozoa from the Oligochaete, *Enchytraeus albidus*. Z Mikrosk Anat Forsch 82(1967)257-269

Reger, J.F.: A Fine Structure Study on Spermiogenesis in the Arachnid *Leiobunum* sp. (Phalangida, Harvestmen). J Ultrastruct Res 28(1969)422-434

Reger, J.F.: Spermiogenesis in the Spider, *Pisuarina* sp.: A Fine Structure Study. J Morphol 130(1970)421-434

Reger, J.F.: A Fine Structure Study on Spermiogenesis in the Ectoproct *Bugula* sp. J Submicrosc Cytol 3(1971)193-200

Reger, J.F.; Florendo, N.T.: Studies on Motile, Non-tubule-containing, Filiform Spermatozoa of Ostracod, *Cypridopsis* sp. I. Spermiogenesis. J Ultrastruct Res 28(1969a)235-249

Reger, J.F.; Florendo, N.T.: Studies on Motile, Non-tubule-containing, Filiform Spermatozoa of the Ostracod, *Cypridopsis* sp. II. Mature Spermatozoa. J Ultrastruct Res 28(1969b)250-259

Retzius, G.: Zur Kenntniss der Spermatozoen. Biol Untersuch 1(1881)77-88

Rogers, B.J.; Morton, B.E.: The Release of Hyaluronidase from Capacitating Hamster Spermatozoa. J Reprod Fertil 35(1973)477-487

Rogers, B.J.; Yanagimachi, R.: Release of Hyaluronidase from Guinea Pig Spermatozoa through an Acrosome Reaction Initiated by Calcium. J Reprod Fertil 44(1975)135-138

Roomans, G.M.; Afzelius, B.A.: Acrosome Vesiculation in the Human Sperm. J Submicrosc Cytol 7(1975)61-69

Roomans, G.M.: Calcium Binding to the Acrosomal Membrane of Human Spermatozoa. Exp Cell Res 96(1975)23-30

Rosati, F.; Baccetti, B.; Dallai, R.: The Spermatozoon of Arthropoda. X. Araneids and the Lower Myriapods. In: Comparative Spermatology, pp. 247-254, ed. by B. Baccetti. Academic Press, New York, 1970

Sandoz, D.: Étude Ultrastructurale et Cytochimique de la Formation de l'Acrosome du Discoglosse (Amphibien, Anoure). In: Comparative Spermatology, pp. 93-113, ed. by B. Baccetti. Academic Press, New York, 1970a

Sandoz, D.: Étude Cytochimique des Polysaccharides au Cours de la Spermatogenèse d'un Amphibien Anoure: le Discoglosse *Discoglossus pictus* (Otth.). J Microsc 9(1970b)243-262

Schincariol, A.L.; Habowsky, J.E.J.; Winner, G.: Cytology and Ultrastructure of Differentiating Interstitial Cells in Spermatogenesis in *Hydra fusca*. Can J Zool 45(1967)590-593

Shay, J.W.: Ultrastructural Observations on the Acrosome of *Lumbricus terrestris*. J Ultrastruct Res 41(1972)572-578

Srivastava, P.N.; Zaneveld, L.J.D.; Williams, W.L.: Mammalian Sperm Acrosomal Neuraminidases. Biochem Biophys Res Commun 39(1970)575-582

Stagni, A.; Lucchi, M.L.: Ultrastructural Observations on the Spermatogenesis in *Hydra attenuata*. In: Comparative Spermatology, pp. 357-361, ed. by B. Baccetti. Academic Press, New York, 1970

Stambaugh, R.: Enzymatic and Morphological Events in Mammalian Fertilization. Gamete Res 1(1978)65-85

Stambaugh, R.; Smith, M.; Faltas, S.: An Organized Distribution of Acrosomal Proteinase in Rabbit Sperm Acrosomes. J Exp Zool 193(1975)119-123

Stambaugh, R.; Smith, M.: Tubulin and Microtubule-like Structures in Mammalian Acrosomes. J Exp Zool 203(1978)135-141

Stanley, H.P.: An Electron Microscope Study of Spermiogenesis in the Teleost Fish, *Oligocottus maculosus*. J Ultrastruct Res 27(1969)230-243

Stanley, H.P.: Fine Structure of Spermiogenesis in the Elasmobranch Fish *Squalus suckleyi*. I. Acrosome Formation, Nuclear Elongation and Differentiation of the Midpiece Axis. J Ultrastruct Res 36(1971)86-102

Starke, F.J.: Elektronenmikroskopische Untersuchung der Zwittergonadenacini von *Planorbarius corneus* L. (Basommatophora). Z Mikrosk Anat Forsch 119(1971)483-514

Summers, R.G.: The Fine Structure of the Spermatozoon of *Pennaria tiarella* (Coelenterata). J Morphol 131(1970)117-130

Summers, R.G.: An Ultrastructural Study of the Spermatozoon of *Eudendrium ramosum*. Z Mikrosk Anat Forsch 132(1972)147-166

Summers, R.G.; Talbot, P.; Klough, E.M.; Hylander, B.L.; Franklin, L.E.: Ionophore A23187 Induces Acrosome Reactions in Sea Urchin and Guinea Pig Spermatozoa. J Exp Zool 196(1976)381-385

Talbot, P.; Franklin, L.E.: Morphology and Kinetics of the Hamster Sperm Acrosome Reaction. J Exp Zool 198(1976)163-176

Talbot, P.; Kleve, M.G.: The Distribution of Actin in Hamster Sperm. J Cell Biol 75(1977)G726, p. 170a

Talbot, P.; Summers, R.G.; Hylander, B.L.; Klough, E.M.; Franklin, L.E.: The Role of Calcium in the Acrosome Reaction: An Analysis Using Ionophore A23187. J Exp Zool 198(1976)383-392

Tandler, B.; Moriber, L.G.: Microtubular Structures Associated with the Acrosome during Spermiogenesis in the Water Strider, *Gerris remigis* (Say). J Ultrastruct Res 14(1966)391-404

Teuchert, G.: Elektronenmikroskopische Untersuchung über die Spermatogénese and Spermatohistogénese von *Turbanella cornuta* Remane (Gastrotriche). J Ultrastruct Res 56(1976)1-14

Thibault, C.: Présence d'une Spermalysine dans le Spermatozoide Maturé (Capacité) du Lapin. Proceedings of the 5th International Congress on Animal Reproduction, Trento, Vol 7, pp. 294-295, 1964

Tillman, W.L.: Enzymology of Spermatozoan Penetration of Mammalian Ova, pp. 1-105. Thesis, University of Georgia, Athens, 1972

Tilney, L.G.: Actin Filaments in the Acrosomal Reaction of *Limulus* Sperm. Motion Generated by Alterations in the Packing of the Filaments. J Cell Biol 64(1975a)289-310

Tilney, L.G.: The Role of Actin in Non-muscle Cell Motility. In: Molecules and Cell Movement, pp. 339-388, ed. by Inoue and Stephens. Raven Press, New York, 1975b

Tilney, L.G.: Polymerization of Actin. V. A New Organelle, the Actomere, that Initiates the Assembly of Actin Filaments in Thyone Sperm. J Cell Biol 77(1978)551-564

Tilney, L.G.: The Polymerization of Actin. I. How Nonfilamentous Actin Becomes Nonrandomly Distributed in Sperm: Evidence for the Association of this Actin with Membranes. J Cell Biol 69(1976a)51-72

Tilney, L.G.: The Polymerization of Actin. II. Aggregates of Non-filamentous Actin and its Associated Proteins: A Storage Form of Actin. J Cell Biol 69(1976b)73-89

Tilney, L.G.; Hatano, S.; Ishikawa, H.; Mooseker, M.S.: The Polymerization of Actin: Its Role in the Generation of the Acrosomal Process of Certain Echinoderm Sperm. J Cell Biol 59(1973)109-126

Tingari, M.D.: Observations on the Fine Structure of Spermatozoa in the Testis and Excurrent Ducts of the Male Fowl, *Gallus domesticus*. J Reprod Fertil 34(1973)255-265

Turquier, Y.; Pochon-Masson, J.: L'Infrastructure de Spermatozoide de *Trypetesa (Alcippe) massarioides* Turquier (Ciripède acrothoracique). Arch Zool Exp Gén 110(1969)435-470

Tuzet, O.; Bogoraze, D.; Lafargue, F.: Recherches Ultrastructurales sur la Spermiogenèse de *Diplosoma listerianum* (Milne-Edwards, 1841) et *Lissoclinum pseudoleptoclinum* (Von Drasche, 1883) (Ascidies Composées, Aplousobranches). Ann Sci Nat Zool 14(1972)177-190

Tuzet, O.; Garrone, R.; Pavans de Ceccatty, M.: Observations Ultrastructurales sur la Spermatogenèse chez la Démosponge *Aplysilla rosea* Schulze (Dendroceratide): Une Métaplasie Exemplaire. Ann Sci Nat Zool 12(1970)27-50

Tyler, A.: Extraction of an Egg Membrane Lysin from Sperm of the Giant Keyhode Limpet (*Megathura crenulata*) Proc Natl Acad Sci USA 25(1939)317

Tyler, A.: Properties of Fertilizin and Related Substances of

Eggs and Sperm of Marine Animals. Am Nat 83(1949)195-219
Vacquier, V.D.; Moy, G.W.: Isolation of Bindin: The Protein Responsible for Adhesion of Sperm to Sea Urchin Eggs. Proc Natl Acad Sci USA 74(1977)2456-2460
Van Deurs, B.: On the Ultrastructure of the Mature Spermatozoon of a Chaetognath, *Spadella cephaloptera*. Acta Zool 53(1972)93-104
Van Deurs, B.: Spermatology of some Pycnogonida (Arthropoda), with Special Reference to a Microtubule-Nuclear Envelope Complex. Acta Zool Stockholm 55(1974)151-162
Villa, L.: An Ultrastructural Investigation of Normal and Irradiated Spermatozoa of a Tunicate, *Ascidia malaca*. Boll Zool 42(1975)95-98
Wada, S.K.; Collier, J.R.; Dan, J.C.: Studies on the Acrosome. V. An Egg Membrane Lysin from the Acrosomes of *Mytilus edulis* Spermatozoa. Exp Cell Res 10(1956)168-180
Waldeyer, W.: Bau und Entwicklung der Samenfänden. Anat Anz 2(1887)345-368
Waldeyer, W.: Die Geschlechtszellen. In: Handbuch der Vergleichenden und Experimentellen Entwickelungslehre der Wirbeltiere. Vol. I, pp. 86-467, ed by O. Hertwig, 1906
Walker, M.H.: Some Unusual Features of the Sperm of *Nucella lapillus* L. In: Comparative Spermatology, pp. 383-391, ed. by B. Baccetti. Academic Press, New York, 1970
Walker, M.; MacGregor, H.C.: Spermatogenesis and the Structure of the Mature Sperm in *Nucella lapillus* L. J Cell Sci 3(1968)95-104
Warner, F.D.: Spermatid Differentiation in the Blowfly *Sarcophaga bullata* with Particular Reference to Flagellar Morphogenesis. J Ultrastruct Res 35(1971)210-232
Weissman, A.; Lentz, T.L.; Barnett, R.J.: Fine Structural Observations on Nuclear Maturation during Spermiogenesis in *Hydra littoralis*. J Morphol 128(1969)229-240
Whitfield, P.J.: The Ultrastructure of the Spermatozoon of the Hoplonemertine, *Emplectonema neesii*. Z Mikrosk Anat Forsch 128(1972)303-316
Wingstrand, K.G.: Comparative Spermatology of a Pentastomid, *Raillietiella hemidactyli*, and a Branchiuran Crustacean, *Argulus foliaceus*, with a Discussion of Pentastomid Relationship. K Danske Vidensk Selsk Skr 19(1972)5-72
Woollacott, R.M.: Spermatozoa of *Ciona intestinalis* and Analysis of Ascidian Fertilization. J Morphol 152(1977)77-88
Yamane, J.: The Proteolytic Action of Mammalian Spermatozoa and Its Bearing upon the Second Maturation Division of Ova. Cytologia 1(1930)394-403
Yanagimachi, R.; Teichman, R.J.: Cytochemical Demonstration of Acrosomal Proteinase in Mammalian and Avian Spermatozoa by a Silver Proteinate Method. Biol Reprod 6(1972)87
Yanagimachi, R.; Usui, N.: Calcium Dependence of the Acrosome Reaction and Activation of Guinea Pig Spermatozoa. Expl Cell Res 89(1974)161-174
Yang, C.H.: Sperm Acrosomal Enzymes Involved in Fertilization, p. 116 Thesis, University of Georgia, Athens, 1972
Yang, C.H.; Srivastava, P.N.: Separation and Properties of Hyaluronidase from Ram Sperm Acrosomes. J Reprod Fertil 37(1974)17-25
Zaneveld, L.J.D.; Dragoje, B.M.; Schumacher, G.F.B.: Acrosomal Proteinase and Proteinase Inhibition of Human Spermatozoa. Science 177(1972b)702-703
Zaneveld, L.J.D.; Polakoski, K.L.; Williams, W.L.: Properties of a Proteolytic Enzyme from Rabbit Sperm Acrosome. Biol Reprod 6(1972a)30-39
Zaneveld, L.J.D.; Polakoski, K.L.; Schumacher, G.F.B.: Properties of Acrosomal Hyaluronidase from Bull Spermatozoa. J Biol Chem 248(1973)564-570
Zaneveld, L.J.D.; Robertson, R.T.; Williams, W.L.: Synthetic Enzyme Inhibitors as Anti-fertility Agents. FEBS Lett 11(1970)345-347
Zaneveld, L.J.D.; Williams, W.L.: A Sperm Enzyme that Disperses the Corona Radiata and its Inhibition by Decapacitation Factor. Biol Reprod 2(1970)363-368
Zahler, W.L.; Doak, G.A.: Isolation of the Outer Acrosomal Membrane from Bull Sperm. Biochim Biophys Acta 406(1975)479-488
Zissler, D.: Die Spermiohistogenese des Süsswasser Ostracoden *Notodromas monacha* O.F. Müller. I. and II. Z Mikrosk Anat Forsch 96(1969)87-133

CONTRIBUTED PAPERS

ULTRASTRUCTURAL STUDY OF SPERMIOGENESIS OF THE ANURAN AMPHIBIAN *BOMBINA VARIEGATA*

R. Folliot

Faculty of Biological Sciences, Laboratory of Cellular Biology, University of Rennes, France

The morphology and the genesis of the peculiar spermatozoon of *Bombina variegata* have been investigated formerly by some of the early cytologists especially Broman (1900) and Champy (1913).

It was soon established that the helically spindle-shaped *Bombina* sperm cell cannot be divided into distinct head and tail parts, and that the motile complex including an undulating membrane effectively extends along the entire length of the head.

A transverse section of the spermatozoon (Fig. 1) shows, at the same level, the nucleus and the flagellum connected to the main body of the cell by an undulating membrane. Champy explained this situation, which is visible with the light microscope, as the young flagellum in the *Bombina* spermatid turning down along the nucleus. This explanation means that the posterior part of the nucleus should be in front of the sperm cell. Recently Furieri (1975) has made an electron microscope study of the morphology of the mature *Bombina* spermatozoon. He showed that the front part of the spermatozoon is actually the acrosome-capped anterior end of the nucleus. Consequently, the origin of the flagellum of the mature spermatozoon, that is the centriolar apparatus, is situated in the anterior part of the cell close to the acrosome. Therefore, the fundamental question concerning the morphogenesis of this spermatozoon is: is the closeness of the acrosome to the centriolar apparatus a permanent arrangement or does it arise from successive migrations of the centriolar apparatus to the posterior part of the nucleus and later back towards the anterior part? There are examples of the latter phenomenon both in invertebrate (*e.g.,* Marchand and Mattei, 1977) and vertebrate (*e.g.,* Boisson *et al.,* 1969) species. Spermiogenesis in *Bombina* has been studied in order to understand the evolution of the different organelles and the morphogenesis of this peculiar spermatozoon.

© 1979 Urban & Schwarzenberg, Inc. Baltimore-Munich *The Spermatozoon,* edited by D.W. Fawcett and J.M. Bedford

MATERIALS AND METHODS

Small pieces of testis were fixed in 2.5% glutaraldehyde in 0.1 M phosphate buffer for 15-30 min at room temperature and postfixed in 2% osmium tetroxide for 90 min or directly fixed in osmium tetroxide. Tissues were embedded in Epon-Araldite mixture. Thin sections were double stained with uranyl acetate for 2 h and lead citrate for 10 min. For experiments with enzyme digestion, thin sections were incubated, after a preliminary oxidation by H_2O_2, in solutions of pronase (Calbiochem, B grade) in distilled water at 37°C.

Testes of *Bombina variegata,* collected in eastern France, contain different stages of spermatogenesis and mature sperm cells throughout the year, but the greatest number of various spermatid stages were found in September.[1]

OBSERVATIONS AND DISCUSSION

In the early spermatid, the Golgi complex gives rise to proacrosomal vesicles (Fig. 2) which later fuse into a large acrosomal vesicle (Fig. 3). This vesicle, except in a few small dispersed dense masses of material, appears almost empty. A similar apparently empty type of acrosomal vesicle has been observed in the bandicoot (Sapsford *et al.,* 1967), the elasmobranch fish *Squalus suckleyi* (Stanley, 1971), the amphibian *Xenopus laevis* (Reed and Stanley, 1972), and the lizard *Lacerta viridis.*[2] In *Bombina* the acrosomal vesicle comes in contact with the nucleus. Within this region, a subacrosomal structure appears as a rod of fibrous material that extends longitudinally for most of its length inside a nuclear canal (Fig. 3). This rod is the axis or perforatorium. It is, in fact, a bundle of fibers that may exhibit in cross

---

[1] The author is indebted to Dr. J. Joly, University of Rennes, for providing the specimens.
[2] Folliot, R.: unpublished

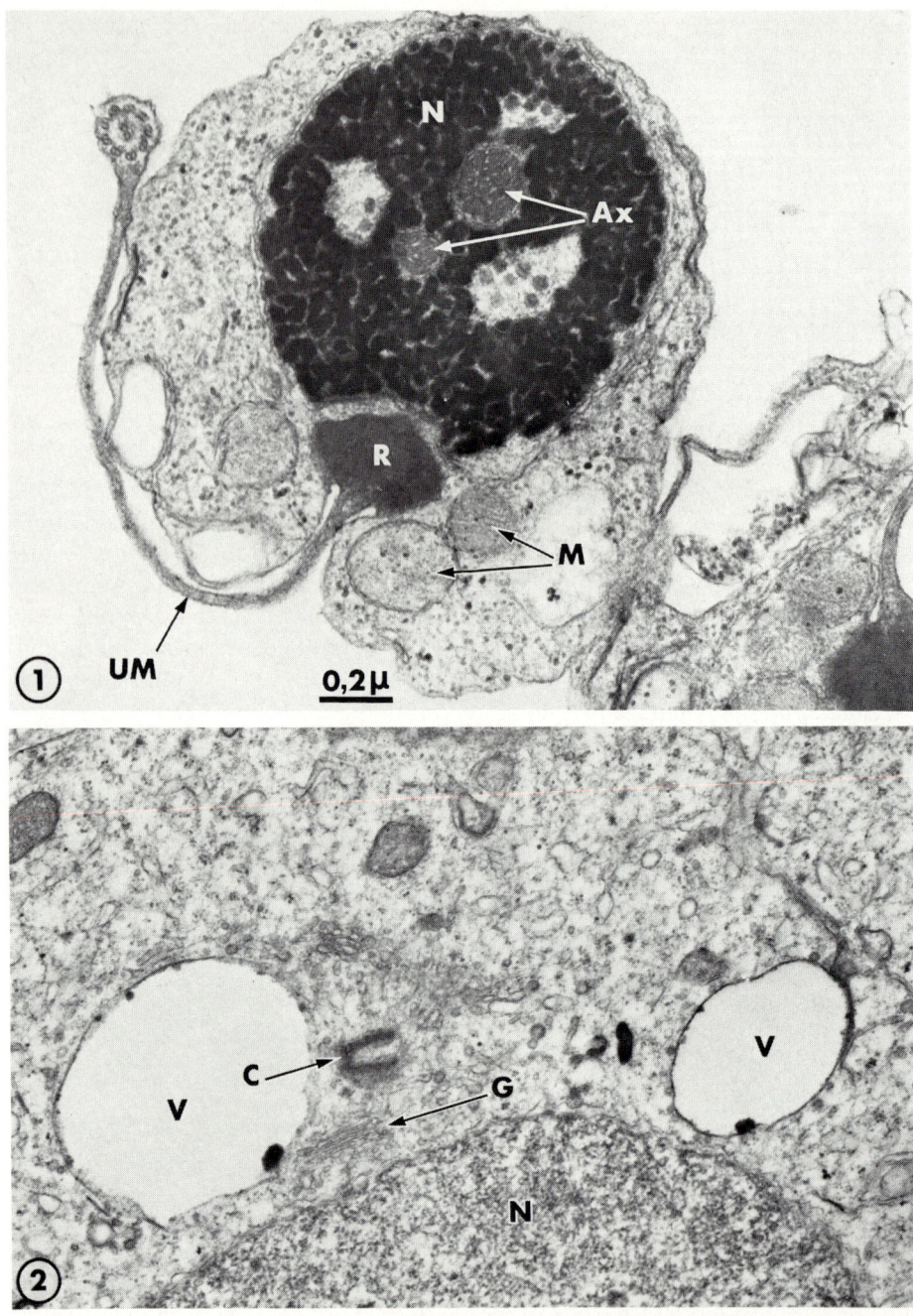

Figure 1. Cross section in the midpiece of a spermatozoon. Ax, axis (divided in two parts); M, mitochondria; N, nucleus; R, rod; UM, undulating membrane. X47,000

Figure 2. Part of a spermatid cell. C, centriole; G, Golgi body; N, nucleus; V, proacrosomal vesicles. X22,750

section a regular honey-combed structure. Sometimes it is divided in two bundles, each in a nuclear envelope-limited canal (Fig. 1 and 9). In the case of *Discoglossus pictus*, Sandoz (1977) has recently suggested that the axis originates from proteinaceous material initially contained and segregated in the acrosomal vesicle. A similar opinion had been discussed by Kaye (1962) for the sperm cell of the house cricket and by Picheral (1972) for that of the newt *Pleurodeles*. In the case of *Bombina*, a great part of the small dense masses mentioned above inside the acrosomal vesicle, is observed aggregated in front of the forming axis (Fig. 3 and 7). In that region, the acrosomal membrane is thickened, especially the two dark bands of the unit membrane.

The clear, conspicuous space of the unit membrane, approximately 35 Å wide, is crossed by very slender trabeculae (Fig. 3'). Later in the morphogenesis the axis protrudes out of the nucleus at the apical end as a large subcylindrical blunt structure. There, it is capped by a rather discrete flat acrosome (Fig. 4). Ordinarily the posterior margin of the acrosome does not overlap the nucleus' anterior material.

At the beginning of *Bombina* spermiogenesis the centrioles are situated close to the Golgi complex (Fig. 2 and 5). Later, the two perpendicular centrioles of a diplosome lie also in the vicinity of the cell plasma membrane. A flagellum arises from the centriole which is perpendicular to this membrane (and shall become the distal centriole). The flagellum protrudes into a cavity that in transverse section looks apparently closed

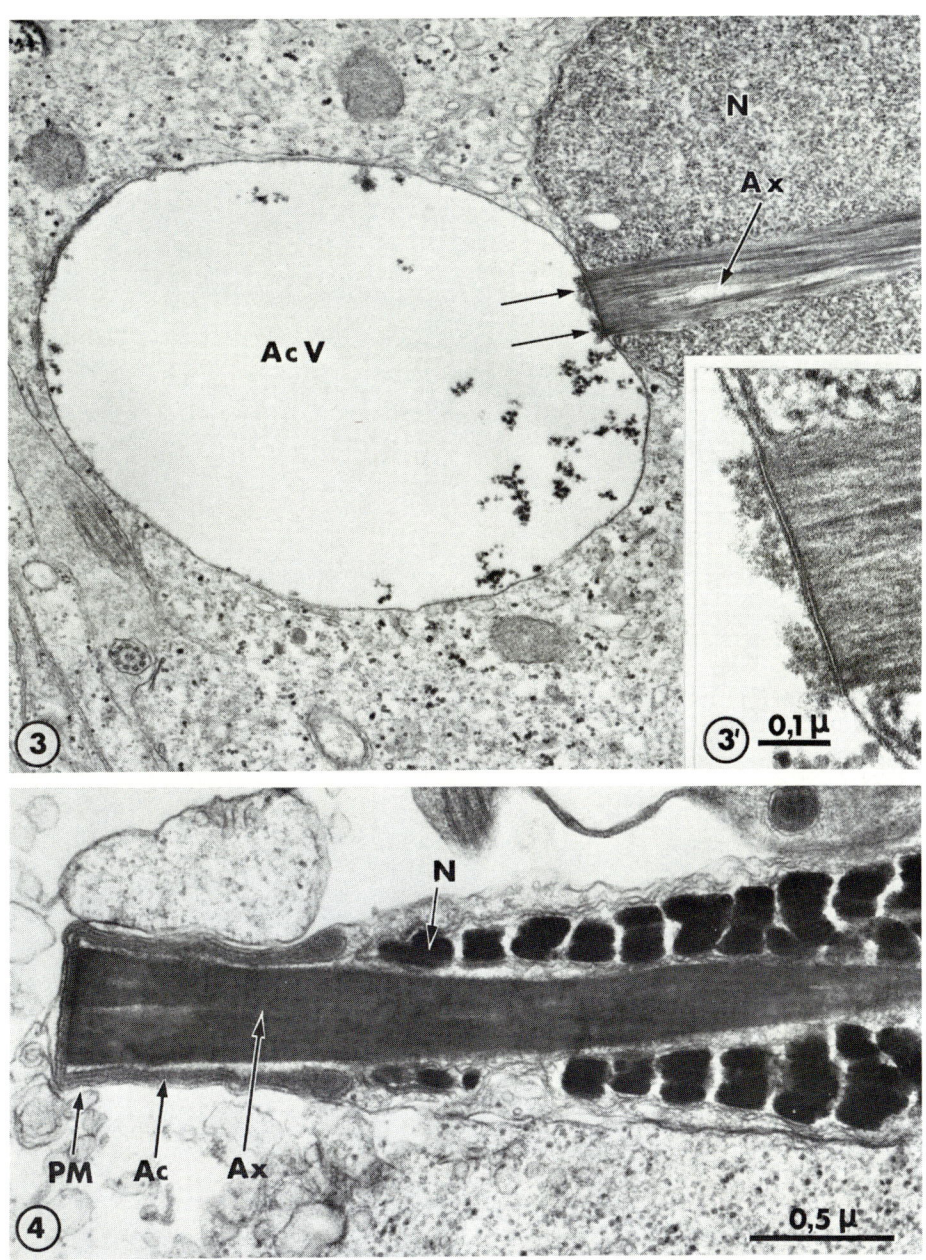

Figure 3. Part of a spermatid cell. AcV, acrosomal vesicle; arrows indicate aggregation of dense masses in front of the axis. Ax, axis; N, nucleus. X22,750
Figure 3'. Enlargement of the site indicated by the arrows in Figure 3. X91,000
Figure 4. Longitudinal section of the anterior part of a spermatozoon. Ac, acrosome; Ax, axis; N, nucleus. X39,000

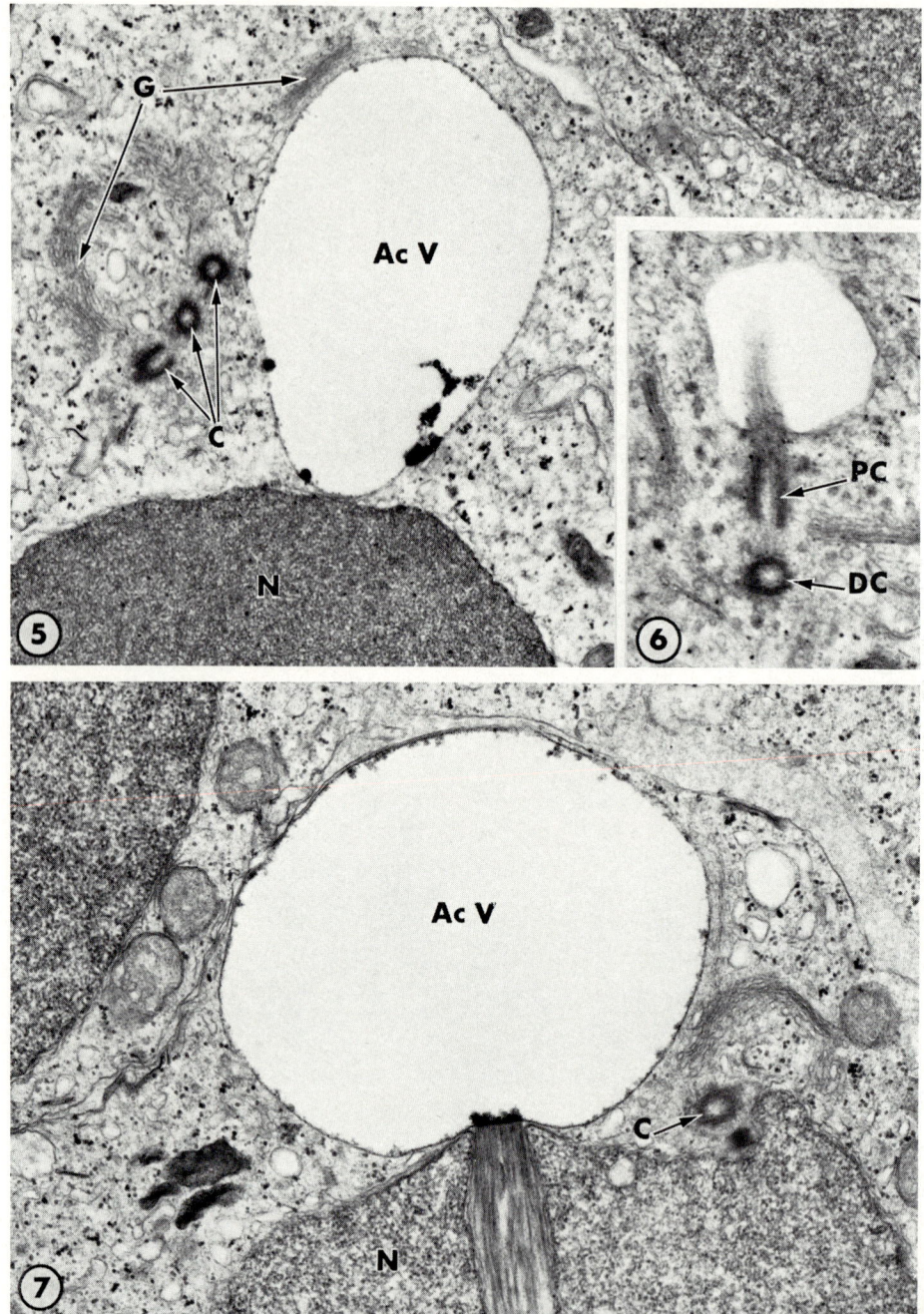

Figure 5. Part of a spermatid cell. AcV, acrosomal vesicle; C, centrioles; G, golgi; N, nucleus. X17,500
Figure 6. Diplosome close to the invaginated plasma membrane. DC, distal centriole; PC, proximal centriole initiating a flagellum. X22,750
Figure 7. Part of a spermatid cell. AcV, acrosomal vesicle; C, centriole in a nuclear indentation; N, nucleus. X22,750

(Fig. 6), but in reality is a tubular cavity of the outer space invaginated in the cytoplasm. This is certainly correlated with a retraction of the diplosome toward the interior of the cell. In fact the centrioles can be seen later in a small indentation in the anterior part of the nucleus near the acrosome (Fig. 7).

In the young spermatids of most species, as in *Bombina*, the acrosome and the centriole(s) are, at first, close to each other. Later the acrosome and the centriole(s) are situated at opposite poles of the nucleus as a result either of a Golgi-centriolar complex migration or of a nuclear rotation (Stanley, 1971). In *Bombina*, this arrangement of the acrosome, nucleus, and centriole in a linear anteroposterior sequence does not occur. Since the *Bombina* spermatozoon finally becomes elongated, it can be deduced that the presence of an acrosome and a centriolar complex at two opposite poles of the nucleus is not necessary for its elongation.

In the implantation fossa of the later elongating nucleus (Fig. 8), the proximal centriole extends transversely, and the distal centriole, in a longitudinal plane, lies at a 35° angle to the sperm cell axis. Consequently

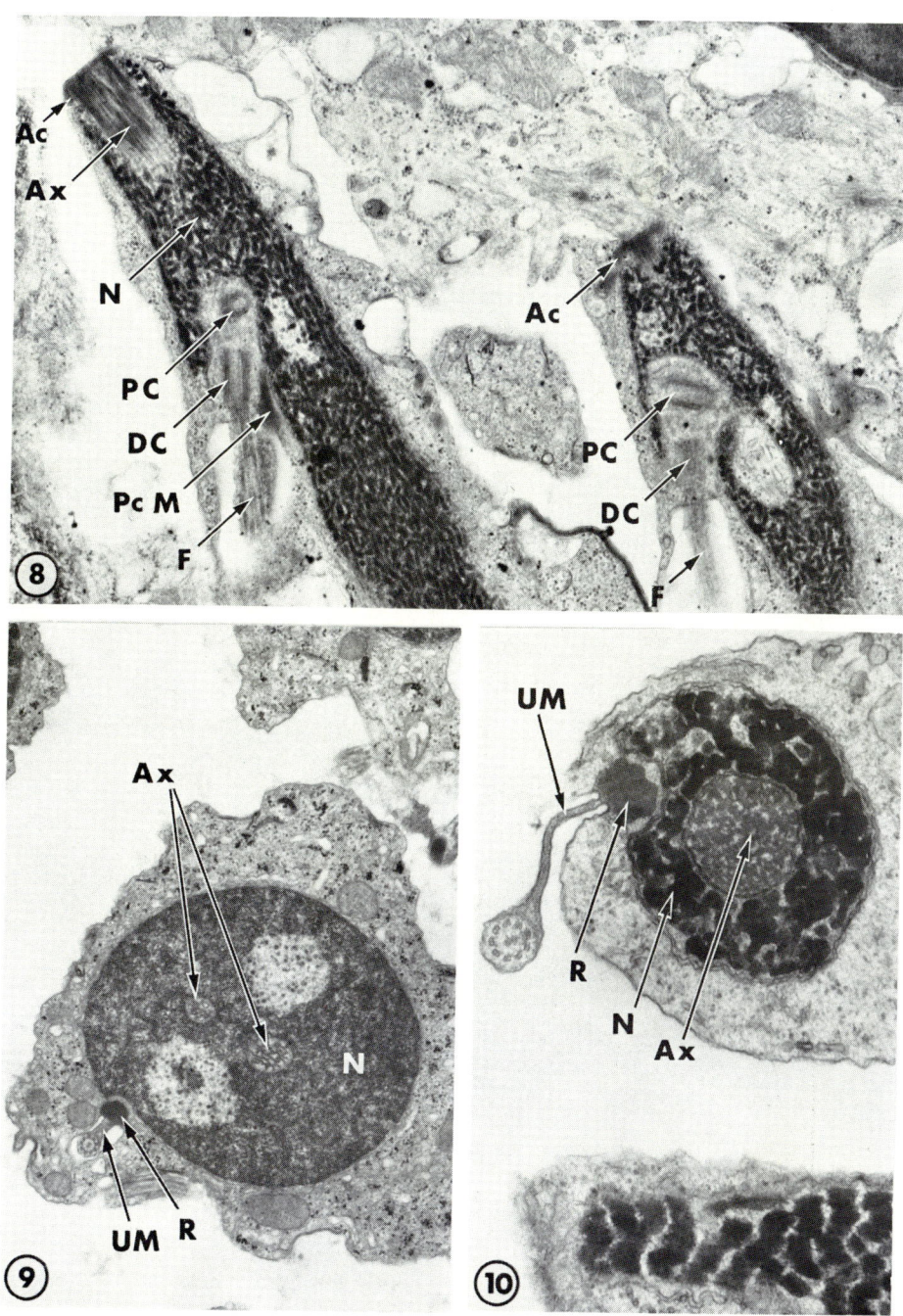

Figure 8. Longitudinal section of two late spermatids. Ax, axis; Ac, acrosome; DC, distal centriole; F, flagellum; N, nucleus; PC, proximal centriole (transverse section in spermatid on left, longitudinal section in spermatid on right); PcM, pericentriolar material. X20,500

Figure 9. Cross section in the anterior part of a spermatozoon. Ax, axis; N, nucleus; R, rod; UM, undulating membrane. X30,750

Figure 10. Cross section in the anterior part of a young spermatid. Ax, axis (divided in two parts); N, nucleus; R, rod; UM, undulating membrane. X15,250

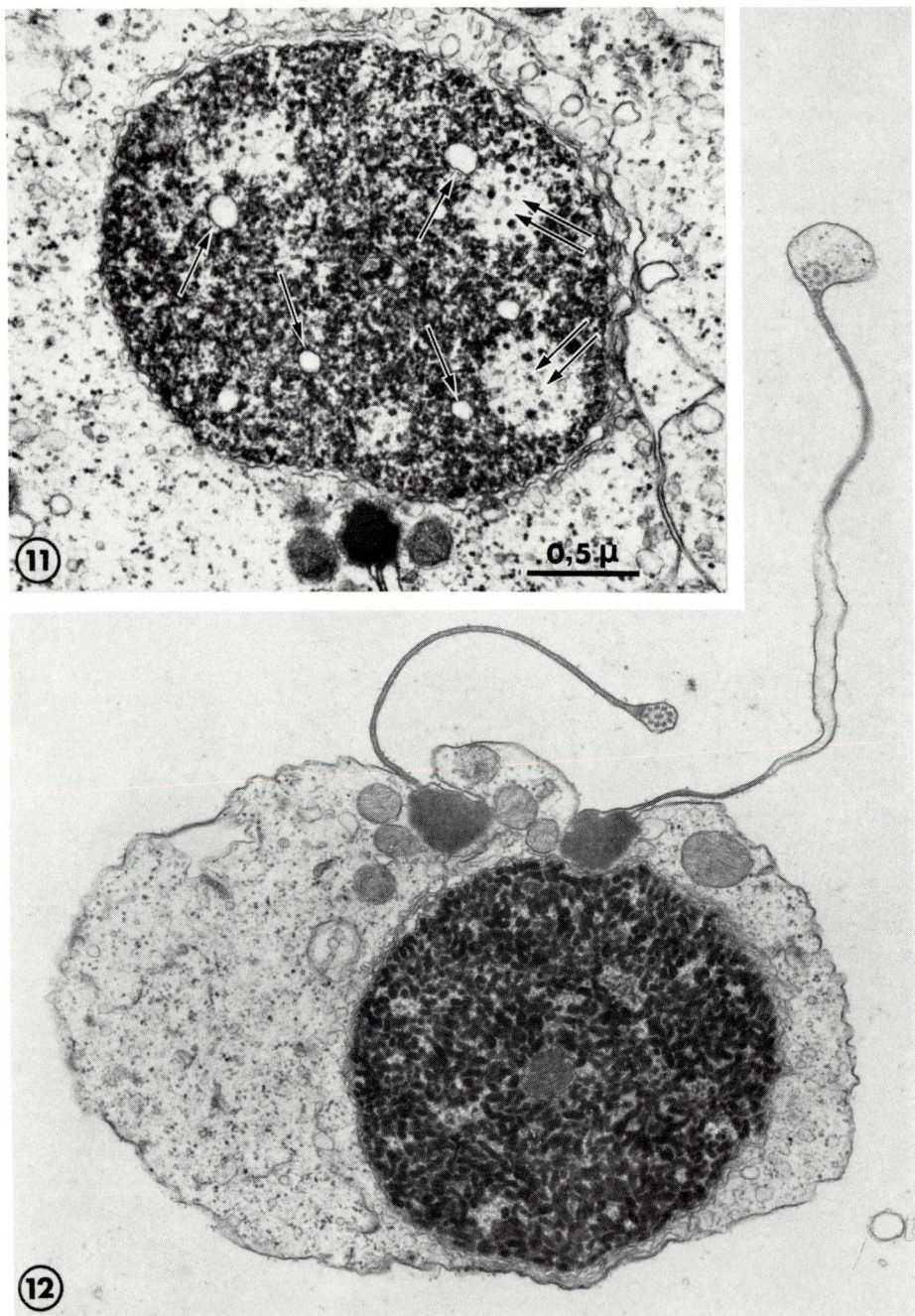

Figure 11. Cross section of a young spermatid nucleus. Single arrows: membrane-limited vacuoles. Double arrows: clear areas with dispersed granules. X29,250

Figure 12. Cross section of a sperm cell with two motile complexes. X20,900

the flagellum continuous with the distal centriole is lateral to the sperm cell. It is held at the level of doublets No. 3 and 4 by an undulating membrane (Fig. 1) connected to the cell's main body in front of a longitudinal rod of dense material. The rod extends partly in a longitudinal groove of the nucleus (Fig. 9 and 10) and is surrounded by mitochondria (Fig. 1). At its anterior it is continuous with a dense mass of pericentriolar material (Fig. 8). The rod can be almost totally digested after incubation of thin sections in a solution of 0.1% pronase for 30 min. This reveals its proteinaceous composition. The rod can be considered as functionally homologous to the postnuclear axial rod of the urodele spermatozoon (Picheral, this volume) and to the postnuclear lateral rod of the toad *Bufo arenarum* sperm cell (Burgos and Fawcett, 1956). *Bombina* sperm cells with two motile complexes are not uncommon (Fig. 12), a fact that can be correlated with the presence of more than two centrioles in some spermatids (Fig. 5).

The nuclear content of the young spermatid consists of fine chromatin granules, clear areas with some dispersed granules and numerous membrane-limited clear vacuoles (Fig. 11). In later spermiogenesis these latter vacuoles disappear and the chromatin granules condense into a number of almost prismatic lumps of the same size which show, in longitudinal sections, a kind of regular arrangement (Fig. 4). Consequently the *Bombina* spermatozoon nucleus, even in sexually mature animals, is never homogeneous and compact as it is in most species. Even in the most mature stages of testicular sperm cells a residual cytoplasm is present.

To sum up, most of the peculiar features of the *Bombina* sperm cell can be related to the fact that the acrosome and centriole complexes remain, throughout the course of spermiogenesis, in closely adjacent positions.

REFERENCES

Boisson, C.; Mattei, X.; Mattei, C.: Mise en Place et Évolution du Complexe Centriolaire au Cours de la Spermiogenèse d'*Upeneus prayensis* C.V. (Poisson, Mullidae). J Microscopie 8(1969)103-112

Broman, I.: Über Bau und Entwicklung der Spermien von *Bombinator ignaeus*. Anat Anz 17(1900)129-145

Burgos, M.H.; Fawcett, D.W.: An Electron Microscope Study of Spermatid Differentiation in the Toad, *Bufo arenarum* Hensel. Biophys Biochem Cytol 2(1956)223-240

Champy, C.: Recherches sur la Spermatogenèse des Batraciens et les Éléments Accessoires du Testicule. Arch Zool Gen Exp 52(1913)13-304

Furieri, P.: The Peculiar Morphology of the Spermatozoon of *Bombina variegata* L. Monit Zool Ital 9(1975)185-201

Kaye, J.S.: Acrosome Formation in the House Cricket. J Cell Biol 12(1962)411-443

Marchand, B.; Mattei, X.: La Spermatogenèse des Acanthocéphales. III. Formation du Dérivé Centriolaire au Cours de la Spermiogenèse de *Serrasentis socialis* Van Cleave, 1924 (Paleacanthocephala, Gorgorhinchidae). J Ultrastruct Res 59(1977)263-271

Picheral, B.: Les Éléments Cytoplasmiques au Cours de la Spermiogenèse du Triton *Pleurodeles waltlii* Michah. I. La Genèse de l'Acrosome. Z Mikrosk Anat H Zellf. 131(1972)347-370

Reed, S.C.; Stanley, H.P.: Fine Structure of Spermatogenesis in the South African Clawed Toad *Xenopus laevis* Daudin. J Ultrastruct Res 41(1972)277-295

Sapsford, C.S.; Rae, C.A.; Cleland, K.W.: Ultrastructural Studies on Spermatids and Sertoli Cells during Early Spermiogenesis in the Bandicoot *Parameles nasuta* Geoffroy (Marsupiala). Aust J Zool 15(1967)881-909

Sandoz, D.: Étude Comparative des Phénomènes Sécrétoires dans L'Appareil Génital de Quelques Vertébrés. Thèse Doctorat d'Etat, Université Paris VI, 1977

Stanley, H.P.: Fine Structure of Spermiogenesis in the Elasmobranch Fish *Squalus suckleyi*. I. Acrosome Formation, Nuclear Elongation and Differentiation of the Midpiece Axis. J Ultrastruct Res 36(1971)86-102

CLASSIFICATION OF ABNORMALITIES IN HUMAN SPERMATIDS BASED ON RECENT ADVANCES IN ULTRASTRUCTURE RESEARCH ON SPERMATID DIFFERENTIATION

A.F. Holstein* and C. Schirren

Departments of Microscopic Anatomy and Andrology, Eppendorf University Hospital, University of Hamburg, Germany

When diagnosing human fertility disturbances only by means of light microscopy, in most cases, the structure of the germinal epithelium was investigated. Provided that biopsy material of the human testis is routinely embedded in Epon, there is the possibility of electron microscopic analysis of human spermatids as part of any diagnostic screening program. Thanks to cooperation among andrologists, dermatologists, and urologists, such material is available at Hamburg University Clinics. In about 50% of the cases studied by this laboratory disturbances of the differentiation of spermatids have been detected. Such an electron microscopic diagnostic procedure appears rewarding, since the patient can be informed, with a high degree of reliability, about the extent and severity of the actual disturbance in the differentiation of spermatids, and a prognosis can be formulated upon which decisions, such as adoption of children, can be based when there is a strong wish for children in the face of a negligible or negative fertility situation in the male.

The basis for our investigations is a detailed knowledge of subcellular structures that play a role in the differentiation of human spermatids. The understanding of several of these structures and their importance in spermatid differentiation is hampered by their rather transient appearance in the process of spermatid maturation. Some of these transient subcellular structures have been characterized by Fawcett (1977). However, at the present time, it is still rather difficult to define which of those structures are regular ones, which are biologically tolerable variants of such normal structures and which are abnormal and, therefore, a possible cause of infertility.

A large scientific exploratory program is required to characterize and evaluate these numerous variants and abnormalities. This chapter presents only a very small selection of the correlative clinical and morphological work the authors have performed in this field.

The individual steps in the process of spermatid differentiation in man are well characterized by Horstmann (1961), De Kretser (1969), Wartenberg and Holstein (1975), and Holstein (1976). In the first diagram (Fig. 1), the most important events are outlined: the formation of the acrosome, the nuclear condensation process, and the establishment of the flagellar structures. The development of spermatids is subdivided into eight stages according to significant cytological features.

Special attention should be focused on only two details: the spindle-shaped body of the tail and the so-called flower-like structures.

The spindle-shaped body consists of wound tubular structures about 200 Å in diameter and which, as a whole, appears as local enlargement of the tail. It is first seen in stage three of the differentiation process (Fig. 2) and which vanishes during stage 6. This transient structure is located at a position corresponding to the midpiece in the mature spermatid; it extends from the distal centriole to the upper portion of the main piece, thus measuring about 4 μm in length. The spindle-shaped body occupies the space of the mitochondrial sheath of the midpiece and may be responsible for the formation of the fibrous sheath of the main piece.

Concomitant with the reduction of the spindle-shaped body, the fibrous sheath is gradually established. Transitions of tubular structures of the spindle-shaped body into ribs of the fibers can be demonstrated (Fig. 3). The relatively short time period during which the spindle-shaped body exists and its characteristic stages in development and involution permit a more precise classification of different forms of spermatids within the complex course of the differentiation of human spermatids than previous classifications based

---

*Supported by grants of the Deutsche Forschungsgemeinschaft
© 1979 Urban & Schwarzenberg, Inc. Baltimore-Munich *The Spermatozoon*, edited by D.W. Fawcett and J.M. Bedford

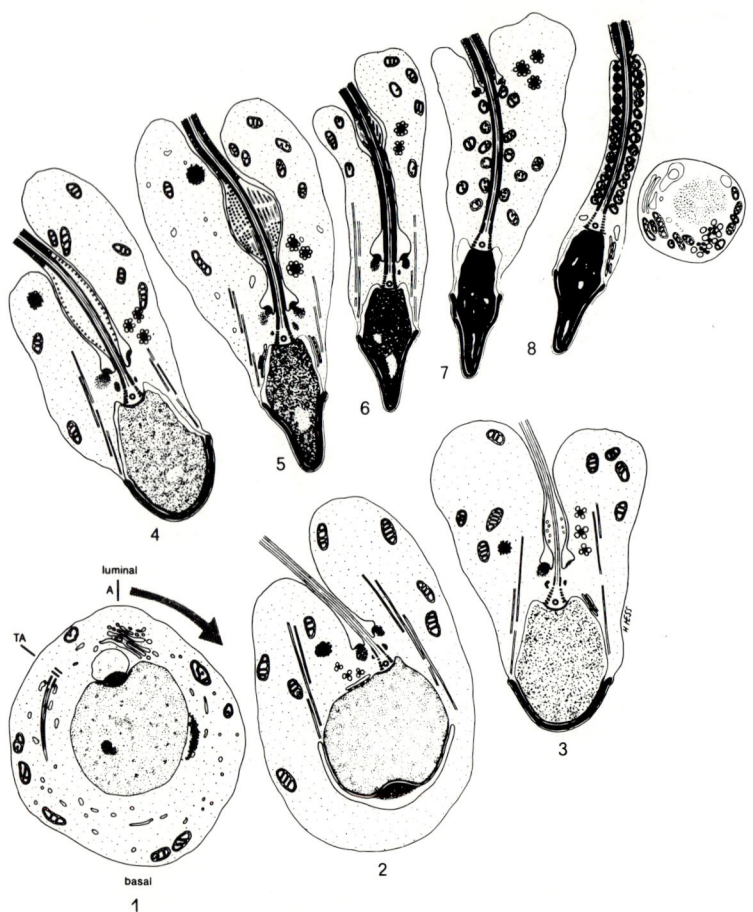

Figure 1. Semischematic drawing of spermatid differentiation. According to the development of the acrosome, the condensation of the nucleus, and the development of tail structures eight stages can be distinguished. Drawing based on electron micrographs.

on evaluations of the shape of the acrosome, the process of nuclear condensation, or shape of the nucleus itself (Clermont 1963; De Kretser 1969).

Another, hitherto neglected structure occurs transiently during the differentiation of spermatids (Fig. 4a): flower-like structures consisting of a central, electron-dense granular core and surrounding vesicle clusters (Fig. 4b). In 1970, Susi and Clermont demonstrated comparable structures in spermatids of rats and considered them derivatives of the chromatoid body. In man, these flower-like structures appear during stage 2 of spermatid development close to the nucleus and the chromatoid body, undergo a sequence of characteristic alterations (Fig. 5), and are finally incorporated into the residual body where they disintegrate (Holstein and Schäfer 1978).

In contrast to the normal spermatid differentiation, a classification of malformations or abnormalities in human spermatids is presented. It is based on electron microscopic investigations of biopsy material from patients suffering from different andrological diseases and of testicular material obtained from castrations of men having committed indecent assault. The testicular samples derived from the latter source were found to have a regular ultrastructure and served as controls. Most of the results will be demonstrated with the help of semischematic diagrams drawn from appropriate electron microscopic pictures.

From all the abnormalities detected so far, malformations of the acrosome are the most frequent. The following types may be distinguished:

1. Malformations of the acrosome attached to the nucleus of the spermatid (Fig. 6). In early spermatids, the following abnormalities are recognized:
   - (1.1) lack of electron-dense material in the acrosome vesicle;
   - (1.2) incorporation of additional vesicles and electron-dense particles into the acrosome vesicle;
   - (1.3-1.4) incorporation of membrane-bound vesicle clusters into the acrosome vesicle;

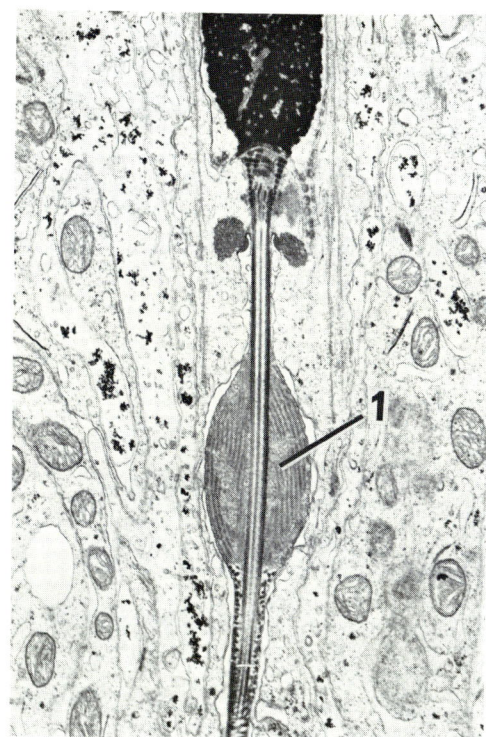

Figure 2. Spindle-shaped body (1) of a spermatid at stage 5 of development. X12,000

(1.5) a partial enlargement of the acrosome;
(1.6) separation of the acrosome from the nucleus and the interposition of vesicles in between both structures;
(1.7) gigantic acrosome vesicles without electron-dense material; and
(1.8) two acrosome vesicles attached to one nucleus.

In later spermatids, similar abnormalities may be found: (Fig. 7):

(1.9) enlargement of the acrosome,
(1.10-1.13) partial invagination of the acrosome into the nucleus of the spermatid;
(1.14) separation of the acrosome from the nucleus of the spermatid;
(1.15) formation of a butt-like enlargement at the upper margin of the acrosome;
(1.16-1.17) an acrosome vacuole partly filled with small vesicles; and
(1.18) incorporation of numerous canaliculi into the acrosome.

2. Malformations of the acrosome, which lacks contact to the nucleus of the spermatid (Fig. 8):

(2.1) lack of attachment of the acrosome vesicle to the nucleus and lack of orientation of the electron-dense material in the vesicle towards the nucleus;
(2.2) acrosome vesicles that consist of small vesicle aggregates;
(2.3) formation of several acrosome vesicles without electron-dense content;
(2.4) splitting of the acrosome into two ring-like structures;
(2.5) formation of an acrosome that consists of a single spherical electron-dense body;
(2.6) vesicle with incorporated clusters of small vesicles;
(2.7) cap-like acrosomes without contact to the nucleus and with interposed vesicles;
(2.8) formation of a vesicle that establishes restricted point-like contact to the nucleus of a spermatid;
(2.9) the acrosome appears as a shell-like structure that resides in the cytoplasm of the spermatid;
(2.10) the nucleus of the spermatid is devoid of an acrosome but instead is surrounded by several membranes; and
(2.11) the acrosome has a cap-like shape, occupying, inside the elongated cytoplasm of the

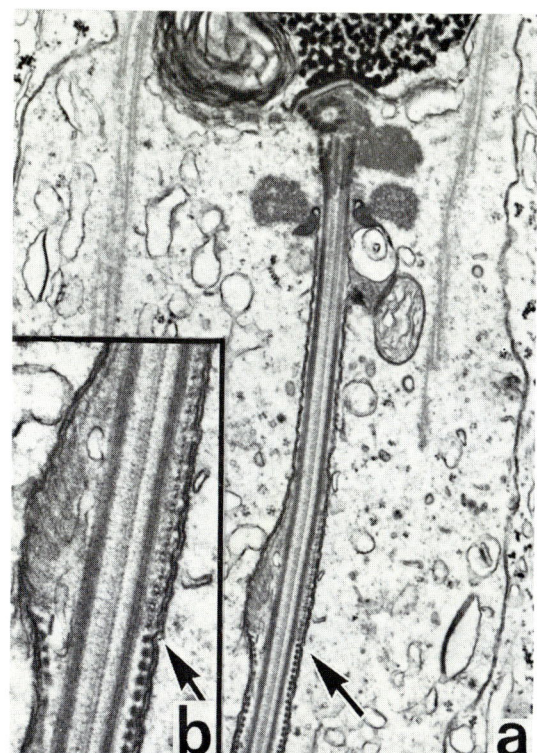

Figure 3. Transition (arrow) of tubular structures of the involuting spindle-shaped body into the ribs of the main piece. a) X16,000, b) X40,000

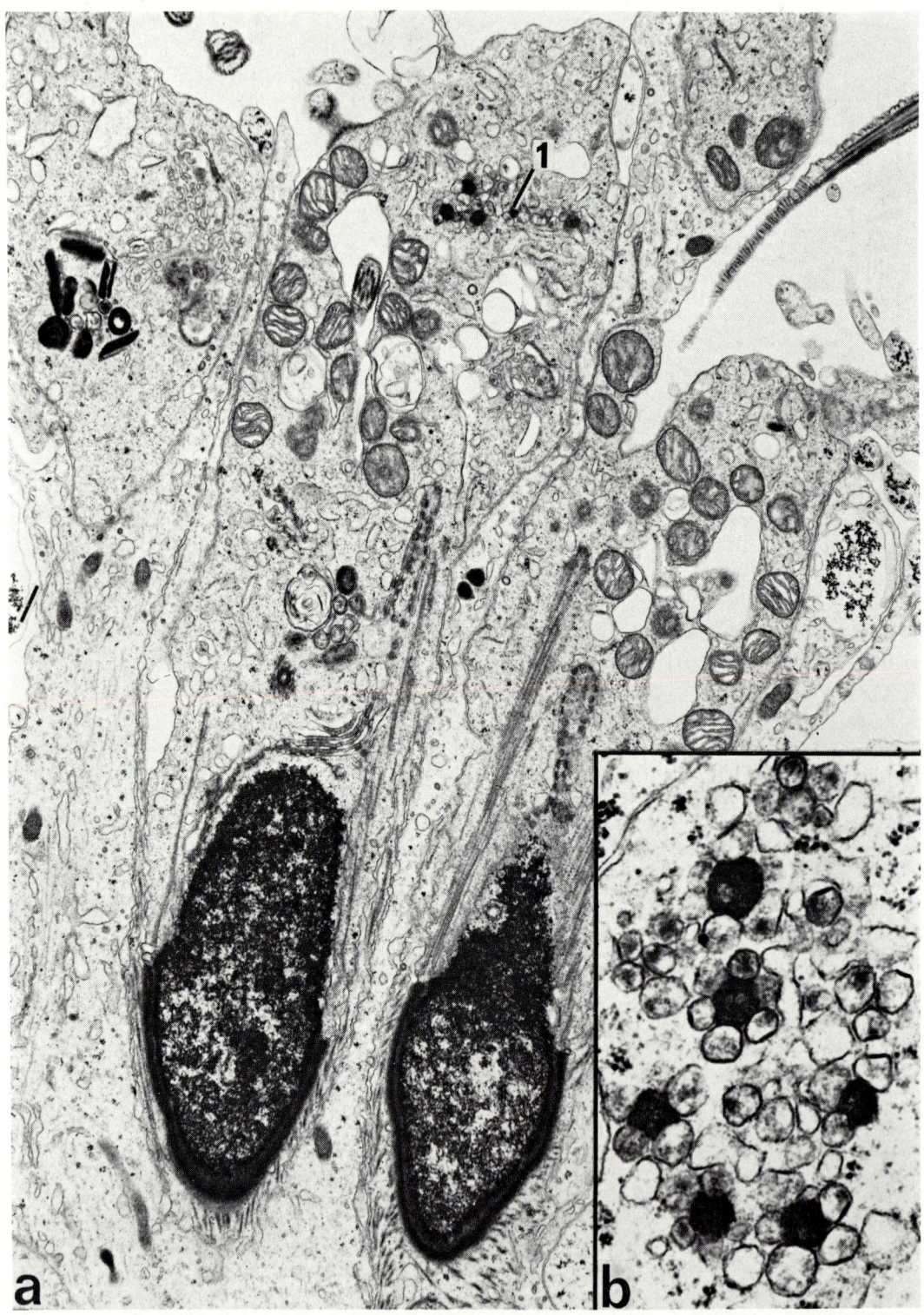

Figure 4. a) Developing spermatids with flower-like structures (1) X13,000. b) Higher magnification of aggregated flower-like structures. X40,000

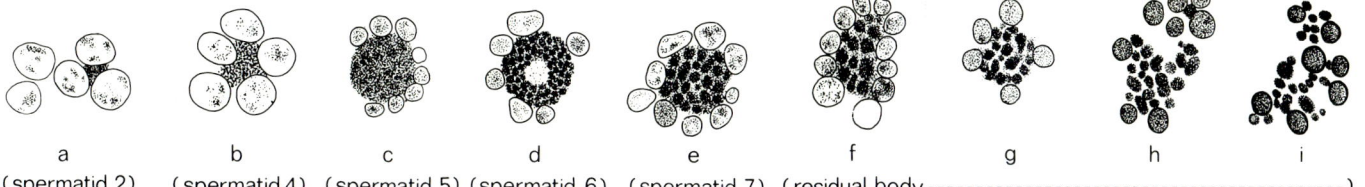

a b c d e f g h i
(spermatid 2) (spermatid 4) (spermatid 5) (spermatid 6) (spermatid 7) (residual body------------------------------)

Figure 5. Summarization of the development of flower-like structures, correlated to the stages of spermatid differentiation.

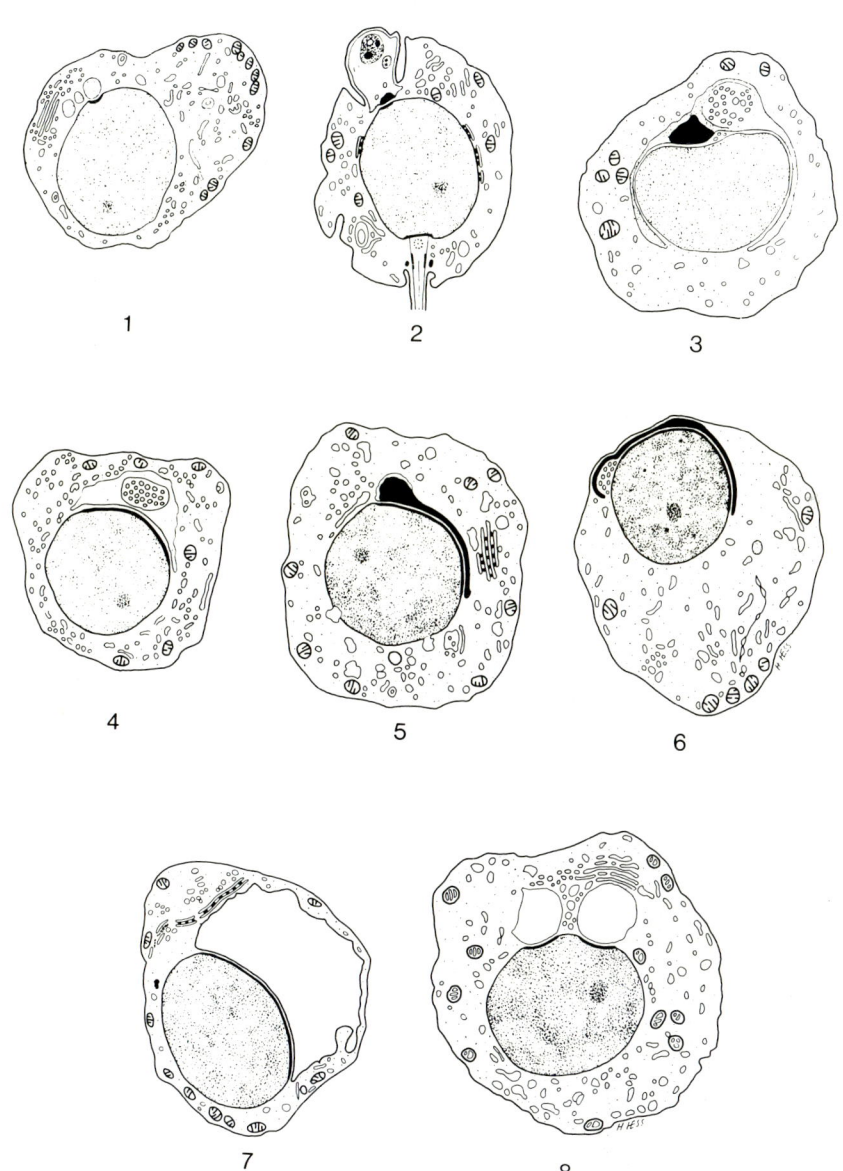

Figure 6. Malformations of the acrosome attached to the nucleus of younger spermatids. For details see text. (Modified from Holstein, 1975)

Classification of Abnormalities in Human Spermatids / 345

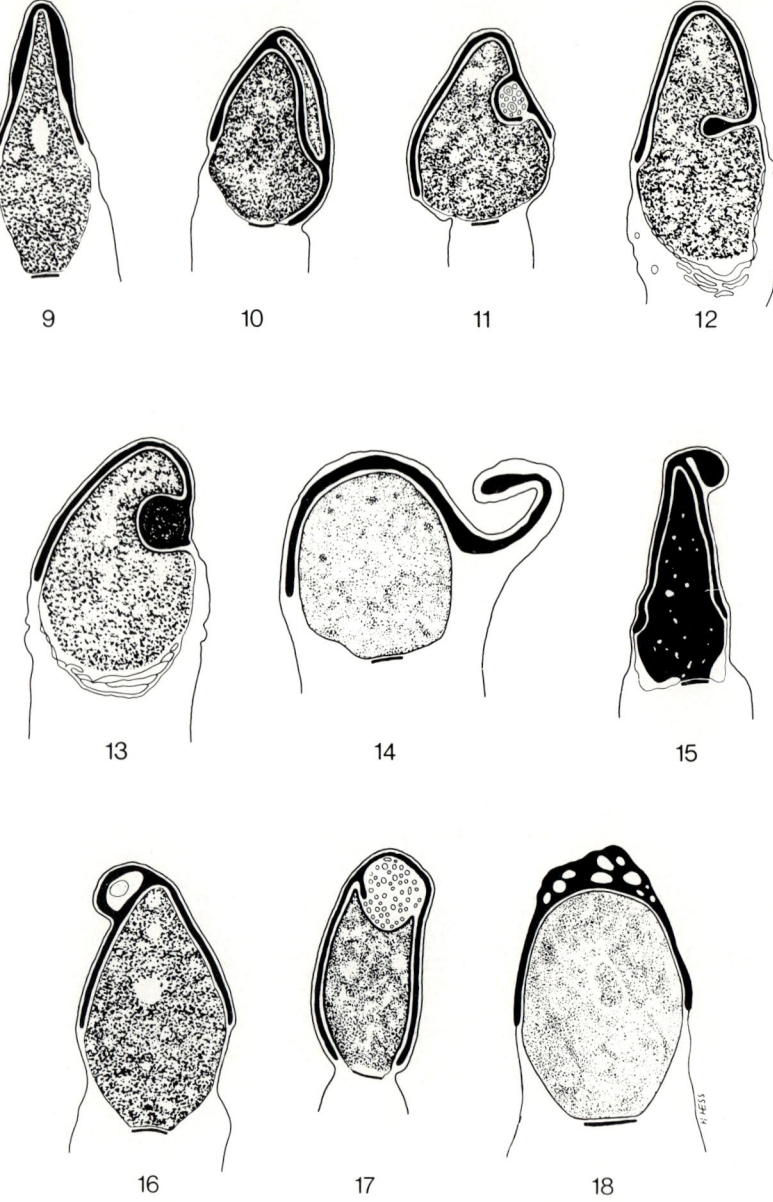

Figure 7. Malformations similar to those in Figure 6, but in more developed spermatids.

spermatid, a position rather remote from the nucleus.

3. Multinucleate spermatids (Fig. 9):
   (3.1) two nuclei are linked by an acrosomal vesicle;
   (3.2) the acrosome contains additional vesicles;
   (3.3) one acrosome covers two nuclei;
   (3.4) a centrally situated acrosome vesicle connects several nuclei;
   (3.5) two or more nuclei are linked together by one acrosome;
   (3.6) in multinucleated spermatids, rather bizarre forms of acrosomes may be found.

4. Nuclear inclusions and disturbances of the nuclear condensation process (Fig. 10):
   (4.1-4.4) several layers of membranes or aggregated tubules are contained in the karyoplasm;
   (4.5) the abundance of membranes may cause a displacement of the nuclear chromatin;
   (4.6-4.7) the nuclear membrane issues surplus membrane systems;

(4.8) the nucleus of the spermatid may have large areas of irregularly condensed DNA;
(4.9) globular inclusions are seen in the nucleus;
(4.10) from the redundant membrane extensive membrane systems are seen to originate, there being no indication for a condensation of the karyoplasm.

5. Malformations of the tail (Fig. 11 and 12). It is sometimes rather difficult to distinguish normal from abnormal structures. This holds in particular for the centrioles and the neck region. Some abnormalities of the midpiece and main piece may be demonstrated in longitudinal sections of spermatids:
   (5.1) lack of mitochondrial sheath;
   (5.2) lack or malformation of the fibrous sheath of the main piece;
   (5.3) dissolution of the axonema; and
   (5.4) an isolated tail anlage without contact to the nucleus of the spermatid.

6. Transverse sections of spermatid tails reveal consistently the following defects:
   (6.1-6.13) suppressed or surplus microtubules and axonemata;
   (6.14) duplicated axonemata, which
   (6.15) may also occur in asymmetric halves, or
   (6.16) which may be localized outside the fibrous sheath;
   (6.19) depicts a strongly enlarged fibrous sheath; and
   (6.20) presents an engulfment of the fibrous sheath by the mitochondrial sheath. To this diagram should be added the malformation described by Afzelius *et al.* (1975) and by Pedersen and Rebbe (1975) in which there is a loss of the lateral arms of the microtubules. Despite careful research the authors failed to detect this particular abnormality.

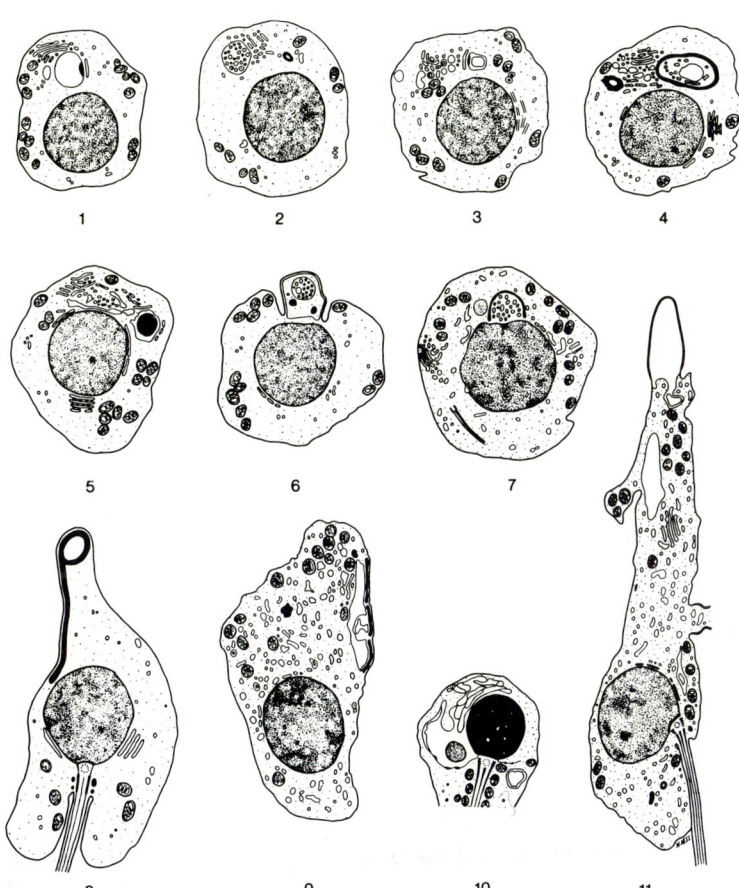

Figure 8. Malformations of the acrosome lacking contact with the nucleus of the spermatid. For details see text. (Modified from Holstein, 1975)

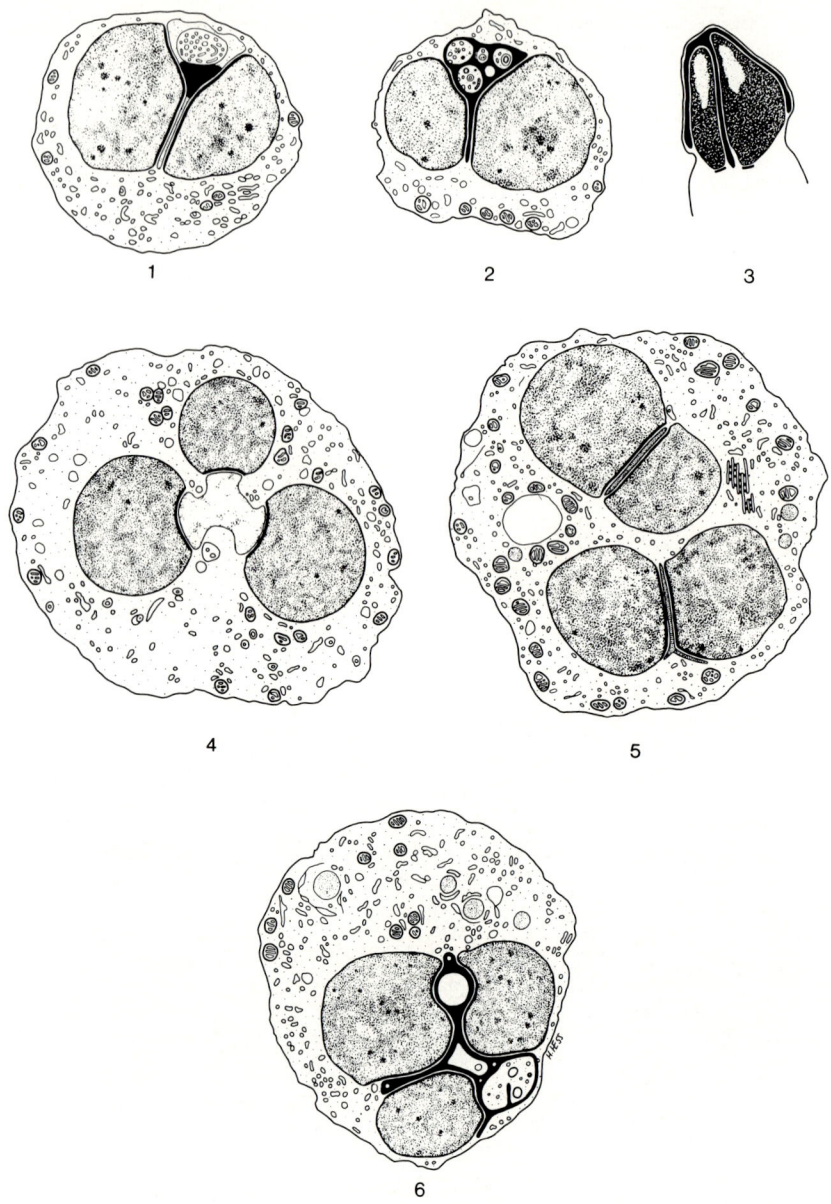

Figure 9. Multinucleated spermatids. For details see text. (Modified from Holstein, 1975)

All of the malformations outlined above may occur as separate abnormalities in individual spermatozoa, or in various combinations. Of special interest are those cases in which all spermatids/spermatozoa derived from the patient are affected by the same type of abnormality. In such cases, the morphogenesis of the malformation can be studied with ease since almost every spermatozoon is in a different developmental stage of its abnormality, and, furthermore, the defect appears to be genetically programmed. So far, however, chromosome analysis has failed to confirm this postulate.

The patients in this study exhibited a total of five different forms of abnormalities that belong to the latter category:

Spermatids with gigantic acrosome vesicles Already in the very early spermatids the acrosome vesicle is conspicuously large. It develops into a gigantic vacuole filled with poorly electron-opaque material that may exceed the nucleus of the spermatid in size. In binucleate spermatids the acrosome vesicle may be particularly large (Fig. 13). Electron-dense acrosomal material occurs only in the more advanced, later stages of differentiation in such spermatids. The outer membrane of this gigantic vacuole shows invaginations incorporating thin tubes of spermatid cytoplasm into the acrosome (Fig. 7 and 18). In later stages of spermatid differentiation there is no regular Sertoli cell membrane with underlying regularly arranged microfilaments facing this gigantic acrosome; rather, the microfilaments occur in sporadic bundles. At the end of their differentiation, such spermatids do have a normally condensed, but spherically shaped nucleus surmounted by a diadem-like acrosome (Fig. 7 and 18). In spread-preparations, these spermatids appear round-headed, however, these should not be confused with the acrosome-less, round-headed spermatids first described by Schirren *et al.* (1971).

Spermatids having no acrosome They lose their acrosome because of the fact that its anlage develops independently of the nucleus. A very early diagnostic criterion for this abnormality is a localization of the acrosomal dense substance which lacks topical relationship to the nucleus (Fig. 14). Even with progressing differen-

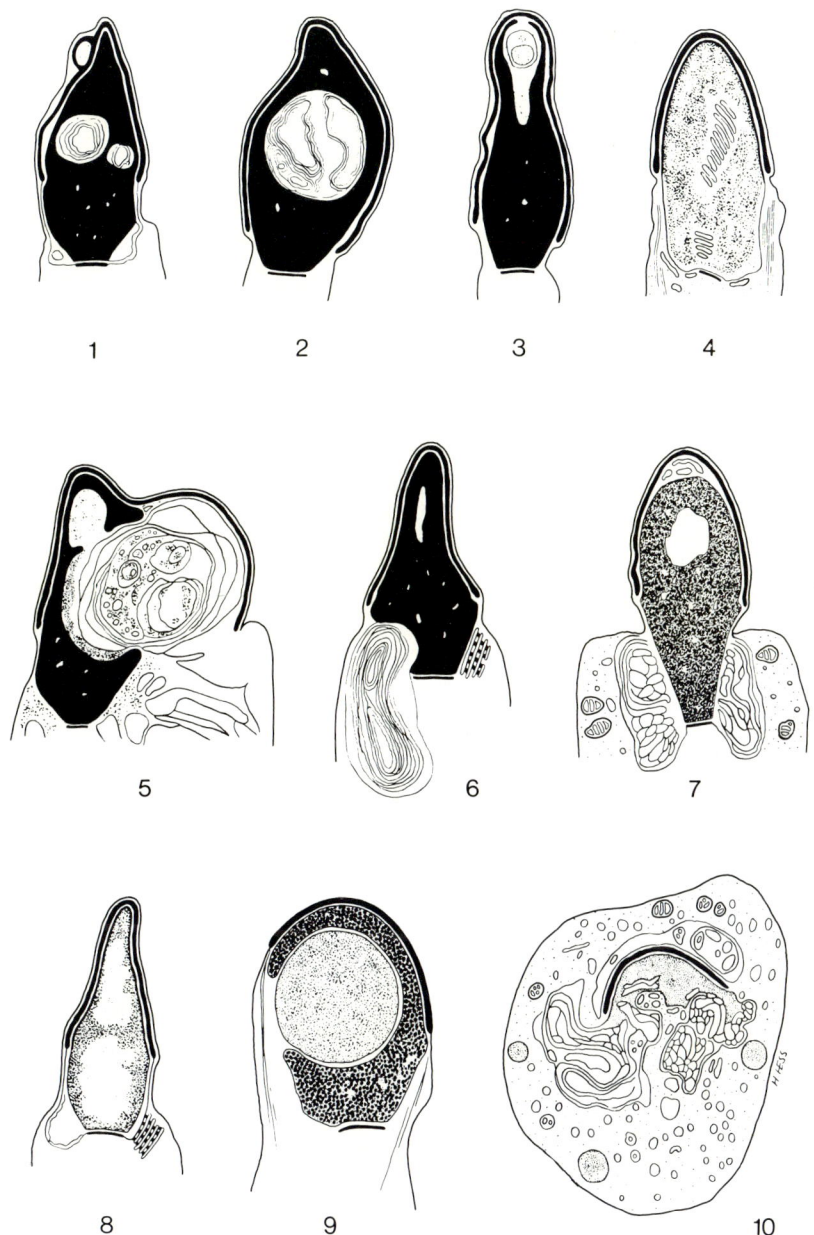

Figure 10. Nuclear inclusions and disturbances of nuclear condensation. For details see text. (Modified from Holstein, 1975)

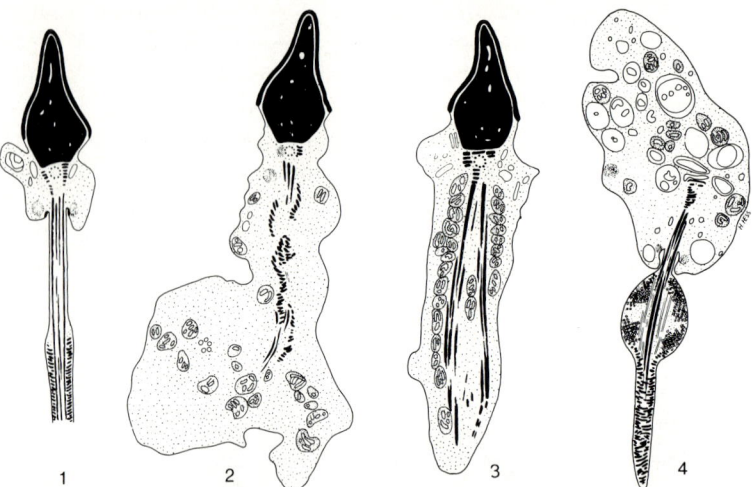

Figure 11. Malformations of the tail of the spermatid. For details see text.

tiation of the spermatids, the acrosome fails to establish close contact with the nucleus and is finally lost (Schirren *et al.*, 1971). Various differently shaped acrosome equivalents are thus formed, but all of them independent from the nucleus. The acrosome remnants are taken over by the Sertoli cell. Spermatids from nine patients were analyzed with this abnormality by means of electron microscopy: the morphogenesis of this abnormality was the same in each case. Among the patients there were additional cases with acrosome-less spermatozoa. No biopsies were taken in these cases, since the absence of acrosin (Fritz *et al.*, 1972) in the sperm in conjunction with the usual spermiogram is an adequate diagnostic indication of this abnormality.

Spoonlike nuclei in spermatids The only conspicuous alteration in this type of malformation is the strange shape of the nucleus and all remaining substructures in the spermatids appear normal. On one side the nucleus is strongly indented and thus resembles a spoon (Fig. 15). On following the development of these spermatids, it is evident that they abandon their contact with the Sertoli cells at the beginning of stage 3 of differentiation. The cell membrane that covers the acrosome borders on the extracellular space, which contains some free glycogen granules. There is no morphologically obvious reason for premature release of these spermatids from the germinal epithelium. The authors suspect that a defect in the Sertoli cell itself may cause this abnormality.

Malformation of the spermatid tail In this abnormality, already recognizable at stage 1 of spermatid differentiation, is a plump drop of cytoplasm instead of a thin cilium in which the tubules of the axonema are clustered. During the subsequent development, no regular spindle-shaped body is established, rather, the annular fibers of the main piece emerge directly from the distal centriole (Fig. 16). In addition, their number is increased. The mitochondria are located outside the fibrous sheath. Both the nucleus and acrosome look normal. All spermatozoa affected with this abnormality are nonmotile.

Multinucleate spermatids Occasionally patients are seen in whom all spermatids produced are multinucleate. As many as eight nuclei are contained in a single spermatid perikaryon. Rather complexly organized forms occur. The nuclei are joined by a centered acrosome vesicle. The electron-dense acrosomal substance is deposited between the nuclei and often contains vesicular inclusions (Fig. 9). Only binucleate spermatids often have several tails with regular structure. Multinucleate spermatids in most cases do not develop tail structures. Therefore they are nonmotile.

In conclusion, a detailed analysis of normal structures in differentiating spermatids and knowledge of the morphogenesis of their abnormalities may assist in understanding this complex and unique process of cell differentiation and may also assist in the exact diagnosis and prognosis of fertility disturbances.

SUMMARY

The foregoing essay includes three parts: 1) A short review of normal spermatid differentiation, with special attention focused on two transiently appearing subcellular structures, *e.g.*, the spindle-shaped body of spermatid tail and the so-called flower-like structures, 2) A classification of malformations of human spermatids, and 3) Particular malformations of spermatids that make up 100% of spermatids in biopsy material of certain patients:

a) spermatids with gigantic acrosome vesicles,
b) spermatids having no acrosome,
c) malformations of the main piece,
d) spoon-like nuclei in spermatids,
e) multinucleate spermatids.

These malformations are accompanied by infertility and may be considered as pathomorphological correlates of certain andrological diseases.

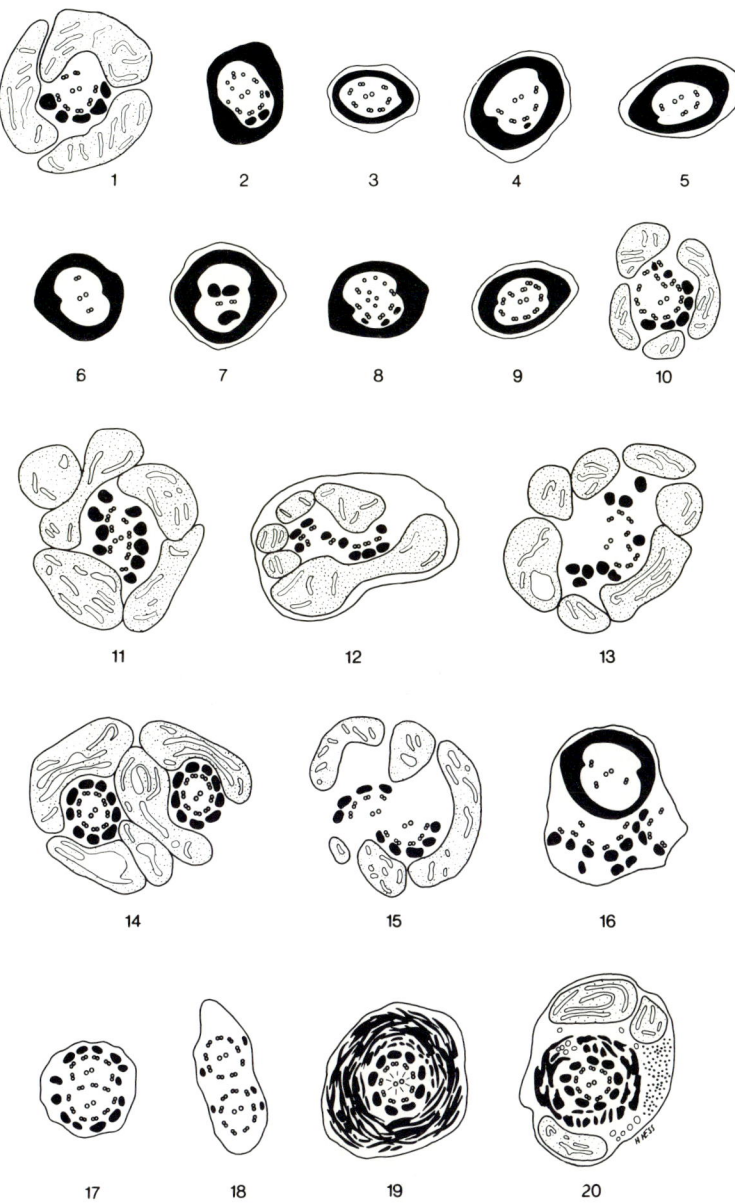

Figure 12. Transverse sections of malformed spermatid tails. For details see text. (Modified from Holstein, 1975)

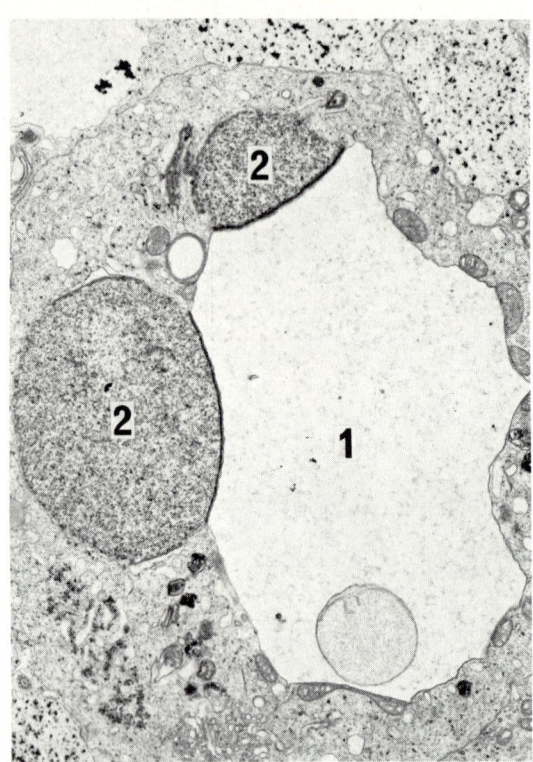

Figure 13. Gigantic acrosome vesicle (1) facing two nuclei (2) X5000

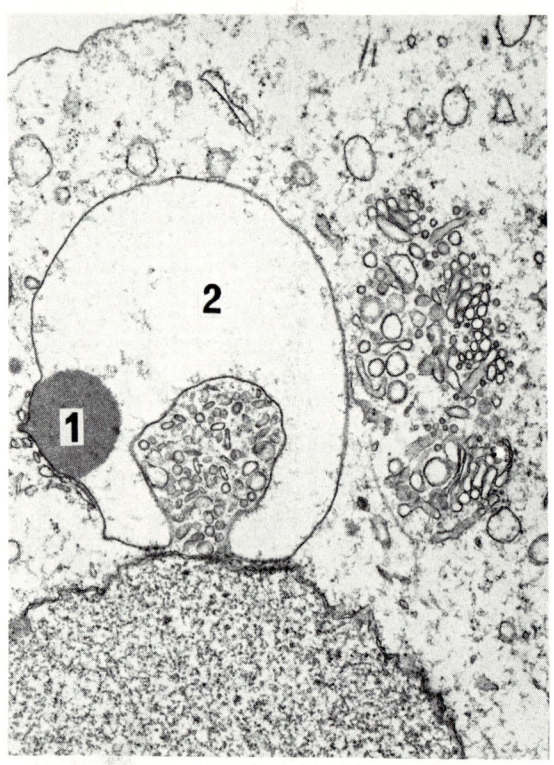

Figure 14. Maloriented electron dense material (1) in the acrosome vesicle (2) as an early indication of round-headed acrosomeless spermatozoa. X16,000

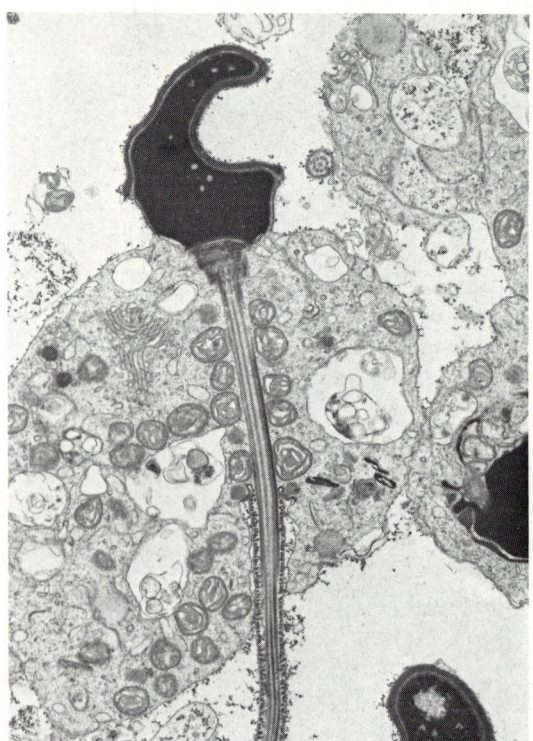

Figure 15. Spoon-like nucleus in a severe case of spermatid malformation. X12,000

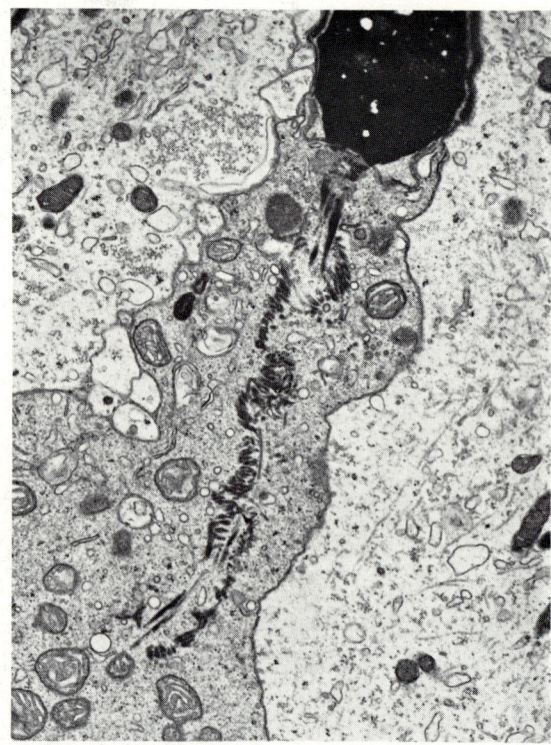

Figure 16. Clustered axonema structures in a special case of malformation of the main piece. X14,000

REFERENCES

Afzelius, B.A.; Eliasson, R.; Johnsen, Ø.; Lindholmer, C.: Lack of Dynein Arms in Immotile Human Spermatozoa. J Cell Biol 66(1975)225-232

Clermont, Y.: The Cycle of the Seminiferous Epithelium in Man. Am J Anat 112(1963)35-51

De Kretser, D.M.: Ultrastructural Features of Human Spermiogenesis. Z Zellfarsch. 98(1969)477-505

Fawcett, D.W.: Unsolved Problems in Morphogenesis of the Mammalian Spermatozoon. In: International Cell Biology, pp. 588-601, ed. by D.R. Brinkley and K.R. Porter. Rockefeller University Press, 1977

Fritz, H.; Förg-Brey, B.; Fink, E.; Meier, M.; Schießler, H.; Schirren, C.: Humanacrosin: Gewinnung und Eigenschaften. Hoppe-Seylers Z Physiol Chem 353(1972)1943-1949

Holstein, A.F.: Morphologische Studien an abnormen Spermatiden und Spermatozoen des Menschen. Virchows Arch [Pathol Anat] 367(1975)93-112

Holstein, A.F.: Ultrastructural Observations on the Differentiation of Spermatids in Man. Andrologia 8(1976)157-165

Holstein, A.F.; Schäfer, E.: A Further Type of Transient Cytoplasmic Organelle in Human Spermatids. Cell Tiss Res 192(1978)359-361

Horstmann, E.: Elektronenmikroskopische Untersuchungen zur Spermiohistogenese beim Menschen. Z Zellfarsch 54(1961)68-89

Pedersen, H., Rebbe, H.: Absence of avrus in the axoneme of immobile human permatozoa. Biol. Reprod. 12(1975)541-544

Schirren, C.G.; Holstein, A.F.; Schirren, C.: Über die Morphogenese rundköpfiger Spermatozoen des Menschen. Andrologie 3(1971)117-125

Susi, F.R.; Clermont, Y.: Fine Structural Modifications of the Rat Chromatoid Body during Spermiogenesis. Am J Anat 129(1970)177-192

Wartenberg, H.; Holstein, A.F.: Morphology of the "Spindle-shaped Body" in the Developing Tail of Human Spermatids. Cell Tiss Res 159(1975)435-443

THE ULTRASTRUCTURE OF THE PROSPERMIUM OF ORNITHODOROS TICKS AND ITS RELATION TO SPERM MATURATION AND CAPACITATION

B. Feldman-Muhsam and B.K. Filshie

Hadassah Medical School, The Hebrew University, Jerusalem, Israel; Commonwealth Scientific and Industrial Research Organization, Division of Entomology, Canberra, Australia

Maturation and capacitation of sperm cells in ticks are accompanied by considerable changes in form. These changes occur in two stages. The first, known as spermateleosis, takes place in the female genital tract, inside the capsules of the endospermatophore and immediately after copulation. The second stage occurs only when the sperm cells migrate out of the capsules to the oviducts, and consists of the evagination of the acrosomal canal which, until then, is concealed within the posterior part of the sperm.

When stored in the vesiculum seminalis ready to be ejaculated during copulation, the sperm cells are generally in the form of relatively short rods which have been called "spermatids" (Nordenskiöld, 1909; Reger, 1961) or "advanced spermatids" (Brinton et al., 1974, or "prospermia" (Oppermann, 1935; Balashov, 1967). In view of the considerable differences between the forms of the sperm cell before and after spermateleosis, it seems appropriate to use different terms for the two stages. Hereafter, the cell in the stage prior to spermateleosis will be referred to as the prospermium, and after, as the spermiophore. The term spermatid is reserved for forms found in the testis. Although, for the mature sperm cell, many authors prefer the term spermatozoon, these authors have adopted the term spermiophore proposed by Tuzet and Millot (1937), because in the tick the enormous cell is certainly not involved, in its entirety, in fertilization.

MATERIALS AND METHODS

Male ticks *Ornithodoros gurneyi* and *O. tholozani* that had a blood meal were dissected in cold 0.9% saline and the vesiculum seminalis transferred to and opened under ice-cold 2.5% glutaraldehyde fixative in 0.05 M cacodylate buffer containing 0.15 M sucrose at pH 7.2.

Impregnated females were similarly dissected, and spermiophores recovered from both endospermatophores and ampullae were fixed to obtain sperm cells at various stages of maturation and capacitation.

After glutaraldehyde fixation, sperm cells were washed in several changes of 0.05 M cacodylate buffer containing 0.15 M sucrose at pH 7.2 and room temperature, post fixed with 1% osmium tetroxide in 0.05 M cacodylate buffer for 2 h at room temperature, dehydrated, and embedded in epoxy resin.

Thin (approximately 50 nm) sections were stained with uranyl acetate and lead citrate and examined in either a Siemens Elmiskop I or a JEOL 100C transmission electron microscope.

RESULTS AND DISCUSSION

Morphology

The morphology of the prospermia has been studied in *Argas miniatus* (Casteel, 1917) and in *A. persicus* (Sharma, 1944). The ultrastructure of *Amblyomma dissimili* has been examined by Reger (1961) and that of *Ornithodoros moubata*, by Breucker and Horstmann (1972). There are, however, several gaps in our knowledge of internal structures and disagreement between authors regarding the functions of organelles of the sperm cell.

The prospermium is an elongated cell 227-247 μm long in *O. gurneyi* and 405-464 μm in *O. tholozani*. It is composed of the same components as the future spermiophore, but folded upon itself like a cuff.

The prospermium (Fig. 1) consists of an inner core surrounded by an outer sheath. The space between the core and the sheath is filled with cytoplasmic material (described below). The inner core and the outer sheath are about equal in length and one is actually a continuation of the other, the continuation being at the posterior end of the prospermium, if the end where the

© 1979 Urban & Schwarzenberg, Inc. Baltimore-Munich *The Spermatozoon*, edited by D.W. Fawcett and J.M. Bedford

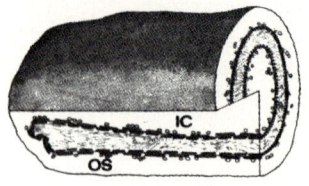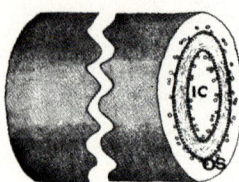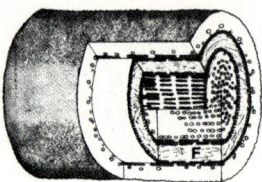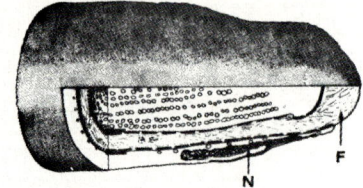

Figure 1. Cutaway diagram of the prospermium. The inner core (IC) and outer sheath (OS) are separated by a space containing a filamentous matrix (F). The nucleus (N) is located in the outer sheath, at the anterior end of the prospermium.

"head" of the inner core lies is considered anterior. The tail end of the outer sheath is therefore at the anterior end of the prospermium, near the "head" of the inner core. At the anterior tip of the prospermium the outer sheath does not surround the inner core entirely. The tail end of the outer sheath is closed by a different membrane, which forms the anterior end of the prospermium. This membrane constitutes an operculum which has been studied by light microscopy by Borut and Feldman-Muhsam (1976). The anterior part of the inner core is roughly hemispherical. It later becomes the "head" of the spermiophore.

Ultrastructure

Head and Collar A low-power transmission electron micrograph of a longitudinal section through the anterior part of the prospermium of *O. gurneyi* is shown in Figure 2. Feldman-Muhsam and Filshie (1976) described the appearance of the head of the spermiophore from scanning electron micrographs. Transmission electron micrographs of tangential sections of the surface of the head of the inner core (Fig. 3) confirm the presence of a hexagonal surface structure. The plasma membrane of the head forms short, mushroom-shaped, cellular processes each with a cylindrical stem and a hexagonal cap (Fig. 3 and 4). The hexagonal caps of the processes form a regular network over the surface of the head. Within processes, electron-dense filaments, oriented parallel to the stem, can be seen in both the cap and the stem. Filaments are cut transversely in tangential sections (Fig. 3). There appears to be one near each corner of the hexagons but others are present throughout the cap. Filaments from the stem penetrate proximally into the cytoplasm of the head to a depth of about 0.14 μm. Similar filaments, oriented perpendicular to the plasma membrane between stems, penetrate the cytoplasm to the same depth (Fig. 4). These filaments could be involved in fine movements of the head of the spermiophore.

Scanning micrographs of the spermiophore show that the head is connected to the body by a special structure which was called a collar by Feldman-Muhsam and Filshie (1976). Transmission electron micrographs of the prospermium demonstrate the complicated internal structure of the collar, which may be divided into two main parts, an anterior neck and a posterior brim. The neck is connected anteriorly to the hexagonal network of the head and is composed of an inner circular unit membrane, and an outer row of strip processes which have a bean-shaped cross section, seen clearly in transverse sections (Fig. 5). These strip processes are about 0.13 μm wide. Each contains a number of electron-dense granules (Fig. 5 and 6).

The brim is composed of a double ring of cellular processes. Those of the anterior ring are about 0.65 μm long, and those of the posterior are much shorter. The brim covers a circular constriction of the inner core. At the posterior end of the constriction, the plasma membrane assumes its typical structure with the attached peripheral layer of cellular processes covering the remaining surface of the spermiophore (Feldman-Muhsam and Filshie, 1976). On its outer surface, the plasma membrane of the constricted part has electron-dense particles ~ 24 nm in diameter connected to the membrane (Fig. 7). To these particles a second row of particles seem to be attached by means of a network of fine filamentous connections (Fig. 7). Particles of both rows appear, at high magnification, to have an unstained core ~ 8 nm in diameter. A network of endoplasmic reticulum is associated with the collar. This network lies within the cytoplasm of the core, at a distance of about 0.3 μm beneath the membrane of the neck and the constriction (Fig. 5 and 6). At the level of the brim there are several branches of the reticulum that are oriented radially toward the brim (Fig. 5-7).

The Inner Core The plasma membranes of the main body of the inner core and outer sheath are continuous with one another and both carry the characteristic cellular processes that have been described by Reger (1961), Breucker and Horstmann (1968), and Feldman-Muhsam and Filshie (1976). There is some disagreement between these authors, in the interpretation of structural details of these processes.

The bulk of the cytoplasm of the inner core is filled

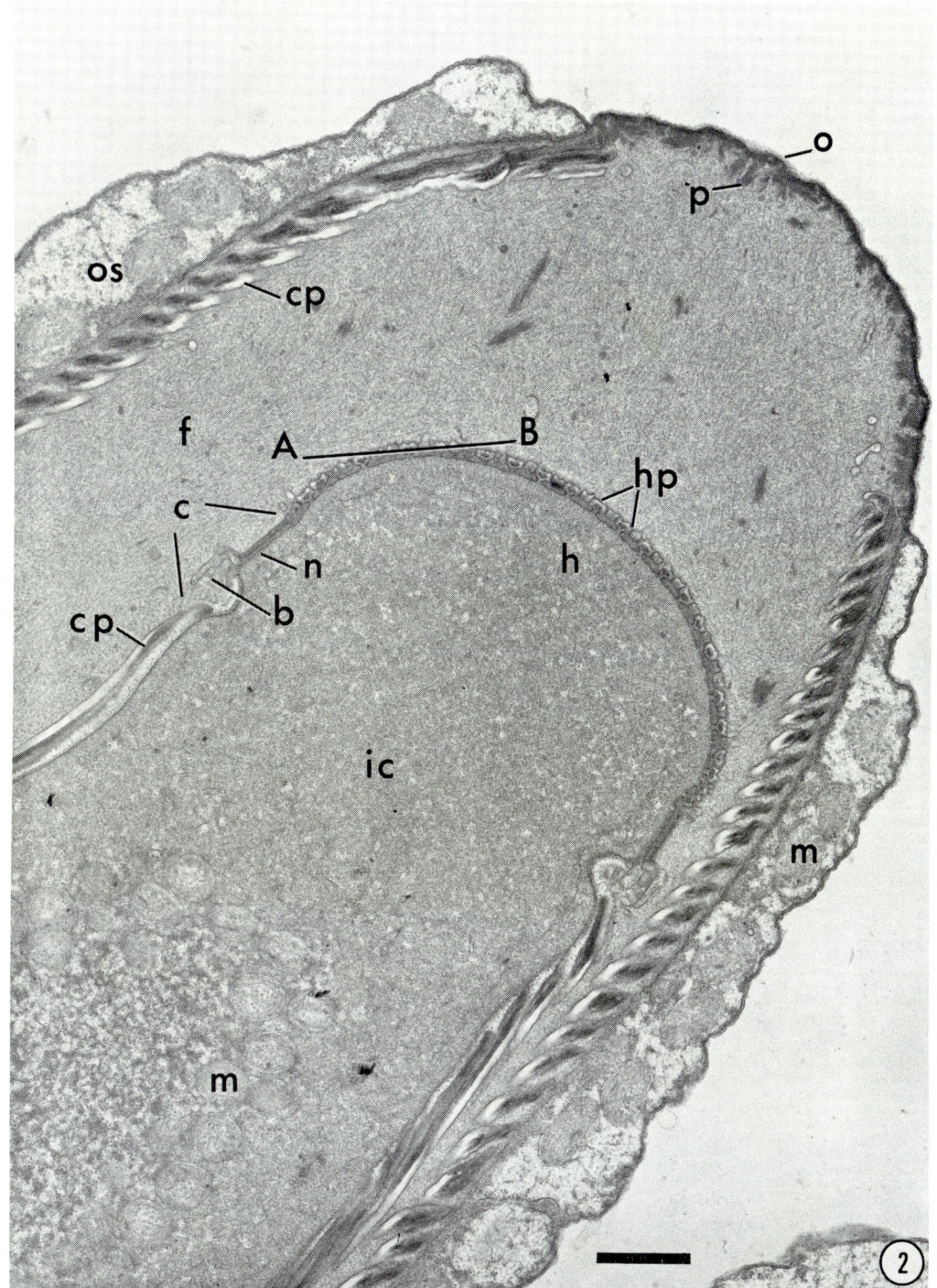

Figure 2. Longitudinal section through the anterior end of the prospermium of *O. gurneyi*. The line AB represents the approximate plane of section of Figure 3. Brim, b; collar, c; cellular processes, cp; filamentous matrix, f; head, h; head processes, hp; inner core, ic; mitochondria, m; neck, n; operculum, o; outer sheath, os; paracrystals, p. Bar = 1 μm. X14,000

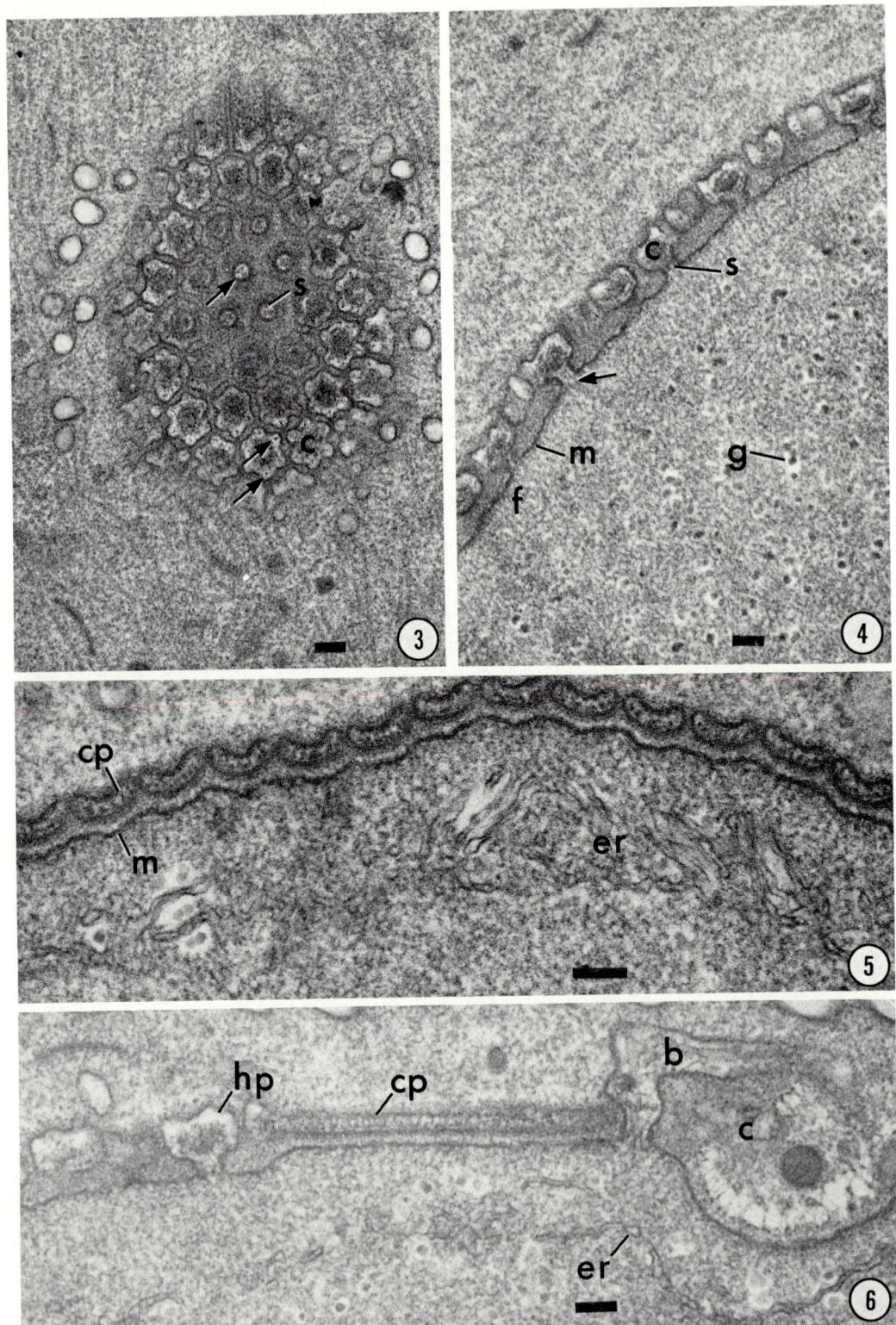

Figure 3. Tangential section of head processes of *O. gurneyi* (section plane similar to AB of Figure 2). Arrows indicate filaments within the caps (c) and stems (s) of the processes. Bar = 100 nm. X42,000

Figure 4. Transverse section of the head processes of *O. gurneyi*. Each process consists of a cap (c) and a stem (s). Radially oriented filaments form a band (f) beneath the plasma membrane (m). Filaments pass into the stem of processes (arrow). Cytoplasm of head contains granules (g) each with an electron lucent-halo. Bar = 100 nm. X50,000

with electron-dense granules (Fig. 4), each surrounded by an electron-lucent halo. The plasmalemmal region, to a depth of ~ 0.25 μm beneath the plasma membrane is relatively electron-dense. Within this layer are fibrils which have been described in the spermiophore by Feldman-Muhsam and Filshie (1976).

In the anterior part of the inner core, starting ~ 2 μm behind the collar there is a mass of mitochondria embedded in the above-mentioned granulated cytoplasm. The mitochondria are arranged in superimposed conical configurations which, in transverse sections, appear as concentric circles and, in longitudinal sections (and *in vivo* under the light microscope), as converging rows (Fig. 8). Toward the anterior part of the mitochondrial aggregation there are, in transverse sections, only one or two concentric circles and the number of circles increases with the distance backward. The aggregation of mitochondria extends over one-third the length of the inner core. Behind this aggregation, in the posterior part of the inner core, there is only one cylindrical layer of mitochondria which lies adjacent to the electron-dense subplasmalemmal zone.

The Outer Sheath At the posterior end of the prospermium the plasma membrane of the inner core folds upon itself, turns inside out, continues toward the anterior end of the prospermium and thereby becomes the plasma membrane of the outer sheath. This membrane reaches the posterior margin of the operculum near the anterior end of the prospermium and just anterior to the head of the inner core (Fig. 2 and 8). Because of this introversion, the components of the two membranes appear to be arranged in the opposite order; for instance, the typical cellular processes of the two membranes face each other.

The outer sheath is composed of several layers of which the first, starting at the mesial side, is the outer layer of cellular processes, followed by the inner plasma membrane, the cytoplasm and the outer membrane of the prospermium, the latter being alternatively referred to by Casteel (1917) as the "gelatinous envelope" and by Oliver and Brinton (1971) as "the peripheral-most membranes." The subplasmalemmal zone of the outer sheath resembles that of the posterior part of the inner core, and a discontinuous layer of mitochondria adheres to it. This layer of mitochondria is the continuation of the single layer found in the posterior part of the inner core (mentioned above). The remainder of the cytoplasm of the outer sheath contains large granules which Reger (1974) showed to be glycogen in *Dermacentor andersoni*.

The Operculum High magnification micrographs show that the outer membrane of the outer sheath is composed of three unit membranes. The outermost of these unit membranes appears to be continuous with the outermost membrane of the operculum, and is the plasma membrane of the whole prospermium. Beneath the plasma membrane of the outer sheath is a flattened cisternum of endoplasmic reticulum that turns back at the anterior margin of the outer sheath (Fig. 9) to cover the inner plasma membrane of the outer sheath for a distance of some 6 μm posteriorly[1]. The importance of this overlap becomes evident only at the last stage of sperm maturation, when the acrosomal canal evaginates.

Beneath the operculum plasma membrane are two fused unit membranes having the characteristic five-layered structure (Fig. 10) reminiscent of similar fused membranes found in the Schwann cell of the mammalian nerve sheath. This five-layered membrane is homologous in position with the inner plasma membrane of the outer sheath. However, the plasma membrane is a unit membrane (three-layered) and carries the characteristic cellular processes, whereas the five-layered membrane is much more electron-dense and lacks the processes. Our micrographs do not create the impression that the fused membrane of the operculum is continuous with the inner plasma membrane of the outer sheath. The fused membrane appears to terminate at the junction of the operculum and the outer sheath (Fig. 9).

To the inner face of the fused membranes of the operculum, an array of paracrystals adheres (Fig. 10). The crystals seem to be composed of relatively long straight fibers that pack together in hexagonal array, with a center-to-center spacing of about 13 nm. Similar paracrystals are scattered elsewhere between the inner core and the outer sheath, but never as concentrated as beneath the operculum.

The Matrix between the Inner Core and the Outer Sheath This matrix is densely interspersed with filamentous components (Fig. 11). Small numbers of filaments tend to orient parallel with one another into bundles, individual bundles being apparently randomly

---

[1] A similar overlap exists in *Ixodidae*, as can be seen in Reger's (1961) micrographs (Fig. 3 and 8-10).

Figure 5. Transverse section of a prospermium of *O. gurneyi* showing cross sections of strip-like processes (cp) of the head in the region of the neck. Endoplasmic reticulum, er; plasma membrane, m. Bar = 100 nm. X85,000

Figure 6. Median longitudinal section of a propermium of *O. gurneyi* showing details of structure of the collar region of the head. Brim, b; constriction, c; strip-like processes, cp; endoplasmic reticulum, er; head processes, hp. Bar = 100 nm. X67,000

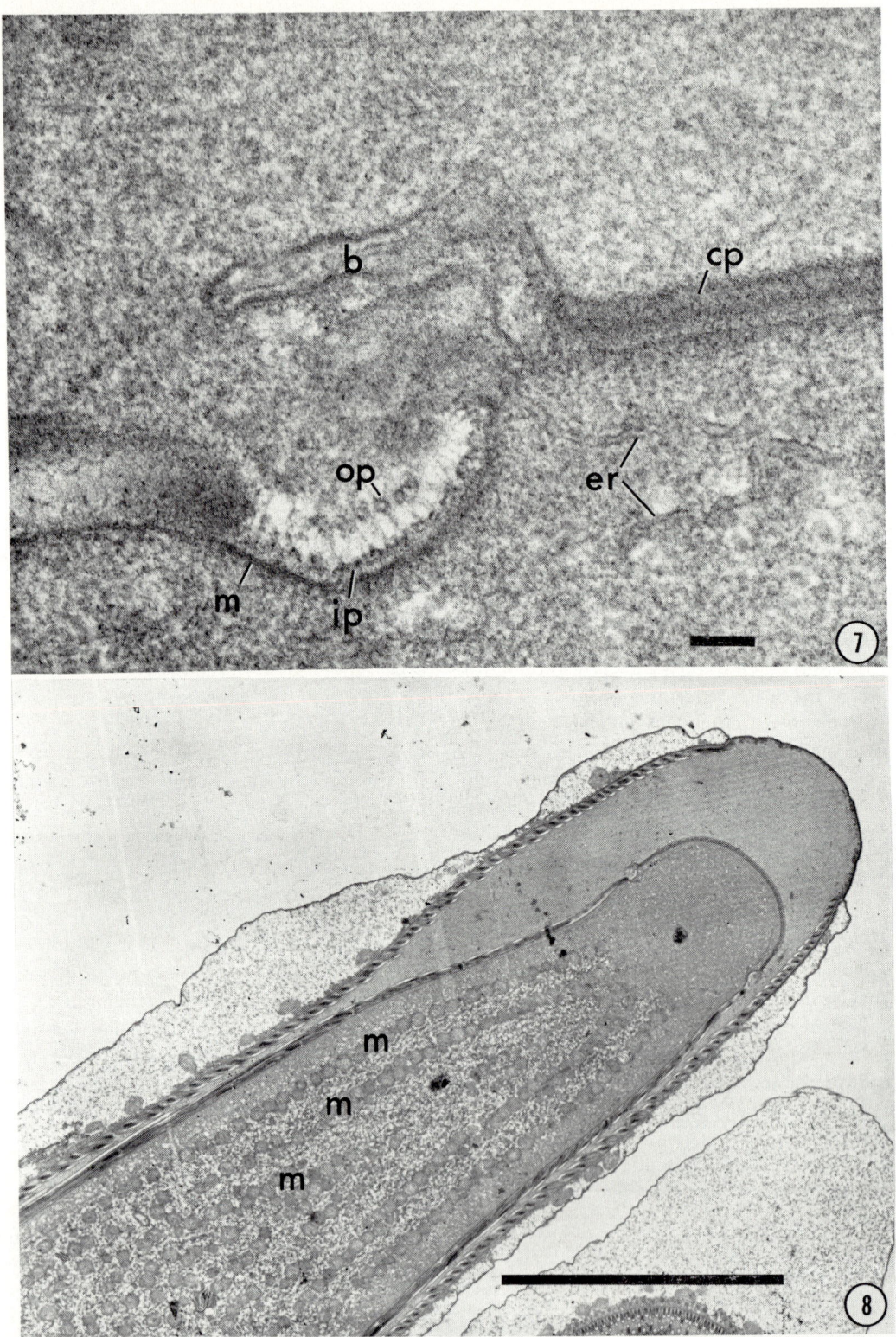

Figure 7. Detail of the brim region of the head (similar section to Figure 6). Cellular process of brim, b; strip-like process of collar, cp; endoplasmic reticulum, er; plasma membrane, m; inner and outer rows of particles, ip and op. Bar = 100 nm.

Figure 8. Median longitudinal section of prospermium of O. gurneyi illustrating the configuration of concentric conical layers of mitochondria (m) in the inner core. Bar = 10 μm.

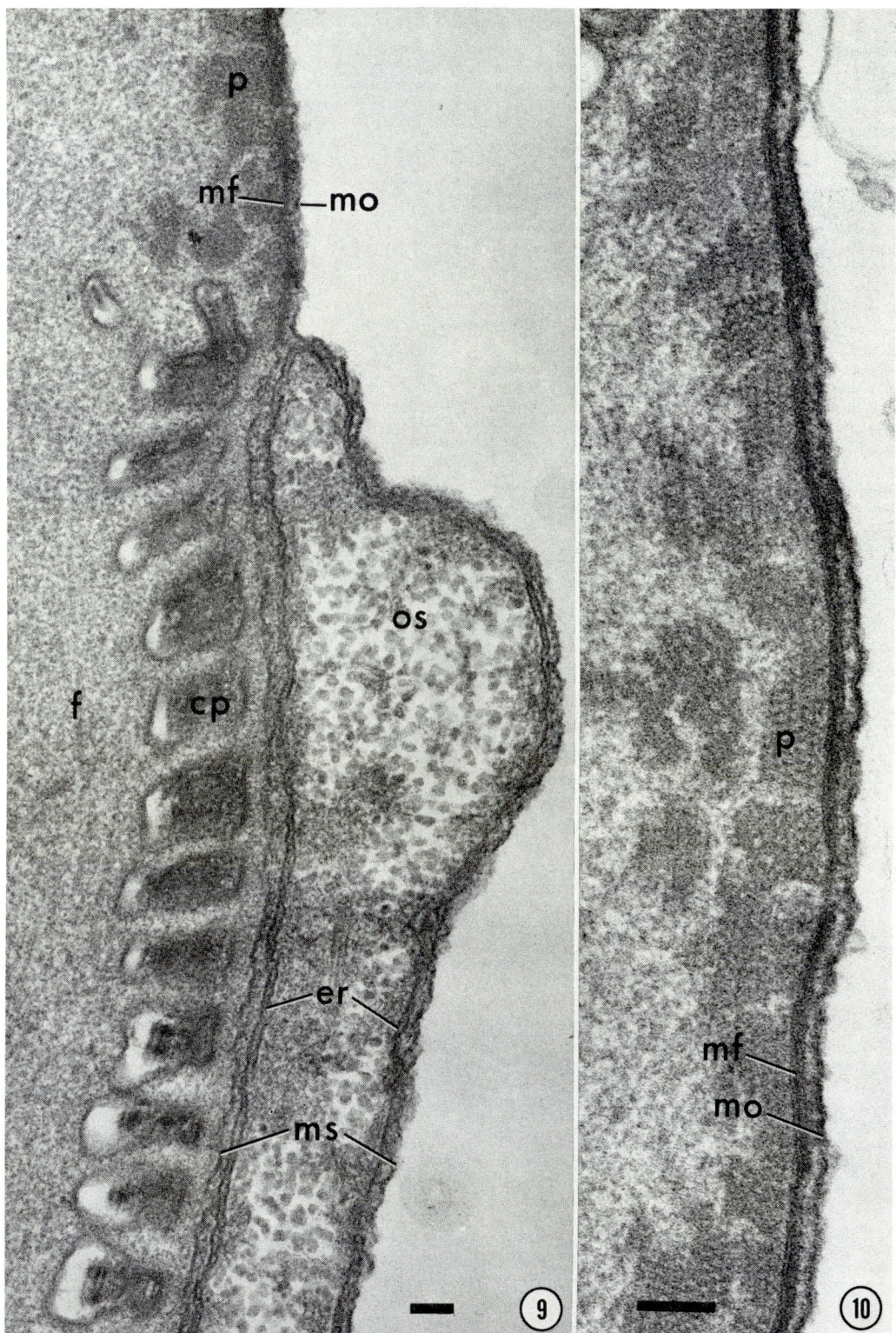

Figure 9. Median longitudinal section of prospermium of O. gurneyi at the junction of the outer sheath (os) and the operculum. Cellular processes, cp; endoplasmic reticulum, er; filamentous matrix, f; fused membranes of operculum, mf; plasma membrane of operculum, mo; plasma membrane of outer sheath, ms; paracrystals, p. Bar = 100 nm.

Figure 10. Median longitudinal section of prospermium of O. gurneyi at the anterior tip of the operculum. Fused five-layered membrane, mf; plasma membrane of operculum, mo; paracrystals, p. Bar = 100 nm.

oriented in the matrix. In any section, bundles may be cut longitudinally, obliquely, or transversely (Fig. 11, upper insert). Each filament is approximately 14 nm in diameter and appears to be composed of an outer ring of sub-filaments and an electron lucent core (Fig. 11, lower insert). Some filaments are at least 0.7 µm long. In high magnification micrographs, longitudinally sectioned filaments sometimes exhibit a beaded appearance (Fig. 11, lower insert). Similar images of filaments in *Neurospora* have been interpreted by Allen *et al.* (1974) as indicating a helical sub-structure.

The Nucleus and Acrosome The nucleus is located in the cytoplasm of the tail end of the outer sheath, that is, very near the anterior end of the prospermium (Fig. 12). It is connected at one end to the acrosomal plate by a stalk and several other structures.

The acrosomal plate is a complex structure. It lies within the cisternum of endoplasmic reticulum found near the anterior end of the prospermium and described above. In *O. gurneyi* is is probably elliptical, about 9 µm wide and at least 11.5 µm long. The plate consists of two relatively thick granular layers (Fig. 13). The outer layer is electron-dense and about 40 nm thick. The inner layer is about the same thickness, but is electron-lucent. There are a few discontinuities in the electron-dense layer forming gaps between 0.15 and 0.4 µm wide. In the region of the acrosomal plate the membranes of the endoplasmic reticulum are closely addressed to the plate, except in some areas, where the inner membrane is deeply invaginated into the cytoplasm of the outer sheath. Between the outer membrane of the reticulum and the outer plasma membrane there is a narrow layer of electron-lucent material in which numerous small electron-dense platelets, about 30 nm in diameter, are embedded (Fig. 13, insert). In the center of the acrosomal plate there is a nipple that is the connecting point of the acrosomal plate and the stalk of the nucleus. In the region of the nipple the two granular layers of the acrosomal plate are absent and, in their place, are a number of membranes oriented parallel to the surface (Fig. 13).

In *O. gurneyi*, the nucleus is a long narrow cylinder about 15 µm long and 1.2 µm wide. It contains a network of chromatin in the form of long anastomosing strips. The strips are electron-dense and contain even more electron-dense and fairly regularly arranged filaments (Fig. 14). The chromatin network is embedded in the granular ground substance of the nucleus. Some large dense granules are also present and these may also be chromatin. The nuclear membrane has numerous nuclear pores (Fig. 14, insert).

The nucleus is connected to the acrosomal plate by a complex structure (Fig. 13). At the connecting locus, the nucleus widens to form a cone with a peripheral, electron-dense flange. The nuclear membrane in the region of the cone and flange adheres closely to the inner membrane of the acrosomal plate. The central nuclear stalk (first described by Breucker and Horstmann, 1968), passes through a central hole in the flange and connects the nucleus with the acrosomal plate by means of the nipple, which lies in the center of the acrosomal plate. The stalk is composed of electron-dense, parallel fibers (Fig. 14) and is surrounded by several layers of endoplasmic reticulum (Fig. 13 and 14). Membranes of the reticulum also surround the nuclear membrane in the region of the cone and the flange.

Spermateleosis

The transformation of the prospermium into the spermiophore has been described by Samson (1909), Casteel (1917), Oppermann (1935), Oliver and Brinton (1971), Brinton *et al.* (1974), and others. All these descriptions state that the first step of spermateleosis is the breaking of the inner core through the outer sheath. Borut and Feldman-Muhsam (1976) observed that this is not true. They showed that even before the "head" of the inner core has started to advance, an operculum opens and, when the head reaches the anterior end of the outer sheath, it passes through an already existing hole. Electron micrographs show that the operculum is not of the same structure as the outer sheath and that at the junction of the two a natural weakness may exist. This weakness may be produced by the termination of the presumably stiff membrane complex of the operculum at the junction. Also, the endoplasmic reticulum which lines the internal face of the outer sheath membrane is turned back at the junction, so that at this point, only a single unit membrane seems to keep the cell intact (Fig. 9).

It has been observed that the operculum separates from the prospermium, as a single piece. The separation always occurs at the same locus, and the shape of the operculum is characteristic for each species (Borut and Feldman-Muhsam, 1976). The mechanism by which the operculum opens is unknown. It may be conjectured that pressure is created at the tip of the prospermium by an enzymatic process, involving assumably the paracrystals concentrated under the operculum. Occasionally it has been observed that an operculum opens, closes immediately, and finally opens permanently.[2]

As spermateleosis proceeds, the inner core advances through the open end of the prospermium, the outer sheath slides back, crumples (Fig. 15), and finally turns

---

[2] Feldman-Muhsam, B.: unpublished

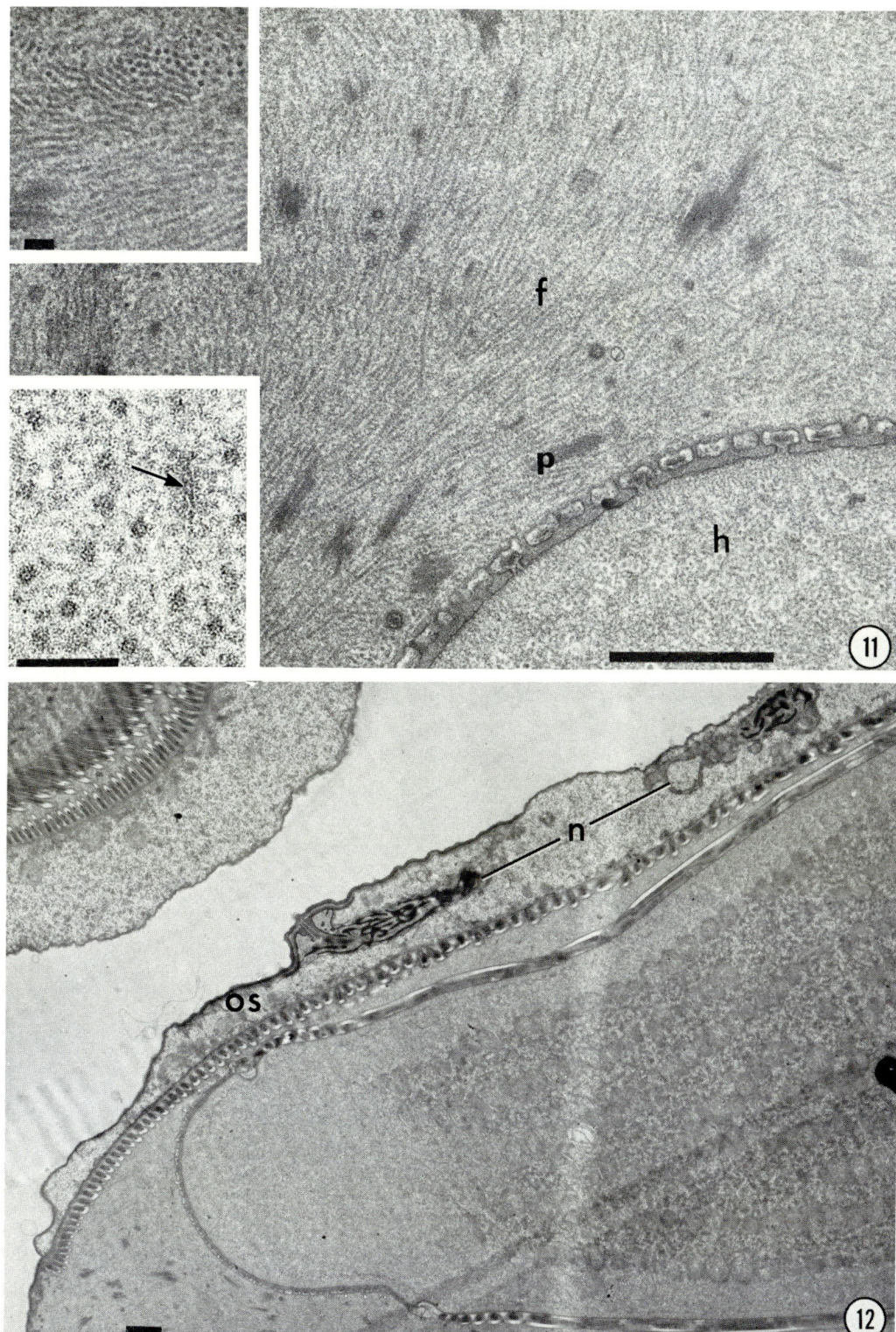

Figure 11. Median longitudinal section of the prospermium of O. gurneyi, showing filaments (f) and paracrystals (p) in the matrix between the outer sheath and the head (h). Bar = 1 μm. Upper insert shows randomly oriented bundles of filaments. Bar = 100 nm. Lower insert shows microtubular substructure of filaments cut transversely and possible helical substructure within a filament sectioned longitudinally (arrow). Bar = 100 nm.

Figure 12. Low magnification, median longitudinal section of the prospermium of O. gurneyi, showing the location of the nucleus (n) at the anterior of the prospermium, i.e. the posterior end of the outer sheath (os). Bar = 1 μm.

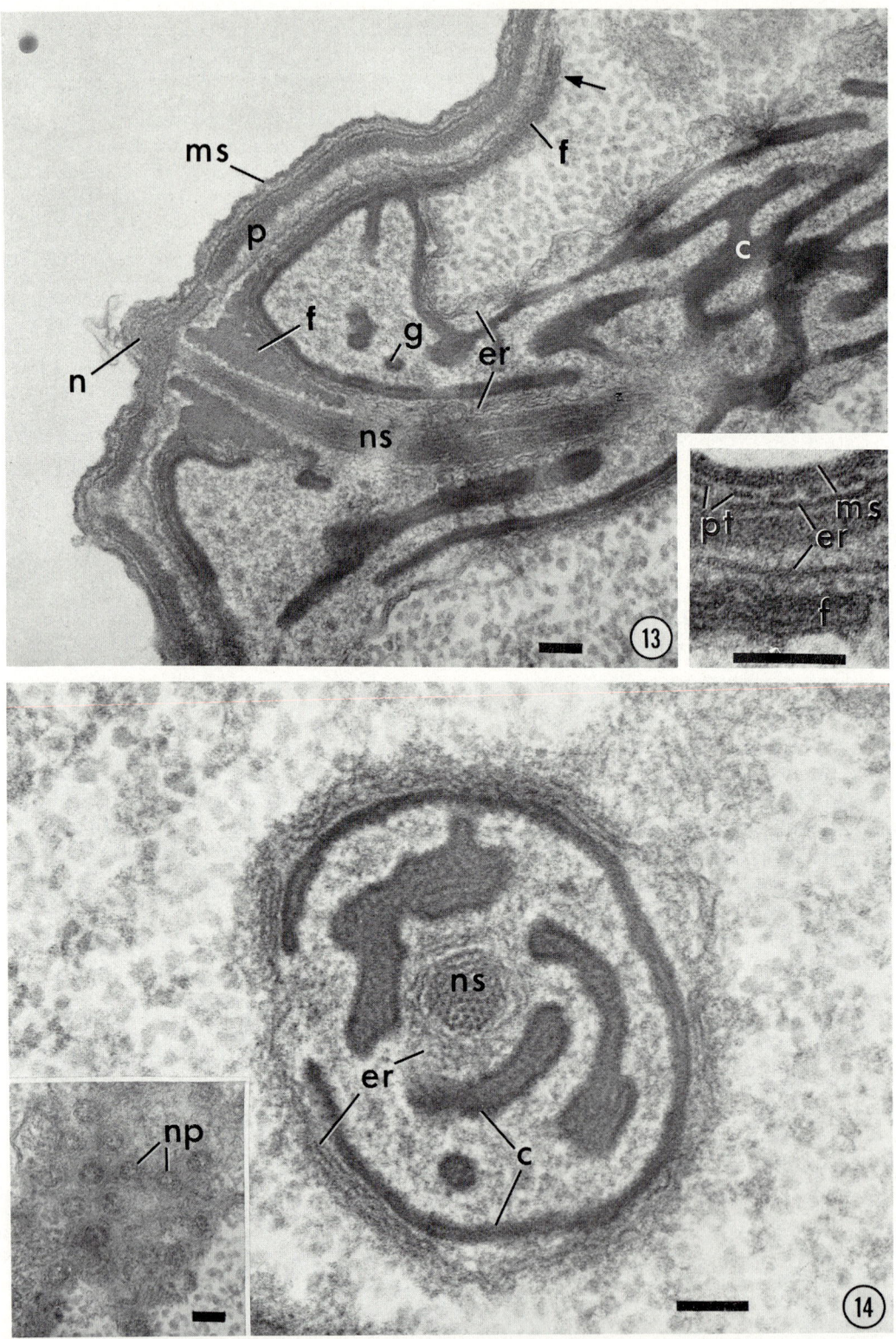

Figure 13. Detail of the region of attachment of the nucleus to the outer sheath in *O. gurneyi*. Chromatin, c; endoplasmic reticulum, er; flange of nucleus, f; chromatin granule, g; outer membrane of outer sheath, ms; nipple, n; acrosomal plate, p; platelets, pt; nuclear stalk, ns. The arrow indicates the relative position of the detail shown in the insert. Bars = 100 nm.

inside out. As a result, the outer sheath becomes the posterior half of the spermiophore, and the length of the spermiophore is, therefore, twice that of the prospermium (Fig. 18). The outer membrane of the prospermium invaginates to become the wall of the acrosomal canal of the spermiophore. This canal opens at the posterior end of the spermiophore, and extends forward over approximately half of its length.

In the spermiophore the acrosomal plate occupies roughly the same area of the acrosomal canal as it did in the outer membrane of the prospermium. Obviously the surface of the wall of the acrosomal canal in the spermiophore is smaller than that of the outer membrane of the prospermium. Thus, during spermateleosis, the outer membrane of the prospermium contracts. At the same time it becomes highly electron dense, so that Breucker and Horstmann (1972) thought "that the whole acrosomal canal is lined by the acrosomal lamella." In fact the fine structure of the wall of the acrosomal canal of the spermiophore is the same as that of the outer membrane of the prospermium, i.e. both are composed of three unit membranes. Furthermore, the endoplasmic reticulum which forms the flattened cisternum of the prospermium and lines the inner plasma membrane of the outer sheath for about 6 µm (Fig. 16) can be seen in the spermiophore to line the posterior end of the plasma membrane for the same length (Fig. 17 and 18). The nucleus remains fastened to the acrosomal plate which in turn remains embedded at the same place of the same membrane which has become the acrosomal canal. Thus during spermateleosis the nucleus moves backward together with the outer sheath, and after completion of the process of invagination it is located in the cytoplasm near the posterior end of the spermiophore.

The whole process of spermateleosis probably cannot be achieved without the action of relatively strong forces. It is evident that the agent that exerts these forces must act simultaneously on both the inner core and the outer sheath, pushing one and pulling the other and must be located between the two. In fact the space between the two contains numerous filaments, which are most likely of a contractile nature. The authors assume that these filaments play a major role in the process of spermateleosis. It is worthwhile noting that the whole matrix between the inner core and the outer sheath is discarded during this process. Thus, whatever its biological function, at the completion of spermateleosis the filamentous matrix has fulfilled its role.

Evagination of the Acrosomal Canal

The spermiophores remain in the capsules of the endospermatophore for either a short or a long time according to whether the female has had a blood meal. If she has fed, the spermiophores leave the capsules and proceed to the oviducts, the ampullae, and the ovaries. At this stage, a further change of form occurs. The acrosomal canal evaginates slowly out of the posterior end of the spermiophore (Fig. 17). The everted acrosomal canal is anchored to the body of the spermiophore by the above-mentioned overlapping membranes.

It will be remembered that in the spermiophore the nucleus is concealed in the interior of the cell, near the acrosomal canal. However, after evagination of the acrosomal canal, the nucleus is brought to the surface of the cell and the acrosomal plate is exposed (Fig. 17). This evagination process is shown diagrammatically in Figure 18.

Spermateleosis and evagination of the acrosomal canal are the most manifest morphological transformations accompanying maturation and capacitation. Many other changes affect the ultrastructure of the nucleus, the acrosomal canal, and other components of the sperm cell. These changes are being studied at present. One conspicuous example is a development affecting the wall of the acrosomal canal, occuring after spermateleosis and before evagination of the canal. At this stage electron-dense granular material accumulates in the cisternum surrounding the acrosomal canal. In certain regions this accumulation forms a swelling (Fig. 19) which may be as large as the lumen of the acrosomal canal. At the same time the innermost layer of the acrosomal wall, i.e. the plasma membrane, becomes rough on the side facing the lumen. After evagination this rough surface becomes the external covering of the everted acrosomal canal (Fig. 20).

REFERENCES

Allen, E.D.; Lowry, R.I.; Sussman, A.S.: Accumulation of Microfilaments in a Colonial Mutant of *Neurospora crassa*. J Ultrastruct Res 48(1974)455-464

Balashov, Y.S.: Bloodsucking Ticks (Ixodoidea)—Vectors of Diseases of Man and Animals. Akad Nauk USSR Zool Inst

---

Figure 14. Cross section of the cylindrical nucleus of O. gurneyi. Chromatin (c) forms a layer round the inside of the nuclear envelope and also forms a network internally. Central stalk (ns) is surrounded by endoplasmic reticulum (er), which also surrounds the nucleus. Bar = 100 nm. The insert is a tangential section of the nuclear envelope showing nuclear pores (np). Bar = 100 nm.

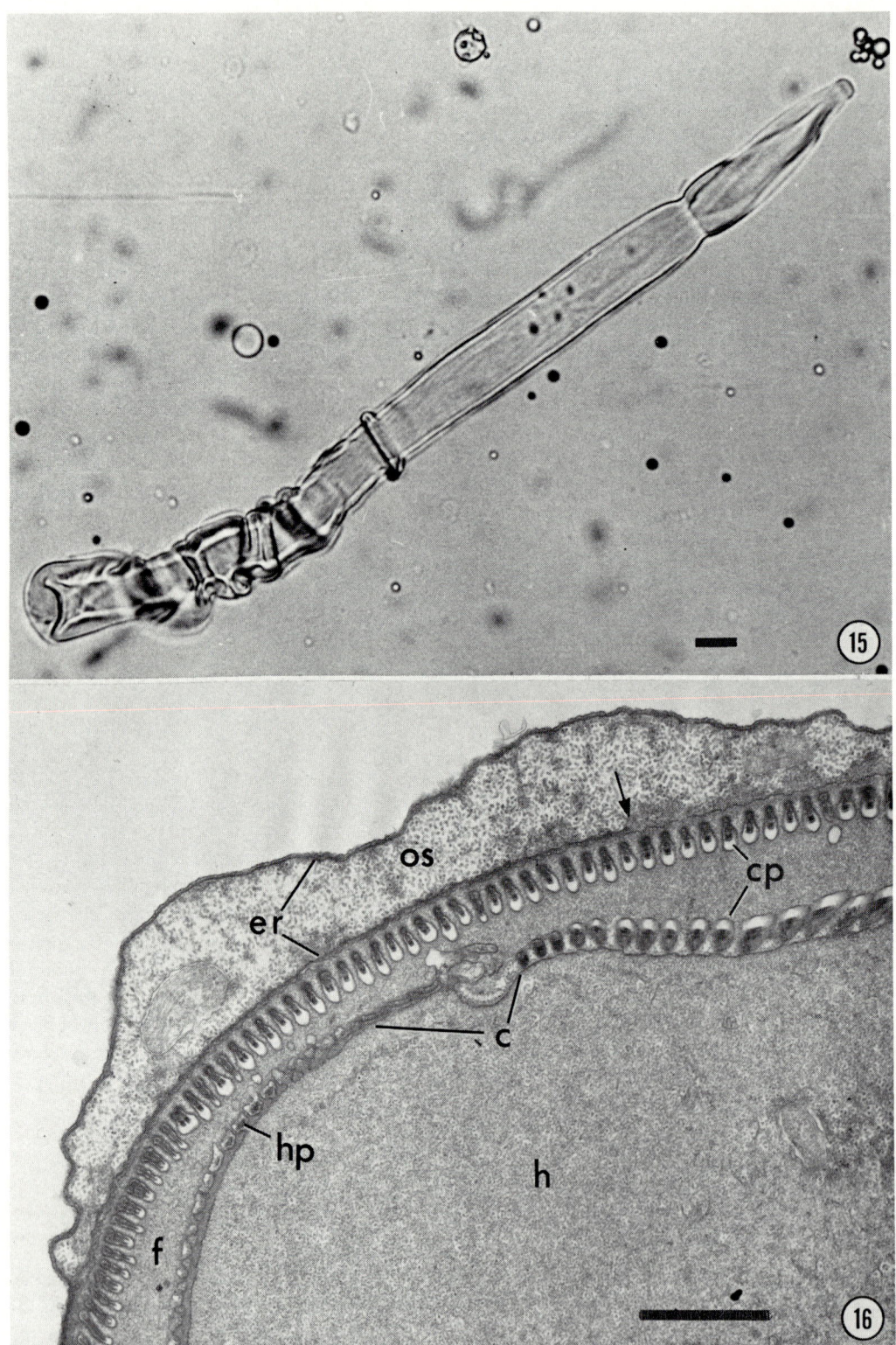

Figure 15. Phase contrast light micrograph of a sperm cell of *Ornithodoros parkeri* taken during spermateleosis. Bar = 10 μm.
Figure 16. Median longitudinal section of the prospermium of *O. gurneyi*. Arrow shows the level at which the endoplasmic reticulum (er) terminates on the internal face of the inner plasma membrane of the outer sheath (os). Collar, c; cellular processes, cp; filamentous matrix, f; head, h; head processes, hp. Bar = 1 μm.

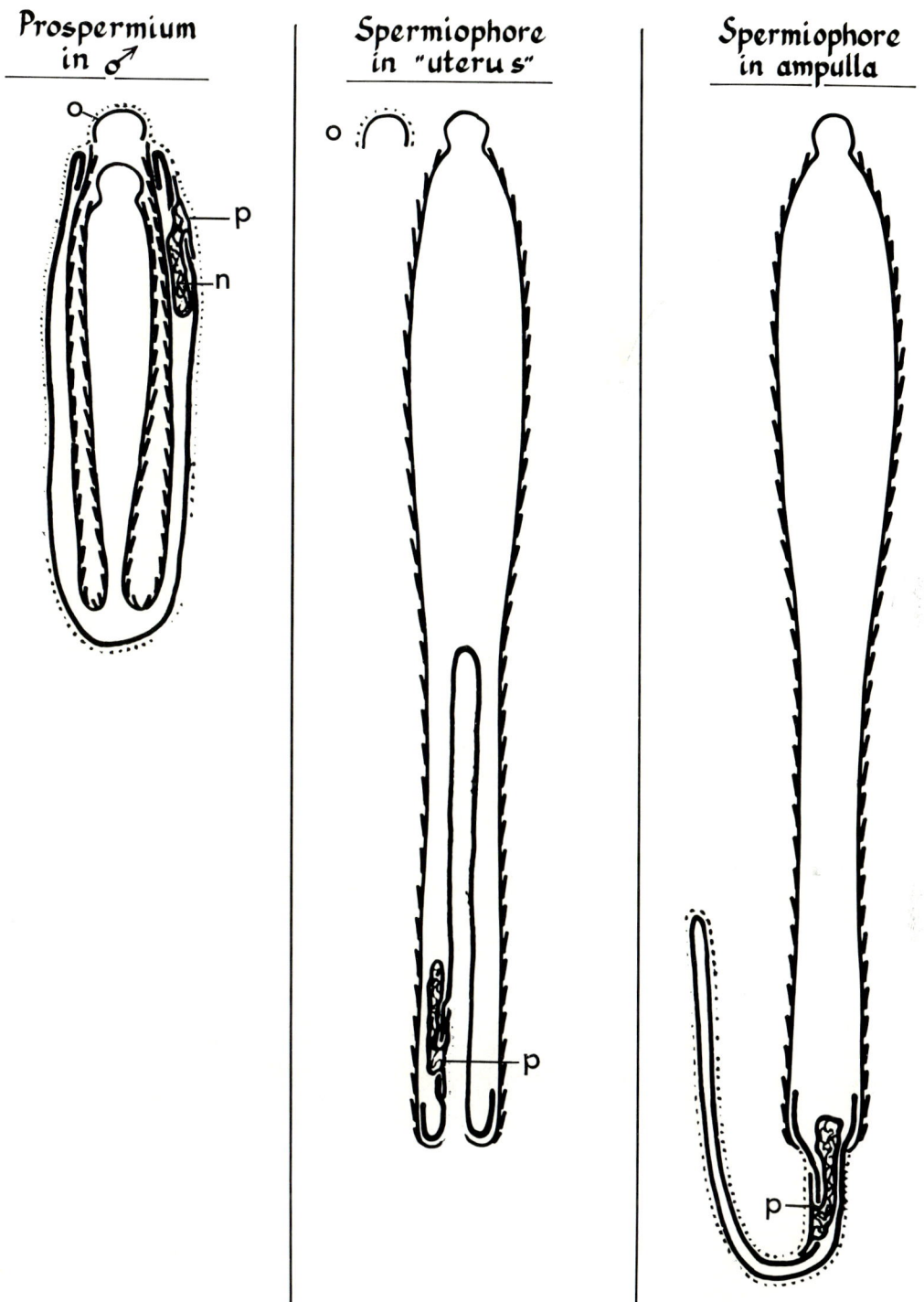

Figure 18. Diagrammatic representations of longitudinal sections of sperm cells in their three main configurations. Note the position of the nucleus (n), the acrosomal plate (p), and the detached operculum (o).

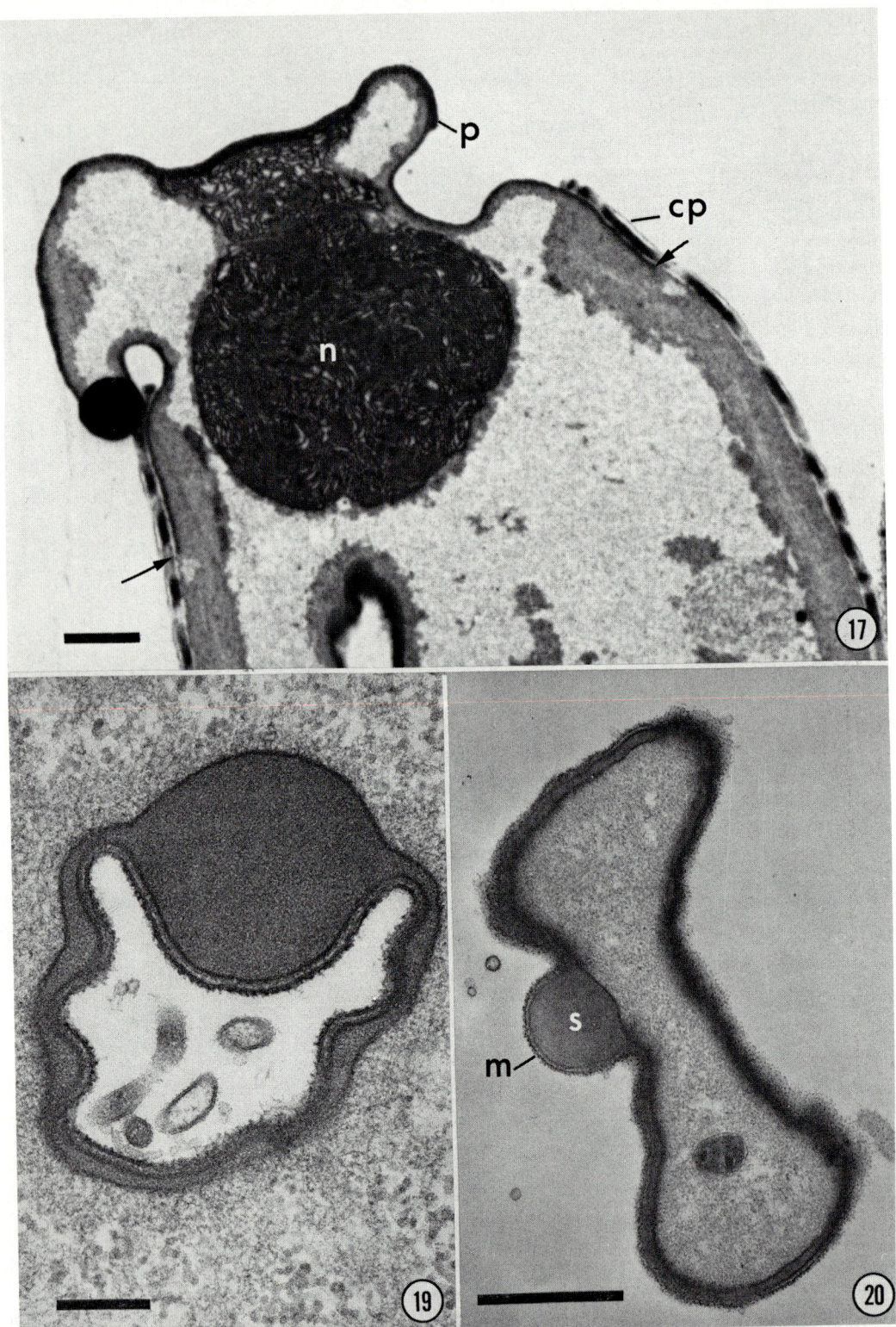

Figure 17. Longitudinal section of the spermiophore of *O. tholozani* after the acrosomal canal has started eversion. Arrows show the level at which the endoplasmic reticulum terminates on the internal face of the plasma membrane. Cellular processes, cp; nucleus, n; acrosomal plate, p. Bar = 1 μm.

Figure 19. Cross section of the acrosomal canal of *O. tholozani* showing a large swelling in the cisternum of endoplasmic reticulum which surrounds the canal. Bar = 1 μm.

Leningrad (1967) Translated by O.G. Strekalovsky in Misc Pubs Ent Soc Am 8(1972)159-376

Borut, S.; Feldman-Muhsam, B.: A New Observation on Spermateleosis in Ticks. J Parasitol 62(1976)318-320

Breucker, H.; Horstmann, E.: Die Spermatozoen der Zecke *Ornithodorus moubata* (Murr.). Z Zellforsch Mikrosk Anat 88(1968)1-22

Breucker, H.; Horstmann, E.: Die Spermatogenese der Zecke *Ornithodorus moubata* (Murr.). Z Zellforsch Mikrosk Anat 123(1972)18-46

Brinton, L.P.; Burgdorfer, W.; Oliver, J.H., Jr.: Histology and Fine Structure of Spermatozoa and Egg Passage in the Female Tract of *Dermacentor andersoni* Stiles (Acari, Ixodidae). Tissue Cell 6(1974)109-125

Casteel, D.B.: Cystoplasmic Inclusions in Male Germ Cells of the Fowl Tick, *Argas miniatus,* and Histogenesis of the Spermatozoon. J Morphol 28(1917)643-683

Feldman-Muhsam, B.; Filshie, B.K.: Scanning and Transmission Electron Microscopy of the Spermiophores of *Ornithodoros* Ticks. An Attempt to Explain Their Motility. Tissue Cell 8(1976)411-419

Nordenskiöld, E.: Zur Spermatogenese von *Ixodes reduvius.* Zool Anz 34(1909)511-516

Oliver, J.H., Jr.; Brinton, L.P.: Sperm Maturation in Ticks: An Example of Capacitation in Invertebrates. In: Daniel, M. and Rosický, B. eds Proceedings of the 3rd International Congress of Acarology, Prague, 1971, W. Junk, The Hague and Accademia, Publishing House of the Czechoslovak Academy of Sciences, Prague, pp. 733-737, 1973.

Oppermann, E.: Die Entstehung der Riesenspermien von *Argas columbarum* (Shaw) (*reflexus* F.). Z Mikrosk Anat Forsch 37(1935)538-560

Reger, J.F.: The Fine Structure of Spermatids from the Tick, *Amblyomma dissimili.* J Ultrastruct Res 5(1961)584-599

Reger, J.F.: The Origin and Fine Structure of Cellular Processes in Spermatozoa of the Tick *Dermacentor andersoni.* J Ultrastruct Res 48(1974)420-434

Samson, K.: Zur Spermiohistiogenese der Zecken. Sber Gesellschaft Naturforsch Freunde Berlin 8(1909)486-499

Sharma, G.P.: Studies on Spermatogenesis in Ticks. Proc Natl Inst Sci India 10(1944)305-316

Tuzet, O.; Millot, I.: Recherches sur la Spermiogenèse des Ixodes. Bull Biol Fr Belg 71(1937)190-205

Figure 20. Cross section of the everted acrosome of O. *tholozani*. Note the rough outer surface of the plasma membrane (m) and the swelling (s) within the acrosomal plate (p). Bar = 1 μm.

APPENDIX

The purpose of this international meeting was to review the present state of knowledge in the subject areas of the symposia and related contributed papers. An important secondary objective was to stimulate discussion and exchange of information on promising research methods. To this end, informal workshops were held on procedures for isolation and biochemical characterization of germ cells and their structural components, and on methods for quantitative assessment of sperm motility. The participants were asked to submit a brief exposition of the procedure presented, together with a critique of its advantages and limitations, and selected references to publications where additional information can be found. These contributions, which vary considerably in depth and format, are assembled in the Appendix. It is hoped that they will prove useful to other investigators and will contribute to progress in the field by encouraging wider use of the methods described.

WORKSHOP ONE
Isolation and Biochemical Characterization of Germ Cells and Their Structural Components

Meaningful biochemical studies of spermatogenesis have long been hampered by the heterogeneity of the cell population in the seminiferous epithelium. Methods that have now been developed for isolation of relatively pure fractions of the several cell types make it possible to study the biochemical correlates of germ cell differentiation. A variety of ingenious procedures are available for biochemical dissection of the spermatozoon and characterization of most of its structural components. These and related methods are responsible for recent rapid advances in our understanding of the biochemistry and physiology of the spermatozoon.

SEPARATION OF MALE GERM CELLS BY SEDIMENTATION VELOCITY

L.J. Romrell

Department of Anatomy, University of Florida College of Medicine, Gainesville, Florida 32610 USA

Velocity sedimentation at unit gravity has been used to separate dissociated cells from a variety of tissues into highly enriched populations of specific cell types (for recent reviews see Pretlow et al., 1975 and Catsimpoolas, 1977). A number of investigators have utilized the STA-PUT velocity sedimentation system of Miller and Phillips (1969) to separate testis cells for the study of events in spermatogenesis. Details of the methodology for the separation of testis cells can be found in the papers of Bellvé et al. (1977), Meistrich et al. (1973), and Romrell et al. (1976). Techniques used for the dissociation of mouse and rabbit testes are summarized in Figures 1 and 2. Table 1 briefly outlines procedures which may be used for the separation of dissociated cell suspensions in commercially available STA-PUT chambers.

Pretlow et al. (1975) have emphasized the importance of the assessment of both the viability and purity of cells in isolated populations when evaluating data from studies of separated cells. These two important factors are discussed below

Assessment of Viability

Isolated cells cannot be critically compared with functioning of the same cells in their natural environment. Therefore, the assessment of viability is somewhat subjective making it essential to assess as many parameters of viability as is reasonably possible.

The following parameters, as well as others, may be considered:
1. Determination of proportion of cells which exclude vital dyes. This must be considered a minimal requirement for viability due to the insensitivity of method.
2. Measurement of residual cellular metabolism (*e.g.*, oxygen consumption, amino acid incorporation) and specific biosynthetic activities. The pitfall here is that the activity measured may only denote the intactness of molecular complexes within the cells. Furthermore, any measurement of metabolic activity represents an average of the cell population and not a measurement of the activity of the individual cells. Cytochemical techniques (*e.g.*, autoradiography or histochemistry) may be used to determine the proportion of cells demonstrating specific biosynthetic activities.
3. Morphological assessment of cellular integrity by light and electron microscopy.
4. Determination of maintenance of normal function. This is difficult to assess in testicular cell fractions because tissue culture techniques that provide the "essential" environment for differentiation to continue *in vitro* are not currently available.

Evaluation of Enriched Cell Populations

The evaluation of studies on enriched cell populations requires that data be presented that characterize the cell populations throughout the isolation procedure.

The following parameters should be considered:
1. Determination of the proportion of cell types in starting suspension (for example, Tables 2 and 3).
2. Determination of the proportion of cells recovered after separation. It is important to determine if significant numbers of cells are lost or damaged. Certain cell types may be particularly vulnerable to the isolation procedures.
3. Determination of the proportion of cells in isolated fractions. The proportion of specific cell types found in each fraction should be determined. A metabolic activity of specific interest may be found to reside in a minor contaminate of an isolated fraction.
4. Identification of cells within fractions using morphological criteria. Electronic counters cannot discriminate pairs or aggregates of small cells from single large cells and usually are not set up to distinguish intact cells from debris (free nuclei, etc.) of similar size.
5. Demonstration of the purity of cell population with photomicrographs. Representative micrographs should be presented. Caution should be taken in presenting such data since sampling "error" may

© 1979 Urban & Schwarzenberg, Inc. Baltimore-Munich *The Spermatozoon*, edited by D.W. Fawcett and J.M. Bedford

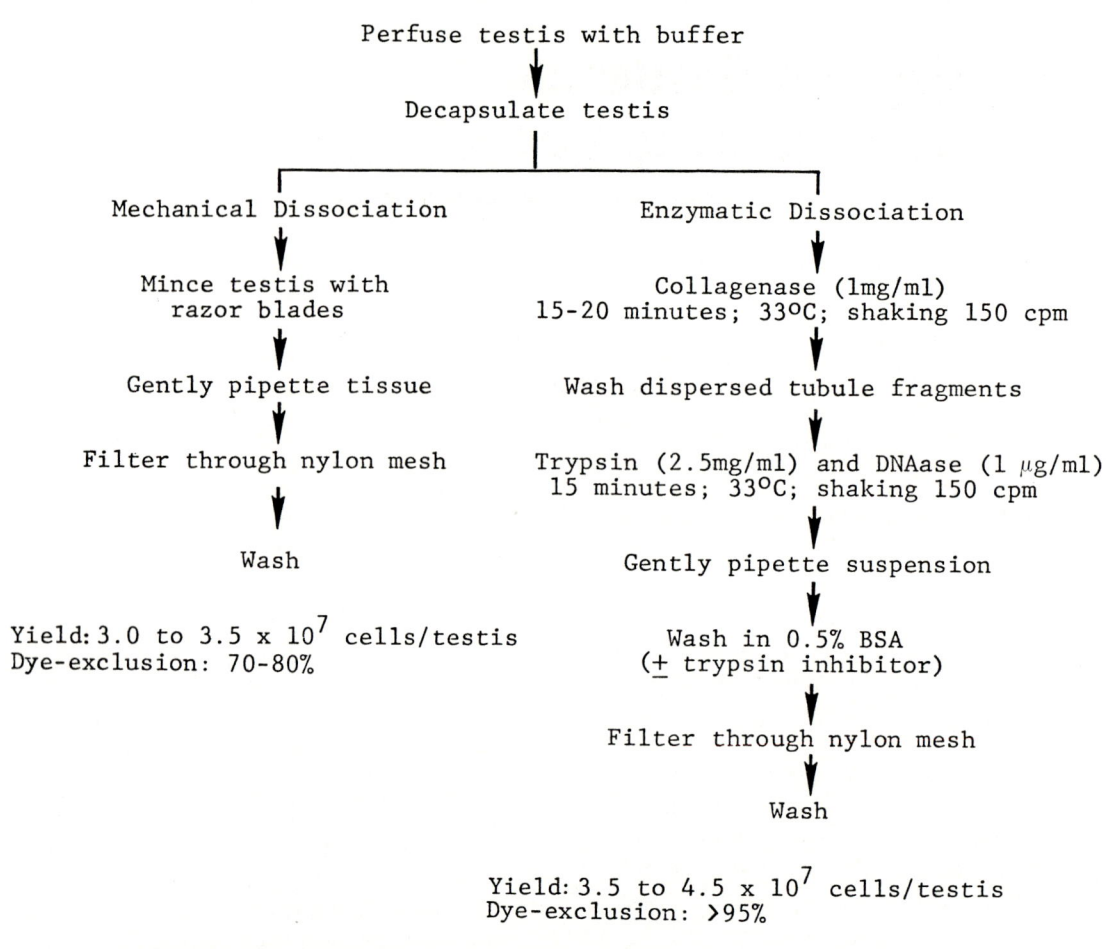

Approximately 20 ml incubation medium/gram tissue

Figure 1. Preparation of testicular cell suspensions (mouse)

occur in sections of pellets; sections should be cut in the long axis of the pellet (meniscus to tip). Because the sedimentation rate is due in part to the size and density of the cells, separation of the cells will occur during centrifugation in the preparation of cell pellets. Separation of cells into enriched populations within different parts of the pellet may occur (*e.g.,* largest cell types at the tip; smallest cell types at the meniscus).

REFERENCES

Bellvé, A.R.; Cavicchia, J.C.; Millette, C.F.; O'Brien, D.A.; Bhatnagar, Y.M.; Dym, M.: Spermatogenic Cells of the Prepuberal Mouse. Isolation and Morphological Characterization. J Cell Biol 74(1977)68-85

Meistrich, M.L.; Bruce, W.R.; Clermont, Y.: Cellular Composition of Fractions of Mouse Testis Cells following Velocity Sedimentation Separations. Exp Cell Res 79(1973)213-227

Miller, R.G.; Phillips, R.A.: Separation of Cells by Velocity Sedimentation. J Cell Physiol 73(1969)191-201

Pretlow, T.G., II; Weir, E.E.; Zettergren, J.G.: Problems Connected with the Separation of Different Kinds of Cells. In: International Review of Experimental Pathology Vol. 14 G.W. Richter and M.A. Epstein. Academic Press, New York, 1975

Romrell, L.J.; Bellvé, A.R.; Fawcett, D.W.: Separation of Mouse Spermatogenic Cells by Sedimentation Velocity. A Morphological Characterization. Dev Biol 49(1976)119-131

Swierstra, E.E., Foote, R.H.: Cytology and Kinetics of Spermatogenesis in the Rabbit. J Reprod Fert 5(1963)309-322

Methods of Cell Separation. Vol. 1, pp. 361, ed. by Nicholas Catsimpoolas. Plenum Press, New York, 1977

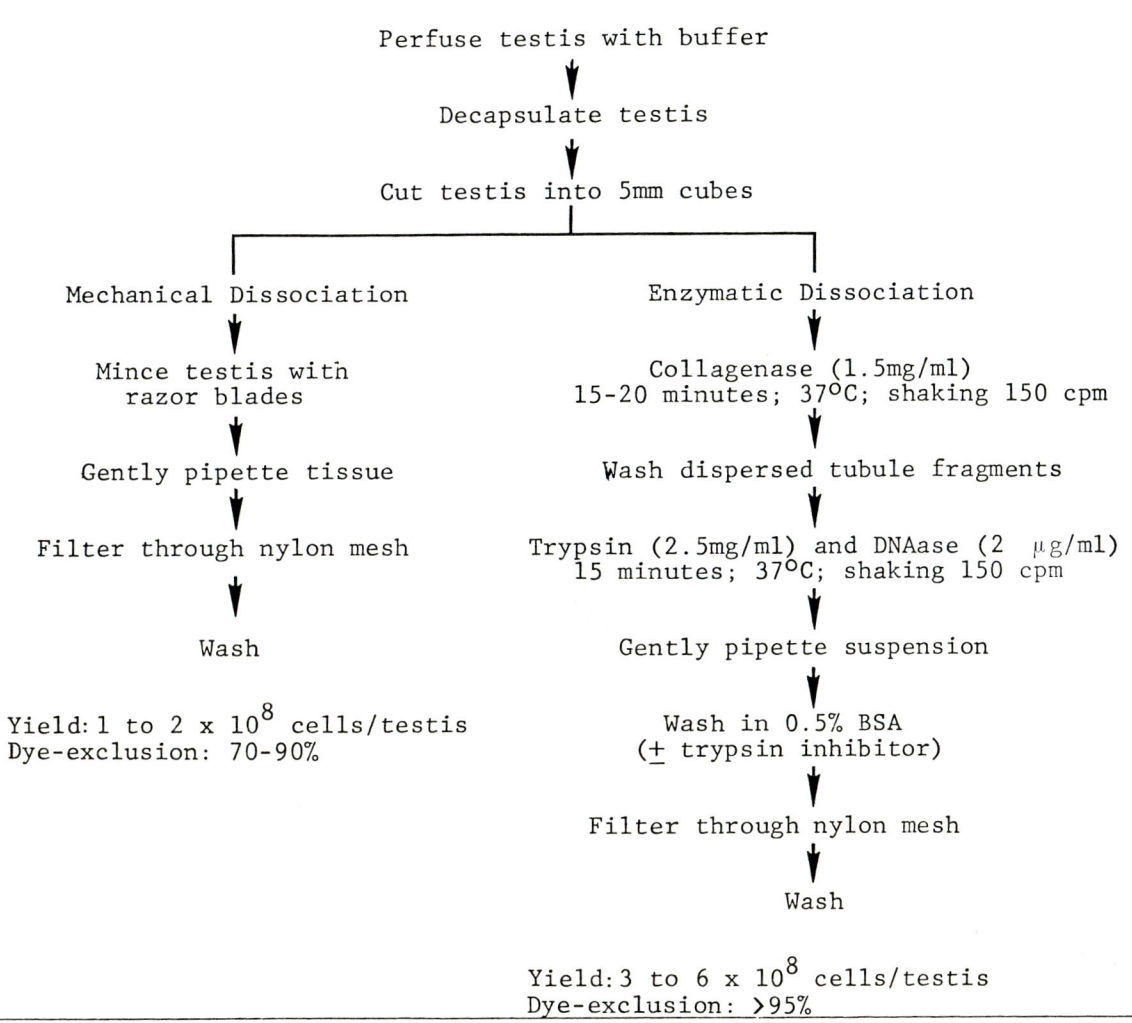

Figure 2. Preparation of testicular cell suspensions (rabbit)

Table 1. Volumes of Solutions Introduced into and Collected from Standard STA-PUT Chambers

Solutions	Chambers		
	Sp-120(10 ml/mm)	SP-180(25 ml/mm)	SP-250(50 ml/mm)
Buffer	20 ml	50 ml	50 ml
Cells in 0.5% BSA (Bovine serum albumin)	10 ml	25 ml	50 ml
2% BSA	275 ml	550 ml	1100 ml
4% BSA	275 ml	550 ml	1100 ml
Sample collected	5 ml	10 ml	10 ml
(Total number of samples)	(116)	(118)	(230)

Sequence of loading:
 1) Buffer
 2) Cell suspension (concentration $2\text{-}10 \times 10^6$ cells/ml)
 3) 2-4% bovine serum albumin gradient
Loading rate—initially 10 ml/min then 5 min after introduction of cell suspension increased to 40 ml/min
Unloading rate—15 ml/min
Total separation time 4 h—0 time is marked at the introduction of the cells into the chamber; collection is completed at 4 h.
 Note. To standardize numbering of the collected tubes it is suggested that the numbering system used by Meistrich (1973) be adopted, i.e. the last tube collected be the reference tube and that tubes be numbered in sequence from that tube. This eliminates variation in sample number of specific cell fractions between runs which results from variable amounts of solutions remaining in the gradient maker and tubing. If the above volumes of solutions are used, the last tube collected is designated 120 for the SP-120 and SP-180 chambers, or 230 for the SP-250 chamber, and the tubes are then numbered in descending order. The STA-PUT apparatus (Velocity Sedimentation Cell Separator) is available from Johns Scientific, 219 Broadview Avenue, Toronto 8, Ontario, Canada.

Table 2. Percentage of Cell Types[a]—Rabbit Testis

	Swierstra & Foote (1963)[b] Intact Testis	O'Rand & Romrell (1977) Cell Suspension
Spermatogonia	3.4 ⎫ 4.1	⎫ 5.5
Preleptotene spermatocytes	0.7 ⎭	⎭
Primary spermatocytes	28.4	26
Secondary spermatocytes	1.2	—
Round spermatids	42.9	49
Elongate spermatids	18.2	12
Sertoli cells	4.8	1.6
Leydig cells	—	5.5

[a]Only nucleated cells were counted in the determination of these percentages.
[b]Percentage calculated from Table 3.

Table 3. Percentage of Cell Types[a]—Mouse Testis

	Meistrich et al. (1973)		Romrell et al. (1976)
	Intact Testis	Cell Suspension	Cell Suspension
Spermatogonia	⎫ 5	⎫ 2.8	⎫ <5
Preleptotene spermatocyte	⎭	⎭	⎭
Primary spermatocyte	17.9	8.7	10-20
Secondary spermatocyte	1.3	1.2	—
Round spermatid	28	41	40-50
Elongate spermatid	38.2	38.6	20-30
Sertoli cells	2.1	1.1	1-3
Leydig cells	3	1.6	<1
Other	5	5.2	5-10

[a]Only nucleated cells were counted in determination of these percentages.

ISOLATION OF MAMMALIAN SPERMATOGENIC CELLS AND CHARACTERIZATION OF CHROMOSOMAL PROTEINS

A.R. Bellvé and D.A. O'Brien

Department of Physiology and Laboratory of Human Reproduction and Reproductive Biology, Harvard Medical School, Boston, Massachusetts 02115 USA

The mammalian testis contains an extensive variety of somatic and germinal cell types. This cellular complexity precludes most direct biochemical research on the ontogenetic processes that are involved in spermatogenesis. Even developmental studies, which take advantage of the temporal inception of spermatogenesis, are confounded by the radical changes that occur in the proportions of testicular cell types (Clermont and Perey, 1957; Bellvé et al., 1977a). In an effort to overcome these limitations, procedures based on sedimentation velocity at unit gravity have been developed to isolate various populations of spermatogenic cells (Lam et al., 1970; Meistrich et al., 1973). This technique, along with recent refinements in cell preparation, facilitates the isolation of relatively homogeneous populations of spermatogenic cells from both the prepuberal (Bellvé et al., 1977a) and adult mouse seminiferous epithelium (Romrell et al., 1976). For the first time, these discrete cell populations now encompass virtually all stages of spermatogenesis from primitive type-A spermatogonia through to the haploid spermatid (Bellvé et al., 1977b).

BASIC PROTOCOL

The procedures used for the preparation of spermatogenic cell suspensions and for cell separation have been recently described in detail (Bellvé et al., 1977b). Preparation of the germ cell suspension involves three fundamental steps. These include: 1) perfusion of the testis *in situ* to remove blood tissue, 2) digestion of the decapsulated testis with collagenase to obtain seminiferous tubules or cords free of interstitial tissue, and 3) dispersion of the seminiferous epithelial cells with trypsin to yield a monodisperse suspension of germ cells. Sertoli cells tend to remain as aggregates and, consequently, can be partially removed by filtering the cell suspension through Nitex nylon mesh (35 μ). This basic procedure of perfusion, sequential enzymatic digestion, and selective filtration has the distinct advantage of effectively eliminating virtually all somatic cells that would otherwise contaminate the germ cell suspension. Moreover, it markedly reduces both the incidence and degree of nucleation of symplasts that can form by the confluence of two or more interconnected germ cells (Romrell et al., 1976). Consequently, the final purities of the pachytene spermatocyte, round spermatid (steps 1-8), and residual body populations are enhanced considerably (Table 1). It is not possible, however, to recover from the adult testis discrete populations of spermatogonia or primary spermatocytes at stages prior to pachytene of meiotic prophase.

Spermatogenesis is reinitiated in the prepuberal mouse four to five days after birth. Thereafter, the germ cells proliferate and undergo differentiation in a well-defined temporal sequence. Aside from Sertoli cells, only primitive type-A spermatogonia are present at day 6, type-A and type-B spermatogonia on day 8, and primary spermatocytes at successive stages of meiotic prophase between days 9 and 20 (Bellvé et al., 1977a). Utilizing this temporal data, it has proven feasible to isolate several discrete populations of spermatogonia and primary spermatocytes from the prepuberal seminiferous cords (Table 1). The purities of the Type-B spermatogonium and leptotene-zygotene spermatocyte populations have been improved recently by reducing the period of tryptic digestion of the seminiferous cords to 10-12 min. This modification leaves a greater proportion of the prepuberal Sertoli cells as aggregates, presumably because of persisting focal tight junctions (Nagano and Suzuki, 1976). These cellular aggregates are then removed, in part, by filtering the initial cell suspension prior to cell separation. However, Sertoli cells still form the principal contaminant of the germ cells isolated from the prepuberal mouse testis (Table 1). It is entirely feasible that this problem could be over-

---

The research and materials required for the preparation of this manuscript were, in part, supported by National Institute of Child Health and Human Development grants HD-08270 and HD-06916. Dr. D.A. O'Brien was the recipient of a Danforth Foundation and a Hoechst-Roussel Fellowship.

© 1979 Urban & Schwarzenberg, Inc. Baltimore-Munich *The Spermatozoon*, edited by D.W. Fawcett and J.M. Bedford

Table 1. Purity and Composition of Cell Populations Isolated from the Mouse Seminiferous Epithelium

Cell Type	Cell Populations (%)								
	PA	A	B[a]	PL	L/Z	P	RS	RB	S
Prim. type-A spermatogonia	90	—	—	—	—	—	—	—	<1
Type-A spermatogonia	—	91	6	—	—	<1	—	—	—
Type-B spermatogonia	—	3	85	1	1	—	—	—	—
Preleptotene spermatocytes	—	—	—	93	7	—	—	—	—
Leptotene spermatocytes	—	—	—	3	39	—	—	—	—
Zygotene spermatocytes	—	—	—	—	28	<1	—	—	—
Pachytene spermatocytes	—	—	—	—	10	89	—	—	—
Secondary spermatocytes	—	—	—	—	—	—	<1	—	—
Round spermatids	—	—	—	—	—	—	87	3	—
Condensing spermatids	—	—	—	—	—	—	1	6	—
Residual bodies	—	—	—	—	—	—	2	89	—
Sertoli cells	10	6	9	3	14	10	—	—	99
Multinucleates	—	—	—	—	<1	—	—	—	—
Others	<1	<1	<1	<1	<1	<1	<10[b]	2	<1

Cell populations include primitive type-A spermatogonia (PA), type-A spermatogonia (A), type-B spermatogonia (B), preleptotene primary spermatocytes (PL), leptotene/zygotene primary spermatocytes (L/Z), pachytene primary spermatocytes (P), round spermatids (RS), residual bodies (RB), and prepuberal Sertoli cells (S). The data are expressed as percent of total cells recovered in each cell population. Those cells (~3-5%) which could not be identified due to unfavorable section are not included.

[a]The population of type-B spermatogonia may contain a low proportion of intermediate spermatogonia which have a greater diameter (~10-11 μm) but cannot always be identified with certainty.

[b]Cells classified as "Others" may include a low proportion of leptotene and zygotene primary spermatocytes.

(Data modified after Bellvé et al., 1977a; reproduced with permission, J Cell Biol.)

come by utilizing a monospecific antibody to induce complement-mediated lysis of the contaminating Sertoli cells. This technique of immune cytolysis has been used effectively to purify erythropoietin-responsive cells from suspensions of fetal mouse liver cells (Cantor et al., 1972).

Since dissociation of the testis necessitates the use of proteolytic enzymes, their possible effect on cellular constituents, particularly membrane components, must be seriously considered. In general, ultrastructural integrity of the isolated germ cells appears to be well preserved (Romrell et al., 1976; Bellvé et al., 1977a; Barcellona and Meistrich, 1977). However, this does not eliminate the possibility of proteolysis apparent only at the molecular level. In an effort to reduce any detrimental effects, the concentration of collagenase and trypsin has been reduced to 0.5-0.1 mg/ml, without compromising the efficacy of the procedure (Bellvé et al., 1977a, b; Chandley et al., 1977). Dissociation of the seminiferous epithelium can also be accomplished by a second incubation with collagenase in the absence of trypsin. However, the period of incubation required is considerably longer and dissociation is most likely induced by the numerous noncollagenous proteases that contaminate the enzyme preparation (Miyoshi and Rosenbloom, 1974). Consequently, this alternative does not proffer any real advantage. Even with the substantially reduced enzyme concentrations, it is still beneficial to add soybean trypsin inhibitor to inactivate trypsin molecules that may be adsorbed to the cell surface (Snow and Allen, 1970). In fact, addition of a trypsin inhibitor is essential for studies involving the biochemical fractionation of cellular constituents.

BIOCHEMICAL FRACTIONATION OF CHROMOSOMAL PROTEINS

The isolation of these discrete cell populations provides an unusual opportunity to study the mechanisms regulating successive stages of mammalian spermatogenesis, including the proliferation of spermatogonia, meiosis, and spermiogenesis. During this differentiation process major transitions in the complement of chromosomal proteins are needed to cope with alterations in nuclear metabolism, to regulate differential gene transcription, and to facilitate rearrangements in the structural conformation of chromatin (review: Bellvé, 1979). Recent studies on somatic cell types have clearly demonstrated that the complexity of histone and nonhistone chromosomal proteins is considerably greater than described previously. For instance, several non-allelic variants of histones 2A, 2B, and 3, three of the four histone species in the nucleosome core, have been characterized (Alfageme et al., 1974; Franklin and Zweidler, 1977; Blankstein et al., 1977). Furthermore, application of two-dimensional polyacrylamide gel electrophoresis has facilitated the resolution of approximately 470 nonhistone proteins from chromatin of HeLa cells (Peterson and McConkey, 1976). This comprises polypeptides of one order of magnitude more than has been detected on one-dimensional sodium dodecyl sulfate (SDS) gels of testicular chromosomal proteins (Kadohama and Turkington, 1974; Mills and Means, 1977). Clearly, an unambiguous resolution of spermatogenic histone and nonhistone chromosomal proteins requires more sophisticated techniques than have been used in the past.

Characterization of Spermatogenic Histones
Developmental studies on the rat testis indicate that at least two atypical histones either increase or are first detectable after the appearance of primary spermatocytes (Grimes et al., 1975; Shires et al., 1975; Mills et al., 1977). One of these unusual histone species, denoted as TH2B or 2S, has an electrophoretic mobility comparable to somatic histone 3 and is therefore difficult to resolve by acetic acid-urea polyacrylamide gel electrophoresis (Branson et al, 1975; Shires et al., 1975). To counteract this problem a two-dimensional electrophoretic technique has been developed that permits resolution of all major spermatogenic histones and their minor variants (Bhatnagar and Bellvé, 1978). In this procedure Lubrol-WX is employed in the second dimension gel. The nonionic detergent causes a differential retardation in the mobility of certain histone variants by interacting with hydrophobic regions in which the helix probability is sensitive to minor amino acid substitutions (Franklin and Zweidler, 1977). When subjected to these electrophoretic conditions, the spermatogenic histones yield a complex profile in comparison with those of the mouse thymus (Fig. 1 and 2). Variant species of histones 2A and 2B occur in the same proportion in both tissues, but an additional variant of histone 3, denoted as H3·5, is evident only in the spermatogenic preparation (Fig. 1). Furthermore, histone 2S is now resolved into two polypeptide species, H2S·1 and H2S·2. The major histone 2S·2 is probably analogous to the cysteine-containing TH2B recently isolated by Shires et al., (1976), while histone 2S·1 may represent a previously undetected variant of the major species. Variants of histone 2B can also be resolved simply by changing the concentration of urea and/or Lubrol-WX (data not shown).

Chromatin of somatic cells and germ cells prior to the condensing spermatid step consists of a duplex strand of DNA that periodically winds in a double turn around a nucleosome particle (review: Kornberg, 1977). The protein core of each nucleosome is comprised of an octameric complex containing two each of the histones 2A, 2B, 3, and 4. The existence of variant forms for three of the major histone species means that at least 54 compositionally different forms of nucleosomes occur in somatic chromatin (Bafus et al., 1978). Whether histones 2S·1 and 2S·2 participate in nucleosome formation during meiosis has not been resolved. Nevertheless, excluding these two histone species, the complexity of variants occurring in spermatogenic cells is still greater than in somatic chromatin. It is reasonable to surmise, therefore, that the germ cells contain an even more diverse population of nucleosomes, although these need not all coexist in any one cell type. Particular variants may be confined exclusively to certain stages of spermatogenesis, in a manner similar to the stage-specific synthesis of variants that occurs during sea urchin embryogenesis (Cohen et al., 1975). The functional significance of such diverse forms of nucleosomes can only be surmised at this time.

Characterization of Spermatogenic Nonhistone Proteins
The technique of two-dimensional polyacrylamide gel electrophoresis developed by O'Farrell (1975) is capable of simultaneously resolving 1,000-5,000 proteins from *Escherischia coli*. However, the resolution obtained with chromatin proteins of eucaryotic cells is restricted by the presence of basic proteins, primarily the histones. These proteins tend to aggregate at the higher pH range of the first dimension isoelectric focusing gel, and hence produce a vertical smear in the second-dimension SDS polyacrylamide gel. This problem can be overcome by the following protocol. Chromatin of spermatogenic cells is dissociated in a medium containing 5 M guanidine hydrochloride (G·HCl), 5mM ethylenediaminetetraacetate (EDTA), 50mM dithiothreitol (DTT), 1mM phenylmethylsulfonyl fluoride in 0.5 M Tris HCl (pH 8.6). The sample is then dialyzed against phosphate buffer (0.1 M, pH 6.8) to reduce the concentration of G·HCl to 0.84 M, and the proteins are subjected to ion exchange chromatography on Bio-Rex 70. Nonhistone chromosomal proteins do not bind to the Bio-Rex 70 and are eluted with 0.84M G·HCl in phosphate buffer (pH 6.8). The appropriate fractions are pooled, dialyzed against 1mM Tris-HCl (pH 7.0), and lyophilized. The histones bind to the cationic resin and can be eluted later by increasing the concentration of G·HCl (Levy et al., 1972; Kolk and Samuel, 1975).

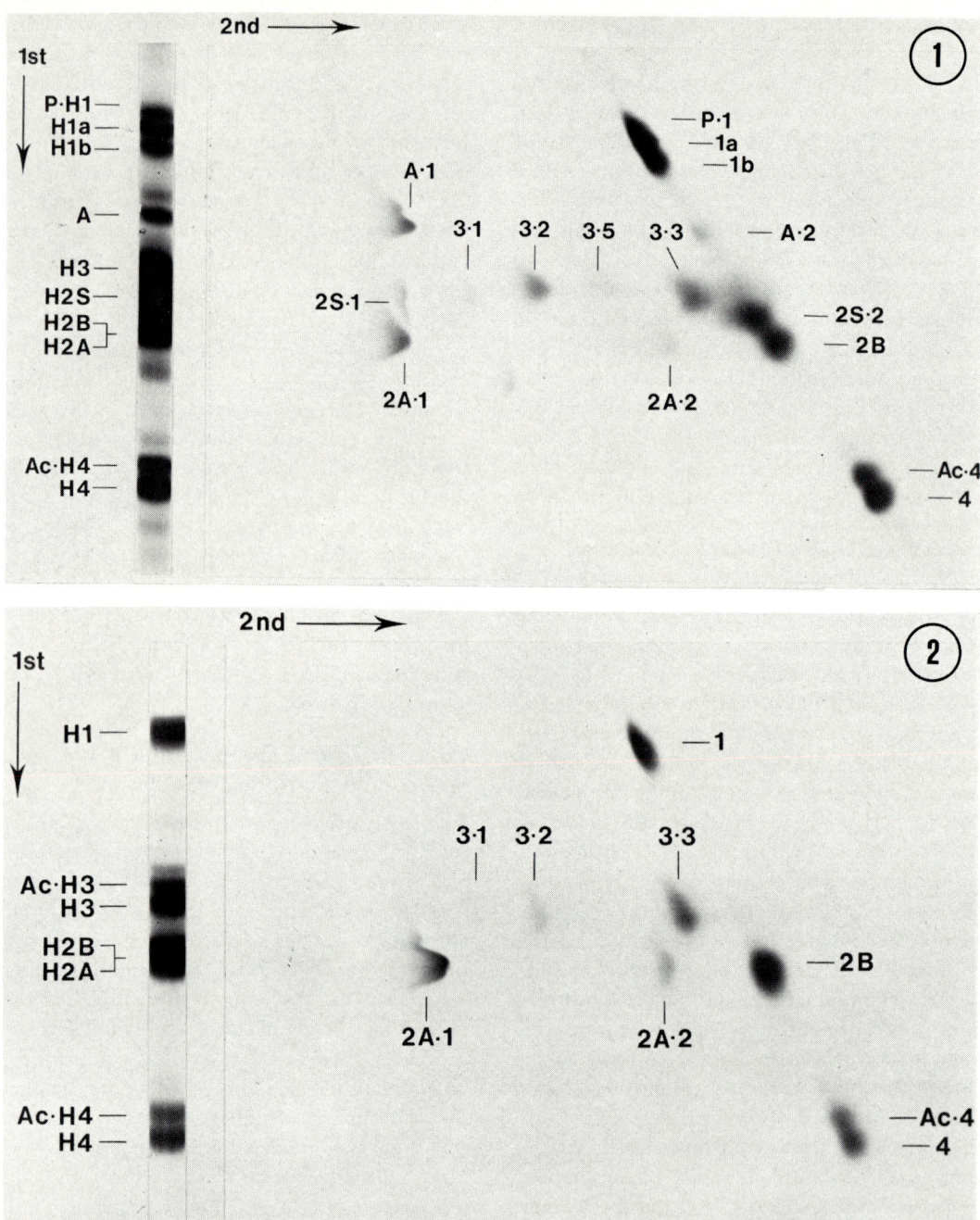

Figure 1. The pattern obtained from mouse spermatogenic histones that were subjected to one-dimensional (vertical gel) and two-dimensional (slab gel) acetic acid-urea polyacrylamide gel electrophoresis. Spermatogenic cells are recovered from the adult mouse testis by sequential enzymatic dissociation. Histones are extracted from germ cell chromatin and separated by electrophoresis on a cylindrical gel (2 mm x 150 mm) in the presence of 6.25 M urea. The cylindrical gel is then placed onto a slab gel (3 x 70 x 100 mm) and the proteins further resolved by electrophoresis in the presence of 6 M urea and 0.4% Lubrol-WX. A complex pattern of spermatogenic histones, comparable to that obtained by other investigators, is evident in the first dimension. However, the presence of nonionic detergent in the second dimension causes a differential retardation in the electrophoretic mobility of certain variants of histones 2S, 2A, and 3. In contrast, under these conditions the mobility of histones 1, 2S·2, 2B, an 4, including acetylated histone 4 (Ac·4), are not affected, and therefore these polypeptides migrate to a diagonal position.

Figure 2. One- and two-dimensional polyacrylamide gel electrophoresis of mouse thymus histones. The electrophoretic pattern obtained for these basic chromosomal proteins is not as complex in either the first dimension (vertical gel) or second dimension (slab gel) in comparison to that observed for spermatogenic histones (Fig. 1). (Figures 1 and 2 reproduced from Bhatnagar and Bellvé, 1978, with permission, Anal Biochem.)

After being prepared in this manner, the nonhistone proteins can be resolved by two-dimensional electrophoresis into more than 150 polypeptides, each differing in their isoelectric point and/or molecular weight (Fig. 3). Undoubtedly, additional polypeptides will be revealed by isotopically labelling the cells with [^{35}S]methionine and subjecting the resulting two-dimensional fingerprint to fluorography. The latter procedure will enable resolution of proteins synthesized *de novo*, providing that each is present at greater than 500 copies per haploid genome (Peterson and McConkey, 1976).

The Transition of Nuclear Proteins during Spermiogenesis

The nucleus of the mammalian spermatozoon generally contains a single species of protamine, an arginine- and cysteine-rich protein of low molecular weight (6.1-7.5k daltons) that is species-specific (Coelingh *et al.*, 1972; Monfoort *et al.*, 1973; Kistler *et al.*, 1973; Bellvé *et al.*, 1975; Calvin, 1976). However, in contrast to other mammals, two distinct species of protamine exist in the human (Kolk and Samuel, 1975) and the mouse spermatozoon (Bellvé *et al.*, 1975; Balhorn *et al.*, 1977). The second protamine species has a higher molecular weight (~8,900 daltons), an extremely high molar ratio of arginine and histidine, and an atypical sequence of basic amino acids at the carboxyterminal end (Bellvé and Carraway, 1978[1]). The mouse spermatozoan nucleus and its surrounding perinuclear material also contain a heterogeneous, but limited, number of nonprotamine proteins, with molecular weights ranging from 14,000-76,000 daltons.[2] Both classes of proteins are synthesized primarily during late spermiogenesis, coincident with the displacement of chromosomal histones and condensation of the spermatid nucleus (Bellvé *et al.*, 1975[3]). This transitional period is also characterized by the transient appearance of several basic nuclear proteins that may be involved in the initiation of condensation of spermatid chromatin (Kistler *et al.*, 1973, 1975; Grimes *et al.*, 1977; Loir and Lanneau, 1978). Concurrently, virtually all of the nonhistone nuclear proteins are eliminated. These dramatic changes in the complement of nuclear proteins during late spermiogenesis are associated with the complete repression of gene transcription, the apparent loss of nucleosome substructure (Kierszenbaum and Tres, 1975), and shaping of the sperm nucleus (Fawcett *et al.*, 1971).

CONCLUSIONS

The complement of chromosomal proteins undergoes a series of major transitions during the course of mammalian spermatogenesis. Characterization of these events has necessitated the development of new techniques for the isolation of discrete populations of germ cells and for the fractionation of nuclear proteins. Undoubtedly, application of these procedures will yield valuable information on the mechanisms that are involved in regulating this differentiative process. It is also reasonable to anticipate that these techniques, in conjunction with procedures for isolating specific nuclear structures, will permit identification and biochemical characterization of proteins that are involved in the assembly of the synaptonemal complex and in shaping of the sperm nucleus.

REFERENCES

Alfageme, C.R.; Zweidler, A.; Mahowald, A.; Cohen, L.M: Histones of *Drosophila* Embryos. J Biol Chem 249(1974)3729-3736

Bafus, N.L.; Albright, S.C.; Todd, R.D.; Garrard, W.T.: A Method for Mapping the Distribution of Modified and Variant Histones among Mono- and Polynucleosomes. J Biol Chem 253(1978)2568-2574

Balhorn, R.; Gledhill, B.L.; Wyrobek, A.J.: Mouse Sperm Chromatin Proteins: Quantitative Isolation and Partial Characterization. Biochemistry 16(1977)4074-4080

Barcellona, W.J.; Meistrich, M.L.: Ultrastructural Integrity of Mouse Testicular Cells Separated by Velocity Sedimentation. J Reprod Fertil 50(1977)61-68

Bellvé, A.R.: The Molecular Biology of Mammalian Spermatogenesis. Oxford Reviews of Reproductive Biology ed. by C.A. Finn. Vol. 1. pp. 159-161 Oxford University Press, Oxford

Bellvé, A.R.; Anderson, E.; Hanley-Bowdoin, L.: Synthesis and Amino Acid Composition of Basic Proteins in Mammalian Sperm Nuclei. Dev Biol 47(1975)349-365

Bellvé, A.R.; Carraway, R.: Characterization of Two Basic Chromosomal Proteins Isolated from Mouse Spermatozoa. J Cell Biol 79(1978)177a

Bellvé, A.R.; Cavicchia, J.C.; Millette, C.F.; O'Brien, D.A.; Bhatnagar, Y.M.; Dym, M.: Spermatogenic Cells of the Prepuberal Mouse. Isolation and Morphological Characterization. J Cell Biol 74(1977a)68-85

Bellvé, A.R.; Millette, C.F.; Bhatnagar, Y.M.; O'Brien, D.A.: Dissociation of the Mouse Testis and Characterization of Isolated Spermatogenic Cells. J Histochem Cytochem 25(1977b)480-494

Bhatnagar, Y.M.; Bellvé, A.R.: Two-dimensional Electrophoretic Analysis of Major Histone Species and Their Variants from Somatic and Germline Tissue. Anal Biochem 86(1978)754-760

---

[1] Bellvé, A.R.; Carraway, R.: Two Basic Chromosomal Proteins of Mouse Spermatozoa. Characterization of a Protamine with an Atypical Carboxyterminal Sequence. J Biol Chem, submitted

[2] O'Brien, D.A.; Bellvé, A.R.: Protein Constituents of the Mouse Spermatozoon. An Electrophoretic Characterization. Dev Biol, submitted.

[3] O'Brien, D.A.; Bellvé, A.R.: Protein Constituents of the Mouse Spermatozoon. II. Temporal Synthesis during Spermatogenesis. Dev Biol, submitted

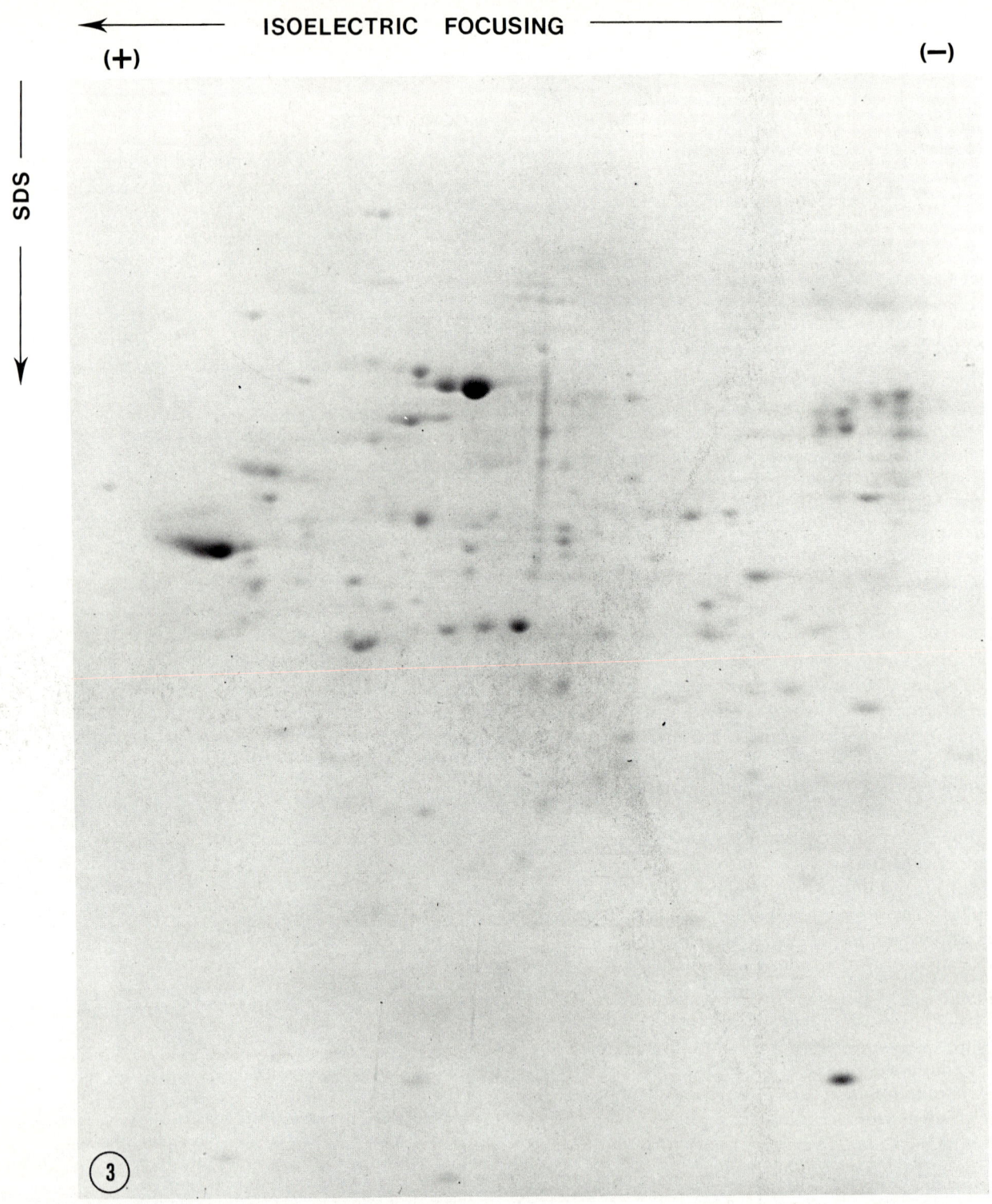

Figure 3. Resolution of mouse spermatogenic nonhistone chromosomal proteins by two-dimensional polyacrylamide gel electrophoresis. Chromosomal proteins are recovered from mouse spermatogenic cells and subjected to ion exchange chromatography on Bio-Rex 70 to remove the histones. Nonhistone chromosomal proteins are partially resolved by electrophoresis on an isoelectric focusing gel (2 x 150 mm). This gel is then embedded onto an SDS slab polyacrylamide gel (2 x 150 x 170 mm) and electrophoresis continued in the second dimension. The procedure permits complete resolution of more than 150 polypeptide species, stainable by Coomassie blue, that differ in their isoelectric point and/or molecular weight. Positive and negative signs indicate electrode polarity.

Blankstein, L.A.; Stollar, B.D.; Franklin, S.G.; Zweidler, A.; Levy, S.B.: Biochemical and Immunological Characterization of Two Distinct Variants of Histone H2A in Friend Leukemia. Biochemistry 16(1977)4557-4562

Branson, R.E.; Grimes, S.R.; Yonuschot, S.; Irvin, J.L.: The Histones of the Rat Testis. Arch Biochem Biophys 168(1975)403-412

Calvin, H.I.: Comparative Analysis of the Nuclear Basic Proteins in Rat, Human, Guinea Pig, Mouse and Rabbit Spermatozoa. Biochim Biophys Acta 434(1976)377-389

Cantor, L.N.; Morris, A.J.; Marks, P.A.; Rifkind, R.A.: Purification of Erythropoetin-responsive Cells by Immune Hemolysis. Proc Natl Acad Sci USA 69(1972)1337-1341

Chandley, A.C.; Hotta, Y.; Stern, H.: Biochemical Analysis of Meiosis in the Male Mouse. I. Separation and DNA Labeling of Specific Spermatogenic Stages. Chromosoma 62(1977)243-253

Clermont, Y.; Perey, B.: Quantitative Study of the Cell Population of the Seminiferous Epithelium in Immature Rats. Am J Anat 100(1957)241-268

Coelingh, J.P.; Monfoort, C.H.; Rozijn, T.H.; Gevers Leuven, J.A.; Schiphof, R.; Steyn-Parvé, E.P.; Braunitzer, G.; Schrank, B.; Ruhfus, A.: The Complete Amino Acid Sequence of the Basic Nuclear Protein of Bull Spermatozoa. Biochim Biophys Acta 285(1972)1-14

Cohen, L.H.; Newrock, K.M.; Zweidler, A.: Stage-specific Switches in Histone Synthesis during Embryogenesis of the Sea Urchin. Science 190(1975)994-997

Fawcett, D.W.; Anderson, W.A.; Phillips, D.M.: Morphogenetic Factors Influencing the Shape of the Sperm Head. Dev Biol 26(1971)220-251

Franklin, S.F.; Zweidler, A.: Non-allelic Variants of Histones 2A, 2B and 3 in Mammals. Nature 266(1977)273-275

Grimes, S.R.; Chae, C-B.; Irvin, J.L.: Effects of Age and Hypophysectomy upon Relative Proportions of Various Histones in Rat Testis. Biochem Biophys Res Commun 64(1975)911-917

Grimes, S.R.; Meistrich, M.L.; Platz, R.D.; Hnilica, L.S.: Nuclear Protein Transitions in Rat Testis Spermatids. Exp Cell Res 110(1977)31-39

Kadohama, N.; Turkington, R.W.: Changes in Acidic Chromatin Proteins during the Hormone-dependent Development of Rat Testis and Epididymis. J Biol Chem 249(1974)6225-6233

Kierszenbaum, A.L.; Tres, L.L.: Structural and Transcriptional Features of the Mouse Spermatid Genome. J Cell Biol 65(1975)258-270

Kistler, W.S.; Geroch, M.E.; Williams-Ashman, H.G.: Specific Basic Proteins from Mammalian Testes. Isolation and Properties of Small Basic Proteins from Rat Testes and Epididymal Spermatozoa. J Biol Chem 248(1973)4532-4543

Kistler, W.S.; Noyes, C.; Hsu, R.; Heinrikson, R.L.: The Amino Acid Sequence of a Testis-specific Basic Protein that is Associated with Spermatogenesis. J Biol Chem 250(1975)1847-1853

Kolk, A.H.J.; Samuel, T.: Isolation, Chemical and Immunological Characterization of Two Strongly Basic Nuclear Proteins from Human Spermatozoa. Biochim Biophys Acta 393(1975)307-319

Kornberg, R.D.: Structure of Chromatin. Ann Rev Biochem 46(1977)931-954

Lam, D.M.K.; Furrer, R.; Bruce, W.R.: The Separation, Physical Characterization, and Differentiation Kinetics of Spermatogonial Cells of the Mouse. Proc Natl Acad Sci USA 65(1970)192-199

Levy, S.; Simpson, R.T.; Sober, H.A.: Fractionation of Chromatin Components. Biochemistry 11(1972)1547-1554

Loir, M.; Lanneau, M.: Partial Characterization of Ram Spermatidal Basic Nuclear Proteins. Biochem Biophys Res Commun 80(1978)975-982

Meistrich, M.L.; Bruce, W.R.; Clermont, Y.: Cellular Composition of Mouse Testis Cells following Velocity Sedimentation Separation. Exp Cell Res 79(1973)213-227

Mills, N.C.; Means, A.R.: Nonhistone Chromosomal Proteins of the Developing Rat Testis. Biol Reprod 17(1977)769-779

Mills, N.C.; Van, N.T.; Means, A.R.: Histones of Rat Testis Chromatin during Early Postnatal Development and Their Interactions with DNA. Biol Reprod 17(1977)760-768

Miyoshi, M.; Rosenbloom, J.: General Proteolytic Activity of Highly Purified Preparations of Clostridial Collagenase. Connect Tiss Res 2(1974)77-84

Monfoort, C.H.; Schiphof, R.; Rozijn, T.H.; Steyn-Parvé, E.P.: Amino Acid Composition and Carboxy-terminal Structure of Some Basic Chromosomal Proteins of Mammalian Spermatozoa. Biochim Biophys Acta 322(1973)173-177

Nagano, T.; Suzuki, F.: The Postnatal Development of the Junctional Complexes of the Mouse Sertoli Cells as Revealed by Freeze-fracture. Anat Rec 185(1976)403-418

O'Farrell, P.H.: High Resolution Two-dimensional Electrophoresis of Proteins. J Biol Chem 250(1975)4007-4021

Peterson, J.L.; McConkey, E.H.: Non-histone Chromosomal Proteins from HeLa Cells. A Survey by High Resolution, Two-dimensional Electrophoresis. J Biol Chem 251(1976)548-554

Romrell, L.J.; Bellvé, A.R.; Fawcett, D.W.: Separation of Mouse Spermatogenic Cells by Sedimentation Velocity. A Morphological Characterization. Dev Biol 49(1976)119-131

Shires, A.; Carpenter, M.P.; Chalkley, R.: New Histones Found in Mature Mammalian Testes. Proc Natl Acad Sci USA 72(1975)2714-2718

Shires, A.; Carpenter, M.P.; Chalkley, R.: A Cysteine-containing H2B-like Histone Found in Mature Mammalian Testis. J Biol Chem 251(1976)4155-4158

Snow, C.; Allen, A.: The Release of Radioactive Nucleic Acids and Mucoproteins by Trypsin and Ethylenediaminetetraacetate Treatment of Baby Hamster Cells in Tissue Culture. Biochem J 119(1970)707-714

ISOLATION OF STABLE STRUCTURES FROM RAT SPERMATOZOA

H.I. Calvin

Department of Human Genetics and Development and Center for Reproductive Sciences, Columbia University, New York, New York 10032 USA

The mammalian spermatozoon possesses a diverse complement of distinct structural elements, many of which have acquired an unusual degree of stability as a consequence of intermolecular disulfide bonding (Bedford and Calvin, 1974a, b). Unlike most somatic cells, the sperm of mammals is only superficially lysed in hypotonic media, which strip off the plasma membrane, but allow metabolic activity to persist (Keyhani and Storey, 1973). Even spermatozoa extracted with Triton X-100 and dithiothreitol (DTT) retain an intact motile apparatus, capable of reactivation with adenosine triphosphate (ATP) (Lindemann and Gibbons, 1975). The isolation of most sperm organelles thus requires relatively severe chemical or physical treatments. The use of such procedures for the isolation of disulfide-bonded structures from the rat spermatozoon is the major subject of this chapter. Where appropriate, alternative methods for the isolation of these or other sperm components are mentioned. Most of the procedures discussed here have been described or reviewed previously (Calvin, 1976).

SEPARATION OF HEADS AND TAILS

A variety of physical methods have been employed to sever the head-tail junction of the mammalian spermatozoon (Calvin, 1976). More recently, emphasis has been placed on chemical lysis of the structural elements which bind the head to the tail (Young and Cooper, 1979).

Prior to the isolation of disulfide-stabilized elements from the heads or tails of the rat spermatozoon in this laboratory, the heads are routinely detached from the tails by sonication and the two major surviving fractions separated by sucrose density gradient centrifugation. It should be noted, however, that procedures for the isolation of keratinoid structures may also begin by selective solubilization of unwanted structures prior to density gradient centrifugation (Olson, 1979).

© 1979 Urban & Schwarzenberg, Inc. Baltimore-Munich *The Spermatozoon*, edited by D.W. Fawcett and J.M. Bedford

Decapitation of rat spermatozoa, expressed with a hemostat from the cauda epididymidis, is carried out by sonication of 3-4-ml sperm suspensions for 2 min in 12-ml conical centrifuge tubes cooled in ice, with a 125 w Bronwill Model IIA sonifier, fitted with a $3/16$-in. microtip and adjusted to a setting of 65% of maximum power (~80 w). This sonication quantitatively severs the head from the tail and fragments the latter into several segments, the largest of which usually includes the entire neck and midpiece regions (Calvin et al., 1973).

Sonicated heads and tails are then separated by sucrose density gradient centrifugation. After the sonicate is mixed thoroughly with concentrated sucrose to attain a final concentration of 1.80 M sucrose, the suspension is adjusted with additional 1.80 M sucrose to a final concentration of $4-8 \times 10^6$ sperm/ml and applied to a stepwise gradient composed of 13-ml layers of 2.05 M and 2.20 M sucrose in a 1-in. x $3\frac{1}{2}$-in. nitrocellulose tube. The pH of all sucrose media is maintained slightly below neutrality by the inclusion of 0.02 M sodium phosphate (pH 6.0), in order to retard oxidation of —SH groups (Calvin et al., 1973). Samples are layered to within $1/8$ in. of the top of the nitrocellulose tube (12-13-ml sample volume) and centrifuged at 22,500 rpm (~91,000 g, r_{max}) for 1 h in a Beckman SW-27 rotor at 2-4°C. As shown in Figure 1, the majority of the particulate material is concentrated at the 1.80 M/2.05 M sucrose interface (tail fragments) and in the pellet (heads). The tail layer is removed with a syringe fitted with an 18-gauge needle, the remainder of the sucrose poured off, and the heads recovered by resuspending the pellet, after carefully wiping the walls of the inverted tube with a damp tissue. Tails are freed of sucrose by dilution with aqueous buffer and recentrifugation. Both heads and tail midpieces are recovered in >70% yield by these procedures. Smaller tail fragments derived from the principal piece and endpiece appear in the same fraction as the midpieces. Heads are consistently >99% free of tail contamination. On the other hand, contamination of the tail fraction approaches one head per 20 tail midpieces.

The presence of heads in the tail fraction results from

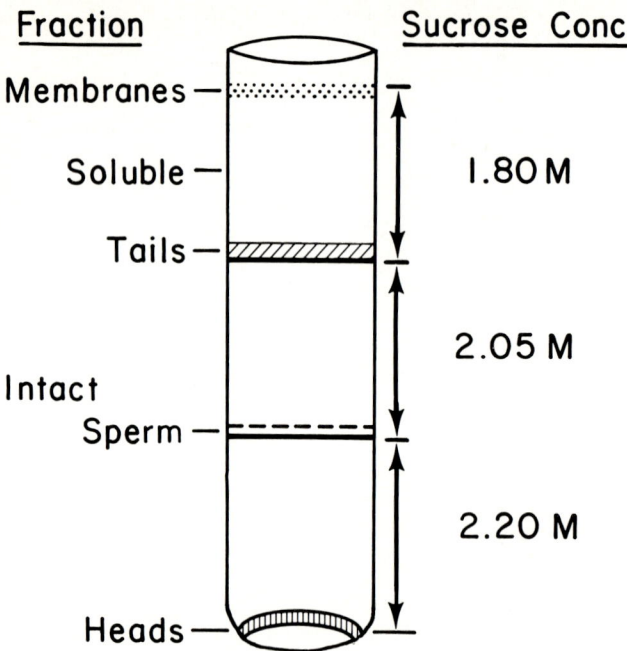

Figure 1. Diagram of gradient separation of rat sperm heads and tails.

their being trapped in the dense band of tail fragments which forms at the 1.80 M/2.05 M sucrose interface. This effect has been partially overcome by applying the sample to the gradient in 1.80 M sucrose, a medium through which the tail fragments centrifuge relatively slowly. Contamination can be further reduced by sonicating the sperm tails into shorter fragments before mixing with the sucrose or, even more effectively, by premixing the sonicate in 2.05 M sucrose and floating the tails upward into 1.80 M sucrose during centrifugation (Calvin, 1976). In any case, purified tails can be relayered over 2.05 M sucrose and recentrifuged to eliminate contamination by heads.

The gradient described in Figure 1 has been employed to isolate relatively intact tails produced by the trypsin cleavage procedure of Millette *et al.* (1973), as noted previously (Calvin, 1976). Its successful modification for the separation of rabbit or human sperm heads and tails, following cleavage by sonication (Calvin, 1976) or by incubation with butylamine (Young and Cooper, 1979), has also been documented.

ISOLATION OF DISULFIDE-STABILIZED STRUCTURES

Sonification of the isolated rat sperm heads in the presence of 0.1% sodium dodecyl sulfate (SDS) either dissolves or detaches essentially all the material surrounding the nuclear chromatin (Calvin, 1976). Increasing the SDS concentration to 1% facilitates this removal. The procedure now recommended for obtaining chromatin is to suspend the sperm heads (repurified once through 2.20 M sucrose) in 1% SDS-0.05 M Tris HCl (pH 7.5) at room temperature and sonicate moderately to lift off the perforatorium (45% of maximum power for 1 min with the Bronwill Model IIA). The sonicate, typically 300×10^6 heads in 2 ml of SDS-Tris, is then diluted with 6 ml of 0.05 M Tris HCl (pH 7.5), cooled to 0-4°C, applied to a gradient of 1.60 M sucrose (25 ml)/2.20 M sucrose (5 ml) and centrifuged for 20 min at 91,000 g, r_{max}. Pure chromatin is found in the pellet. The surviving perinuclear material, which sediments at the boundary between the two layers, appears to consist almost entirely of perforatorium, as judged by its appearance under the electron microscope. A well-characterized preparation of rat perforatorium has been obtained by an alternative approach, in which nuclear chromatin is selectively solubilized by sarkosyl-DTT (Olson *et al.*, 1976; Olson, 1979). In addition, alternative procedures for the isolation of mammalian sperm chromatin have been reported (Calvin, 1976).

Incubation of the tails in 1% SDS leaves a substantial residue, composed of the connecting piece, dense fibers, fibrous sheath, and mitochondrial ghosts (Bedford and Calvin, 1974a). The individual conformations and the arrangement of these structures are virtually undisturbed by SDS.

Subsequent incubation at room temperature overnight in 1% SDS-0.2mM DTT $-$0.05 M Tris HCl (pH 7.4), or in the same medium at pH 8.5 for 2-3 h, leaves the dense fibers and connecting piece relatively intact, while dissolving the fibrous sheath and loosening the attachments between the mitochondrial remnants. A fraction consisting of dense fibers and connecting pieces may be isolated from such partially digested preparations by mild sonication (45% setting with the Bronwill Model IIA sonifier for 2 min) and centrifugation at 10,000 g for 10 min (Calvin *et al.*, 1975; Calvin, 1976). The residue is washed twice with water or dilute SDS (0.02%) to free the dense fiber-connecting piece fraction of mitochondrial vesicles, which appear in the supernatant, together with fine, short fragments of dense fibers (Calvin and Cooper, 1979). Contaminating sperm heads may still be removed at this point, by layering the product over 2.05 M sucrose and centrifugation for 20 min at 91,000 g. Due to the heterogeneity of the dense fiber fragments, they have not been resolved completely either from the mitochondrial remnants in the supernatant fraction or the connecting pieces in the residue. However, a significant proportion of those fibers that distribute with the mitochondrial remnants can be resolved from the latter by centrifugation through 1.60 M sucrose. The isolation of intact mitochondria or mitochondrial ghosts from bull spermatozoa is discussed elsewhere in this volume (Pallini), as is the isolation of fibrous sheath from rat spermatozoa (Olson).

Isolation of sperm structures which are relatively unstable, such as the acrosome, cyctoplasmic droplet, or plasma membrane, is incompatible with the methodology outlined above. For progress made in this area, the reader is referred to publications concerned with purification of plasma membrane (Lunstra et al., 1974), outer acrosomal membrane (Zahler and Doak, 1975), cytoplasmic droplet (Roberts et al., 1976), and acrosomal vesicles (Multamaki, 1973).

REFERENCES

Bedford, J.M.; Calvin, H.I.: Changes in —S—S—linked Sperm Tail Structures during Epididymal Maturation, with Comparative Observations in Sub-mammalian Species. J Exp Zool 187(1974a)181-203

Bedford, J.M.; Calvin, H.I.: The Occurrence and Possible Functional Significance of —S—S— Crosslinks in Sperm Heads, with Particular Reference to Eutherian Mammals. J Exp Zool 188(1974b)137-156

Calvin, H.I.: Isolation and Subfractionation of Mammalian Sperm Heads and Tails. Methods Cell Biol 13(1976)85-104

Calvin, H.I.; Cooper, G.W.:

Calvin, H.I.; Hwang, F.H.F.; Wohlrab, H.: Localization of Zinc in a Dense Fiber-connecting Piece Fraction Analogous Chemically to Hair Keratin. Biol Reprod 13(1975)228-239

Calvin, H.I.; Yu, C.C.; Bedford, J.M.: Effects of Epididymal Maturation, Zinc (II) and Copper (II) on the Reactive Sulfhydryl Content of Structural Elements in Rat Spermatozoa. Exp Cell Res 86(1973)280-285

Keyhani, E.; Storey, B.T.: Energy Conservation Capacity and Morphological Integrity of Mitochondria in Hypotonically Treated Rabbit Epididymal Spermatozoa. Biochim Biophys Acta 305(1973)557-569

Lindemann, C.B.; Gibbons, I.R.: Adenosine Triphosphate-induced Motility and Sliding of Filaments in Mammalian Sperm Extracted with Triton X-100. J Cell Biol 65(1975)147-162

Lunstra, D.D.; Clegg, E.D.; Morre, D.J.: Isolation of Plasma Membrane from Porcine Spermatozoa. Prep Biochem 4(1974)341-352

Millette, C.F.; Spear, P.G.; Gall, W.E.; Edelman, G.M.: Chemical Dissection of Mammalian Spermatozoa. J Cell Biol 58(1973)662-675

Multamaki, S.: Isolation of Pure Acrosomes by Subcellular Fractionation of Bull Spermatozoa. Int J Fertil 18(1973)193-205

Olson, G.E.; Hamilton, D.W.; Fawcett, D.W.: Isolation and Characterization of the Perforatorium of Rat Spermatozoa. J Reprod Fertil 47(1976)293-297

Roberts, M.L.; Scouten, W.H.; Nyquist, S.E.: Isolation and Characterization of the Cytoplasmic Droplet in the Rat. Biol Reprod 14(1976)421-424

Zahler, W.L.; Doak, G.A.: Isolation of the Outer Acrosomal Membrane from Bull Sperm. Biochim Biophys Acta 406(1975)479-488

SEPARATION OF THE HEAD AND TAIL OF MAMMALIAN SPERMATOZOA BY PRIMARY AMINES: EVIDENCE FOR THEIR JUNCTION BY SCHIFF BASES

R.J. Young and G.W. Cooper

Laboratory of Reproductive Biology, Department of Obstetrics and Gynecology, Cornell University Medical College, New York, New York 10021 USA

Dissociation of the structural components of mammalian spermatozoa allows the study of their macromolecular composition and how these structures are assembled. The authors have been interested particularly in the nature of the associations between nuclear chromatin, the nuclear envelope, and the connecting piece of the sperm tail that collectively form the fulcrum for motility. To determine how these are connected, spermatozoa have been treated with a variety of reagents, including primary amines, aldehydes, and mercaptans, and changes in ultrastructure induced by these have been correlated with their reactivity. Herein is presented a summary of studies on a specific type of sperm head-tail detachment induced by primary amines. A preparative method for the isolation of the heads and tails of rabbit spermatozoa after treatment with n-butylamine is given in Figure 1. Ultrastructural analysis of the site of head detachment and experiments testing possible mechanisms by which primary amines induce this are presented in Figures 2-4 and Tables 1-4. These observations are based on rabbit spermatozoa, but amine-induced sperm head detachment is a general phenomenon which occurs in a comparable manner in mice, guinea pigs, men, and an ascrotal mammal, *Octodon degus*.

All primary amines tested (Table 1) detach the heads and tails of rabbit spermatozoa (Cooper and Young, 1977). Detachment occurs at the level of the nuclear envelope over the tail implantation fossa by separation of the inner and outer nuclear membranes (Fig. 2 and 3). Their close apposition is bridged there by periodic,

---

The authors wish to thank Ms. K. Sweeny and Ms. Miu-Ying Fong for their skillful technical assistance. This work was supported in part by the Rockefeller Foundation and N.I.H. Grants HD-10230 and HD-09215.

© 1979 Urban & Schwarzenberg, Inc. Baltimore-Munich *The Spermatozoon*, edited by D.W. Fawcett and J.M. Bedford

---

electron-dense structures (Fig. 4); see Fawcett (1975) for a review of the ultrastructure of the head and neck of mammalian spermatozoa. The site of head-tail detachment induced by primary amines thus clearly differs from that resulting with other reagents (Calvin, 1976). For example, trypsin, with or without prior treatment with dithiothreitol, detaches sperm heads and tails by cleavage of the fibrous structures that join the basal plate to the capitulum of the connecting piece (Millette *et al.*, 1973).

The mechanism of n-butylamine action was revealed by assaying different compounds for their ability to induce head-tail detachment (Table 1). Primary amines were highly effective, whereas the percent detachment decreased when these were substituted by a phenyl or hydroxyl group, as with benzylamine or ethanolamine (Table 1). Alcohols, acetylated amines, secondary and tertiary amines, or diamines were inactive. Detachment induced by n-butylamine also depended on pH, with a maximum percentage occurring at the pK_a (10.7) of the amine (Table 2). The requirement that the amine group of a primary amine be unprotonated suggested that primary amines induced head detachment by transimination in intermolecular Schiff bases. Since detachment occurs between the inner and outer membranes of the nuclear envelope, the periodic structures found between these membranes at the tail implantation fossa should be the sites of intermolecular Schiff base formation.

Schiff bases are formed by the condensation of primary amines with aldehydes, *e.g.*, R^1—CHO + H_2N—$R^2 \longrightarrow R^1$—CH=N—R^2 + H_2O. The resulting —C=N— or aldimine bond is reactive and can undergo displacement with a second primary amine to form a new Schiff base, thus releasing the first amine, *e.g.*, R^1—CH=N—R^2 + R^3—$NH_2 \longrightarrow R^1$—CH=N—R^3 + H_2N—R^2. Head detachment induced by n-

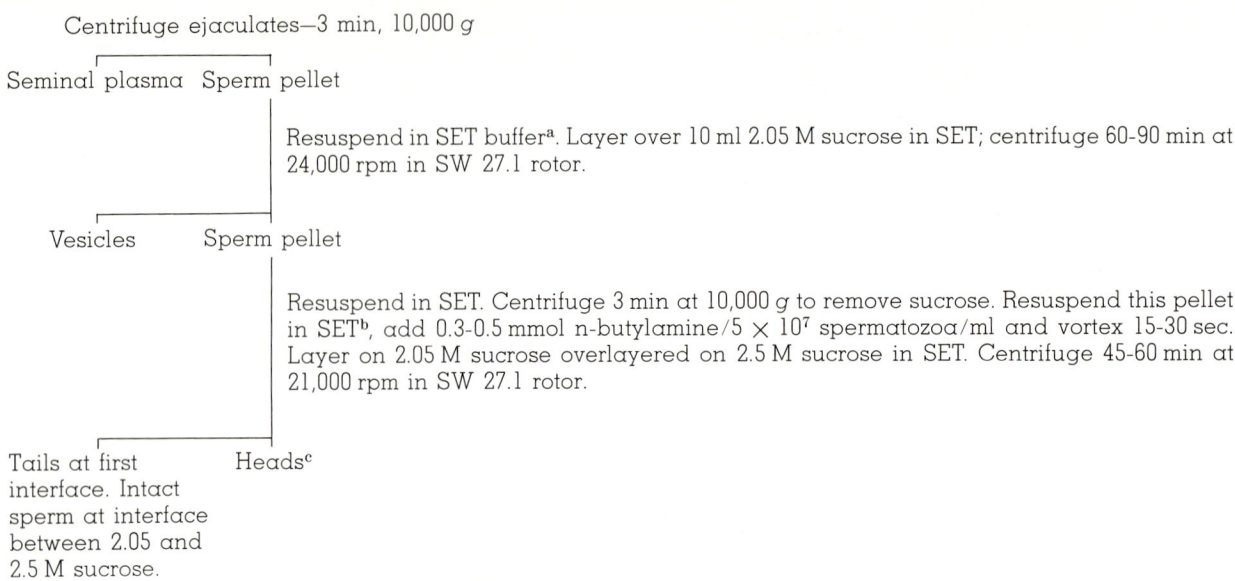

Figure 1. Preparative Procedure for the Isolation of the Heads and Tails of Rabbit Spermatozoa. a) SET = 0.1 M Tris HCl (pH 7.2), 0.15 M NaCl, 0.005 M EDTA. b) Acrosomes are detached after this centrifugation. The wall of the centrifuge tubes should be washed with buffer and wiped dry before resuspending the sperm pellets to avoid contamination with acrosomal enzymes and material from seminal plasma. c) Siliconized glassware was used as detached heads have a tendency to aggregate and stick to glass. Head aggregation can also be reduced by a repeat centrifugation through 2.05 M sucrose before amine treatment, by using the minimum amount of amine needed for detachment, and by including 2-5% Sarkosyl in the sucrose solutions. A second centrifugation through the discontinuous sucrose gradient reduces tail contamination to 1-2%, with an 80-90% overall yield of heads.

butylamine can therefore be represented as an amine displacement reaction that separates by transimination all proteins linked by Schiff bases. To determine whether aldimine bonds do indeed crosslink proteins in the inner and outer membranes of the nuclear envelope, the authors took advantage of the fact that amine displacement will not occur if Schiff bases are converted to secondary amines by reduction, e.g., $R^1-CH=N-R^2 + 2H \longrightarrow R^1-CH_2-NH-R^2$. Table 3 shows that rabbit spermatozoa are resistant to head detachment by n-butylamine if they were first reduced at pH 5.0 with sodium cyanoborohydride ($NaCNBH_3$). This reagent is specific for the reduction of aldimine bonds under mild conditions (Lane, 1975), and the resistance of spermatozoa to head detachment by primary amines after reduction is evidence that aldimine bonds initially linked proteins at the detachment site, i.e. the nuclear envelope.

Intermolecular crosslinking by Schiff base formation occurs in elastin (Franzblau, 1971), collagen (Tanzer, 1976), and in structures containing collagen-like molecules (Kefalides, 1975). The chemical, physical, and mechanical properties of elastin and collagen change on aging as a result of the spontaneous conversion of aldimine bonds to more stable crosslinks (Franzblau, 1971; Tanzer, 1976). Similar conversion of the intermolecular bonds linking the sperm head and tail might be expected to occur as spermatozoa age in vivo. Such conversion does not occur to a significant extent in the male reproductive tract, as evidenced by the effects of primary amines on epididymal and ejaculated spermatozoa, but more than 75% of rabbit spermatozoa recovered from the vagina, uterus, or oviducts of female rabbits within 6 h of mating were resistant to head detachment by n-butylamine. In vitro stabilization of the head-tail linkages of rabbit spermatozoa requires incubation temperatures in the range of rabbit body temperature (39.8°C), as well as cations. Rabbit spermatozoa were resistant to n-butylamine detachment after incubation at 37°C for 16-24 h but were not stabilized in vitro at 22°C (Table 4). Addition of divalent cations (Cu, Zn, Mg, or Ca), at concentrations equivalent to those in female reproductive tract fluids, increased the rate of stabilization, with that catalyzed by cupric ions approaching the kinetics of head-tail stabilization in the female rabbit (Table 4).

These experiments show that the spermatozoan tail is linked to the head via aldimine bonds crosslinking proteins in the membranes of the nuclear envelope. In the rabbit, these aldimine bonds are transformed to more stable structures during sperm transport in the female preceding ovulation, i.e. before 9.5-10 h after

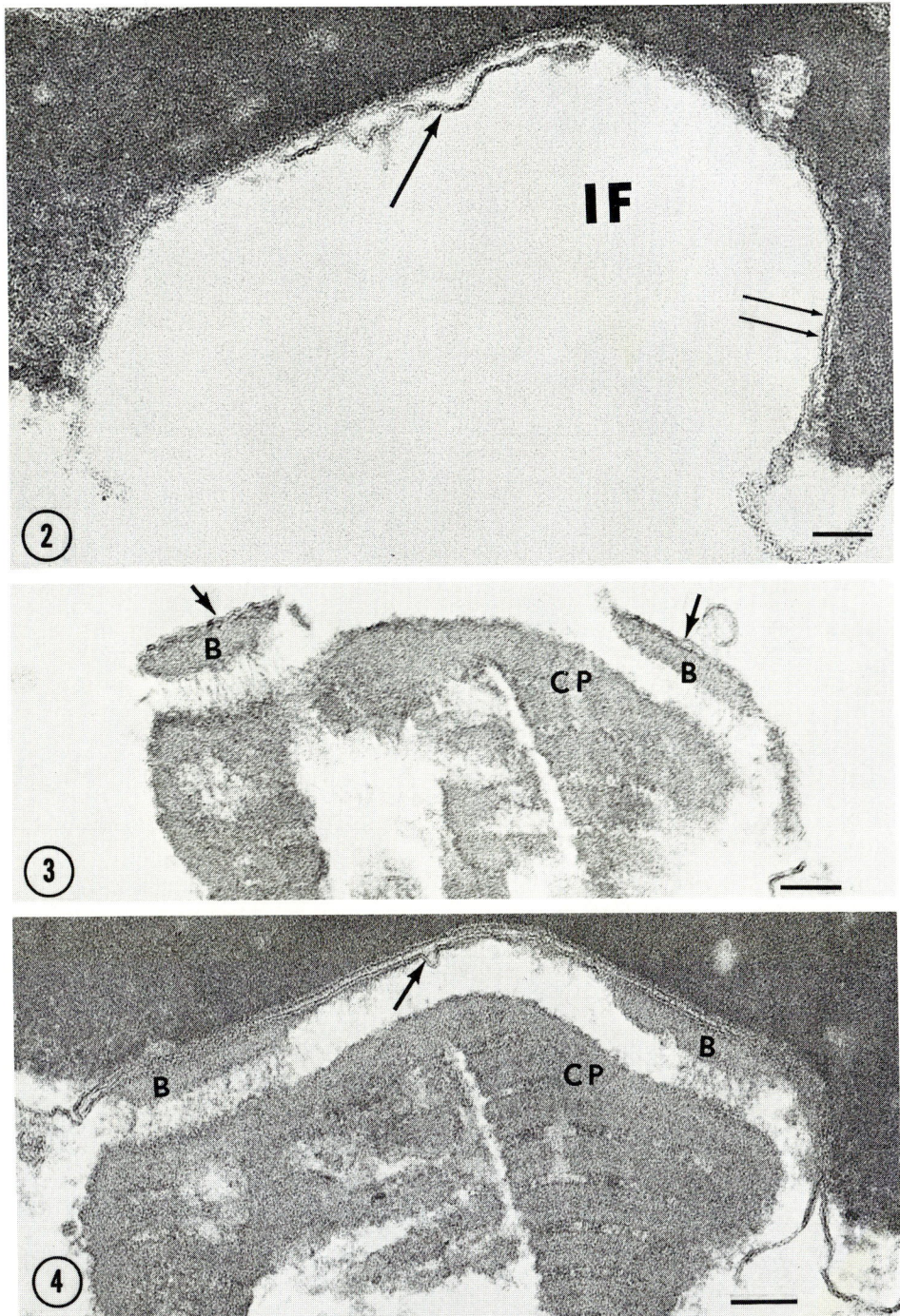

Figure 2. Base of rabbit sperm head after tail detachment by n-butylamine treatment in SET buffer (final pH = 10.7) and vortexing 30 sec. Frontal section through the implantation fossa (IF). The sperm tail has detached across the nuclear envelope, leaving the inner membrane (small arrows) attached to the nuclear chromatin. Large arrow points to a remnant of the outer membrane of the envelope which has not pulled away with the basal plate of the tail connecting piece. Bar = 100 nm. X115,000

Figure 3. Tail detached by n-butylamine treatment, as in Figure 2. Frontal section through tail connecting piece. Fibrous strands join the basal plates (B) to the capitulum of the connecting piece (CP). Large arrows point to portions of the outer membrane of the nuclear envelope associated with the basal plates. Bar = 100 nm. X112,000

Figure 4. Control spermatozoon incubated in phosphate buffer (pH 11.0) and vortexed 30 sec. Frontal section through the head-tail junction; basal plates (B), capitulum of the connecting piece (CP). The membranes of the nuclear envelope are bridged by "cross-ties" oriented normal to the inner and outer membranes. These periodic structures are best seen here over the right basal plate. Bar = 100 nm. X102,000

Table 1. Head-Tail Detachment of Rabbit Spermatozoa[a]

Compound	Mean % Detachment
n-butylamine	>90
sec-butylamine	90
iso-butylamine	82
t-butylamine	80
cyclohexylamine	62
n-amylamine	19
ethanolamine[b]	22
benzylamine	10
3,4-dimethoxyphenylethylamine	10
di-n-butylamine	5
tri-n-butylamine	5
di-pentylamine	5
N,N,N',N¹-tetramethylethylenediamine	0
n-butylacetamide	0
n-butyl alcohol	0
ethyl alcohol	0

[a] 0.4-0.5 mmol of each reagent was added to $3\text{-}5 \times 10^7$ spermatozoa/ml SET buffer and vortexed 15-30 sec. SET = 0.1 M Tris HCl (pH 7.2), 0.15 M NaCl, 0.005 M ethylenediamine tetracetate (EDTA). Mean % detachment in Tables 1-4 is based on the mean of triplicate counts of intact and dissociated spermatozoa minus the mean % background dissociation. The latter ranged from 1-10%.
[b] 0.7 mmol/ml.

Table 2. Effect of pH on Head-Tail Detachment by N-Butylamine[a]

Buffer	Final pH	Mean % Detachment
0.1 M phosphate (pH 10.5)	10.5-11	87
0.1 M carbonate (pH 9.0)	9.0-9.5	32
1.0 M Tris-HCl (pH 7.2)	7.0-8.0	15
1.0 M citrate (pH 5.0)	5.0-6.0	5

[a] 0.1 mmol n-butylamine/ml of the above buffers; $3\text{-}5 \times 10^7$ spermatozoa/ml.

Table 3. Head-Tail Detachment After NaCNBH₃ Reduction[a]

NaCNBH$_3$ (mg/ml)	Mean % Detachment
—	97
10	71
20	26
50	8

[a] $0.5\text{-}1.0 \times 10^7$ spermatozoa/ml in 1.0 M citrate (pH 5.0) for 1 h at 22°C. Spermatozoa were washed in SET buffer before treatment in SET with 0.15 mmol n-butylamine/ml.

Table 4. Stabilization In Vitro of Head-Tail Linkages[a]

Incubation Time (h)	Divalent Cation	Concentration (mM)	Mean % Detachment
0	—	—	80->90
16-24[b]	—	—	80->90
16-24	—	—	4-20
2.5	Cu	0.01	29
5	Cu	0.01	<5
5	Mg	0.1	37
16	Mg	0.1	5-10
6	Zn	0.1	43
16	Zn	0.1	5-10
6	Ca	5.0	55
16	Ca	5.0	5-10

[a] Incubation at 37°C: $0.5\text{-}1.0 \times 10^7$ spermatozoa/ml in 0.1 M Tris-HCl + 0.15 M NaCl. Spermatozoa were treated with 0.3-0.5 mmol n-butylamine in SET buffer.
[b] Incubation at 22°C.

mating. Whether aging changes at this level of sperm structure have any consequences for sperm motility in the female tract is unknown.

REFERENCES

Calvin, H.I.: Isolation and Subfractionation of Mammalian Sperm Heads and Tails. In: Methods in Cell Biology. Vol. XIII, pp. 85-104, ed. by D.M. Prescott. Academic Press, ew York, 1976

Cooper, G.W.; Young, R.J.: Mammalian Sperm are Dissociated into Heads and Tails by Primary Amines: Demonstration of Intermolecular Covalent Bonds between the Nuclear Membranes and Basal Plate of the Tail Connecting Piece. Anat Rec 187(1977)556A

Fawcett, D.W.: The Mammalian Spermatozoon. Dev Biol 44(1975)394-436

Franzblau, C.: Elastin. In: Comprehensive Biochemistry. Vol. 26C, pp. 659-712, ed. by M. Florkin and E.H. Stotz. Elsevier Publishing Co., New York, 1971

Kefalides, N.A.: Basement Membranes: Structural and Biosynthetic Considerations. J Invest Dermatol 65(1975)85-92

Lane, C.F.: Sodium Cyanoborohydride—A Highly Selective Reducing Agent for Organic Functional Groups. Synthesis (1975)135-146

Millette, C.F.; Spear, P.G.; Gall, W.E.; Edelman, G.M.: Chemical Dissection of Mammalian Spermatozoa. J Cell Biol 58(1973)662-675

Tanzer, R.L.: Crosslinking. In: Biochemistry of Collagen, pp. 137-162, ed. by G.N. Ramachandran and A.H. Reddi. Plenum Press, New York, 1976

ISOLATION OF THE FIBROUS SHEATH AND PERFORATORIUM OF RAT SPERMATOZOA

G.E. Olson

Department of Anatomy, Vanderbilt University, Nashville, Tennessee 37232 USA

The functional role of several spermatozoan organelles such as the outer dense fibers, connecting piece, fibrous sheath, and perforatorium remain to be identified. Many efforts have focused on developing fractionation techniques so that these structures can be biochemically characterized. Early work established that some sperm components are incredibly resistant to solubilization by many of the commonly employed protein solvents and that some of these sperm components are composed of sulphur-rich, keratin-like proteins (review: Mann, 1964). This was later confirmed by correlated biochemical-ultrastructural approaches that identified specific sperm organelles including the nuclear chromatin, perforatorium, midpiece mitochondria, outer dense fibers, connecting piece, and fibrous sheath as containing a high content of disulphide bonds (Bedford and Calvin, 1971).

Recently several laboratories have devised fractionation schemes utilizing techniques of sonication, differential centrifugation, and selective organelle solubilization to isolate reasonably clean preparations of the outer dense fibers, fibrous sheath, perforatorium, and nuclear chromatin. It should be stressed that although these fractionation procedures yield homogeneous organelle fractions suitable for analysis of structural proteins, they each involve steps that are harsh and that can denature or dissociate any native enzymatic activity associated with the organelle *in vivo*. The following account will detail procedures for isolation of the predominant structural proteins of the fibrous sheath and perforatorium of rat spermatozoa (Olson *et al*, 1976a, b). An effort has been made to design a scheme in which the relative purity of various sperm fractions can be monitored both quickly and accurately by phase contrast photomicroscopy; ultrastructural data is only included to validate the results of the fractionation protocol.

© 1979 Urban & Schwarzenberg, Inc. Baltimore-Munich *The Spermatozoon*, edited by D.W. Fawcett and J.M. Bedford

FIBROUS SHEATH

The fibrous sheath is restricted to the principal piece region of the spermatozoan where it surrounds the dense fiber-axonemal complex. It is composed of two longitudinally oriented continuous columns that course parallel to axonemal doublet tubules No. 3 and 8 and ribs that wrap halfway around the flagellum and fuse to the continuous columns (Fig. 3).

The scheme employed for the isolation of the fibrous sheath involves a set of extraction steps designed to solubilize specific flagellar components as well as a differential centrifugation step to separate sperm heads from flagellar elements:

Fractionation Protocol for Fibrous Sheath (All Steps Performed on Ice at 0-4°C)

1. Suspend cauda epididymal sperm with phosphate buffered saline, then centrifuge 500 g for 5 min to pellet sperm.
2. Extract pellet twice, 15 min each, with: 1% Triton X-100, 2mM dithiothreitol (DTT), 50mM Tris-HCl (pH 9.0). Centrifuge 1000 g for 10 min.
3. Wash pellet twice by resuspension in 50mM Tris-HCl (pH 9.0) and centrifugation 1000 g for 10 min.
4. Extract pellet either for 2 h with 6 M urea, 5mM DTT, and 50mM Tris-HCl (pH 8.0) or overnight (18 h) with 4 M urea, 5mM DTT, and 50mM Tris-HCl (pH 9.0).
5. Spin suspension 200 g for 5 min to remove any aggregates.
6. Layer 200 g supernatant over cushion composed of 75% sucrose, 25mM Tris-HCl (pH 8.0) and centrifuge 100,000 g (Rmax) for 60 min.
7. Fractionate band at interface and dilute with 4 M urea, 5mM DTT, 50mM Tris-HCl and pellet by centrifugation at 100,000 g for 30 min.

There are several easy modifications of the above protocol which can be employed and still yield a step 7 pellet that has a high purity of isolated fibrous sheath. One modification is to resuspend the step-1 sperm pellet

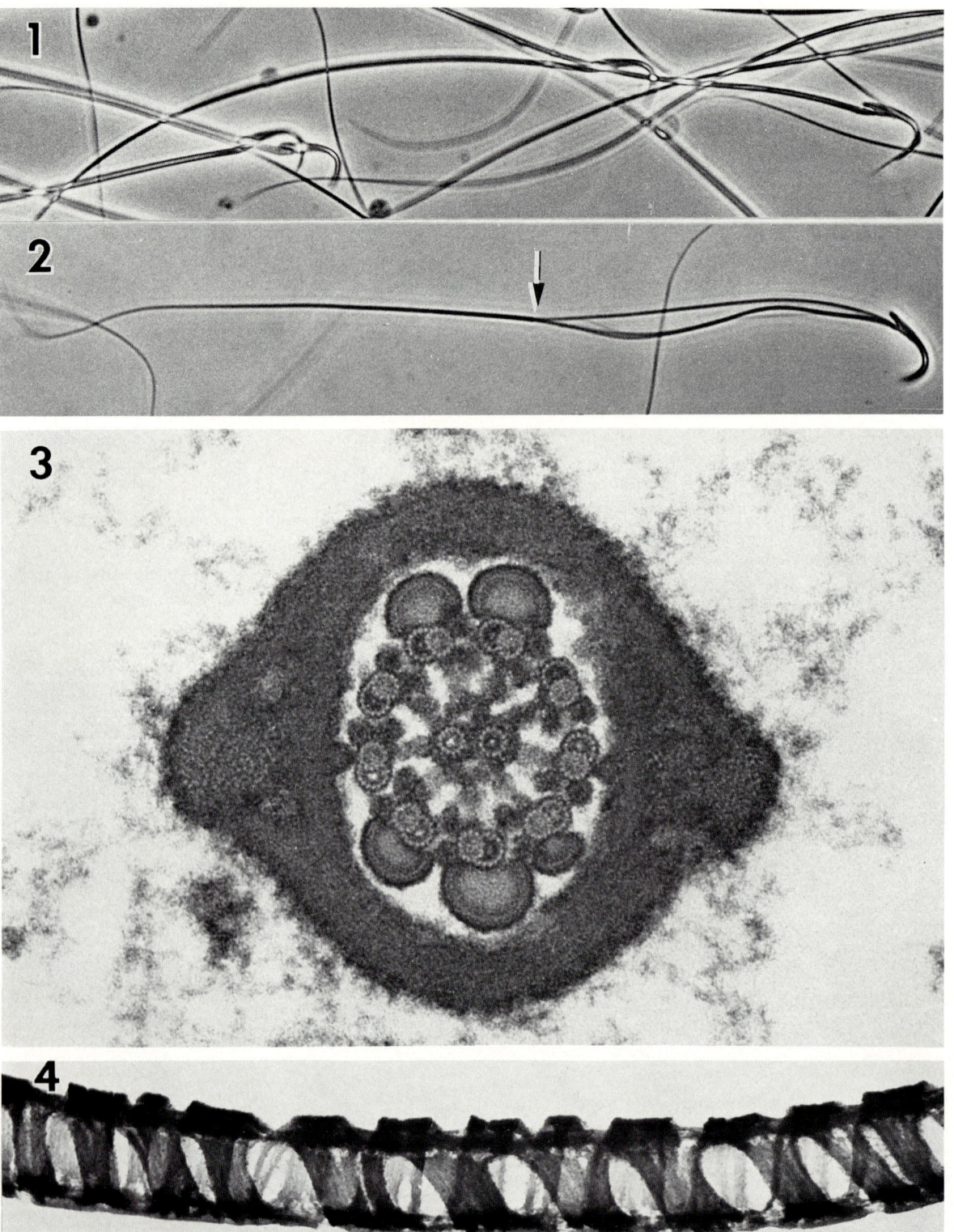

Figure 1. Phase contrast photomicrograph of intact rat spermatozoa.
Figure 2. Phase contrast photomicrograph of Triton-DTT extracted spermatozoa. This preparation was vigorously pipetted so that the outer dense fiber-doublet microtubule complexes in the midpiece region have frayed apart making the proximal end of the principal piece region easy to identify (arrow).
Figure 3. Cross section of principal piece region of Triton-DTT extracted spermatozoon. The axoneme and fibrous sheath appear intact. 170,000X.

in phosphate buffered saline and at this stage separate the sperm heads from the tails by the protocol described in the next section. The fractionated tails can then be pelleted by centrifugation and utilized at step 2 of the above protocol and then steps 5, 6, and 7 can be omitted. In this case the step-4 urea extract is centrifuged at 100,000 g for 30 min to pellet the nonsolubilized fibrous sheath.

Each of the extraction steps in the above procedure results in the solubilization of specific flagellar organelles. These morphological changes can be correlated by biochemical methods, such as sodium dodecyl sulfate (SDS) polyacrylamide gel electrophoresis, to show sequential loss of specific flagellar proteins (Fig. 11). Extraction of spermatozoa with the step-2 solution, Triton-DTT, results in the solubilization of the plasma membrane, midpiece mitochondria, and annulus; the structural components of the flagellum including the axoneme, connecting piece, outer dense fibers, and fibrous sheath appear to remain intact (Fig. 1-4). During the urea extraction there is a progressive solubilization of flagellar components including the axoneme, connecting piece, and outer dense fibers. An interesting feature of the progressive solubilization of the outer dense fibers is that after about 30 min in the 4 M urea, they undergo a remarkably ordered coiling resulting in a spiral appearance to the midpiece (Fig. 5). As the solubilization proceeds the coils become progressively tighter and it appears that the outer dense fibers ultimately retract from the lumen of the fibrous sheath so that detached coils are observed. Eventually these coils dissolve so that the only visible remaining flagellar organelle is the fibrous sheath (Fig. 6). The fibrous sheath isolated from the urea extract appears morphologically intact possessing both the continuous columns and ribs (Fig. 7). At the lower urea concentrations, DTT concentrations, or pH some material remains within the fibrous sheath lumen which is probably dense fiber remnants.

PERFORATORIUM

The perforatorium is located at the anterior end of the sperm head, interspersed between the acrosome and nucleus. In thin section electron micrographs it has a homogeneous electron-dense appearance. When detached from the sperm nucleus and viewed by phase contrast or whole-mount electron microscopy the perforatorium appears somewhat rigid since it retains the curved shape characteristic of the intact sperm head (Fig. 8-10).

When testing several detergents for their capacity to solubilize sperm organelles it was noted that sodium lauroryl sarcosine (sarkosyl) caused the perforatorium to detach from the nucleus of rat spermatozoa. Sarcosyl also has rather specific effects on flagellar organelles and the connecting piece-outer dense-fiber complex appears to be the most resistant flagellar structure (Fig. 8). This detergent was employed to isolate these flagellar components as well as the structural protein of the perforatorium.

The first step in the isolation of the structural protein of the perforatorium is to separate the sperm heads from flagellar components and this is easily accomplished by centrifugation of sonicated sperm suspension on a sucrose step gradient. Sperm suspended in physiological saline are subjected to the minimal amount of sonication required to decapitate greater than 95% of the spermatozoa. The sonicated suspension is then diluted with 6-7 volumes of 70% sucrose, $1mM$ ethylenediaminetetraacetate (EDTA), $20mM$ $NaPO_4$ (pH 6.5). A step gradient is then formed using equal volume steps of 1) sperm suspension, 2) 65% sucrose, 3) 70% sucrose, and 4) 75% sucrose. This is centrifuged at 100,000 g for 60 min and the gradients fractionated. The sperm tails layer at the 65-70% interface whereas the heads form a pellet at the bottom of the tubes.

An extraction protocol with an ionic detergent is then employed to differentially solubilize sperm head components. The isolated sperm heads are suspended in a solution of 1% sarkosyl, $2mM$ DTT, and $5mM$ Tris-HCl (pH 9.0) and then monitored by phase contrast microscopy. Within 10-15 min the sperm nucleus begins to decondense and the perforatorium begins to detach from the anterior end of the nucleus (Fig. 9 and 10). Within 30 min the only sperm head components noted by electron microscopy are the perforatorium and decondensed chromatin. At early stages of chromatin decondensation the nucleus has a heterogeneous appearance with dense granular areas noted with the nuclear matrix, but after 45-60 min the nucleus is fully decondensed and no granularity is obvious. The perforatorium remains intact after the chromatin is fully decondensed and at this stage can be pelleted by centrifugation at 100,000 g for 20 min.

The pellet is washed once with the sarkosyl solution and then recentrifuged at 100,000 g for 20 min. SDS gel electrophoresis of this perforatorium fraction shows a single low molecular weight polypeptide band (Fig. 11).

Figure 4. Whole mount electron micrograph of fibrous sheath which shows the three dimensional relationship between the continuous columns and ribs. 41,000X.

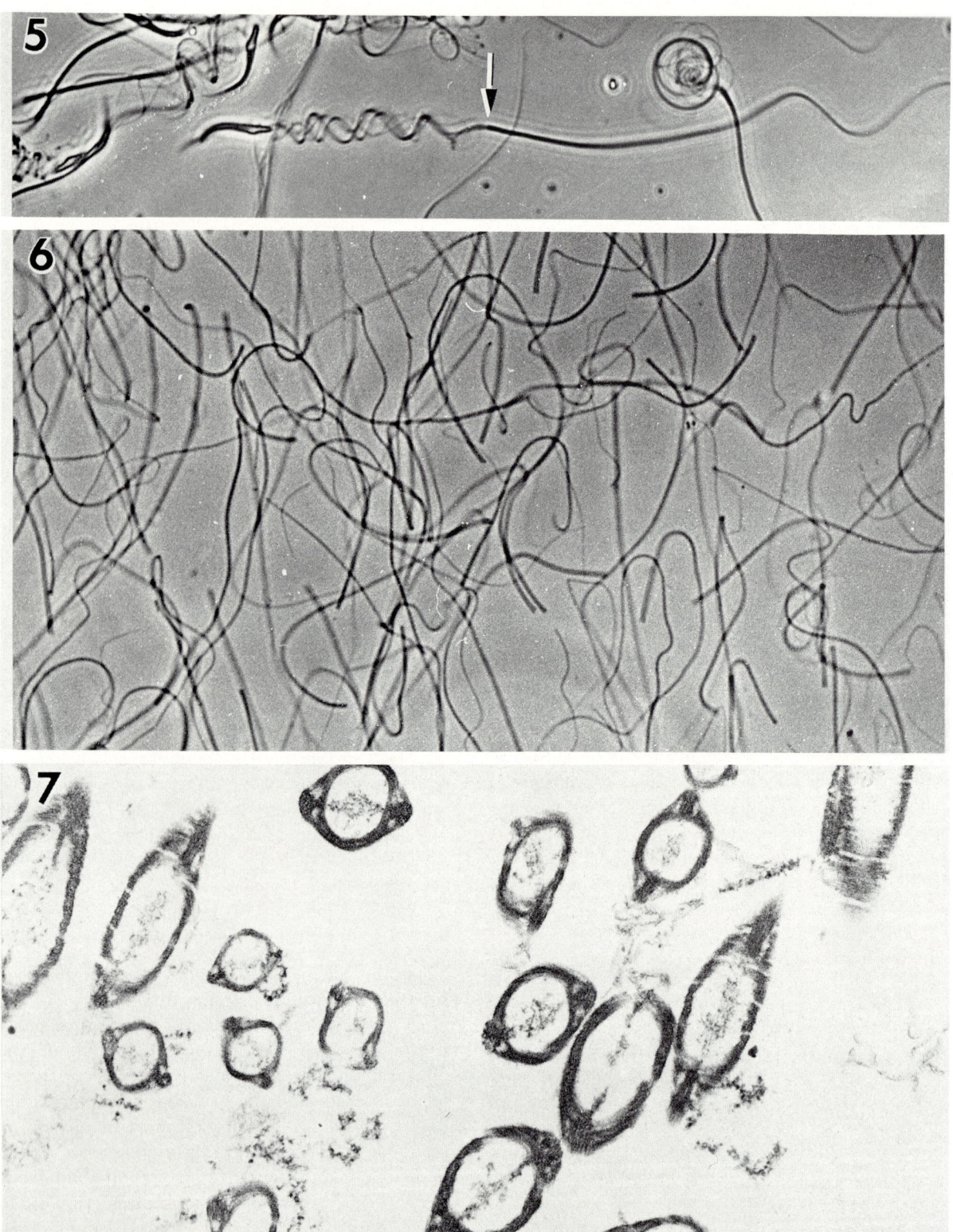

Figure 5. Phase contrast photomicrograph of rat spermatozoon in 4 M urea extracting solution. The outer dense fibers of the midpiece region have assumed a helical configuration. The arrow marks the beginning of the principal piece region.
Figure 6. Phase contrast photomicrograph of fibrous sheath fractionated from a sucrose step gradient.
Figure 7. Thin-section electron micrograph of isolated fibrous sheath. 22,000X.

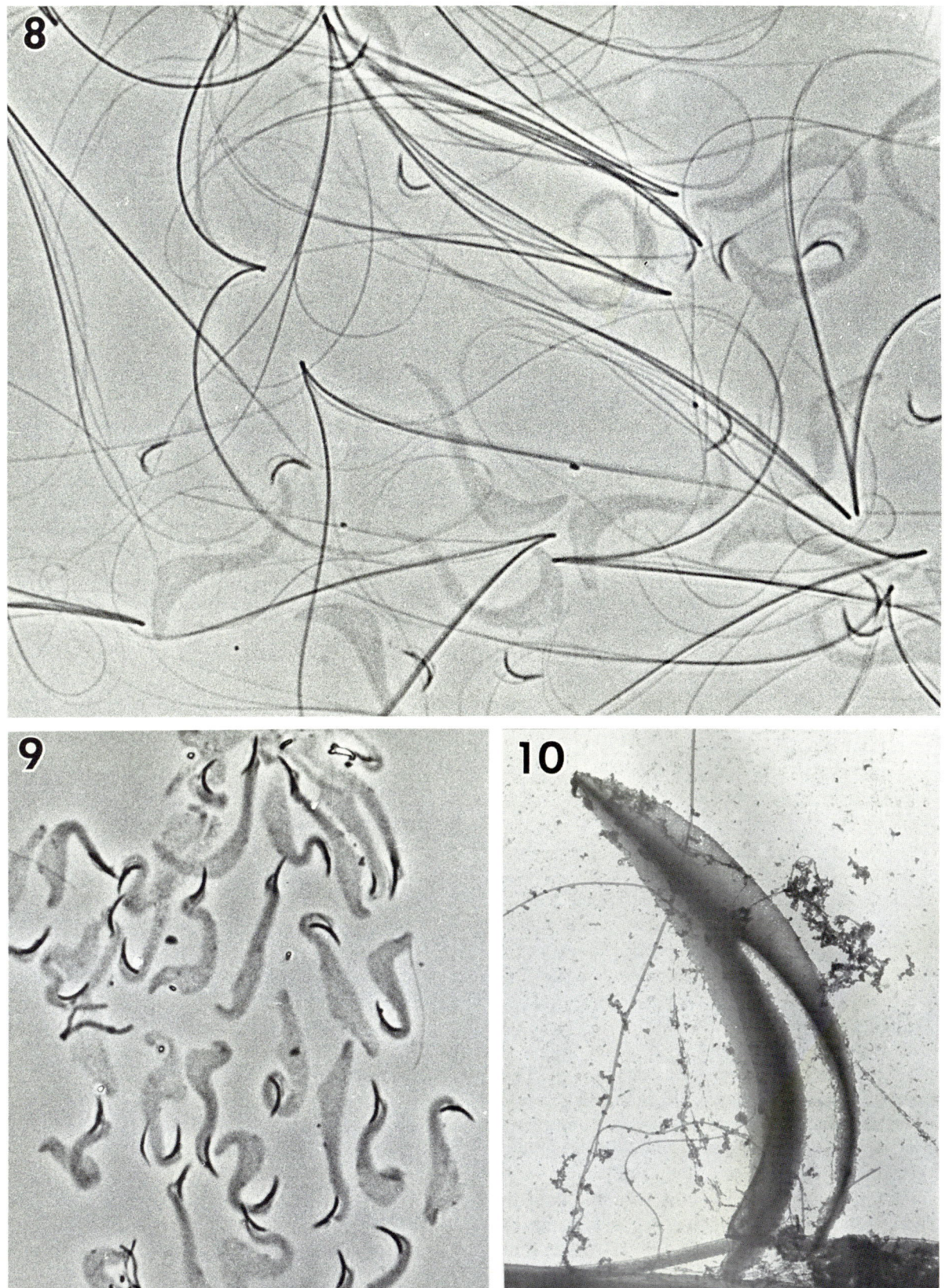

Figure 8. Phase contrast photomicrograph of rat spermatozoa after 15 min extraction in 1% Sarkosyl +2mM DTT pH 9.0. Connecting piece-outer dense-fiber complexes, decondensed nuclei, and detached perforatorium are the only noted structures.
Figure 9. Isolated nuclei in sarkosyl solution showing detachment of perforatorium.
Figure 10. Whole-mount electron micrograph showing morphology of detached perforatorium. 20,000X.

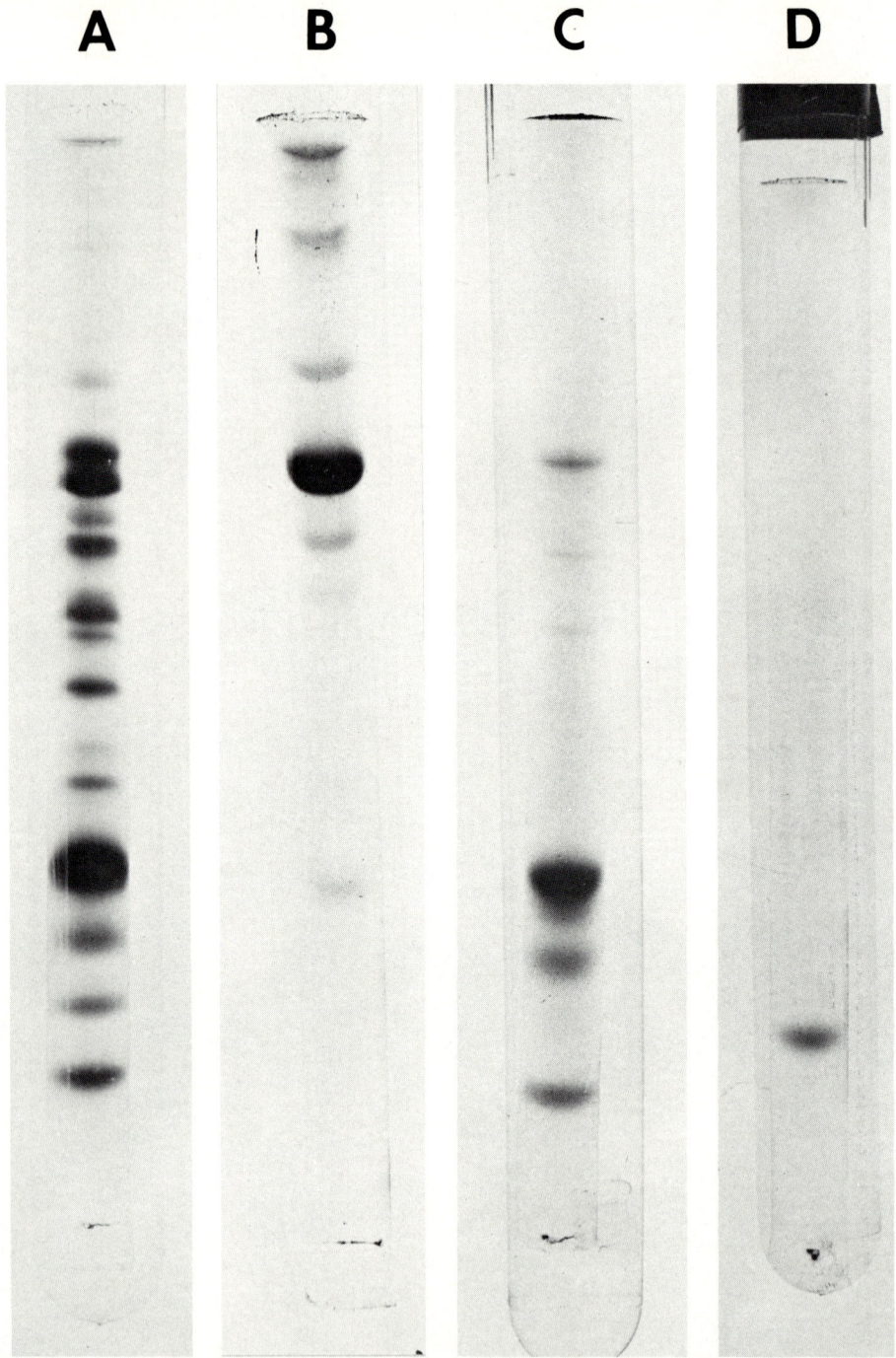

Figure 11. SDS-polyacrylamide gel showing polypeptide profile in: A) Triton-DTT extracted rat spermatozoa; B) Isolated fibrous sheath fraction, the predominant polypeptide has a molecular weight of about 80,000. C) Isolated dense fiber fraction from sarkosyl extracted sperm. D) Perforatorium fraction from sarkosyl extracted sperm.

REFERENCES

Bedford, H.I.; Calvin, J.M.: Formation of Disulfide Bonds in the Nucleus and Accessory Structures of Mammalian Spermatozoa during Maturation in the Epididymis. J Reprod Fertil Suppl 13(1971)65-75

Mann, T.: The Biochemistry of Semen and of the Male Reproductive Tract. John Wiley and Sons, New York, 1964

Olson, G.E.; Hamilton, D.W.; Fawcett, D.W.: Isolation and Characterization of the Fibrous Sheath of Rat Epididymal Spermatozoa. Biol Reprod 14(1976)517-530

Olson, G.E.; Hamilton, D.W.; Fawcett, D.W.: Isolation and Characterization of the Perforatorium of Rat Spermatozoa. J Reprod Fertil 47(1976b)293-297

ISOLATION OF MITOCHONDRIA FROM BULL EPIDIDYMAL SPERMATOZOA

V. Pallini

Institute of Zoology, University of Siena, Siena 53100 Italy

Fractionation procedures have recently been developed that have allowed the characterization of several mammalian sperm structures, *i.e.* plasma and acrosomal membranes (Morré et al., 1974; Zahler and Doak, 1975; Clegg, 1979), accessory fibers (Baccetti et al., 1973; Calvin et al., 1975; Baccetti et al., 1976a, b), fibrous sheath (Olson et al., 1976a), and perforatorium (Olson et al., 1976b; review: Calvin, 1976).

Until quite recently, no methods have been available for the isolation of mammalian sperm mitochondria. However, the structure and function of these organelles have received considerable attention: besides electron microscopic observations (*e.g.*, Elfvin, 1968; Fawcett, 1970; Bedford and Calvin, 1974; Phillips, 1977), biochemical studies have been performed on isolated midpieces (*e.g.*, Mohri et al., 1965), or on whole spermatozoa (*e.g.*, Keyhani and Storey, 1973; Storey and Keyhani, 1973; Premkumar and Bhargava, 1972; Van Dop et al., 1977).

Further investigations of both structure and function would certainly benefit from the availability of isolation methods. The isolation of bull sperm mitochondria has been reported in preliminary form (Robinson and Forrester, 1974, quoted by Calvin, 1976); subsequently, Bartoov and Messer (1976) have reported the detachment of mitochondria from ram spermatozoa by treatment with a disulfide-reducing agent (dithiothreitol) followed by homogenization; the purification of the organelles was performed by passage through a sand column and differential centrifugation.

More recently, by using digestion of bull sperm with pepsin and differential centrifugation, Hrudka (1978) has obtained preparations of mitochondria that have allowed a detailed study of the inner membrane structure.

This chapter describes a procedure in which bull epididymal sperm mitochondria are detached by sonication and purified by isopycnic centrifugation. Some morphological and chemical characteristics of the isolated organelles are reported and compared with those of mitochondria detached by use of disulfide-reducing reagent.

METHODS

Collection of Spermatozoa and Detachment of Mitochondria

Bull spermatozoa were collected within 3-5 h after the bulls were slaughtered by teasing the ductules of the cauda epididymidis in ice-cold 0.12 M NaCl, 0.01 M Tris-HCl pH 7.5 (TBS); the resulting sperm suspension was filtered through cheese-cloth, the cells sedimented at 1200 g at 2°C, weighed, and suspended in 9 volumes of cold TBS containing phenylmethyl-sulfonyl fluoride (0.2 mg/ml).

In order to detach mitochondria, a 25-ml aliquot of 10% (W/V) sperm suspensions was placed in a glass beaker (4-cm diameter) and subjected to 15 bursts (20 sec each, separated by 40-sec intervals) of the Biosonik IV sonifier (Bronwill) equipped with the $14\frac{1}{2}$-in. tip and operated at 40% of maximum power. During the whole procedure the beaker was cooled in an ice bath and the temperature of the sperm suspension oscillated between 0°C and 15°C.

Alternatively, 10% sperm suspensions in TBS were vigorously stirred for ~4 h at 0°C in the presence of 0.01-0.05 M mercaptoethanol.

Isopycnic Centrifugation

For preparative purposes, continuous linear density gradients of 27 ml total volume were prepared by mixing 25% sucrose (d = 1.11 at 5°C) with 62% sucrose (d = 1.31 at 5°C) in cellulose nitrate tubes of the SW 27 Beckman rotor. Sucrose solutions were checked by refractometry and contained 0.2 M NaCl, 0.01 M Tris-HCl at pH 7.5; 12-ml aliquots (corresponding to a maximum of 1.2 g of packed cells) of sonicated or mercaptoethanol-treated sperm suspensions were layered over the gradients and centrifuged at 83,000 g (average)

This investigation was supported by the C.N.R (Centro Nazionale delle Ricerche), project "Biology of Reproduction."

The author gratefully acknowledges the technical assistance of Mario Barbetti.

© 1979 Urban & Schwarzenberg, Inc. Baltimore-Munich *The Spermatozoon*, edited by D.W. Fawcett and J.M. Bedford

at 5°C for at least 6 h. Material from the bands was collected with a Pasteur pipette, diluted with TBS, and sedimented at 83,000 g.

SDS-polyacrylamide Gel Electrophoresis

The high pH, discontinuous method of Laemmli (1970) was applied employing 0.5 x 12 cm separation gels consisting of 12% acrylamide. Prior to electrophoresis, mitochondrial suspensions were mixed with equal volumes of 0.12 M Tris-HCl pH 6.8, 4% sodium dodecyl sulfate (SDS), 10% mercaptoethanol, 10% glycerol, 0.01% bromphenol blue, and heated at 100°C for 2 min. Electrophoresis was carried out at 1 mA per gel until the tracking dye had reached the bottom of the gels. Staining was performed with 0.2% Coomassie blue in 50% methanol, 7% acetic acid and destaining was obtained with 20% and 10% methanol, 7% acetic acid. Molecular weight scales were constructed by calibrating the gels with the following reference proteins: cytochrome C (11,700 M_r), IgG light chain (23,500 M_r), rabbit muscle actin (45,000 M_r), IgG heavy chain (50,000 M_r).

Chemical Methods

Cytochrome oxidase activity was measured, and units defined, after Cooperstein and Lazarow (1951); total protein was determined with the Lowry method (1951) using bovine serum albumin as a standard. The procedure of Schneider (1957) was used to fractionate acid-soluble RNA and DNA phosphate; phospholipids were extracted with chloroform-methanol according to Folch et al. (1957); total phosphate was determined as indicated by Ames (1966).

Electron Microscopy

Samples of mitochondria were fixed in Karnovsky's fixative for 1 h at 4°C, washed in cacodylate buffer 0.1 M pH 7.2 overnight, postfixed in 1% OsO_4 in the same buffer for 30 min at 4°C, dehydrated, and embedded in Epon. In some experiments 2% tannic acid was added to the fixative. Sections were stained with uranyl acetate and lead nitrate.

The material was negatively stained with 1% PTA (phosphotungstic acid) in 0.4% saccharose, pH 7.

All the samples were examined with a Philips EM 301 electron microscope.

RESULTS

Mitochondria Detached by Sonication

Subcellular structures of sonicated spermatozoa were reproducibly separated into four fractions banding at different densities (Fig. 1). Band 1 (d: 1.14) was found to consist of smooth vesicles of various sizes; band 2 was always formed by two closely spaced bands (2A, d: 1.19 and 2B, d: 1.20) and contained mitochondria; band 3 (d: 1.26) was formed by more or less damaged flagella, some of them still containing segments of mitochondrial sheath, and by fragments of accessory fibers, microtu-

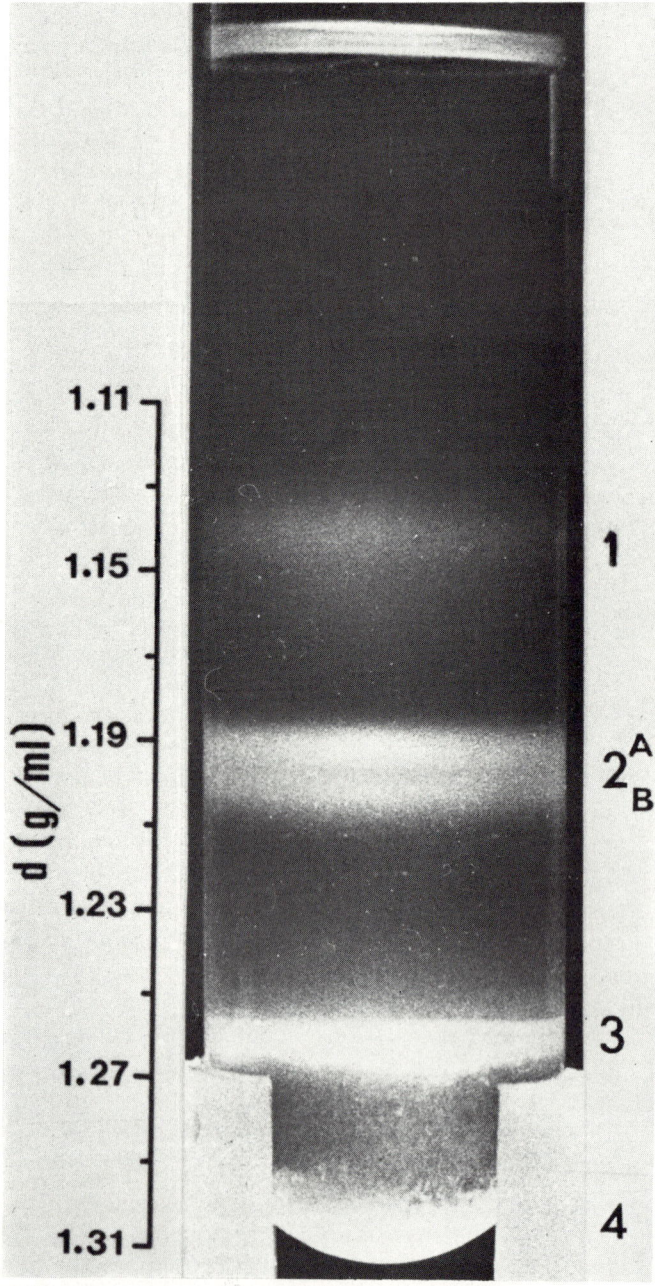

Figure 1. The centrifuge tube after isopycnic equilibration of sperm sonicate. For description of bands (numbers on the right side), see text. The density scale describes the initial shape of the gradient.

bules, and fibrous sheath; the sediment, 4, consisted of sperm heads and some whole spermatozoa. The solution layered above the sucrose gradient (supernatant fraction) contained the soluble proteins of the spermatozoon.

As demonstrated by electron microscopy (Fig. 2 and 3), bands 2A and 2B collected together consisted essentially of pure mitochondria separated from other midpiece structures. Minor contamination by smooth vesicles and microtubular fragments were occasionally observed; if required, these contaminants could be removed by a second passage through the density gradient. Sonication-detached and purified mitochondria preserved their peculiar crescent shape and membrane fine structure and were frequently still connected to form long segments of mitochondrial helix; their outer membrane retained the typical multilaminar appearance (Fig. 4). By negative staining it was found that bands 2A and 2B consisted of different types of mitochondria: most mitochondria in band 2A had a smooth, extended inner membrane (Fig. 5), whereas those in band 2B had a wrinkled inner membrane (Fig. 6); the rare broken mitochondria usually belonged to the first type and were found in band 2A.

The extent of purification and the yield of sperm mitochondria was quantitatively assessed by measuring the protein content and the cytochrome oxidase activity of the density gradient fractions. The data reported in Table 1 indicate that this enzyme was not influenced by sonication of spermatozoa; the activity recovered in the gradient fractions accounted for more than 80% of the total activity originally present in spermatozoa; fraction 2 alone contained more than 30% of total sperm activity; band 3 and the sediment together accounted for a relatively high percentage, conceivably related with mitochondria still attached to flagella or to whole spermatozoa; the supernatant fraction and band 1 contained a relatively small amount of enzyme in soluble form or carried by small vesicles deriving from mitochondrial damage during sonication. Cytochrome oxidase-specific activity was 8-9-fold higher in purified mitochondria than in whole spermatozoa.

In several chemical determinations, sperm mitochondria were found to contain 8.0-9.5 μg of lipid phosphorus per mg protein and 1.1-1.4 μg of RNA phosphorus per mg protein. In one complete analysis, the lyophylized weight of sperm mitochondria consisted of 83% protein, 15.8% phospholipids, and 1.2% RNA. Acid-soluble and DNA phosphorus were constantly below the sensitivity limit of the determination method; the latter result rules out any significant contamination of the mitochondrial fraction by sperm heads.

The polypeptide composition of sonication-detached, purified sperm mitochondria was analyzed by electrophoresis on 12% SDS-polyacrylamide gels (Fig. 7); 16 major bands were reproducibly observed; samples analyzed on gels 1 and 5 of Figure 7 represent different preparations of mitochondria and show essentially the same pattern of major bands; differences in band intensity, as well as the partial resolution of band 8 into subbands, are probably attributable to differences in gel loading and extent of destaining.

Gels 3 and 4 (Fig. 7) show the polypeptide composition of bull heart and liver mitochondria prepared by differential centrifugation (Bartoov et al., 1970) and then subjected to isopycnic centrifugation as described above. At least at the level of the major bands there is very little, if any, correspondence among mitochondria of different cell types of the same organism. The most intense bands of sperm mitochondria, bands 8 and 9 (30,000M_r) and band 12 (20,000M_r), are absent, or present in minor amounts in mitochondria from heart and from liver.

Mitochondria Detached by Disulfide Reduction

When spermatozoa treated with mercaptoethanol (as described above) were subjected to isopycnic centrifugation, the resulting band pattern was quite similar to that produced by sonicated sperm as shown in Figure 1. Band 2 was comparatively less intense, never resolved into subbands, and consisted of round organelles still recognizable as mitochondria after negative staining. Electron microscopic sections showed that mitochondria detached with mercaptoethanol have greatly altered membrane structure and staining properties (Fig. 8 and 9). In some preparations, the mitochondrial structure was completely destroyed with the formation of enlarged vesicles and amorphous material. The enzymatic properties of these structures were not tested.

By SDS-polyacrylamide gel electrophoresis, it was possible to demonstrate that mercaptoethanol-detached, round mitochondria possess a polypeptide composition remarkably similar with that of sonication detached mitochondria (cf. gels 1 and 2 of Fig. 7); as the only interesting exception, band 12 was comparatively less intense in mercaptoethanol-detached mitochondria.

DISCUSSION

In the above-described procedure for the isolation of bull sperm mitochondria, the detachment of organelles is achieved by sonication and their purification, by isopycnic banding on a continuous density gradient.

The data presented indicate that sonication under the conditions described releases segments of mitochondrial helix or individual organelles, preserving their

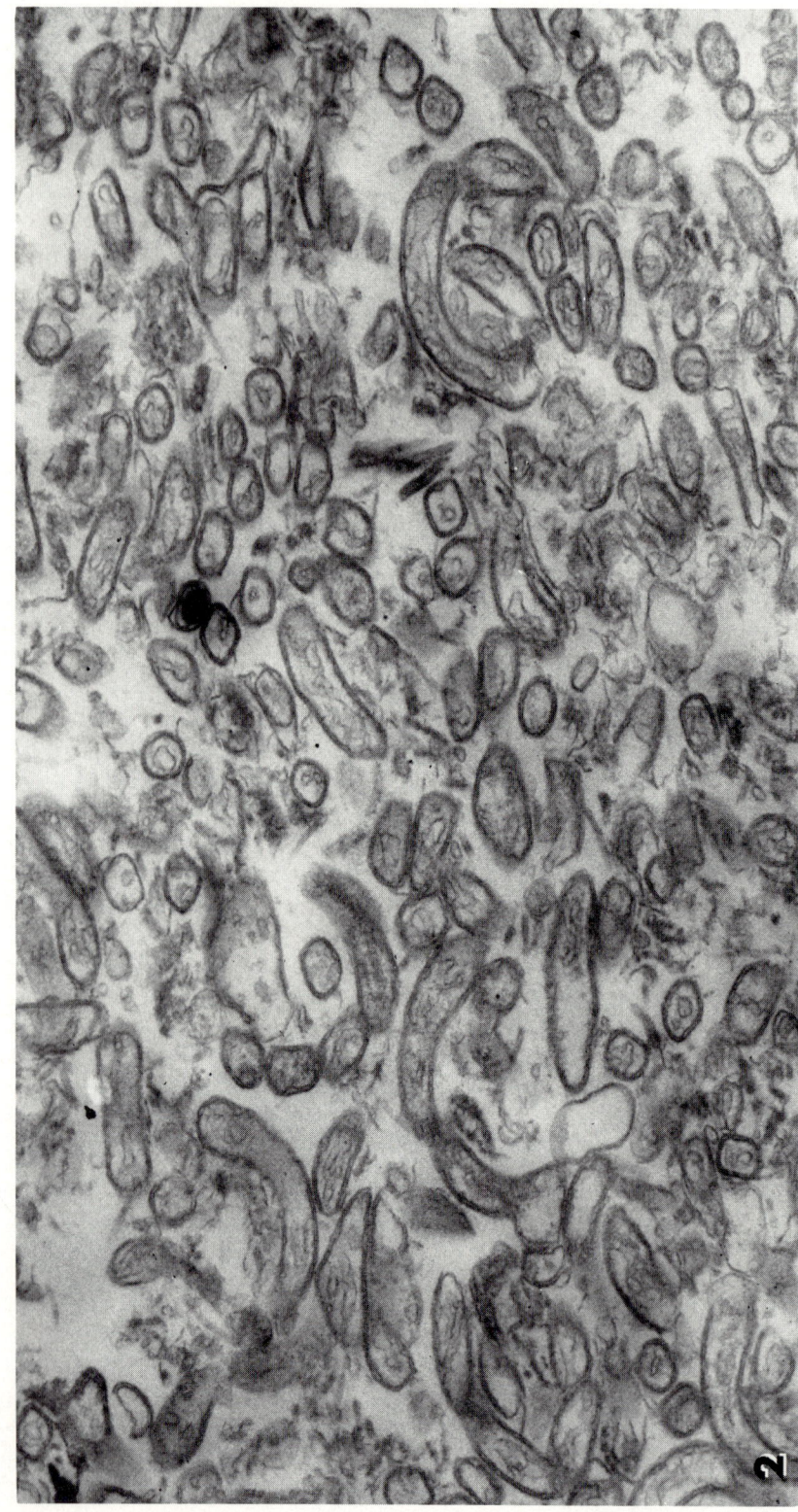

Figure 2. Electron microscopic sections of pellets of purified, sonication-detached mitochondria, X45,000.

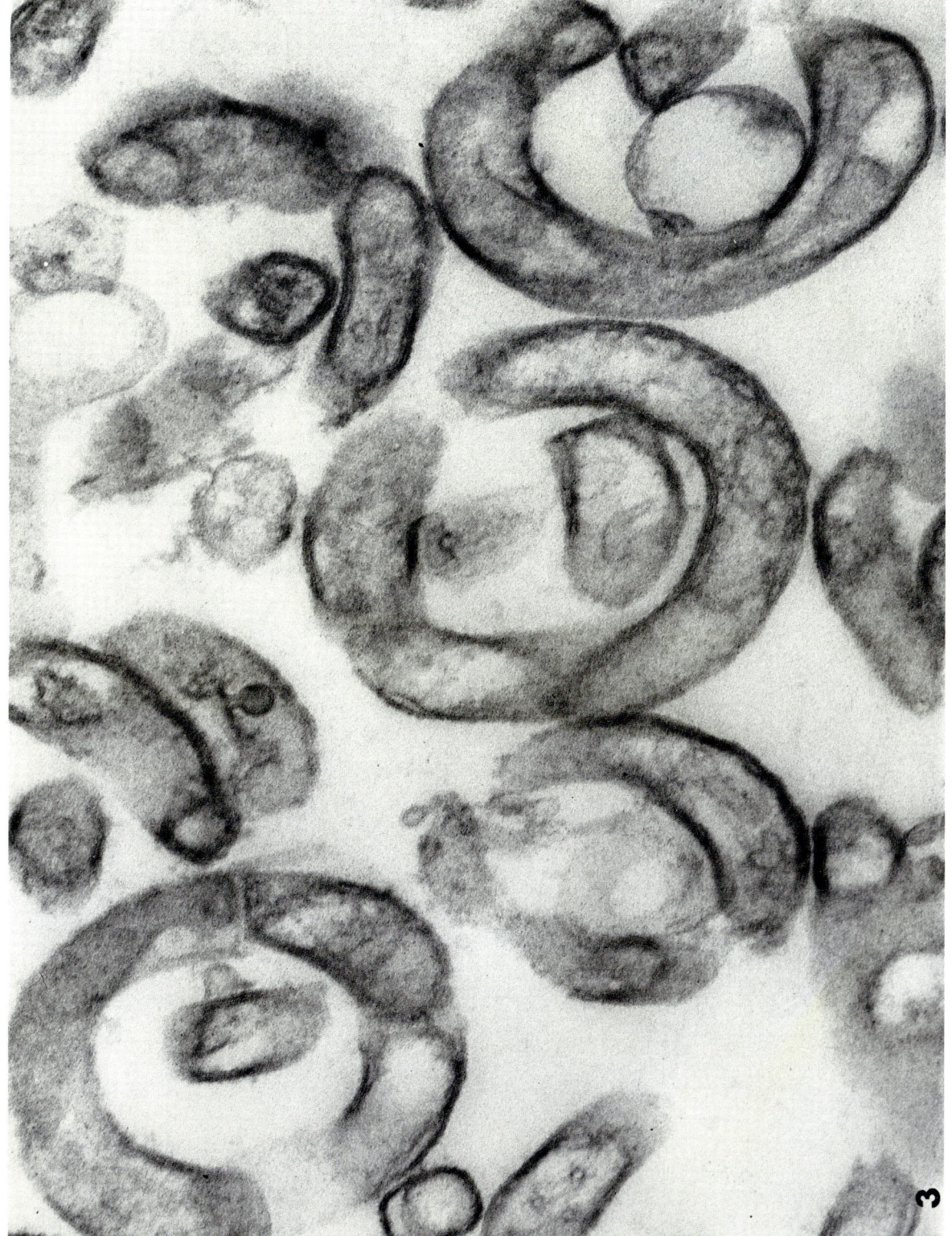

Figure 3. Electron microscopic sections of pellets of purified, sonication-detached mitochondria, X102,000.

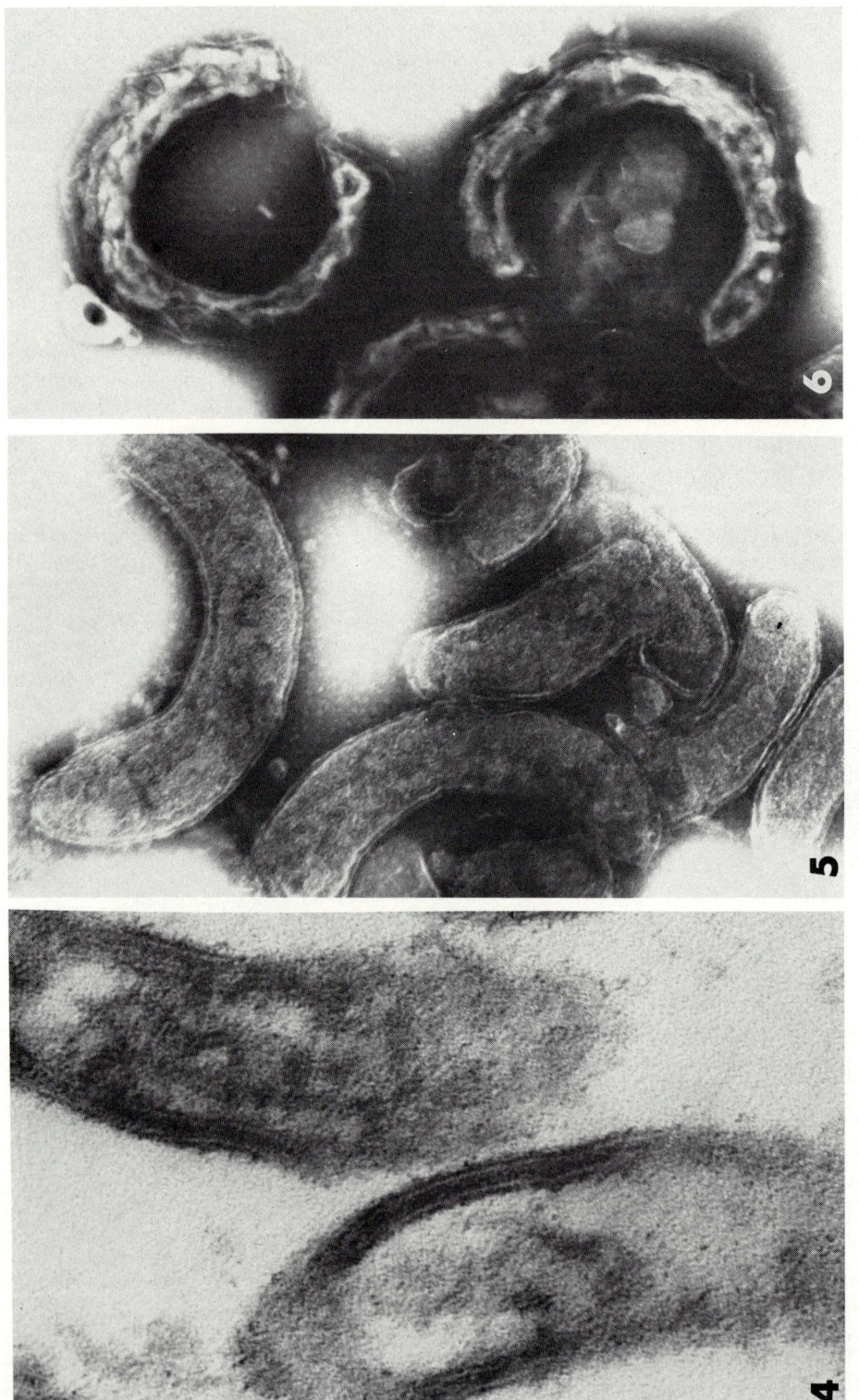

Figures 4-6. Ultrastructure of purified, sonication-detached mitochondria. Figure 4, thin section, impregnation with tannic acid, X285,000; Figure 5, typical mitochondria of band 2A, negative staining, X85,000; Figure 6, typical mitochondria of band 2B, negative staining, X85,000

Table 1. Results of a Typical Fractionation Experiment[a]

	Total Protein (mg)	Total Cytochromeoxidase (units)	Specific Activity (units/mg protein)
Native sperm	495	340	0.69
Sonicated sperm	500	354	0.71
Supernatant fraction	85	16	0.19
Fraction 1	19	6	0.32
Fraction 2	20	126	6.30
Fraction 3	88	61	0.69
Fraction 4	198	82	0.41
Recovery	410	291	
	82%	82.2%	

[a] On each of six gradients 5 g of packed cells were fractionated.

crescent shape and fine structure. Broken mitochondria are rarely observed. In addition, the relatively small percentage of cytochrome oxidase in the supernatant fraction or carried by light membranes (band 1) provides further proof that no extensive mitochondrial damage has occurred.

On the other hand, treatment of spermatozoa with mercaptoethanol, a disulfide-reducing reagent, releases round organelles, or even more damaged structures, which show a greatly altered morphology and which have lost a single specific polypeptide chain. In this connection, it is interesting to note that an analogous reagent, dithiothreitol, has been reported to detach and eventually to disintegrate, mouse epididymal sperm mitochondria (Millette et al., 1973).

As for the isolation step, isopycnic procedures may be the method of choice in dealing with sperm structures. As a matter of fact, the same fibrous or helical structure (e.g. microtubules, accessory fibers, fibrous sheath, the mitochondrial helix itself) tends, upon homogenization or sonication, to break down into segments of very different sizes that sediment at very different rates and, therefore, are distributed in high speed as well as in low speed fractions upon differential centrifugation. On the contrary, a method based on density differences, rather than on differences in the sedimentation rate, will collect in the same fraction pieces of different sizes deriving from the same sperm substructure. Segments of mitochondrial helix, as well as individual organelles, will equilibrate together in a band (band 2) essentially free from contaminants, since the density of mitochondria is markedly different from that of other cell membranes (band 1) and of sperm proteinaceous structures (band 3). These considerations are substantiated by the relatively high recovery and specific activity of cytochrome oxidase, the mitochondrial marker, in band 2, and by the purity of this fraction as revealed by electron microscopy. The resolving power of the isopycnic method is high enough to separate two mitochondrial populations of differing morphologies (bands 2A and 2B); their occurrence has been noted by other authors (Bartoov and Messer, 1976; Hrudka, 1978), but their origin is as yet not clear.

Cytochrome oxidase-specific activity of bull sperm mitochondria was higher than that reported by other authors for liver mitochondria (Bartoov et al., 1970). This characteristic may be related to the metabolic properties of bull spermatozoa. On the basis of the cytochrome oxidase-specific activity, mitochondria were calculated to account for 15-17% of total sperm protein.

Isolated bull sperm mitochondria contain relatively less phospholipids and more protein than mitochondria of somatic cells (Fleischer et al., 1967). This may be due to the existence in sperm mitochondria of a disulfide-stabilized proteinaceous shell, first noticed by Bedford and Calvin (1974) and recently studied in some detail in this laboratory (Pallini et al., 1979).

As to the RNA content, the values obtained with sperm mitochondria compare well with those reported for other cell types (e.g., Bartoov et al., 1970). The failure to measure sperm mitochondrial DNA may indicate that these organelles, similar to mitochondria of other cell types, possess several times more RNA than DNA (Bartoov et al., 1970).

The complexity of the mitochondrial polypeptide composition certainly demands more advanced techniques than monodimensional SDS polyacrylamide gel electrophoresis. However, the data presented indicate that some major bands are peculiar to sperm mitochondria and that the profound morphological alterations induced by the detachment with mercaptoethanol correspond to a comparatively low and very selective modification of the electrophoretic pattern.

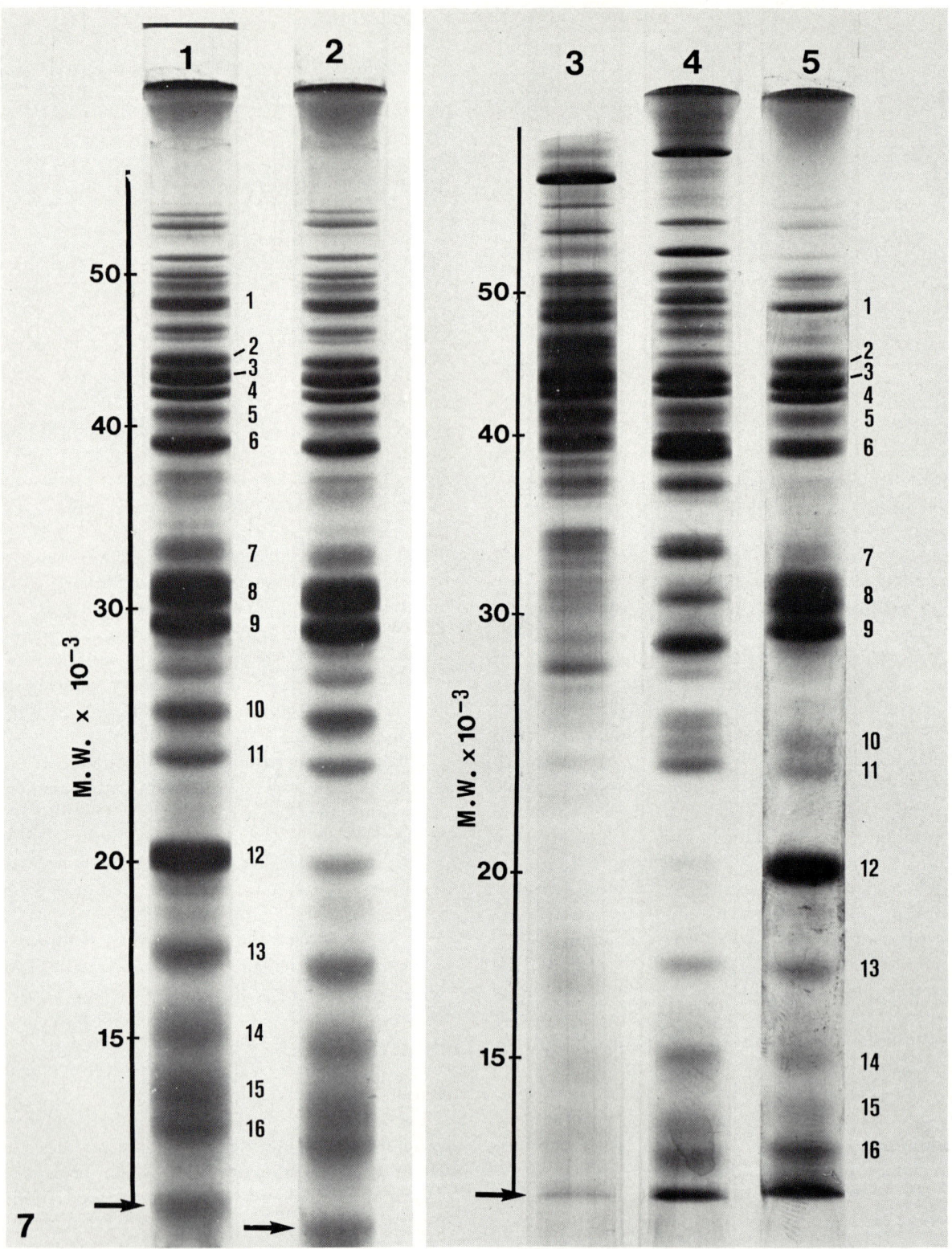

Figure 7. SDS-polyacrylamide electrophoresis of purified mitochondrial preparations. Gel 1, sonication-detached bull sperm mitochondria, 75 μg total protein; gel 2, mercaptoethanol-detached bull sperm mitochondria, 75 μg total protein; gel 3, bull heart mitochondria, 80 μg total protein; gel 4, bull liver mitochondria, 80 μg total protein; gel 5, sonication-detached bull sperm mitochondria, 60 μg total protein.

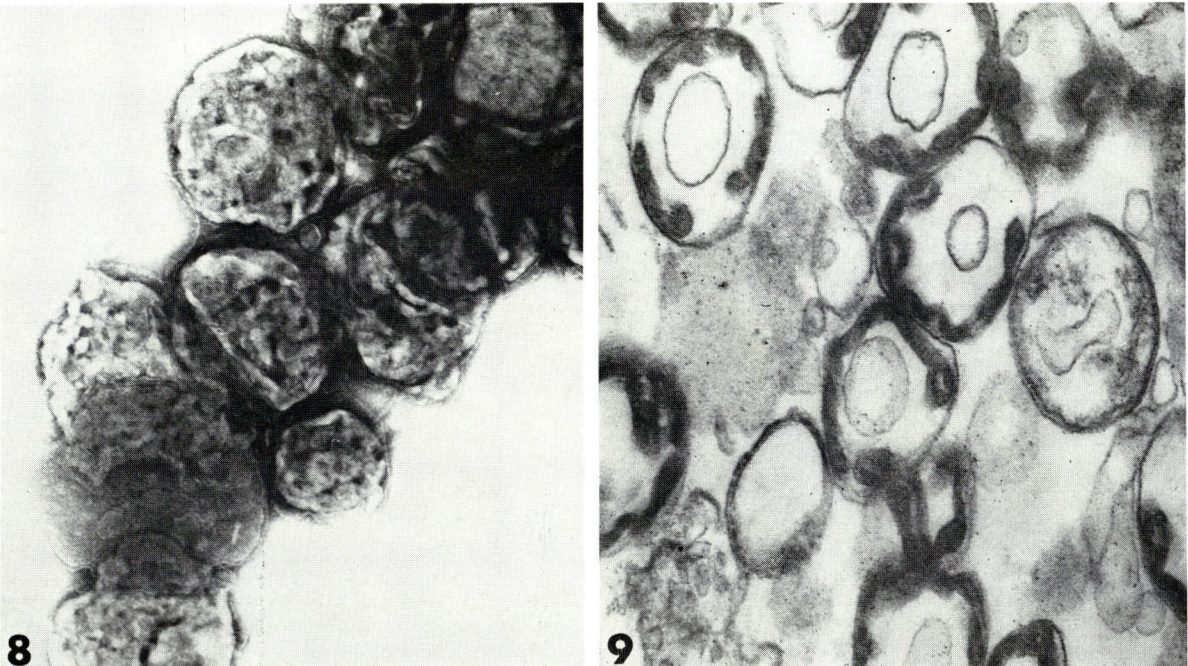

Figures 8-9. Purified preparations of mercaptoethanol-detached mitochondria. Figure 8, negative staining, X51,000; Figure 9, thin section of a pellet, X51,000

SUMMARY

Bull sperm mitochondria are detached by sonication and purified by centrifugation on a continuous density gradient. The isolated organelles preserve their native crescent shape and membrane fine structure and are essentially free from contaminants visible in the electron microscope. More than 30% of total sperm cytochrome oxidase is present in the mitochondrial fraction with a 8-9-fold increase in specific activity. Isolated mitochondria contain 8.0-9.5 µg of lipid phosphorus and 1.1-1.4 µg of RNA phosphorus per mg protein. As demonstrated by SDS-polyacrylamide gel electrophoresis, the predominant polypeptides of sperm mitochondria are absent or present in comparatively minor amounts in bull heart and liver mitochondria. When mitochondria are detached from spermatozoa by using a disulfide-reducing reagent, profound morphological alterations occur which are accompanied by the loss of a specific polypeptide.

REFERENCES

Ames, B.N.: Assay of Inorganic Phosphate, Total Phosphate and Phosphatases. In: Methods in Enzymology. Vol. VIII, pp. 115-118, ed. by E.F. Neufeld and V. Ginsburg. Academic Press, New York-London, 1966

Baccetti, B.; Pallini, V.; Burrini, A.G.: The Accessory Fibers of the Sperm Tail. I. Structure and Chemical Composition of the Bull Coarse Fibers. J Submicrosc Cytol 5(1973)237-256

Baccetti, B.; Pallini, V.; Burrini, A.G.: The Accessory Fibers of the Sperm Tail. II. Their Role in Binding Zinc in Mammals and Cephalopods. J Ultrastruct Res 54(1976a)261-275

Baccetti, B.; Pallini, V.; Burrini, A.G.: The Accessory Fiber of the Sperm Tail. III. High-Sulfur and Low-Sulfur Components in Mammals and Cephalopods, J Ultrastruct Res 57(1976b)289-308

Bartoov, B.; Messer, G.Y.: Isolation of Mitochondria from Ejaculated Ram Spermatozoa. J Ultrastruct Res 57(1976)68-76

Bartoov, B.; Mitra, R.S.; Freeman, K.B.: Ribosomal-type Ribonucleic Acid from Rodent Mitochondria. Biochem J 120(1970)455-466

Bedford, J.M.; Calvin, H.I.: Changes in —S—S—linked Structures of the Sperm Tail during Epididymal Maturation, with Comparative Observations in Sub-mammalian Species. J Exp Zool 187(1974)181-204

Calvin, H.I.: Isolation and Subfractionation of Mammalian Sperm Heads and Tails. In: Methods in Cell Biology. Vol. XIII, pp. 85-104, ed. by D.M. Prescott. Academic Press, New York, San Francisco, London, 1976

Calvin, H.I.; Hwang, F.H.F.; Wohlrab, H.: Localization of Zinc in a Dense Fiber-Connecting Piece Fraction of Rat Sperm Tails Analogous Chemically to Hair Keratin. Biol Reprod 13(1975)228-239

Clegg, E.D.: this symposium

Cooperstein, S.J.; Lazarow, A.: A Microspectrophotometric Method for the Determination of Cytochrome Oxidase. J Biol Chem 189(1951)665-670

Elfvin, L.S.: An Ultrastructural Difference between the

Outer and Inner Membrane of the Middle Piece Mitochondria in Rat Spermatozoa. J Ultrastruct Res 24(1968)259-268

Fawcett, D.W.: A Comparative View of Sperm Ultrastructure. Biol Reprod 2(1970)90-127

Fleischer, S.; Fleischer, B.; Stoeckenius, W.: Fine Structure of Lipid-depleted Mitochondria. J Cell Biol 32(1967)193-208

Folch, J.; Less, M.; Sloane Stanley, G.H.: A Simple Method for the Isolation and Purification of Total Lipides from Animal Tissues. J Biol Chem 226(1957)497-509

Hrudka, F.: A Morphological and Cytochemical Study on Isolated Sperm Mitochondria. J Ultrastruct Res 63(1978)1-19

Keyhani, E.; Storey, B.T.: Energy Conservation Capacity and Morphological Integrity of Mitochondria in Hypotonically Treated Rabbit Epididymal Spermatozoa. Biochim Biophys Acta 305(1973)557-569

Laemmli, U.K.: Change of Structural Proteins during the Assembly of the Head of Bacteriophage T_4. Nature 227(1970)680-685

Lowry, O.M.; Rosebrough, N.J.; Farr, A.L.; Randall, R.J.: Protein Measurement with the Folin Phenol Reagent. J Biol Chem 193(1951)265-275

Millette, C.F.; Spear, P.G; Gall, W.E.; Edelman, G.M.: Chemical Dissection of Mammalian Spermatozoa. J Cell Biol 58(1973)662-675

Mohri, H.; Mohri, T.; Ernster, L.: Isolation and Enzymic Properties of the Midpiece of Bull Spermatozoa. Exp Cell Res 38(1965)217-246

Morré, D.J.; Clegg, E.D.; Lunstra, D.D.; Mollenhauer, H.H.: An Electron-dense Stain for Isolated Fragments of Plasma and Acrosome Membranes from Porcine Sperm. Proc Soc Exp Biol Med 145(1974)1-6

Olson, G.E.; Hamilton, D.W.; Fawcett, D.W.: Isolation and Characterization of the Fibrous Sheath of Rat Epididymal Spermatozoa. Biol Reprod 14(1976a)517-530

Olson, G.E.; Hamilton, D.W.; Fawcett, D.W.: Isolation and Characterization of the Perforatorium of Rat Spermatozoa. J Reprod Fertil 47(1976b)193-297

Pallini, Baccetti, Burrini: A Peculiar Cystein-rich Polypeptide Related to Some Unusual Properties of Mammalian Sperm Mitochondria. In: The Spermatozoon, ed. by D.W. Fawcett and J.M. Bedford. Urban & Schwarzenberg, Baltimore, 1979.

Phillips, D.M.: Mitochondrial Disposition in Mammalian Spermatozoa. J Ultrastruct Res 58(1977)144-154

Premkumar, E.; Bhargava, P.M.: Transcription and Translation in Bovine Spermatozoa. Nature [New Biol] 240(1972)139-143

Schneider, W.C.: Determination of Nucleic Acids in Tissues by Pentose Analysis. In: Methods in Enzymology. Vol. III, pp. 680-684, ed. by S.P. Colowick and N.O. Kaplan. Academic Press, New York, 1957

Storey, B.T.; Keyhani, E.: Interaction of Calcium Ion with the Mitochondria of Rabbit Spermatozoa. FEBS Lett 37(1973)33-36

Van Dop, C.; Hutson, S.M.; Lardy, H.A.: Pyruvate Metabolism in Bovine Epididymal Spermatozoa. J Biol Chem 252(1977)1303-1308

Zahler, W.L.; Doak, G.A.: Isolation of the Outer Acrosomal Membrane from Bull Sperm. Biochim Biophys Acta 406(1975)479-488

WORKSHOP TWO
Quantitative Assessment of Sperm Motility

The subjective nature of visual assessment of sperm motility is a persistent problem for those engaged in the clinical examination of infertile man. There is often little consistency in judgement of motility on successive visits of the same patient, and considerable variance among different technicians scoring the same sample. Objective appraisal of sperm motility is no less troublesome for laboratory scientists attempting to compare treated and control samples. There is therefore a pressing need for reliable quantitative methods that can provide information on overall motility, percentage of motile sperm, and one that can distinguish ineffective vibratile motion, or circling, from progressive locomotion. This workshop presents a variety of approaches to the problem ranging from relatively simple and inexpensive photographic techniques to sophisticated and costly computer-assisted optical instruments.

BIOPHYSICAL ASPECTS OF HUMAN SPERM MOVEMENT

D.F. Katz and J.W. Overstreet

Department of Obstetrics and Gynecology and Department of Human Anatomy, University of California School of Medicine, Davis, California 95616 USA

The movements of a spermatozoon during swimming are the hydrodynamic consequence of the kinematics of flagellar undulations, *i.e.* the time-dependent details of the beat, the morphology of the sperm body, the rheological properties of the fluid medium which surrounds the sperm, and the morphology and kinematics of other solid objects with which the sperm interacts. Flagellar activity is initiated, modulated, and terminated by physiological alterations in the sperm cell during the processes of maturation, transport, capacitation, and fertilization. Although considerable scientific attention has been focused on sperm motility, the chemistry and physics of this activity remain to be integrated with the biological events of sperm transport in the male and female. This situation is likely to improve as more objective and quantitative methods for assessing sperm movement are incorporated into studies of sperm physiology in the male and female reproductive tracts. In this chapter several approaches for quantitative description of the movement of spermatozoa are outlined. The comprehensiveness of these levels of description is discussed, as are the physiological interpretations appropriate to each. Experimental methodologies are mentioned, and preliminary data for human spermatozoa are presented. The biophysical interaction between human spermatozoa and cervical mucus is then considered.

LEVELS OF DESCRIPTION OF THE MOVEMENT CHARACTERISTICS OF SPERMATOZOA

The movement characteristics of a sperm suspension can be described on a number of levels of increasing detail, the choice of which depends upon the objectives of the study. These levels of description, and the methods of measurement which they require, can be distinguished according to their abilities to:

1. Describe sperm movement on a per-sperm basis.
2. Describe sperm movement on a time-dependent basis.
3. Distinguish the shape of a swimming trajectory from the net displacement of a spermatozoon.
4. Distinguish swimming speed from flagellar beat frequency and various parametric measures of beat shape.
5. Determine the detailed kinematics of the flagellar beat.

A gross level of description focuses exclusively on the percentage of motile sperm, and the mean swimming speed of a sperm suspension. This level is sufficient for a general assessment of sperm vitality and survival, for example in response to exogenous pharmacological agents. A number of experimental methodologies have been used for quantitation of sperm movement at this level including single time-exposure photomicrography (*e.g.*, Rothschild and Swann, 1949; Janick and MacLeod, 1970; Katz and Dott, 1975; Overstreet *et al.*, 1979), high-speed cinemicrography (*e.g.*, Rikmenspoel, 1957; Van Duijn *et al.*, 1971; Katz and Dott, 1975), laser-Doppler spectroscopy (*e.g.*, Jouannet *et al.*, 1977; Hallet *et al.*, 1978), real-time image analyzing computers (Katz and Dott, 1975), and computerized scanning of video tape records (Liu and Warme, 1977). Further discussion of these methods can be found in this appendix.

An intermediate level of description of sperm movement focuses on a variety of parametrical characteristics sampled on a per-sperm basis. A summary of these characteristics, as defined and measured in our laboratory, is contained in Table 1. Description of sperm movement at this level has been incorporated into investigations of sperm physiology, including relationships between motility and metabolic activity, (*e.g.*, Brokaw and Benedict, 1968a, b; Rikmenspoel *et al.*, 1969; Gibbons and Gibbons, 1972; McGrady and Nelson, 1976), sperm movement during capacitation and the acrosome reaction (Katz *et al.*, 1978a), and the interaction of spermatozoa with cervical mucus (Katz *et al.*, 1978b).

Photomicrographic approaches are the only methods capable of accurately recording the diversity of sperm movement characteristics required for this level of description. Considerable information can be obtained from a single time-exposure photomicrograph. Figure 1

© 1979 Urban & Schwarzenberg, Inc. Baltimore-Munich *The Spermatozoon*, edited by D.W. Fawcett and J.M. Bedford

Table 1. Levels of Description of the Movement Characteristics of Spermatozoa

I. Gross Classification of Sperm Motility
  A. Percent motility
  B. Mean swimming speed
II. Parametric Description of the Movements of Individual Spermatozoa
  A. Directly measured characteristics
    1. Swimming speed
      a. Progressive V_P (μm/s)
      b. Total V_T (μm/s)
    2. Beat frequency f (Hz)
    3. Beat amplitude b (μm)
    4. Beat wavelength λ (μm)
  B. Derived movement characteristics
    1. Progressiveness ratio V_P/V_T
    2. Kinetic efficiency V_P/fL
  C. Attribute movement characteristics
    1. Rolling
    2. Yawing
    3. Intermittancy
    4. Circular trajectory
III. Detailed Description of the Movements of Individual Spermatozoa
  A. Kinematic characteristics—direct measurement
    1. Beat shape
      a. Position coordinates along flagellum
      b. Slope angle along flagellum
    2. Beat velocity
      a. Linear velocity along flagellum
      b. Angular velocity along flagellum
    3. Velocity field in medium about sperm
  B. Hydrodynamical characteristics—derived computation
    1. Power output
    2. External bending moment distribution along flagellum
    3. Thrust produced by flagellar beat

depicts the negative of a one-second photomicrographic exposure of human semen in dark field illumination. The diversity of movement patterns is characteristic of human spermatozoa. The flagella of freely swimming spermatozoa do not scatter enough light to be visible, and the "tracks" observed represent the paths traversed by the sperm heads. The length of a track recorded over a known interval is a direct measure of the swimming speed of a single sperm. Rolling motions of the sperm head about its axis of translation result in consecutive, discrete images that are superimposed on the track. These are visually apparent as the characteristic "flash" of the sperm head. Spermatozoa that "yaw" during swimming produce a tortuous track on the negative, with periodic lateral excursions about the axis of propulsion. Spermatozoa whose heads do not roll produce tracks of continuous density. When spermatozoa are not progressing, their flagellar movements are apparent on a time-exposure photomicrograph. These motile but stationary sperm can be clearly distinguished from immotile sperm, which have well-defined, nonblurred flagella. The authors' standardized protocol for analyzing such photomicrographs is designed to furnish quantitative information on percent motility, swimming speed as sampled from all motile spermatozoa and from those swimming at a speed of 25 μm/sec or more ("progressive" sperm), the straightness of the swimming trajectories, and the tendency of spermatozoa to roll and/or yaw while swimming (Overstreet et al., 1979). A quantitative description of sperm movement in four human semen samples, as obtained by this method, is given in Table 2. As evidenced in Table 2, the time-exposure photomicrographic method is capable of describing quantitatively the variety of patterns characteristic of the swimming trajectories of human spermatozoa, as well as providing information on percent motility and swimming speed. The four semen samples illustrated were classified as "normal" based upon contemporary criteria for sperm numbers and percent motility (Freund, 1968; Eliasson, 1975). Nevertheless, there were substantial differences among these samples in both the swimming speeds and the geometric attributes

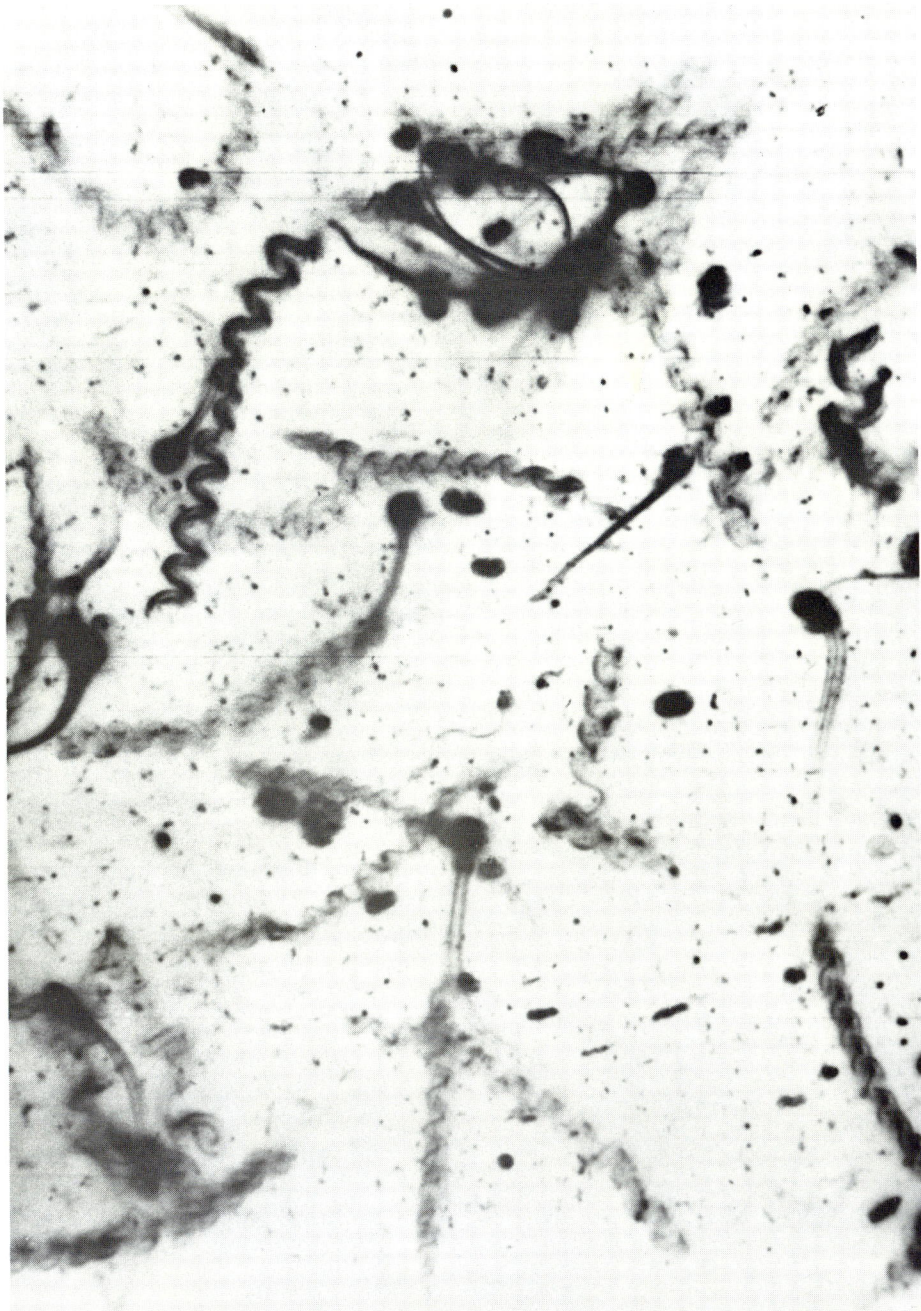

Figure 1. The negative of a one-second photomicrographic exposure of human semen. The different "tracks" reflect various patterns of speeds of human sperm movement. (X1000).

of the swimming trajectories. Such a result cautions against reliance upon knowledge of concentration and percent motility in assessing the quality of a suspension of human spermatozoa in semen.

The individual flagellar beat patterns responsible for the different movement attributes depicted in Table 2 cannot be determined with the time-exposure photomicrographic technique. High-speed cinemicrography is the only current method capable of recording the details of flagellar movement. The capability for obtaining information on flagellar beat frequency and shape is of particular advantage. Table 3 summarizes data obtained by cinemicrographic analysis of fresh semen samples obtained from four additional men. The move-

Table 2. Typical Values of Movement Characteristics of Human Spermatozoa in Semen at 37°C, as Determined by Single Time-Exposure Photomicrography

Exp. No.	Motile Sperm (%)	Gross Swimming Speed (μm/sec)	Translating Sperm (%)	Translating Swimming Speed (μm/sec)	Straight Swimming Sperm (%)	Rolling Sperm (%)	Yawing Sperm (%)
1	80	32.80 ± 4.68	60	46.87 ± 2.13	80	100	0
2	88	52.87 ± 4.67	87	59.66 ± 2.09	80	58	7
3	66	18.93 ± 3.10	33	33.33 ± 3.54	33	33	0
4	76	35.13 ± 2.98	87	38.07 ± 1.95	47	40	53

Values of gross swimming speed and translating swimming speed are expressed as mean ± s.e.m. Translating sperm are defined as swimming at a speed of 25 μm/sec or greater.

ment characteristics presented in Table 3 are summarized below. The direct characteristics are:

1. Beat frequency—obtained over at least 20 consecutive beats.
2. Beat amplitude—obtained as one-half the maximum transverse displacement of the flagellum with respect to an effective centerline.
3. Total swimming speed—the total displacement per unit time of the junction of the sperm head and midpiece during at least 2 s of elapsed real time.
4. Progressive swimming speed—the displacement per unit time measured along the straight line connecting the initial and final points of the preceding trajectory.

The derived characteristics are:

1. Progressiveness ratio—the ratio of progressive swimming speed to total swimming speed.
2. Kinetic efficiency—progressive swimming speed/ (beat frequency x sperm length).

Thus, progressiveness ratio is a measure of the straightness of the swimming trajectory, while kinetic efficiency depicts the number of sperm body lengths swum per beat. From a fundamental hydrodynamic point of view, kinetic efficiency may be regarded as a dimensionless swimming speed. As such it reflects beat shape, sperm morphology, the presence of nearby solid objects, and, in some instances, rheological properties of the suspending medium.

The data presented in Table 3 were based upon the random sampling of at least 20 spermatozoa per suspension. Such randomized determination of progressive swimming speed is comparable to the "gross" swimming speed obtained by our single time-exposure method. As can be seen in comparing of Tables 2 and 3, the range of values obtained by the two methods is similar. Like the results presented in Table 2, the cinemicrographic data indicate significant differences among the four semen samples' direct movement characteristics. In comparison, the values of progressiveness ratio and of kinetic efficiency did not vary significantly. Because of the small sample size, such a lack of variation cannot presently be regarded as common to human semen in general. However, the variability of these two derived characteristics is worthy of further study since, in comparison with that of the direct characteristics, it might prove useful in the fundamental and clinical discrimination among sperm suspensions.

The third, and most comprehensive level of description of sperm movement focuses upon the detailed kinematics of the flagellar beat. Hydrodynamically, it is also appropriate to consider the velocity field in the

Table 3. Values of Movement Characteristics of the Spermatozoa From Four Additional Men, in Semen at 37°C, as Obtained by High-Speed Cinemicrography

Exp. No.	Flagellar Beat Frequency f (Hz)	Flagellar Beat Amplitude b (μm)	Progressive Swimming Speed V_P (μm/sec)	Total Swimming Speed V_T (μm/sec)	Progressiveness Ratio V_P/V_T	Kinetic Efficiency $(V_P/fL) \times 10^2$
1	8.58 ± 0.54	4.44 ± 0.33	36.29 ± 2.71	54.36 ± 3.31	0.63 ± 0.06	8.85 ± 0.76
2	12.87 ± 0.42	4.40 ± 0.28	56.67 ± 5.33	91.14 ± 4.77	0.68 ± 0.05	8.92 ± 0.80
3	6.96 ± 0.61	5.80 ± 0.39	31.02 ± 2.56	46.08 ± 2.59	0.66 ± 0.04	9.26 ± 0.60
4	9.66 ± 0.65	5.38 ± 0.29	41.77 ± 2.82	59.65 ± 6.11	0.72 ± 0.03	9.19 ± 0.62

Values are expressed at mean ± s.e.m.

fluid around a spermatozoon. Studies of the flagellar contraction mechanism utilize experimental data obtained at this level, (*e.g.,* Brokaw, 1970; Brokaw and Josslin, 1973; Brokaw, 1975; Lubiner and Blum, 1972; Rikmenspoel, 1978). Such data serve as input to systems of differential equations that describe the generation and propagation of flagellar waves in terms of properties of the flagellum and its environment. The ensuing calculations include determination of the distribution of external hydrodynamic bending moments acting on the flagellum. The hydrodynamic rate of working, or power output can also be computed using data obtained at this level or, less accurately, at the preceding one. This measure of sperm behavior is germane to studies of the energetics and metabolic activity of spermatozoa.

The accuracy of all mathematical computations based on observations of flagellar movement is dependent upon the accuracy with which both the instantaneous shape of the flagellum and the local velocity distribution along it are determined. In general, the flagellar velocity distribution is the more difficult to measure accurately. A new, improved method for obtaining the flagellar shape and velocity distributions from photo- or cinemicrographs has been developed recently in the authors' laboratory (Mills, 1978). In this method a local cubic "spline" curve is used to describe analytically the instantaneous shape of a flagellum. The spline curve is fitted to experimental data by linear programming (Gass, 1958). Time derivatives, *i.e.* velocities, are then obtained numerically by a five-point parabolic weighted least squares curve fit. An example of the application of this method to a human spermatozoon in semen is given in Figure 2. As illustrated in Figure 2, the flagella of human spermatozoa in various media undergo a number of changes in the derivatives of the slope angle α with respect to transflagellar distance s. Visually, such changes appear more common to the thinner, distal portions of the flagellum than to the thicker midpiece. They may be the consequence of reduced stiffness in the distal flagellum, as has been hypothesized for other mammalian spermatozoa (Phillips, 1972). Mathematical models of the flagellar contraction mechanism, applicable to the human or other mammalian spermatozoa, must therefore allow for such variation in stiffness, (Rikmenspoel, 1965). The computation of the external hydrodynamic bending moment, displayed in Figure 2 was based upon "resistive force theory" (Gray and Hancock, 1955; Lighthill, 1976), as applied to the local, experimentally determined distributions of beat shape and velocity. While this theory represents a mathematical approximation, recent studies have demonstrated that it can be quite accurate in application to the beats of real flagella (Dresdner *et al.,* 1979; Johnson and Brokaw, 1979).

THE INTERACTION OF HUMAN SPERMATOZOA WITH CERVICAL MUCUS

In attempting to understand the biophysics of sperm transport through the mammalian cervix, a distinction must be made between those species with abundant cervical mucus (*e.g.,* ruminants, primates), those with scant cervical mucus (*e.g.,* rabbits), and those whose cervix presents little or no barrier to sperm transport (*e.g.,* pigs, horses, dogs, rodents). When abundant cervical mucus is present, the ascending spermatozoa must interact mechanically with it, and almost certainly with the ciliated cervical epithelium as well. The kinetics of sperm entry into the human cervix and their subsequent migration through this region therefore depend upon: the intrinsic movement and morphological characteristics of the spermatozoa; the micro- and macrophysical characteristics of the cervical mucus; the geometry of the cervical canal including the pattern of mucosal folding and distribution of cilia; and the activity of the female reproductive tract, including the ciliary beat and muscular contractions of the viscera. Hydrodynamic interactions among these factors, with physical and chemical modulation at the molecular level, determine the swimming behavior of spermatozoa during passage through the cervix. At present, those mechanisms responsible for sperm transport through the cervix are only beginning to be elucidated.

Investigations of the biophysics of the sperm-mucus interaction must take into account both the movement characteristics of the spermatozoa and the microscale properties of the mucus as experienced by the spermatozoa. An initial study of human spermatozoa in fresh, ovulatory human cervical mucus has demonstrated fundamental differences in sperm movement in comparison with semen or their behavior in simple balanced-salt solutions (Katz *et al.,* 1978b). The results of this investigation are summarized in Table 4 and Figure 3. Specifically:

1. The sperm flagella beat at higher frequencies in the mucus than in either the parent semen or Tyrode's solution.
2. The progressive swimming speeds did not differ in the three media.
3. The distances swum per beat (kinetic efficiency) were lowest in the mucus.
4. Individual spermatozoa swam along straighter tra-

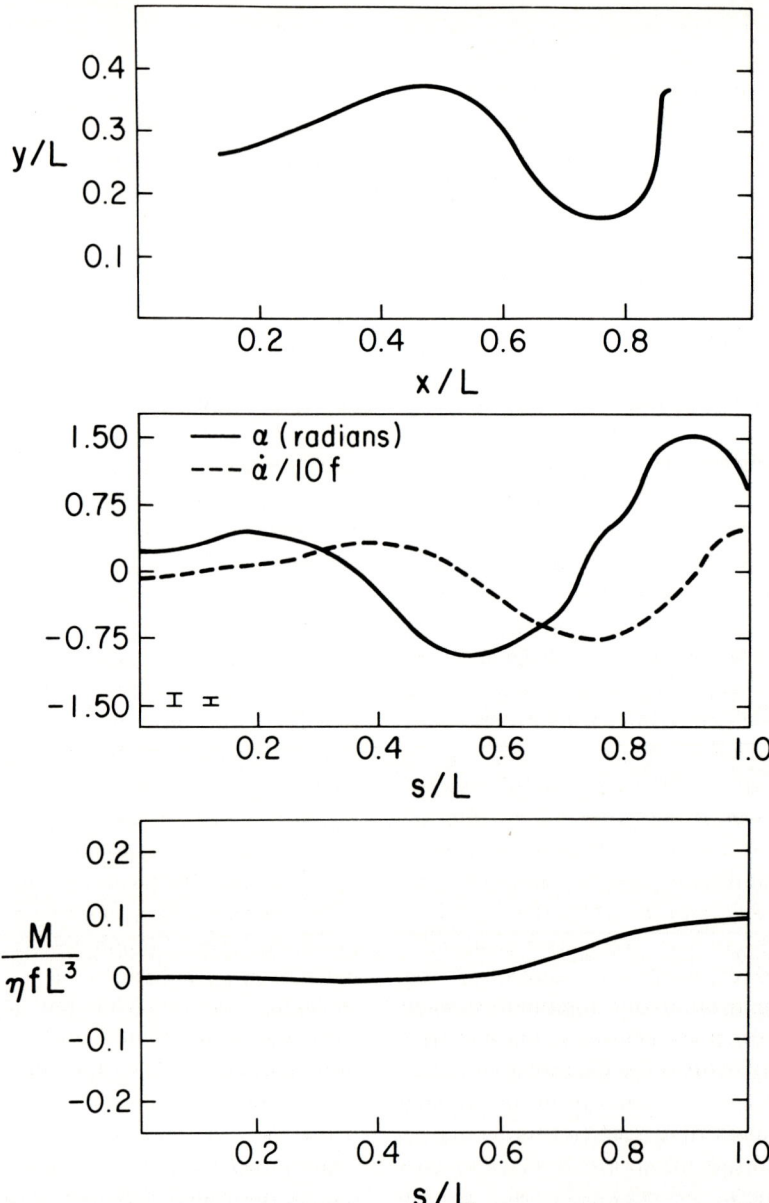

Figure 2. Detailed cinemicrographic analysis of the movement of a human spermatozoon in semen at a particular instant. The symbols are as follows: (x,y) are position coordinates of a point on the flagellum; L is the length of the sperm body; s is a distance coordinate as measured locally along the flagellum; α and $\dot{\alpha}$ are respectively the local slope angle of the flagellum and its time derivative; f is flagellar beat frequency; M is the local external hydrodynamic bending moment acting on the flagellum; and η is the viscosity of the suspending medium. In the middle drawing, the large bracket indicates the experimental error for $\dot{\alpha}$, and the small bracket gives the error for α.

jectories in the mucus, even though no bulk stretching of the mucus had occurred.

5. The flagellar beat shape in the mucus was qualitatively and quantitatively different from that in the simple media (cf Figure 3). The principal bending was confined to the distal portion of the flagellum, and was characterized by lower amplitude and wavelength than in semen or Tyrode's (figure-eight flagellar oscillation).

These differences between sperm movement in semen and in cervical mucus can be attributed largely to the effect of hydrodynamic interactions between the sperm body and the mucous microstructure. Recent studies of

Table 4. Movement Characteristics of Human Spermatozoa in Different Media at Two Temperatures

Exp.	Medium	Temp. (°C)	Number of Observations	Flagellar Beat Frequency f (Hz)	Progressive Swimming Speed V_P (μm/sec)	Total Swimming Speed V_T (μm/sec)	Progressiveness Ratio V_P/V_T	Kinetic Efficiency $(V_P/fL) \times 10^2$
1	Semen	21	10	5.84 ± 0.59[a]	21.39 ± 2.71[a]	25.99 ± 2.57[a]	0.81 ± 0.04[a]	7.40 ± 0.77[a]
	Tyrode	21	10	4.11 ± 0.43[b]	21.54 ± 3.82[b]	37.23 ± 4.87[b]	0.59 ± 0.07[b]	10.78 ± 0.92[b]
	Cervical mucus	21	35	7.72 ± 0.37[c]	18.44 ± 1.15[c]	20.46 ± 1.22[c]	0.91 ± 0.02[c]	4.90 ± 0.30[a]
2	Semen	21	14	4.15 ± 0.50[a]	18.58 ± 2.07[a]	28.81 ± 2.67[a]	0.65 ± 0.06[a]	8.54 ± 0.69[a]
	Tyrode	21	13	4.58 ± 0.50[a]	22.66 ± 2.73[a]	46.64 ± 4.76[b]	0.53 ± 0.07[a]	9.89 ± 0.68[a]
	Cervical mucus	21	20	9.52 ± 0.54[b]	22.45 ± 2.00[a]	24.65 ± 2.10[a]	0.91 ± 0.01[b]	4.84 ± 0.41[b]
3	Cervical mucus	37	13	17.42 ± 0.50	36.44 ± 3.78	39.21 ± 4.35	0.89 ± 0.02	4.30 ± 0.50
4	Cervical mucus	37	23	15.13 ± 0.72	34.11 ± 3.45	35.64 ± 3.62	0.96 ± 0.01	4.36 ± 0.32

Values are mean ± s.e.m.
Within an experiment means with different subscripts are significantly different ($P < 0.05$).
From Katz et al. (1978b).

the mucus (Katz and Berger, 1978; Tam *et al.*, 1978) suggest that human spermatozoa swim in apposition to closely spaced, filamentous structures. This characterization of the macromolecular architecture of native cervical mucus is somewhat different from the classical one, (*e.g.*, Odeblad, 1973), owing to the absence of large "channels" through which spermatozoa migrate. As a consequence, strong hydrodynamic interactions occur between a sperm and the mucus (Katz and Singer, 1978). In some instances, human spermatozoa may actually shear their way through the mucous microstructure. The details of the sperm-mucus interaction vary, owing to the naturally occurring polydispersity and heterogeneity of the mucus. Externally induced shearing of the mucus may alter not just the microstructure, but also the kinetics of sperm migration

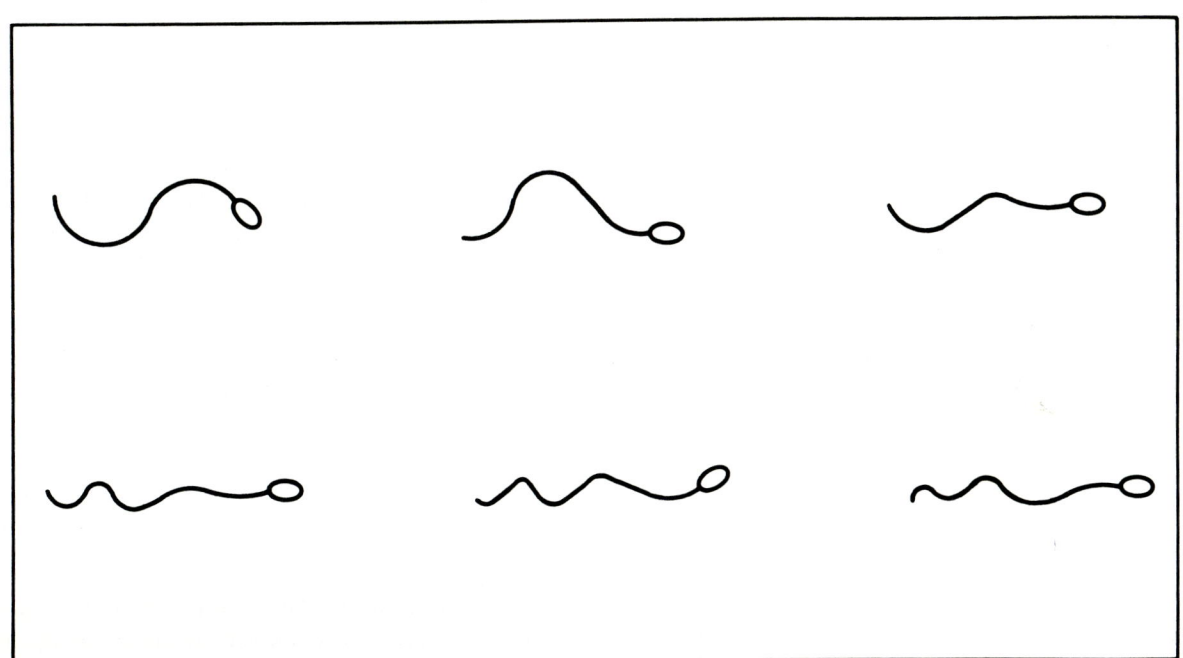

Figure 3. Typical flagellar beat shapes of human spermatozoa in semen (upper) and ovulatory human cervical mucus (lower). From Katz et al. (1978b).

through it. Prolonged sperm residence within regions of mucus appears to be associated with an alteration of the mucous microstructure (Katz and Overstreet, unpublished). It should be appreciated that the local properties of cervical mucus *in vivo* depend upon the age of mucus following secretion and possibly the site of secretion within the cervical epithelium. Consequently, the three-dimensional mosaic of the mucus within the cervical canal must be regarded as a time- and space-dependent entity. Elucidation of the effect upon sperm transport of the sperm-mucus interaction should therefore take such time- and space-dependence into account.

REFERENCES

Brokaw, C.J.: Bending Moments in Free Swimming Flagella. J Exp Biol 53(1970)445-464

Brokaw, C.J.: Effects of Viscosity and ATP Concentration on the Movement of Reactivated Sea Urchin Sperm Flagella. J Exp Biol 62(1975)701-709

Brokaw, C.J.; Benedict, B.: Mechanochemical Coupling in Flagella. I. Movement Dependent Dephosphorylation of ATP by Glycerinated Spermatozoa. Arch Biochem Biophys 125(1968a)770-778

Brokaw, C.J.; Benedict, B.: Mechanochemical Coupling in Flagella. II. Effects of Viscosity and Motility of Ciona Spermatozoa. J Gen Physiol 52(1968b)283-299

Brokaw, C.J.; Josslin, R.: Maintenance of Constant Wave Parameters by Sperm Flagella at Reduced Frequencies of Beat. J Exp Biol 59(1973)617-628

Dresdner, R.D.; Katz, D.F.; Berger, S.A.: The Propulsion by Large Amplitude Waves of Uniflagellar Microorganisms of Finite Length. J Fluid Mech, in press

Eliasson, R.: Analysis of Semen. In: Progress in Fertility, pp. 691-713, ed. by S.J. Behrman and R.W. Kistner, Little Brown, Boston, Mass., 1975

Freund, M.: Semen Analysis. In: Progress in Infertility, pp. 593-627, ed. by S.J. Behrman and R.W. Kistner, Little Brown, Boston, Mass., 1968

Gass, S.I.: *Linear Programming*, McGraw-Hill, New York, 1958

Gibbons, B.H.; Gibbons, I.R.: Flagellar Movement and Adenosine Triphosphate Activity in Sea Urchin Sperm Extracted with Triton X-100. J Cell Biol 54(1972)75-97

Gray, J.; Hancock, G.J.: The Propulsion of Sea Urchin Spermatozoa, J Exp Biol 32(1955)802-814

Hallet, F.R.; Craig, T.; Marsh, J.: Swimming Speed Distributions of Bull Spermatozoa as Determined by Quasielastic Light Scattering. Biophys J 21(1978)203-216

Janick, J.; MacLeod, J.: The Measurement of Human Spermatozoan Motility. Fert Steril 21(1970)140-146

Johnson, R.E.; Brokaw, C.J.: Flagellar Hydrodynamics: A Comparison Between Resistive Force Theory and Slender Body Theory. Biophys J, in press

Jouannet, P.; Volochine, B.; Deguent, P.; Serres, C.; David, G.: Light Scattering Determination of Various Characteristic Parameters of Spermatozoa Motility in a Series of Human Sperm. Andrologia 9(1977)36-49

Katz, D.F.; Dott, H.M.: Methods of Measuring Swimming Speed of Spermatozoa. J Reprod Fert 45(1975)263-272

Katz, D.F.; Berger, S.A.: Flagellar Propulsion of Sperm in Cervical Mucus. Presented at the Third International Congress of Biorheology, La Jolla, Aug. 28-Sept. 1, 1978

Katz, D.F.; Yanagimachi, R.; Dresdner, R.D.: Movement Characteristics and Power Output of Guinea Pig and Hamster Spermatozoa in Relation to Activation. J Reprod Fert 52(1978a)167-172

Katz, D.F.; Mills, R.N.; Pritchett, T.R.: The Movement of Human Spermatozoa in Cervical Mucus. J Reprod Fert 53(1978b)259-265

Katz, D.F.; Singer, J.R.: Water Mobility in Bovine Cervical Mucus. Biol Reprod 18(1978)843-849

Lighthill, M.J.: Flagellar Hydrodynamics. S.I.A.M. Rev. 18(1976)161-230

Liu, Y.T.; Warme, P.K.: Computerized Evaluations of Sperm Cell Motility. Comp Biomed Res 10(1977)127-138

Lubliner, J.; Blum, J.J.: Analysis of Form and Speed of Flagellar Waves According to a Sliding Filament Model. J Mechanochem Cell Motil 1(1972)157-167

McGrady, A.V.; Nelson, L.: Cholinergic Effects on Bull and Chimpanzee Sperm Motility. Biol Reprod 15(1976)248-253

Mills, R.N.: Experimental Studies of the Hydrodynamics of Human Spermatozoa. Ph.D. Thesis, University of California, Berkeley, 1978

Odeblad, E.: Biophysical Techniques of Assessing Cervical Mucus and Microstructure of Cervical Epithelium. In: Cervical Mucus In Human Reproduction, pp. 58-74, ed. by M. Elstein, K.S. Moghissi and R. Borth, Scriptor, Copenhagen, 1973

Overstreet, J.W.; Katz, D.F.; Hanson, F.W.; Fonseca, J.R.: A Simple, Inexpensive Method for Objective Assessment of Human Sperm Movement Characteristics. Fert Steril 31(1979)162-172.

Phillips, D.M.: Comparative Analysis of Mammalian Sperm Motility. J Cell Biol 53(1972)561-573

Rikmenspoel, R.: Photoelectric and Cinematographic Measurements of the "Motility" of Bull Sperm Cells. Thesis, Utrecht, 1957

Rikmenspoel, R.: The Tail Movement of Bull Spermatozoa. Observations and Model Calculations. Biophys J 5(1965)365-392

Rikmenspoel, R.: Movement of Sea Urchin Flagella. J Cell Biol 76(1978)310-322

Rikmenspoel, R.; Sinton, A.C.; Janick, J.J.: Energy Conversion in Bull Sperm Flagella. J Gen Physiol 54(1969)782-805

Rothschild, Lord; Swann, N.N.: The Fertilization Reaction in the Sea Urchin Egg. A Propagated Response to Sperm Attachment. J Exp Biol 30(1949)178-184

Tam, P.Y.; Katz, D.F.; Berger, S.A.: Flow Permeation Studies of Cervical Mucus. Presented at the Third International Congress of Biorheology, La Jolla, Aug. 26-Sept. 1, 1978

Van Duijn, Jr., C.; Van Voorst, C.; Freund, M.: Movement Characteristics of Human Spermatozoa Analysed from Kinemicrographs. Europ J Obstet Gynec 4(1971)121-135

A REVIEW OF THE SPECTROPHOTOMETRIC QUANTITATION OF SPERMATOZOAN MOTILITY

R.W. Atherton

Department of Zoology and Physiology, University of Wyoming, Laramie, Wyoming 82070 USA

Sperm motility may be quantitatively assayed by analyzing spectrophotometrically the optical anisotropic characteristic of motile sperm in a flow. The advantage of this procedure is that it satisfies the following criteria which are of value in any system that is to be adopted for analysis of sperm motility. Specifically any selected system should:

1. be based upon sound physical or chemical phenomena;
2. use, if possible, existing materials and equipment to reduce costs;
3. be suitable for use with numerous species;
4. reduce interpersonal variability by simplicity of operation and objectivity in analysis; and
5. analyze at least one relevant parameter of sperm motility.

The spectrophotometric procedure for quantitation of sperm motility is based upon the optical anisotropic phenomenon of motile sperm in a flow (Walton, 1952; Glover, 1968). Briefly, when saline-diluted semen is placed in a syringe and passed through a flow cell by an infusion pump at a constant rate, an absorbance is recorded that is proportional to sperm concentration. When the flow is stopped, sperm reorientation (the optical anisotropic characteristic of sperm) is recorded as a time-dependent decline in absorbance which can be used as an objective and quantitative assay of sperm motility.

The first spectrophotometric application of this technique analyzed the motility of sea urchin sperm (Timourian and Watchmaker, 1970). Later equipment requirements were simplified to quantitate rooster sperm motility by the adoption of a B and L Spec 20 colorimeter and by the choice of 475-nm wavelength (Wall and Boone, 1973). Equipment costs for this procedure are minimal since the conversion time necessary to alter an existing spectrophotometer is limited only to the time required to replace the standard cuvette with the special flow cell and subsequent rezeroing of the instrument.

Application of this procedure to bulls (Atherton, 1975a), another species of sea urchin (Atherton, 1975b), trout (Atherton, 1977a), rooster (Wall and Boone, 1973; Atherton, unpublished), and man (Atherton et al., 1977; Atherton et al., 1978a) confirmed its validity for analysis of sperm motility in numerous species having either external or internal fertilization.

Simplicity and objectivity of the procedure with minimal interpersonal variation of data processing are comparable, respectively, to the use and resolving power of the spectrophotometer.

This optical anisotropic-based description of sperm motility has been correlated with "the percent of active or motile sperm" in the sea urchin (Timourian and Watchmaker, 1970) and rooster (Wall and Boone, 1973). A significant correlation exists between this spectrophotometric analysis of human sperm motility and both a double blind subjective ranking of progressive sperm motility and to the percentage of dead sperm in the sample. In addition this motility analysis is independent of final sperm concentration and can be correlated to various semen parameters in fathers (Atherton et al., 1978a).

MATERIALS AND METHODS

Materials

A recording spectrophotometer or colorimeter forms the nucleus of the required equipment while the flow cell can be constructed for a cost of approximately $50. Recently the flow cell design was further simplified from its original description by using coverslips with parafilm gaskets instead of quartz windows and teflon ring gaskets (Atherton, 1975a). Commericially produced flow cells (Hellma) are available which are acceptable (Robert Foote, personal communication). This is espe-

---

The author acknowledges the expert technical assistance of Dr. R. M. Kitchen, Mr. F. Jackson, Mr. G. Bond, and Mr. E. W. Radany. This work was supported in part by the University of Wyoming, Division of Basic Research.

© 1979 Urban & Schwarzenberg, Inc. Baltimore-Munich *The Spermatozoon*, edited by D.W. Fawcett and J.M. Bedford

cially useful when using a wavelength of 475 nm and further simplifies the flow cell because the thinness of the coverslip does not require countersinking the steel holding plates. When the coverslips become dirty they are simply discarded. The flow cell inlet is firmly attached by teflon tubing to an 18-gauge needle on a 10-ml syringe fitted to an infusion pump. An infusion pump may not be required if careful and constant manual pressure is applied to the syringe. The effluent passes from the flow cell by teflon tubing into a fraction collector or series of test tubes. Sperm are maintained at the desired temperature by a water-jacketed cuvette holder.

Methods

Undiluted semen from the species of choice is allowed to liquify completely. If the sample is relatively free of cellular debris and crystals the semen is next diluted drop-wise into saline until an absorbance is recorded of 0.7-0.9 units.

Rarely semen samples may be initially unsuitable for spectrophotometric analysis because of one or more of the following features: an abnormally high viscosity, a high concentration of crystals, or disproportionately large numbers of dead cells. These interfering features may be eliminated by filtering semen through columns of glass wool. This effectively removes dead cells, debris, and also enriches the percentage of motile sperm in the sample (Paulson and Polakoski, 1977). When such a filtering procedure was applied to human semen, previously unusable viscous semen could be spectrophotometrically analyzed (Atherton et al., 1977a).

When semen has been prepared and diluted, it is pumped at a constant rate (7 ml/min) through the flow cell to remove air bubbles in the system. When a stable baseline of 0.7-0.9 absorbance units is obtained at 475 nm the flow is discontinued. Immediately a decline in absorbance is recorded as a function of time. This decline in absorbance represents the optical anisotrophic characteristic of sperm which approximates the "relaxation time of elongate particles in a flow" (Walton, 1952). In practice a Spectrophotometric Sperm Cell Motility Index (SMI) is calculated as follows:

$$SMI = \frac{\text{initial absorbance} - \text{final absorbance}}{\text{initial absorbance}} \times 100$$

Initially in sea urchins a 30-s decline in absorbance was recorded from the moment at which the flow was stopped. However, better resolution is obtained when the absorbance decline is followed for 1 min. Because of the optical properties of various semen-diluting media, the proper selection of wavelength is important in obtaining a good spectrophotometric resolution of sperm motility. As an example, at 254 nm, analysis of sea urchin sperm motility is based upon maximal UV recognition of the sperm's cellular components in a low background absorbance media (saline). But in mammals at 254 nm, UV absorption by noncellular seminal plasma components considerably increases background absorbance. This increased optical interference reduced the ability to correlate the spectrophotometric analysis of sperm motility to a qualitative ranking of sperm motility (Atherton, 1975). This background absorbance is eliminated in roosters (Wall and Boone, 1973) and in man (Atherton et al., 1978a) by selection of a 475-nm wavelength.

To determine sperm velocity, sperm track lengths (Janick and Macleod, 1970) were obtained by photographing the flow cell effluent. Kodak Tri-X film was used with 2-s exposures and a range of 15-25 fields photographed per sample. Negatives were projected onto large sheets of paper at a final magnification of X880; a minimum of 300 sperm tracks were traced with the position of nonmotile sperm recorded for each sample. Only the first 300 motile sperm tracks were observed and measured with a dual-scale map measure. Sperm velocity ($\mu m/s$) was then calculated from these sperm tract measurements. Selective inhibition of velocity was studied by incubating sperm in varying concentrations of benzamidine hydrochloride, which was found to inhibit progressive sperm motility (Polakoski, personal communication).

Rabbit sperm motility was quantitated in egg-yolk glycerine cryopreservation extender (EYG) as previously reported for both fresh and thawed cryopreserved bull sperm (Atherton et al., 1978a). This was accomplished by fitting a double beam spectrophotometer with two flow cells and zeroing the absorbance at 475 nm with 10 ml saline:4 drops EYG. Next semen was added drop-wise to the sample side until 0.7-0.9 absorbance units were recorded. The basic procedure is then continued as described above.

Unless otherwise indicated, because large volumes of semen were needed, at least three samples were pooled. Experiments were then repeated a minimum of three times on different pooled samples. All experiments were done at room temperature ($22°C \pm 1°C$).

RESULTS AND DISCUSSION

Correlation of the SMI to Progressive Sperm Motility

The correlation between human and rabbit SMI and the percent progressive sperm motility is presented in Table 1. Progressive sperm motility was determined by

Table 1. Correlation of the Sperm Cell Motility Index (SMI) With Progressively Motile Sperm

Human Semen in Baker's		
% Heat Killed Sample	$\bar{X}$ SMI ± SD	% Progressive Motility
100	0.00 ± 0.00	0.0
80	1.83 ± 0.26	4.5
60	3.86 ± 0.94	6.0
50	4.90 ± 1.48	25.0
40	5.00 ± 0.66	25.5
20	6.60 ± 0.49	39.0
0	8.78 ± 1.40	41.5

Correlation coefficient (r) between SMI and % progressive motility is 0.92.
Correlation coefficient (r) between SMI and % heat-killed cells is −0.92.

Rabbit Semen in Baker's		
100	0.00 ± 0.00	0.0
80	2.83 ± 0.75	10.5
60	5.67 ± 0.57	11.5
50	6.60 ± 1.12	27.0
40	8.13 ± 2.17	36.5
20	9.57 ± 0.97	54.0
0	17.33 ± 3.22	63.0

Correlation coefficient (r) between SMI and % progressive motility is 0.93.
Correlation coefficient (r) between SMI and % heat-killed cells is −0.97.

Modified from Atherton et al. (1978a).

scoring 200 sperm per slide in a double blind experiment. As also shown, the SMI correlated to the percent of dead sperm in the sample. This was done by heating an aliquot of semen at 50°C for 15 min to kill all the sperm. This sample was then cooled and recombined with live sperm to give a solution containing the various percentages of dead sperm as shown. Sperm concentration was constant. These results show that for both human and rabbit sperm, the percent of progressively motile sperm and the percent of dead sperm are highly correlated to the SMI.

It can be observed that when the two species are compared, an SMI of 6.6 gives a percent progressive motility of 39% in man and 27% in rabbit. This difference between species may reflect unique optical properties related to species specific morphology or uniqueness of samples that had to be pooled in order to have enough semen to do the experiment.

Effect of In Vitro Aging on the Human SMI

Table 2 demonstrates the correlation between the human SMI and the percent of progressive motility as a function of two different types of *in vitro* aging. In the first experiment (fresh dilution) 3-5 drops of undiluted semen were diluted with 10 ml of Baker's saline and the SMI determined. This procedure was repeated with fresh dilutions at each indicated time interval. In the second experiment (single dilution) sperm motility was analyzed sequentially on only the original dilution at the selected time intervals.

The results in Table 2 indicate that the fresh dilution retain motility values 2-3 times greater than that of a single dilution. This difference is most probably due to undiluted sperm living longer than diluted sperm. By establishing such a profile for a given semen sample the relative "health" of the sample can be quickly established. Importantly experimental protocols involving sperm motility can be rapidly compared with their respective control values as an experiment progresses.

Effect of Sperm Dilution on the SMI

As shown in Table 3, in both humans and rabbits the SMI was shown to be independent of the final sperm concentration in the flow cell. These data were obtained by determining the SMI on sequentially diluted semen samples. This observation that the SMI is independent of dilution over the range studied might imply that the problem of sperm adhesion to glass, as commonly observed in the microscope, may not be an important factor affecting the SMI. Experiments are in progress to determine the relationships between the SMI and progressive motility at various dilutions.

Table 2. Effect of *In Vitro* Aging on the Human SMI

	Time (min)	$\bar{X}$ SMI ± SD	Progressive Motility (%)
Fresh dilution	0	11.57 ± 2.44	58.5
	5	10.45 ± 1.05	40.5
	15	8.73 ± 1.65	27.5
	30	8.70 ± 1.36	26.0
	60	6.40 ± 1.04	30.5
	90	6.03 ± 0.68	12.5
		(r = 0.86)	
Single dilution	0	11.57 ± 2.44	58.5
	5	10.45 ± 1.05	40.5
	15	5.23 ± 0.95	20.5
	30	4.47 ± 0.40	4.0
	60	3.63 ± 0.38	6.5
		(r = 0.95)	

Correlation coefficient (r) between SMI and percent progressive motility.
Modified from Atherton et al. (1978a).

Table 3. Effect of Dilution on the SMI

Concentration of Sperm Drops/ml-Dilution	Absorbance	Cell No.[a] $\bar{X}$ 10^6/ml	$\bar{X}$ SMI ± SD
Human Semen in Baker's			
15/5—1:6.7	1.57	14.3	4.70 ± 0.56
8/5—1:12.5	1.10	9.6	4.03 ± 0.40
4/5—1:25	0.50	5.0	4.63 ± 0.44
2/5—1:50	0.35	2.5	4.26 ± 0.04
Rabbit Semen in Baker's			
2.0/5.0—1:50	1.49	11.75	31.78 ± 2.09
1.5/5.0—1:67	1.17	6.15	31.15 ± 4.13
1.0/5.0—1:100	0.79	4.68	33.52 ± 1.52
0.5/5.0—1:200	0.39	1.83	29.27 ± 2.81

[a]*Final concentration analyzed*

Rabbit SMI Obtained in Egg-yolk Glycerine Cryopreservation Extender (EYG)

In Table 4 the SMI of rabbit semen in EYG is presented. It should be noted that a high correlation between the SMI and percent progressive motility was obtained ($r = 0.97$). Comparisons between the SMI and progressive motility obtained in Baker's saline (Table 1) do not compare with values obtained in EYG. This could be due to a number of factors. First, these preliminary data were not obtained from the same semen sample. Also the strikingly different physical properties of saline and saline-EYG solutions (viscosity, pH, chemical composition, osmolarity) may preclude obtaining direct relationships between motility values spectrophotometrically in such optically different solutions. Nevertheless, from these data it would appear that this procedure would be valuable in the rapid evaluation of semen motility before and after cryopreservation. Experiments are in progress with very large pooled samples to determine the SMI and progressive motility relationships in saline and EYG.

Table 4. Analysis of Rabbit Sperm Motility Index (SMI) in Egg-Yolk Glycerine Extender

Egg-Yolk Glycerine Extender	
$\bar{X}$ SMI ± SD	Progressive Motility (%)
29.37 ± 1.43	66
24.17 ± 0.47	41
20.06 ± 1.23	37
12.63 ± 0.70	23
11.20 ± 0.49	17

Correlation coefficient (r) between the SMI and percent progressive motility is 0.97.

The Correlation between Sperm Velocity and the SMI

In Table 5 as the concentration of benzamidine hydrochloride was increased, both the SMI and sperm velocity decreased. Although the mechanism is not known by which benzamidine hydrochloride reduces sperm motility, it was a useful compound for these experiments because unlike other treatments (heating and formalin) it could be washed away and the recovery of motility documented (Table 5). Consequently this study indicates that a strong correlation exists ($r = 0.96$) between the SMI and sperm velocity.

Table 5. Correlation of Rabbit Sperm Motility (SMI) to Sperm Velocity in Baker's Saline

Benzamidine Hydrochloride Concentration	$\bar{X}$ SMI ± SD	Sperm Velocity (μM/s)
Control	20.34 ± 3.85	51.6
1mM	18.77 ± 2.86	37.4
5mM	13.30 ± 2.17	28.2
10mM	10.50 ± 0.93	18.9
25mM	4.45 ± 1.00	10.8
50mM	2.88 ± 0.31	9.4

Correlation between $\bar{X}$ SMI and sperm velocity $r = 0.96$.

Reversibility of Benzamidine Hydrochloride Inhibition of Rabbit Sperm Motility

Treatment	$\bar{X}$ SMI ± SD	Velocity (μM/s)
Control	25.07 ± 1.44	39.4
50mM benzamidine	1.34 ± 0.44	<7.6
Washed control	26.02 ± 5.29	39.9
Washed 50mM benzamidine	25.63 ± 3.15	36.7

General Conclusions

In this study the spectrophotometric sperm cell motility index (SMI) clearly satisfies the four criteria established in the introduction. Another type of analysis of this spectrophotometric absorbance change may yield even further data. Specifically the rate of absorbance change is being investigated in comparison with the SMI calculation. Specifically the SMI correlates with the percent of progressively motile sperm, percent of dead sperm, and the *in vitro* age of sperm. Additionally the SMI is independent of sperm concentration over commonly used ranges suitable for spectrophotometric analysis, and has been shown suitable for use with semen diluted into saline-egg yolk glycerine cryopreservation extenders. Compounds such as caffeine, theophylline, arginine, and acetylcholine have been used in the author's laboratory with diverse species to enhance sperm motility. In all cases increased SMI values are correlated to increased visual motility. Finally, for the first time, the SMI has been shown to correlate with sperm velocity.

These encouraging characteristics of this sperm cell motility evaluation system make further documentation of it appear worthwhile. Specifically individual semen samples can now be rapidly analyzed for the effects of diverse physical and chemical treatments on sperm motility. Also a renewed interest in the biophysical properties of sperm in a stopflow system such as this would appear valuable in gaining further information on sperm motility (Atherton, 1977b).

REFERENCES

Atherton, R.W.: A Tentative Hypothesis to Explain the Neurochemical Regulation of Sperm Motility. In: Advances in Invertebrate Reproduction. Vol. I, 120-129, ed. by K.G. Adiyodi and R.G. Adiyodi. Peralam-Kenoth, Karivellur, Kerala 670521, India, 1977a

Atherton, R.W.: Evaluation of Sperm Motility. In: Techniques of Human Andrology. Vol. 1, 173-187, ed. by E.S.E. Hafez. Elsevier/North-Holland, Amsterdam, The Netherlands, 1977b

Atherton, R.W.; Radany, E.W.; Polakoski, K.L.: Quantitation of Human Sperm Motility. In: Techniques of Human Andrology. Vol. 1, 447-449, ed. by E.S.E. Hafez, Elsevier/North-Holland, Amsterdam, The Netherlands, 1977

Atherton, R.W.; Radany, E.W.; Polakoski, K.L.: Spectrophotometric Quantitation of Mammalian Spermatozoan Motility. I. Human Biol Reprod 18(1978a)624-628

Atherton, R.W.; Jackson, F.J.; Bond, G.S.; Radany, E.W.; Kitchin, R.M.: Spectrophotometric Quantitation of Mammalian Sperm Motility in Saline and Egg-yolk Glycerine Cryopreservation Extenders. Presented at the 11th Society for the Study of Reproduction Meeting. Carbondale, Ill., August 8-10, 1978b

Atherton, R.W.: An Objective Method for Evaluating Angus and Hereford Sperm Motility. Int J Fertil 20(1975a)109-112

Atherton, R.W.: Neurochemical Effects on Sperm Motility in *Strongylocentrotus purpuratus*, the Purple Sea Urchin. Comp Biochem Physiol 50C (1975b)21-26

Glover, F.A.: Physical Method of Measuring the Mobility of Bull Spermatozoa. Nature 219(1978)1263-1264

Janick, J.; MacLeod, J.: The Measurement of Human Spermatozoan Motility. Fertil Steril 21(1970)140-145

Paulson, J.D.; Polakoski, K.L.: A Glass Wool Column Procedure for Removing Extraneous Material from the Human Ejaculate. Fertil Steril 28(1977)178-181

Timourian, H.; Watchmaker, G.: Determination of Spermatozoan Motility. Dev Biol 21(1970)62-72

Wall, K.A.; Boone, M.A.: Objective Measurement of Sperm Motility. Poultry Sci 52(1973)657-660

Walton, A.: Flow Orientation as a Possible Explanation of "Wave-motion" and "Rheotaxis" of Spermatozoa. J Exp Biol 24(1952)520-531

MEASUREMENT OF HUMAN SPERM MOTILITY BASED ON AN OPTICAL DOPPLER EFFECT

P. Jouannet

Histology-Embryology Laboratory, Centre Hospitalo-Universitaire de Bicêtre, Université Paris-Sud, 94270 KzemPin-Bicêtre, France

Laser Doppler Velocimetry (LDV) is the determination of the velocity of microscopic particles from the Doppler shift of scattered light. In biology and medicine, this technique has been applied in numerous ways among which are the study of fluids or airflow carrying cells or particles, protoplasmic streaming and self-propelled organisms like bacteria or spermatozoa.[1-2] Spermatozoa motility was first studied using LDV by Berge et al. (1967).

PRINCIPLE OF THE METHOD

The frequency shift Δv of light scattered by spermatozoa is related to incident light frequency vo according to Doppler formula:

$$\Delta v = vo \frac{2v}{c} \cos \alpha \sin \frac{\theta}{2} \quad (1)$$

where c is light velocity, v spermatozoa velocity, θ the angle between the incident beam and the direction in which the scattered light is observed, α the angle between the direction of spermatozoa movement and the exterior bissector of θ.

If θ, α, and v have a single value, $v = Kv \cos \alpha$ has only one value (K being constant). If all spermatozoa are moving in the same direction (α fixed) but at different speeds spread around a mean velocity according to a distribution N(v) which gives the variation of the number N of spermatozoa moving at velocity v as a function of v, the scattered light spectrum is a sum of frequency peaks, each being related to the frequency vo and the velocity v which induced it. The height of every elementary peak is proportional to N(v). In this case the spectrum $S(v)$ represents exactly the outline of N(v).

In semen, the spermatozoa move in all directions. However, if we could isolate those that have the same velocity the optical spectrum should have the same spectral intensity for all frequencies from $v' = vo$ to $v' = vo + \Delta v$. But if one takes into account the entire spermatozoan population with a velocity distribution N(v), the frequency shift gives a more complex spectrum that is the "composition" of N(v) with the above described spectrum. In this case N(v) is represented by the function

$$v \frac{dS(v)}{dv} \quad (2)$$

Human spermatozoan have slow velocities so the frequency shifts are under 100 Hz, that is to say 10^{12} less than frequency of light. Such small frequency changes are very difficult to detect and the spectroscopy photon beating technique (hétérodyne) is used. A phototube receives simultaneously both scattered light and a small part of the incident beam (local oscillator). Beats between these two beams give rise to fluctuations in the photocurrent at frequency Δv. The analysis of these fluctuations by a Fourier analyser gives $S(v)$ directly which is distributed around $v = O$.

INSTRUMENTATION

Figure 1 diagrams the apparatus. The light source is a low power He-Ne laser. Its beam is split into two parts by the slide L_1:

- One provides an incident beam (I), the intensity of which can be controlled by a polarizer (P_1). The scattering angle chosen is 8° under which condition the photomultiplyer PM receives primarily light scattered by the heads of the spermatozoa.
- The other part of the laser beam (II) is directed onto a cylindrical mirror which acts as the local oscillator. This beam is reflected on a slide L_2 in such a way that it and the scattered light (III) are mixed entering the PM.

The intensity of the scattered light is measured by a millivoltmeter and is proportional to the number of scattering centers. The spectrum integrator is a passband filter that allows one to measure the intensity of the frequency spectrum produced by motile spermatozoa. A real-time wave analyser gives the Doppler shifted frequency spectrum on a XY recorder. The semen sample is placed in a cylindrical optical glass cell, 100 μm deep and with a volume of 17 mm³.

© 1979 Urban & Schwarzenberg, Inc. Baltimore-Munich *The Spermatozoon*, edited by D.W. Fawcett and J.M. Bedford

BLOCK DIAGRAM OF EXPERIMENTAL APPARATUS

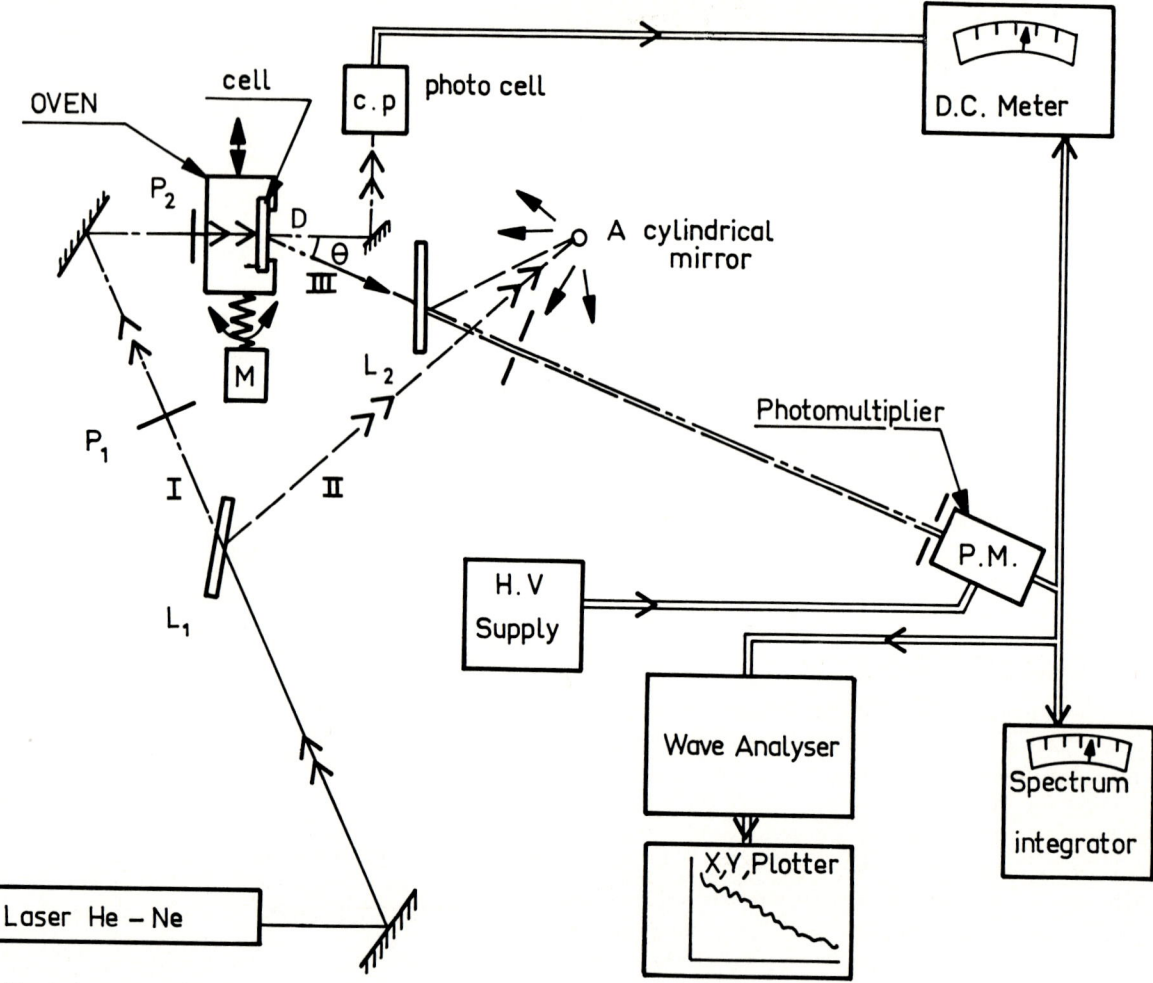

Figure 1. Block diagram of experimental apparatus.

PARAMETERS MEASURED

Spermatozoa concentration. The intensity of the scattered light is proportional to the number of scattering centers. The correlation with the number of spermatozoa is good if there are not too many interference factors.

Concentration of motile spermatozoa is obtained from the integral of the frequency power spectrum $S(v)$.

The percentage of motile spermatozoa is given by the ratio of the integral of the spectrum due to motile spermatozoa to the integral of the total spectrum of the light scattered by the entire population of scattering centers (*i.e.* spermatozoa dead and alive). This last integral is easily obtained by an induced, controlled translational movement of the cell containing the sperm.

Velocity distribution $P(v)$ can be obtained from the Doppler spectrum $S(v)$ derived point to point (Eq. 2).

In nearly all cases, the spermatozoa moving in seminal plasma induce a Doppler spectrum which is exponential[4] (Fig. 2A). The distribution calculated from this spectrum is shown in Figure 2B, it is wide and POISSON-like. In this case, the spectrum in semilogarithmic coordinates is linear and its slope permits rapid calculation of the characteristic velocity V_c: Mode of the population.[3]

The comparison of these results with those obtained with microcinematographic analysis shows that the velocity distribution measured by LDV correlates well with the instantaneous velocity of the spermatozoa and not with their overall rate of progression.

Different types of spectra can be obtained by changing physicochemical conditions of the media in which the spermatozoa move. Figure 2 shows the spectra of frequencies obtained with spermatozoa from the same sample moving in seminal fluid (———) and after migra-

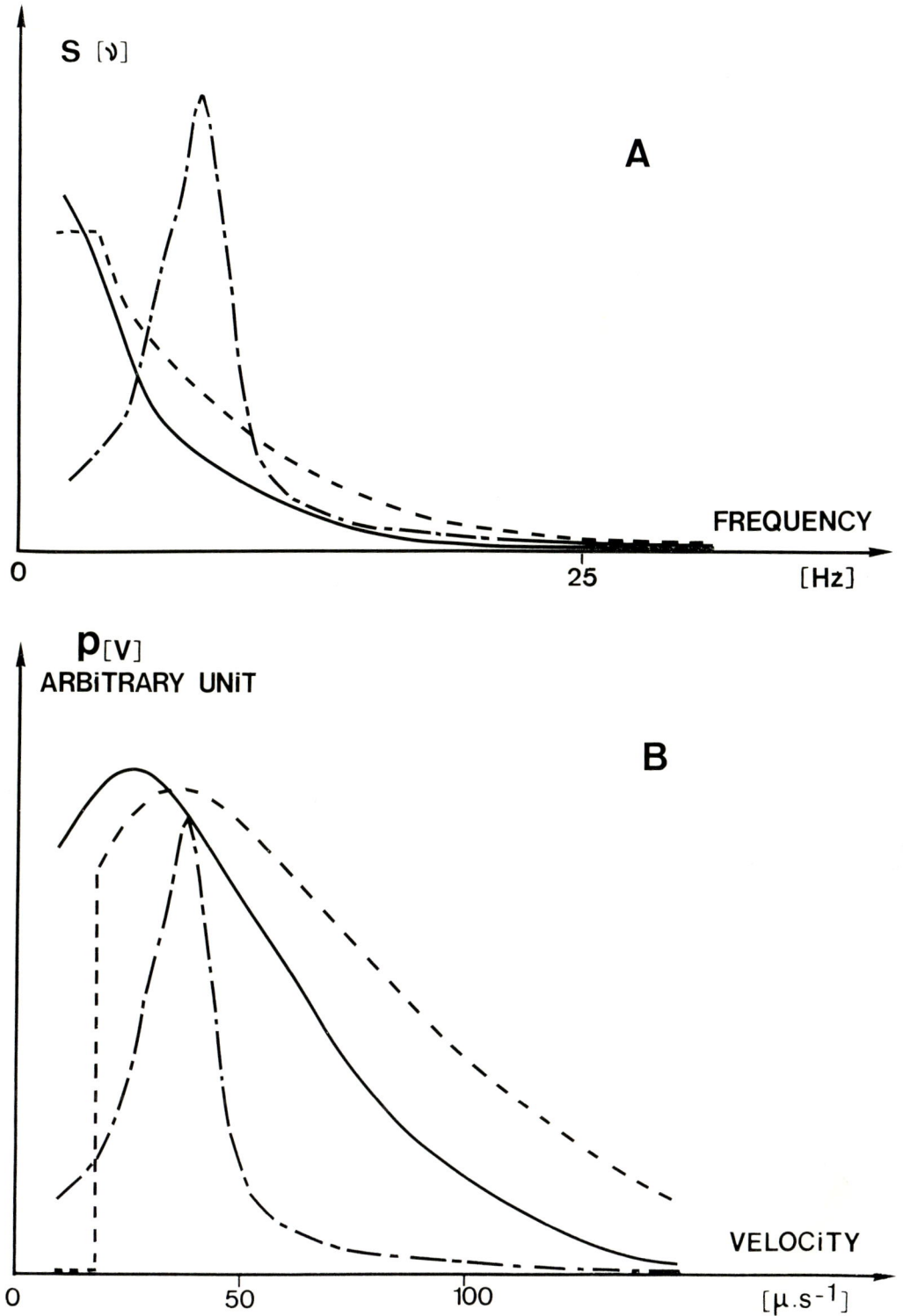

Figure 2. Frequency spectrum of the light scattered (A) and corresponding velocity distribution (B) of spermatozoa from the same sample moving in: seminal plasma (———), BSA solution (- - - -), and midcycle cervical mucus (— – · –).

tion into bovine serum albumine (BSA) solution (– – –) or ovulatory cervical mucus (– · –). In BSA solution, the specrum is exponential but at low frequencies, the slope is zero and represents a velocity threshold. This demonstrates that in BSA, there has been a selection for the most motile spermatozoa and that they move in all directions.

In the cervical mucus, the spectrum is a remarkably well defined peak at a frequency shifted away from 0. This type of spectrum signifies an oriented, unidirectional movement. In this case, the spectrum yields directly the velocity distribution of spermatozoa population.

ADVANTAGES AND WEAKNESSES

A simple, easily applied method for the objective measurement of spermatozoa motility has been long sought. LDV is a method by which the velocity and motility of a population of spermatozoa can be measured without need of a microscope and thus, the human eye.

Measurements are made using a very small volume of semen and dilution is not necessary. The procedure requires only a few minutes and the results are immediate. This technique can be used without modification over a large range of spermatozoa concentrations. However with very low concentrations (below 3.10^6 spermatozoa/ml) or with elevated levels of interference elements (cellular debris, microorganisms, crystals, etc.) as sometimes occurs in case of male sterility, the test becomes less accurate.[4]

LDV does not provide information on motility of the individual spermatozoa for which microcinematography is presently irreplaceable. On the other hand, its greatest interest lies in the objective and quantitative measurement of the effect of various factors—physical, chemical, pharmacologic, immunologic—that may inhibit or stimulate spermatic motility.

TO FIND MORE DETAILED INFORMATION

LDV in General

[1] Cummins H.Z.: Intensity Fluctuation Spectroscopy of Motile Microorganisms. In: Photon Correlation Spectroscopy and Velocimetry, pp. 200-225, ed. by H.Z. Cummins and B.R. Pike. Plenum Publishing Co., New York, 1977

[2] Ware B.R.: Applications of Laser Velocimetry in Biology and Medicine. In: Chemical and Biochemical Applications of Laser, Vol II, pp. 199-239. Acad. Press Inc., New York, 1977

Described Method and Results

[3] Dubois, M.; Jouannet, P.; Berge, P.; Volochine, B.; Serres, C.; David, G.: Méthode et Appareillage de Mesure Objective de la Mobilité des Spermatozoïdes Humains. Ann Phys Biol Méd 9(1975)19-41

[4] Jouannet, P.; Volochine, B.; Deguent, P.; Serres, C.; David, G.: Light Scattering Determination of Various Characteristic Parameters of Spermatozoa Motility in a Series of Human Sperm. Andrologia 9(1977)36-49

COMPUTERIZED MEASUREMENTS OF SPERM VELOCITY AND PERCENTAGE OF MOTILE SPERM

R.P. Amann

Dairy Breeding Research Center, The Pennsylvania State University, University Park, Pennsylvania 16802 USA

It has been estimated that the 95% confidence interval for a single subjective estimation of the percentage of motile sperm is ±30-60 percentage units. Obviously, precise and accurate objective methods for measuring the percentage and velocity of motile sperm, free from observer bias, are essential for research, to train personnel, and to establish standards among laboratories. Therefore, our research group studied procedures for observing a semen sample and developed an analytical computer program that provides information on each sperm observed.

To obtain data on individual sperm, a thin suspension of sperm is viewed using phase-contrast optics and the image is fed into a computer for analysis. The depth of field of a 10X objective is restricted. To ensure that all sperm remain within the field of view, special chambers were fabricated locally. These chambers, similar to a hemacytometer chamber, have a central viewing area and lateral shoulders prepared by sputtering a 5-μm layer of germanium onto the 1-mm thick glass slide. A cover glass serves as the upper side of the chamber. For sperm suspended in salt solutions, 0.5% gelatin is included to minimize adhesion of sperm to the glass; heated skim milk or egg-yolk extenders also can be used. The suspension should contain 30-40 x 10^6 sperm/ml.

An inverted microscope equipped with an electrically heated stage, 10X phase-contrast objective, 25X ocular, and a super-8 movie camera are used to record (at 18 frames/sec) an 8-sec scene on black and white film. If five scenes are recorded and evaluated for each of two slides representing one sample, the predicted standard deviation will be <5.5 percentage units for motility and <9.8 μm/sec for velocity. The computer program (Liu and Warme, 1977) has the following capabilities and advantages:

1. Velocities of ≤45 cells may be evaluated simultaneously; each cell is automatically classified as motile or nonmotile according to a preset velocity cutoff (typically 35 μm/sec for bull sperm).
2. Analysis requires less than 3 min for each scene.
3. Data are collected off line so that evaluation of samples from a remote location and convenient scheduling of computer time are possible.
4. All image analysis equipment is commercially available at a reasonable cost.
5. Software is written almost entirely in Fortran, requires less than 16 K of core memory, and can be adapted to run on most minicomputers.

The complete system for computer evaluation of sperm motility is depicted in Figure 1 and components are listed in Table 1. The microscope image initially is recorded on super-8 film which is projected with a single-frame-advance projector onto a screen for viewing by a video camera. [Use of video tape was rejected because registration from frame-to-frame was impossible in a stop-action mode. Direct video coupling provides information at too high a rate for the computer.] Each frame from the TV camera consists of 256 horizontal rasters and a video compressor scans vertically from left to right, under computer control, across the rasters in 256 cross sections. A gray scale intensity for each point of intersection of a vertical cross section and the horizontal rasters is stored. Since the image viewed by the TV camera remains motionless, the video compressor can scan the video image (actually a series of identical images) slowly and without exceeding the input limit of the computer. Data for one cross section are compared with those for the two previous cross sections to identify segments of a common cell. Vertical coordinates of the sperm head on the cross section are stored. When the right-hand edge of a cell is encountered, the X and Y

This research was a collaborative effort with Dr. Roy H. Hammerstedt. Dr. Paul K. Warme supervised computer programming. Supported by Atlantic Breeders Cooperative, Lancaster, Pennsylvania; Sire Power Inc., Tunkhannock, Pennsylvania; NSF Grant BM574-15221; and PHS Grants GM-20742 and HD-05859.

© 1979 Urban & Schwarzenberg, Inc. Baltimore-Munich *The Spermatozoon*, edited by D.W. Fawcett and J.M. Bedford

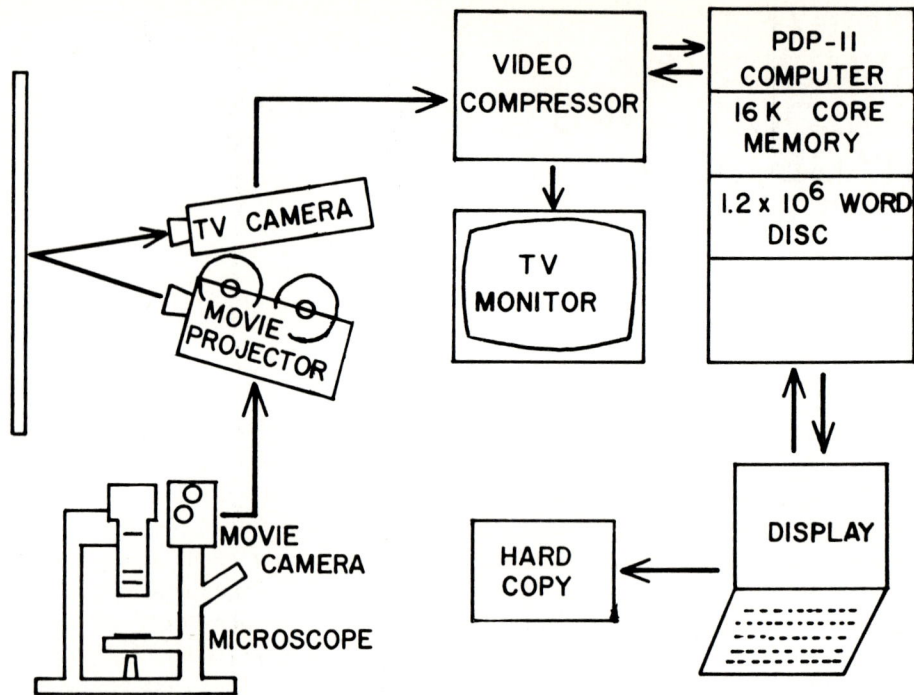

Figure 1. A computerized method for evaluation of sperm motility.

coordinates of the center of that cell are calculated. Adjustable thresholds for background and size filter out the sperm tails and particles differing in size from a sperm head. Filters on the X and Y axes can be adjusted commensurate with the size of the sperm head.

The image of the first frame in a series (Fig. 2) is projected on the computer display and can be compared with the sample image as viewed on the TV monitor. To identify moving sperm and to calculate their velocities, the position of each sperm in frame 1 is compared by the computer with their positions in subsequent frames. The superimposed images of four successive frames are depicted in Figure 3. The correlation of cell location in successive frames is based on the principle of minimum distance of the previously calculated sperm centers. The velocity of each cell is obtained by averaging the distances moved between each pair of successive frames (Fig. 4) and multiplying by the frame rate. Typical output from the printer is shown in Figure 5 and, if desired, data for each individual sperm can be obtained in printed form (Fig. 6) or as punched paper tape.

Rigorous evaluations of the accuracy and precison of this approach reveal that some nonmotile sperm are classified as motile. This error is a consequence of

Table 1. Components of System

Chamber:	fabricated from a 1 x 25 x 75 mm glass slide by etching two parallel groves and sputtering a 5-μm layer of germanium on the lateral surfaces. Use with standard hemacytometer cover glass.
Buffer:	salt solution containing 0.5% gelatin.
Microscope:	Leitz Diavert with modified electric thermostage, 10X phase-contrast objective, 25X occular, Leicina super-8 movie camera, and 100 W tungsten-halogen lamp with KG-1 infrared filter.
Projector:	Kodak Ektagraphic MFS-8 stop-action projector and Dalite screen.
Video:	Sony AVC-3210 camera, Shibaden VM-172U monitor, and Colorado Video Inc. 260 video compressor.
Computer:	Digital Equipment Corp PDP-11 (E-10) computer with 16K core memory, RK-11 1.2 x 10^6 word cartridge disc system, dual cassette drive, Tektronix 4010 storage display terminal, Tektronix 2610 hard copier, and Teletypewriter.
Software:	see Computers Biomed. Res. 10:127-138. 1977.

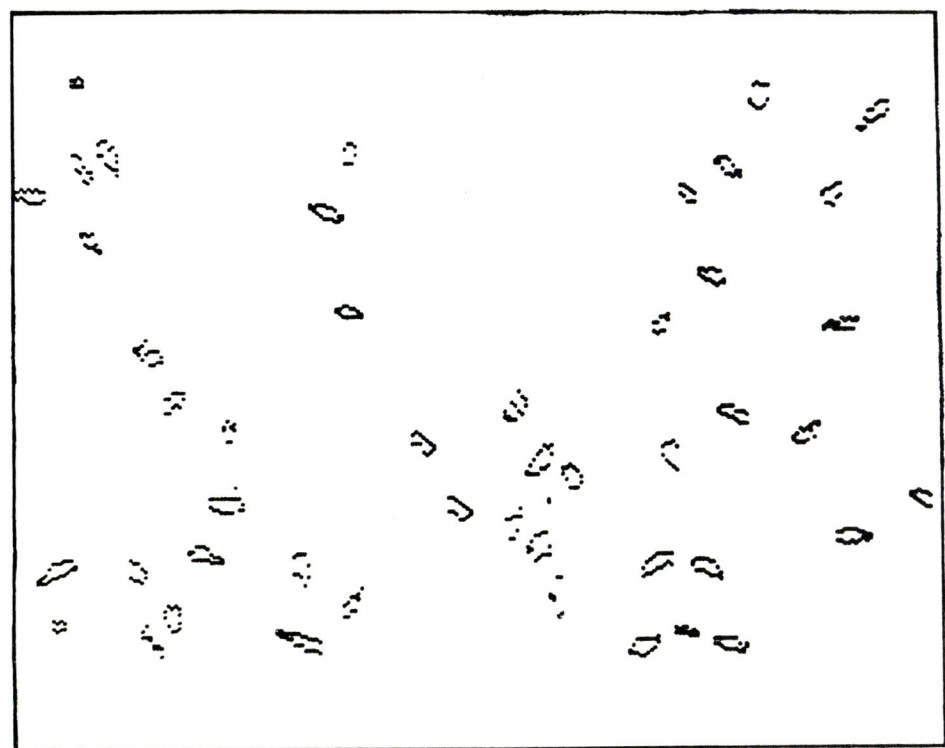

Figure 2. Display of the computer-determined outlines of sperm heads in the first frame of a scene.

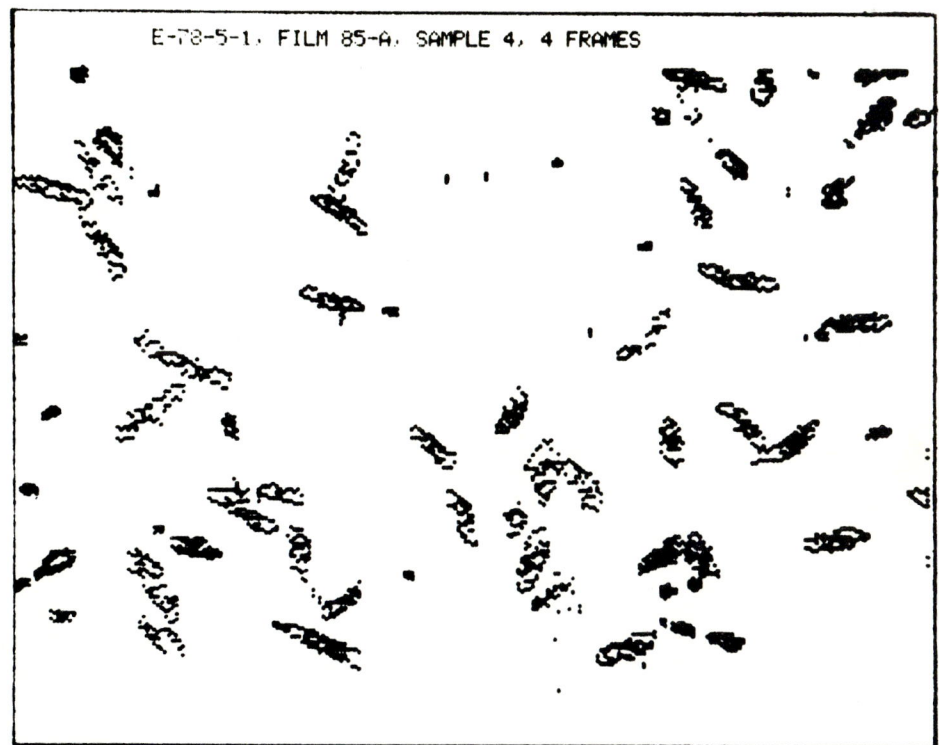

Figure 3. Display of the computer-determined outlines of sperm heads in four successive frames.

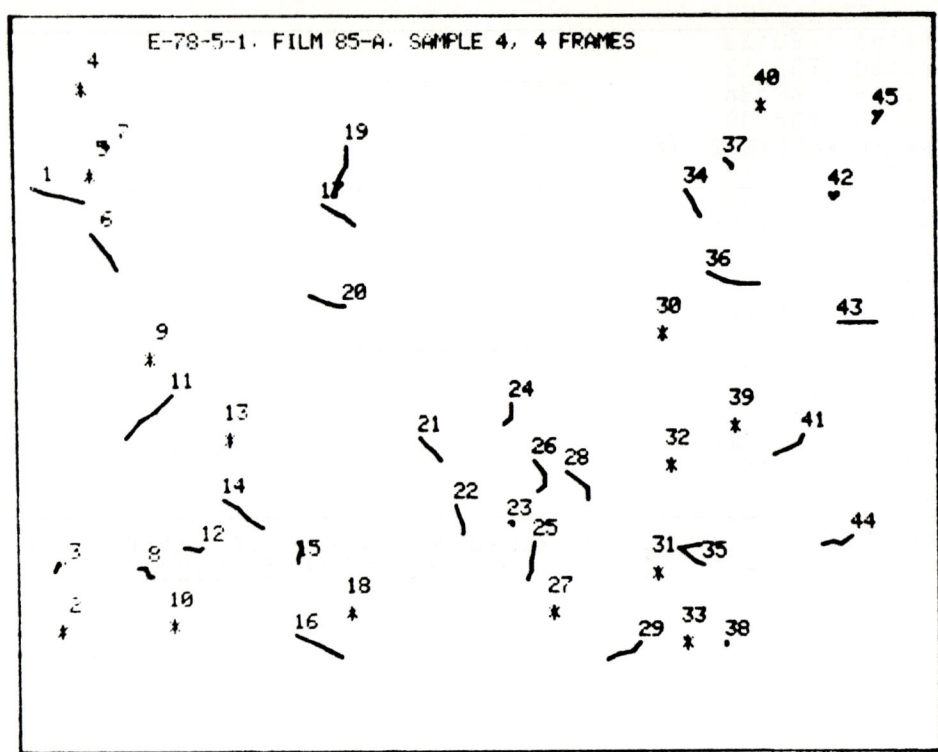

Figure 4. Computer-plotted trace connecting the midpoints of sperm heads in the four successive frames depicted in Figure 3.

E-78-5-1. FILM 85-A, SAMPLE 4, 4 FRAMES

SPERM TYPE	VEL RANGE (MICRONS/SEC)	NO. SPERM	PERCENT DEF	PERCENT ALL	VEL +/− SEM (SD) (MICRONS/SEC)
SPERM WITH VELOCITY $\geq$2 SD OF MEAN	>132.3	1	3		
MOTILE (DEFINED)	35.0 − 132.3	24	77		78.7 +/− 4.8(23.5)
MOTILE (DEFINED+ UNDEFINED)	−	39		87	N.D.
NONMOTILE	<35.0	6	19	13	N.D.
TOTAL SPERM EVALUATED		45			
UNDEFINED SPERM		14			

Figure 5. Routine hard-copy output of a computer analysis of a scene (Fig. 4) for which four successive frames were analyzed. A total of 45 sperm were detected in the first frame and 31 of these sperm were "defined" or followed through the succeeding frames. Sperm with a velocity <35 μm/sec were considered nonmotile (a predefined threshold). One sperm had a velocity of 135 μm/sec which was more than two standard deviations above the mean value for other motile sperm. Excluding this cell, the mean velocity for 24 sperm was 78.7 ± 4.8 μm/sec. Of the defined sperm, 77% were motile and when nondefined sperm (primarily sperm that rotated and were lost in one or more frames) were included, 87% of the 45 sperm were considered to be motile.

```
          E - 78 - 5 - 1, FILM 85 - A, SAMPLE 4, 4 FRAMES
     *** QUANTITATIVE ANALYSIS OF SPERM / FRAME 1 TO FRAME 4 ***

 #  MOTILE  DIST    SPEED
 1  YES     18.41   110.44
 2          ** DISAPPEARED **
 3  NO       4.32    25.89
 4          ** DISAPPEARED **
 5          ** DISAPPEARED **
 6  YES     15.96    95.77
 7  NO       2.64    15.81
 8  YES      7.08    42.48
 9          ** DISAPPEARED **
10          ** DISAPPEARED **
11  >2 SD   22.57   135.42
12  YES      6.79    40.76
13          ** DISAPPEARED **
14  YES     17.33   104.00
15  YES      7.72    46.34
16  YES     18.30   109.78
17  YES     13.47    80.79
18          ** DISAPPEARED **
19  YES     19.44   116.66
20  YES     13.43    80.61
21  YES     11.15    66.89
22  YES     10.60    63.62
23  NO       2.28    13.66
24  YES      8.32    49.91
25  YES     13.57    81.43
26  YES     13.64    81.82
27          ** DISAPPEARED **
28  YES     13.78    82.67
29  YES     13.39    80.34
```

Figure 6. Hard-copy output of data for each individual sperm in the scene shown in Figures 2-4. Each sperm is classified as motile, nonmotile, or undefined (disappeared in one or more frames) and the distance traveled and velocity of each sperm are indicated.

inconsistency in defining the limits of each sperm head by the video compressor-computer and the resulting variation in the location of the assigned midpoint of a nonmotile object. The system will discriminate among samples containing different percentages of motile sperm or sperm whose modal velocity differs. Precision of the system is excellent.

Weaknesses of the total system include a possible "wall effect" of the chamber on motile sperm, the time required to develop the motion picture film, and an overestimation of the percentage of motile sperm. Strengths of this objective method include availability of data for each individual sperm, high precision, nontediousness, and reasonable cost. This system has potential for use in research or in establishing standards for use in training technicians or performing quality control checks among laboratories. The method is impractical for routine use in a clinic or bull stud.

REFERENCE

Liu, Y.T. and Warme, P.K.: Computerized Evaluation of Sperm Cell Motility. Computers Biomed Res 10(1977) 127-138.

INDEX

A

Acrosin, 320, 350
Acrosomal canal
  evagination (*See under* Maturation and Capacitation)
  origin, 364
  relationship, nucleus, 364
Acrosomal organization
  and centriole, 336–339
  in spermiogenesis, 11–12, 17
  and vesicles, 305–306, 333
Acrosome (*See also* Evolution of Acrosome)
  ferritin-lectin localization, 188
  formation, malformation, 341–343, 349–351
  gigantic vesicle, 343
  isolation, 389
  protease activity, 297
  in marsupials, 290–294, 300–302
  nomenclature, 305
  in prospermium, 362
Androgens
  antiandrogen, effect, 57–63
  dihydrotestosterone (DHT), 38
  epididymal, 37
  role in maturation, 16, 38 (*See also under* Viability)
  testosterone, 38
Antibody-antigen binding, 178–180 (*See also under* Plasma Membrane)
ATP assay, 129–130
ATPase(s) (*See under* Dynein)
ATP-dependent sliding, 103
Atypical spermatozoa, insects
  evolutionary trends, 253, 257–258, 263
  phylogenetic aspects, 253
  variable morphology, 255–263
Axial fiber, Urodele, spermatozoon, 267–268, 271–274
Axial spacings, 100, 106
Axoneme(s)
  components, 81–82, 99, 106
  lacking central pair (9+0), 103
  in relation to motility, 99–114
  phosphorylation, 129
  in relation to bend asymmetry, 75–76
  torsion, 71–73

B

Bombina variegata, spermiogenesis, 333–339
Bridge, doublet, 5–6, 103, 121

C

Capacitation (*See also* Maturation)
  and intramembranous particles, 197
  postacrosomal region, 195–202
  and membrane proteins, lateral mobility, 196–197
  sperm-female interaction, *Companularia, Musca, Rana*, 195–196
  surface components, removal, 196
  as surface phenomenon, 195–203
Cell surface (*See under* Plasma membrane)
Central bridges, 105
Central pair
  in ciliary axonemes, 82
  complex, 99–101
  microtubule apparatus, 99, 113–114
  in rat sperm, 106–109
  in squid sperm, 109–114
Central sheath
  in ciliary axonemes, 105
  projections, 105–106
Cilia
  axonemes, *Tetrahymena*, 81–84, 101–105
  central pair, 82, 105
  dynein arms, 82
  microtubule projections, 105–106
  motility, mode of action, 81–82
  9+2 pattern of microtubules, 81, 103
  rapid fixation, movement, 71
  spokes, gill cilia, 100
Chemotaxis, 153
Chromatin isolation, mammalian, 388
Chromosomal proteins, isolation, 380–381
Colchicine, 130
Concanavalin A, 188–189
Connecting piece, fractionation, 388
Corona-radiata-penetrating enzyme (CPE), 320
Cytoplasmic droplet
  isolation, 389
  loss, migration, 7, 11, 17, 291

D

Decapacitation factors, 196, 202
Dense fibers
  fractionation, 388
  influence on wave form, 69
  mammalian, cephalopod, 99
  and selenium, 136, 139
Disulfide-bonded structures, isolation, 387–389
Ductuli efferentes, 35
Ductus epididymidis
  androgen-dependent activity, 7, 18–19
  maturation, storage, functions, 7–19
  sperm passage, 10–12
Dynein (*See also* Dynein 1, 2)
  arm(s), arm cycle, 85–88, 119
  ATPase, 85, 101, 132
  chemistry, 82, 85, 87
  enzymology, myosin, 87
  force generation by, 84
  inner, outer, arms, 99, 101, 120, 123–126
  latent activity, 85
  localization in flagella (*See under* Flagella)
Dynein 1
  21 S ATPase peak, 92
  in flagella, sea urchin, 119–120
  latent activity form, 91–92
    functional activity, 92
    KCl-extracted, 91–93
    molecular weight, 92

437

in outer arms, 121
and plasma membrane, 122
recombination with KCl-extracted axonemes, 91
and sliding-tubule mechanism, 123
Dynein 2
in flagella, sea urchin, 119
and sliding-tubule mechanism, 123
vanadate inhibited, 93

E

Epididymal environment and metabolic rate, 23
Epididymal fluid (See also Epididymal Plasma, Biochemistry)
caput, cauda corpus, 35–40
concentration of Ions:
Ca^{2+}, Mg^{2+}, P, S, 36–40
Na^+ to K^+ ratio, 36–40, 61
cyclic AMP, 37
electron probe microanalysis, 37, 40
glycerophosphorylcholine, 37
osmolality, 35–36
Epididymal maturation
colloidal iron hydroxide binding, 187
in marsupials, 289–292, 301–302
and mediated agglutination, 188
and microtubule phosphorylation, 129–133
sperm surface changes, 187–193
storage function, evolution, 7–19
Epididymal plasma, biochemistry
acetyl carnitine, carnitine, 29–30
amino acids, glutamate, 30
glycerol, glycerolphosphorylcholine, 24
inositol, 26
lactic acid, 24
lipids, 26–27
oxygen tension, 23
reducing sugars, glucose, 23–24
Epididymis (See also Rete Testis)
electrolyte, H_2O transport, 57–63
caput, cauda, 187–188
lecithin, 27–28
microperfusion technique, 57–58
and sperm maturation, 35–40, 187–193, 205, 210–215
Evolution of acrosome
in relation to morphology, content
acrosome reaction enzymes, 319–321
ATPase, 309
in aquatic sperm, 307–310

involution, pseudo-acrosome, 313, 322
lysins, hyaluronidase, 309–310, 317–322
membranes, 319–320
nomenclature, 305
subacrosomal space, 311, 321–322
vesicle origin, 305
Evolution of acrosome
in relation to phyla
internal fertilization phyla, 313–314, 316
mammalian, 318–322
terrestrial invertebrates, 313–317
terrestrial vertebrates, 317–322
Evolution of perforatium
in relation to morphology, content
actin storage, 312
aquatic sperm, 310–311
basic proteins, 313
myosin, 317
nomenclature, 305
profilactin, filamentous actin, 312–313, 322
Pseudoperforatium, 322

F

Fertility (See also Human Spermatid Abnormalities)
antiandrogens, effect, 62–63
biopsy, diagnosing, 341–342, 350–351
Fertilization
changes in capacity, 187
evolution, insects, 253, 258, 263
fate of membrane components, 219–229
reaction, Lilly 1919, 195
Fibrous sheath
isolation procedure, 395–397
and selenium, 136
and spindle-shaped body, 341
Flagella
and anti-Fragment 1 A serum, 119–121
localization of dynein, 119–126
9+2 pattern (See under Microtubules)
Flagellar movement (See also Motility listings)
bend asymmetry, 74–76
bend propagation, 153
calcium-induced asymmetry, 153–156

dark-ground illumination, 71–72
demembranated, reactivated sperm, 119–120, 122–126
inhibition, 122–124
mode of action, 81–82
and rapid-fixation, 71
sea urchin sperm studies, 91–96, 119–126
transient wave forms, symmetry, 95–96
wave form in mammals, 69
Forward motility factor
index (FMI), 45–52
protein (FMP), 47–52
and vasectomized monkeys, 49–51

G

Glutathione peroxidase, rat, 138–140

H

Head-tail detachment
and nuclear membranes, 391
pH dependence, 391
primary amine transamination, 391–392
separation procedure, 387–388, 391–392
Head-tail stabilization
by cyanoborohydride, metal cations, 392
In Vivo observations, 392, 394
–SH oxidation during transit, 12
temperature dependence, 392
Histones
2-dimensional gel electrophoresis, 381
variants, nucleosomes, 381, 383
Human semen (See also under Motility)
interaction, cervical mucus, 77–78, 417–420
movement diversity, 414–416
Human spermatid abnormalities
acrosome malformation (See under Acrosome)
axoneme dissolution, 347
multinucleate, 346, 350
nuclear inclusions, 346–347
round-headed, 349
tail malformation, 347, 350
Human spermatid differentiation
chromatoid body, 342
flower-like structures, 342

flagellar structures, 341
nuclear condensation, 341–342
spindle-shaped body, 341

I

Initial segment, 35

L

Lectins, 188–189
Loligo pealei (*See* squid sperm *under* Central pair)

M

Marginal filament (*See under* Urodele sperm cell)
Marsupial sperm studies
  comparison with eutherians, 289–290, 294–295, 301–302
  comparison with monotremes, platypus, 294–297, 301
  epididymal transit and maturation, 11–13, 289–292, 297, 301–302
  evolution, 294, 297, 301
  function, 290–291
  maturation changes, spermiogenesis, 289–302
  morphological characteristics, 289–302
  special features, *Trichosurus*, 289–292, 301–302
Marsupial sperm survey (*See also* above)
  in relation to Australian species
    family Dasyuridae, 297–300
    family Macropodidae, 394
    family Peramelidae (bandicoot), 297–300
    family Petauridae, 292–294
    family Phalangeridae (brush-tailed possum), 289–292, 301–302
    family Phascolarctidae (koala, wombat), 294, 297
  in relation to American species
    family Didelphidae, 300–301
Maturation and capacitation
  stages in ticks
    acrosomal canal evagination, 364
    spermateliosis, 355, 362, 364
Maturation pattern
  eutherian, therian, subtherian, 8–19
  evolution studies, 7, 15–19
  motility development, 8–9, 15–16, 19

changes during spermiogenesis (*See under* Marsupial sperm studies)
Metazoan sperm structure survey
  lower phyla: Hydrozoa, Scyphozoa, Anthozoa, Ctenophora, 244
  intermediate phylum: Brachiopoda, 250
  higher phyla: (lower protostomes) Sipuniela
    Aschelmintha, Platyhelmintha, Nemerteria, 244
  (higher protostomes) Mollusca, Echiura, Annelida, Arthropoda, 244
  (deuterostomes) Hemichordata, Echinochordata, Urochordata, Cephalochordata, 249
Microtubule(s)
  n-butylamine, 158
  in cilia, flagella, 103
  3-dimensional model, 105
  doublet structure, 99–105
  9+2 pattern, 81
  phosphorylation, 129–133
  selective dissolution, 158
  sliding, 82, 153–156
Mitochondria
  chemical determinations, 142, 402
  cysteine-rich polypeptide, 141
  cytochrome oxidase-specific activity, 407
  electrophoretic studies, 142, 145, 402, 407
  "ghosts", remnants, isolation, 388
  swelling, 142–143, 149
Mitochondrial outer membrane(s)
  component studies, 141–149
  polypeptides, bull sperm, 143–149
  selenium recovery, 135–136
  selenopolypeptides, rat sperm, 135–140
Mitochondrial sheath, 341, 347
Motility (*See also* Flagellar movement, Motility listings)
  biophysical aspects, human, 413–420
  ciliary, flagellar, 99
  cyproterone acetate, effect, 58–63
  elimination of dilution effect, 169–171
  hydrodynamics, 416–419
  methodology critique, 430, 432, 435
  movement characteristics, 413–416
  profiles, excurrent duct, 9
Motility changes (*See also* Flagellar movement, Motility listings)
  acrosome reaction, "activation", 78

analysis, sea urchin sperm, 153–156
  and cyclic AMP, 44
  in epididymal transit, 43, 129
  phosphodiesterase inhibitors, 44, 50
  phosphorylation modification, 129–132
Motility inhibition by ranadate
  in cilia, demembranated, reactivated, 93
  and dynein 2, 93
  and dynein ATPase, 93
  in flagella, 93
  in human sperm, 94
Motility pattern
  in cervical mucus, 77–78
  of early spermatids, 77
  of epididymal spermatozoa, 77
  rotatory behavior, 76–78
  sperm from oviduct, uterus, 78
Motility quantitation
  cinemicrography, 413, 415–416
  computerized measurements, 431–435
  Laser-Doppler velocimetry, 427–428
  percentage estimation, 428–431
  photomicrography, 413–415
  predicted standard deviation, 431
  spectrophotometric procedure, 421–422
  various methods, 413
  velocity determination, 422, 431
  velocity distribution P (v), 428
Motility-stimulating substances
  catecholamines, 170–171
  "sperm motility factor" (SMF), 170–171

N

Negative-stain, accessory structures, 100
Nexin fibers, 99–101, 104
Nonhistone chromosomal proteins, resolution 381–383
Nonprotamine proteins, synthesis, 383
Nuclear membranes
  intermolecular aldemic bonds, 392
  Schiff base formation, 391–392
  sperm-tail junction, 391

O

Optical diffraction
  accessory structures, 100
  microtubule complex, 106
  C_1, C_2 tubules, 108
  orthophosphate uptake, 129–130

P

Pecten maximum (*See* scallop sperm under Radial spokes)
Perforatium, isolation, 388, 395–397
pH, intraluminal, 35
Phosphatase(s), 132
Phosphorylation, microtubules, (*See* under Microtubule(s))
Phosphotransferase, 132
Phylogeny, lower metazoa, 243–250
Plasma membrane
  annulus, zipper, isolation, 157–166
  bound proteins, 187
  and cholesterol, 157–160
  digitonin, filipin, use, 158–162
  isolation, 389
  membrane receptors, spermatocyte, 177
  surface antigens, 177–185
Primitive spermatozoon, 243
Prospermium, *Ornithodoras* ticks
  defined, 355
  head and collar, 356
  inner core, outer sheath, 355–356, 359
  matrix filaments, 359, 362
  morphology, size, 355
  nuclear pores, acrosomal plate, 362
  operculum, 356, 359
Protamine, species-specificity, 383
Protein(s)
  androgen-binding, 35, 38–39
  cysteine-rich, rat sperm, 139
  kinase(s), 129, 132
  membrane proteins, 132
  phosphorylation, phosphoproteins, 129–132

R

Radial spoke(s)
  arrangements, 99–101, 107
  interaction, central sheath, 105, 107–109
  and sliding, 81–82
  triplet, scallop sperm, 100
Rete testis
  cannulation technique, 35
  contents, fluid: amino acids, 30
    reducing sugars, glucose, 23–24
    lactic acid, 24

S

Scruin, 312–313
Sedimentation velocity
  germ cell separation, 375–377
  at unit gravity, 178, 379
Selenium, selenocysteine (*See* under Mitochondrial outer membrane(s))
Seminiferous epithelium
  dissociation, trypsin, 380
  trypsin inhibitor, 380
Seminiferous tubules, fluid, 35–39
Sertoli cells, 177, 178, 379
Sialic acid, 189–191
Sliding microtubule demonstrability
  Chlamydomonas, Tetrahymena, 82
  dark-field microscopy, 82
  invertebrate sperm, 82
  mammalian, metazoan, 82
  model, 81–82
Sliding microtubules (*See also* under Microtubule(s))
  cilia, flagella, 81
  force generation, polarity, 88
  restriction, regulation, 88–89
    central-complex, spoke, deficient, 88
    in chlomydomonas mutants, 88
  trypsin action, 88–89
Sperm autoantisera, 197, 202
Sperm motility index (SMI)
  aging, dilution, effects, 423
  calculations, 422
  progressive motility, correlation, 422–423
  velocity, correlation, 424
Sperm subcompartments, defined, 210
Spermateliosis (*See* Maturation *and* capacitation)
Spermatogenesis
  cell surface roll, 177–180 (*See also* Plasma membrane)
  selenium requirement, rat, 135
Spermatogenic cell suspensions (*See also* Seminiferous epithelium, Testis cell preparations)
  populations isolated, 379
  purity, 379–380
  separation procedures, 379–380
Spermatozoa, biochemistry of metabolism
  acetylcarnitine, carnitine, 28–30
  glutamate, 30
  glycerol kinase, 25–26
  glycerolphosphorylcholine, 27
  inositol, 26
  lipids, fatty acids, 26–27
Spermiogenesis studies (*See Bombina variegata*)
Spermiophore
  defined, 355
  head movements, 356
Surface characterization
  caudal, ejaculated, testicular, 205–215
  electron-spin resonance, 206–208, 210–215
  species differences, 210, 214–215
  whole-cell isoelectric focusing, 209, 214–215
Surface component labelling
  antibody preparation, 223–224
  fluorescein isothiocyanate (FITC), 219–229
  galactose oxidase, 190–192
  I-diI-FITC, 223–229
  sea urchin, hamster, sperm, 210–229
Surface heterogeneity, 219
Symmetry, Pleurodeles, 272

T

T/t locus antigens, 231–237 (*See also* Antibody-antigen binding)
Tail dissassembly
  freeze-fracture technique, 157–158
  guinea pig, 157–167
Tail keratin, rat, 138
Testis cell preparations (*See also* Spermatogenic cell suspensions)
  adult prepuberal, mouse, 379–380
  collagenase dissociation, 380
  perfusion, digestion, procedures, 379–380
  testes dissociation, 375–377
  and spermatogenesis, 380–383
Transport functions (*See* under Epididymis)
Trichosurus, Brush-tailed possum (*See* under Marsupial sperm survey)
Tubule(s) A, B, C_1, C_2, 100–101, 103, 106, 110–114
Tubule extrusion, ATP-driven, 120, 122–126
Tubulin, 99, 130–132, 321

U, V, W

Urodele sperm
  birefringence, nucleus, 269–271
  marginal filament, 267, 271–272
  morphology, 267–272
  movement, 272–273
  phylogeny, tail homologies, 273–274

undulating membrane, 267, 271–272
Viability
  androgen mediated, 7, 12–16, 18–19
  assessment, 375
  and orchidectomy, 13
  and sperm storage, 7, 12–15
Waveform (*See under* Flagellar movement)
Wheat germ agglutinin, 188–189
Wolffian duct epithelium (*See* Ductus epididymidis)

X

X-ray diffraction, accessory structures, 100